PROGRESS IN BRAIN RESEARCH

VOLUME 136

CHANGING VIEWS OF CAJAL'S NEURON

EDITED BY

EFRAIN C. AZMITIA

*Departments of Biology and Psychiatry, Center for Neural Science, New York University,
100 Washington Square East, New York, NY 10003, USA*

JAVIER DeFELIPE

Instituto Cajal (CSIC), Avenida Dr. Arce 37, E-28002 Madrid, Spain

EDWARD G. JONES

Center for Neuroscience, University of California, 1544 Newton Court, Davis, CA 95616, USA

PASKO RAKIC

Department of Neurobiology, Yale University School of Medicine, New Haven, CT 06520, USA

CHARLES E. RIBAK

*Department of Anatomy and Neurobiology, University of California, College of Medicine,
Irvine, CA 92697, USA*

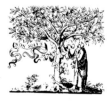

ELSEVIER
AMSTERDAM – BOSTON – LONDON – NEW YORK – OXFORD – PARIS – SAN DIEGO
SAN FRANCISCO – SINGAPORE – SYDNEY – TOKYO
2002

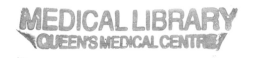
ELSEVIER SCIENCE B.V.
Sara Burgerhartstraat 25
P.O. Box 211, 1000 AE Amsterdam, The Netherlands

First edition 2002

Library of Congress Cataloging in Publication Data
A catalog record from the Library of Congress has been applied for.

ISBN (this volume): 0 444 50815 5
ISBN (Series): 0 444 80104 9   1 0 0 2 8 0 0 3 6 9
ISSN: 0079 6123
⊖ The paper used in this publication meets the requirements of ANSI/NISO Z39.48-1992 (Permanence of Paper).
Printed in The Netherlands.

Dedication

This book is dedicated to His Majesty Don Juan Carlos I, The King of Spain, for his support of Santiago Ramón y Cajal's scientific legacy and coincides with the commemoration of the 150th birthday of Santiago Ramón y Cajal on May 1, 2002.

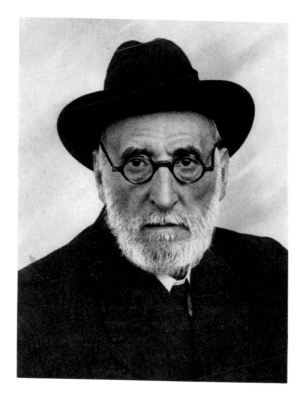

Santiago Ramón y Cajal
(from the private collection of Luis Ramón y Cajal)

Introduction

The neuron is the primary cell of the brain. Typically, it has a well-developed nucleus, abundant cytoplasm, complex dendrites and a long axon that makes numerous synapses. The concept of a neuron was first formulated by Santiago Ramón y Cajal in the Neuron Doctrine, which won him the Nobel Prize in 1906. Cajal's work on the neuron involved many aspects of what is now regarded as neuroscience. Cajal studied neural circuitry, development and degeneration, and considered the role of chemotaxis and neurotropic influences in the formation of functional circuits and in repair of the injured brain. From his research emerged a concept of a highly dynamic immature neuron, struggling to make appropriate connections with the aid of chemical factors. The circuits, once established, were permanent unless there was some form of injury. In these latter instances, Cajal showed that mature neurons of the CNS would try to regenerate, but instead slowly succumbed to degeneration and death. Today, his pioneering research efforts have become disciplines with many of their own concepts and assumptions. Although the specific properties of the neurons studied by each sub-area is different, the general concept remains the stable, synaptic circuit involving the fully mature neuron.

The last three decades have seen the emergence of neuroplasticity, molecular biology and imaging as major foci of work. Researchers investigating the details of synaptic function may not be aware of the dynamic properties of dendrites, and discoveries made using *Aplysia* may fail to consider the evolutionary innovations inherent in human neuronal circuits. Today, many growth factors have been discovered, originating from neurons, glia and other cells, and they can function on mature as well as immature neurons. Another important discovery is that neurogenesis occurs in certain regions of adult brains. Further, apoptosis, programmed cell death, is a key event in development, and also in aging and in certain diseases. Dendrites and spines of mature neurons are mobile, quickly changing in response to chemicals and hormones. Synapses disappear with the withdrawal of postsynaptic parts of the target neuron. These new findings have had a tremendous impact on the clinical development of therapeutic treatments for a variety of human neurological diseases.

Despite these many specific discoveries, the central role of the neuron appears to have been overlooked. This failure to consider the neuron as a whole is not merely of historical significance, but of potential importance to the development and direction of clinically relevant strategies. After all, it is the neuron which is central to the functioning of the brain. It is remarkable that little attention has been given to forming a coherent model of this specialized cell in contemporary neuroscience. The goal of this book is to bring together leading neuroscience researchers in a variety of complementary areas to discuss their own research contributions on the topic of the changing concept of the neuron. It is appropriate that this important task be organized around the original concepts of Cajal, who first proposed the central role of the neuron in brain functioning.

Santiago Ramón y Cajal was born on May 1, 1852 in Petilla de Aragón, a small village in the north of Spain, and died on October 17, 1934 in Madrid. Cajal is the real founder of modern neuroscience and stands prejudged as the greatest neurohistologist of all time. Most fundamental knowledge about the neuron and its interactions with other neurons and with the sensory and motor end organs in the adult, developing and injured nervous system derives from Cajal's seminal work. Today's neuroscientists can profit from returning to Cajal's global theories, armed with the detailed and extensive knowledge and methodologies of the present time. An integrated concept of brain structure and function embodied his work, and his theoretical framework can serve as the organizing principle to develop a dialogue between basic and clinical scientists from different disciplines. To compare the early hypotheses of Cajal with the results obtained during the last few decades of the twentieth century is extremely useful for guiding the progress in the neurosciences for the next millennium.

This volume of Progress in Brain Research contains chapters contributed by the participants of the first joint Cajal Club and Cajal Institute International Meeting on "Changing Views of Cajal's Neuron" held in Madrid, Spain, between May 25–27, 2001. We provide a collection of articles that cover the important issues raised by Cajal, including the following: the structure of the nerve cell; the nature of intracellular communication; the structure and organization of the synapse; trophic actions in development and regeneration; and neuronal plasticity. It is only fitting and proper that the two organizations involved with this meeting both carry the torch of Cajal's knowledge and writings. The Cajal Club, established in 1947 by several neuroanatomists at an annual meeting of the American Association of Anatomists, is the world's oldest scientific society devoted to research on the nervous system. The Cajal Institute, tracing its origins to Cajal's own laboratory, still maintains several themes of research in Cajal's areas and manages a library of Cajal's microscope slides, drawings and books. It was only proper that the King of Spain, Don Juan Carlos I, accepted a special Cajal Club Krieg Achievement Award at this meeting. The award was donated by Roberta Krieg in memory of her husband, Dr. Wendell J.S. Krieg, a founding member of the Cajal Club and its first president. This award was presented to the Minister of Science, Doña Anna M. Birulés i Bertran, at a special reception in the Ministry of Science and Technology in Madrid. The meeting opened with a welcome from Efrain Azmitia (Meeting Co-organizer), Ricardo Martínez Murillo (Cajal Institute Director), Charles Ribak (Cajal Club President) and Dr José Pío Beltrá, the Vice President of the Consejo Superior de Investigaciones Cientificas (CSIC). It was held in an excellent auditorium of the CSIC. Javier DeFelipe (Meeting Co-Organizer) closed the meeting.

This volume is organized into sections based mainly on the order of papers presented at the meeting. The chapters are all based on examining Cajal's original concepts and reviewing the pertinent work which has occurred since to elaborate, and even change, his original concepts. The first chapters addressed issues dealing with Cajal's views on development, evolution and neuronal morphology, including the cytoskeleton, dendrites and synapses. The middle section of this volume is involved with Cajal's views of specific neurons and neuroplastic mechanisms. The last portion of the book includes topics on neuronal organization, brain systems and mental diseases. The chairs for the scientific sessions at this international meeting have also contributed comments to introduce each section of the book. Each of them is a distinguished scholar in a specific area of Cajal's work, and include Facundo Valverde (Cajal Institute), Pedro and Tauba Pasik (Mount Sinai, NY), Patricia Whitaker-Azmitia (Stony Brook, NY), Enrico Mugnaini (Chicago, IL), Ricardo Martínez Murillo (Cajal Institute) and Luciano Angelucci (Rome, Italy). The opportunity to hear from these experts in the field about the evolving concepts of Cajal's neuron makes this volume more interesting.

Several special social events occurred during this meeting, including a visit to Cajal's Madrid home, meeting three of his grandchildren, a wonderful reception at the Royal Botanical Gardens adjacent to the Prado Museum sponsored by Elan Pharmaceuticals and a stunning Flamenco dancing display with a dinner. The venue of Madrid for this meeting was most exciting with late night sidewalk cafés and spirited pedestrians walking throughout the city into the early morning hours.

The primary purpose of this book is not to be a historical review of Cajal's work. Historical perspectives tend to look back and their primary purpose is to review past discoveries. Our agenda is different. We intend to use Cajal's coherent views to help interpret the significance of contemporary research and provide a direction for future progress in neuroscience. Scientific breakthroughs are dependent on technical and methodological innovations, which provide a new source of knowledge for interpreting nature. New concepts are utilized to guide the development of basic research in the laboratory and to stimulate clinical application to treat human diseases. The massive information explosion of the last thirty years has fragmented many areas of neuroscience. As we enter the twenty-first century, we are attempting to develop a mechanism for integrating our current research discoveries into a coherent package that might provide unique and unexpected outcomes in planning future research strategies. It can be argued that a general book of this type will not succeed because the field has already become too large and complex. We acknowledge this difficulty, and recognize that our efforts may be viewed as overly grandiose. However, the mind of Cajal provided concepts which unified centuries of neuroscience research that occurred before the twentieth century. His personal visions laid a general framework, which has spawned a century of research on the brain. The topics we have selected for this book are rooted in the discoveries of Cajal, and are also recognized as areas of future development for the next century.

The major problem to be addressed in this book is how our views of the neuron are changing, and how this impacts on our own research strategy for future research. When Cajal formulated his concept of a neuron, he was mainly using a Golgi method and light microscopy. Today, the problems investigated by individual researchers use a variety of sophisticated methods. These include molecular techniques, electron microscopy, computer-assisted morphometrics, tissue culture, immunocytochemistry, electrophysiology, tract-tracing molecules and imaging. Cajal never saw a synapse, or a receptor, or a PET scan. These innovations have had a profound influence on how we view the neuron, and little attempt has been made over the last fifty years to merge these divergent views into a coherent whole. For example, if the dendrites of a neuron are plastic, what does this do to synaptic connections? If neurons function together as networks, how do individual neurons code information? If apoptosis of neurons is blocked, how does this influence cortical development? If neurogenesis of dentate gyrus neurons is increased in the adult hippocampus, how does this affect our treatment of epilepsy? If neuronal trophic factors are reduced in schizophrenia and Alzheimer's disease, how should these molecules be restored or replaced? It becomes clear that a new view of a neuron is emerging from a variety of new research findings, but it is unclear whether a single view can again be proposed to replace the neuron envisioned by Cajal. It is hoped that the present book illustrates the many insights provided by the participants of the Madrid meeting.

Contemporary research is specialized. Every aspect of the neuron has attracted tremendous interest and study. The synapse, axon, membrane, cytoskeleton, nucleus, dendrites and spines are immensely intricate. The interaction between neurons is approached from a variety of developmental and physiological approaches, and the resultant circuitry is more intertwined than ever imagined. Neurotransmitters, receptors, transporters and molecules all combine to produce complex functions. Trophic factors exist for nearly every type of neuron and glial cell, and produce sequential and concurrent effects on survival, maturation and connectivity. The etiology of neuronal diseases and the repair of damaged neurons hold exciting promise. All these individual advances and approaches would benefit from a more contemporary view of the neuron. We provide these views in this book with the hope that a new concept of Cajal's neuron will emerge.

The Editors

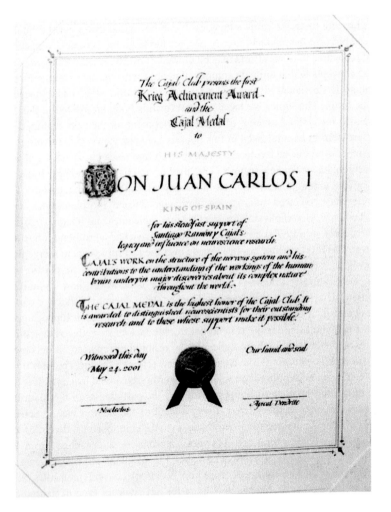

Certificate presented to His Majesty Don Juan Carlos I, King of Spain.

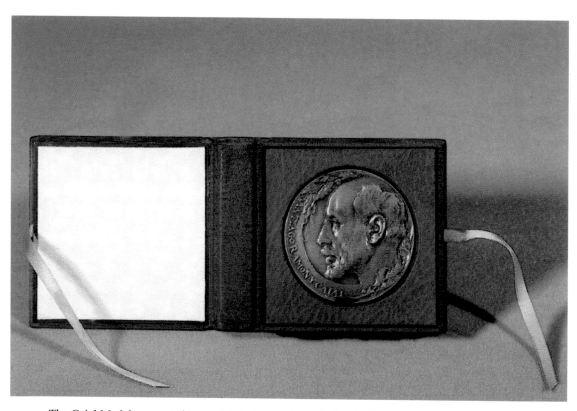

The Cajal Medal, presented to His Majesty Don Juan Carlos I, King of Spain, by the Cajal Club.

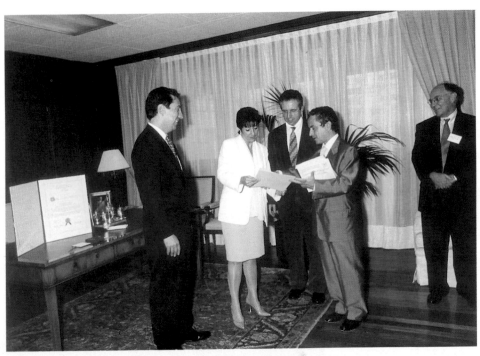

Presentation of the Certificate and Medal to the Minister of Science and Technology. From left to right: Certificate and Medal on desk, Charles E. Ribak, Anna M. Birulés i Bertran, Ramón Marimón Suñol, Ricardo Martínez Murillo and Efrain Azmitia.

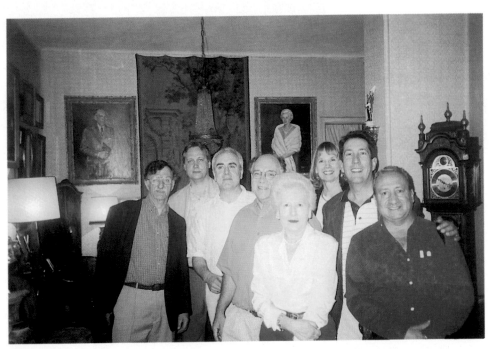

From left to right: Edward Jones, Tamas Freund, Javier DeFelipe, Efrain Azmitia, Cajal's granddaughter (María Ángeles Ramón y Cajal Junquera), Vivien Casagrande, Charles Ribak and Alfredo Feria-Velasco.

List of Contributors

P. Alifragis, Department of Anatomy and Developmental Biology, University College London, London WC1E 6BT, UK

A. Angelucci, Department of Ophthalmology and Visual Science, Moran Eye Center, University of Utah, 50 North Medical Drive, Salt Lake City, UT 84132, USA

L. Angelucci, University La Sapienza, Pharmacology 2, Fac. de Med. & Chirurgia, Piazzale Aldo Moro 5, 00185 Rome, Italy

V. Arango, Department of Neuroscience, New York State Psychiatric Institute, 1051 Riverside Drive, Box 42, New York, NY 10032, USA

E.C. Azmitia, Departments of Biology and Psychiatry, Center for Neural Science, New York University, 100 Washington Square East, New York, NY 10003, USA

M.V.L. Bennett, Department of Neuroscience, Albert Einstein College of Medicine, 1300 Morris Park Avenue, Bronx, NY 10804, USA

A.B. Butler, Krasnow Institute for Advanced Study and Department of Psychology, George Mason University, Fairfax, VA 22030, USA

M.E. Cantino, Department of Physiology and Neurobiology, 3107 Horsebarn Hill Road, U-4156, Storrs, CT 06269, USA

V.A. Casagrande, Department of Cell Biology, Vanderbilt Medical School, Medical Center North C2310, Nashville, TN 37232-2175, USA

E. Charych, Department of Physiology and Neurobiology, 3107 Horsebarn Hill Road, U-4156, Storrs, CT 06269, USA

S.B. Christie, Department of Physiology and Neurobiology, 3107 Horsebarn Hill Road, U-4156, Storrs, CT 06269, USA

S.B. Daniels, Department of Physiology and Neurobiology, 3107 Horsebarn Hill Road, U-4156, Storrs, CT 06269, USA

K. Dashtipour, Department of Neurology, Southern Illinois University, School of Medicine, Springfield, IL 62794-9637, USA

A.L. De Blas, Department of Physiology and Neurobiology, 3107 Horsebarn Hill Road, U-4156, Storrs, CT 06269, USA

J. DeFelipe, Instituto Cajal (CSIC), Avda. Doctor Arce 37, 28002 Madrid, Spain

A.R. del Angel, Division of Neurosciences, CIBO, I.M.S.S., Guadalajara, Jal., Mexico

R. Djavadian, Department of Neurophysiology, Nencki Institute of Experimental Biology, 3 Pasteur Street, 02-093 Warsaw, Poland

G.N. Elston, Vision, Touch and Hearing Research Centre, Department of Physiology and Pharmacology, The University of Queensland, St. Lucia, Qld. 4072, Australia

A. Fairén, Instituto de Neurociencias, Consejo Superior de Investigaciones Cientificas and Universidad Miguel Hernández, Campus de San Juan, Apartado 18, 03550 San Juan de Alicante, Spain

A. Feria-Velasco, CIATEJ, Division of Pathology, Av. Normalistas 800, 44270 Guadalajara, Jal., Mexico

J.M. Frade, Instituto Cajal (CSIC), Avda. Doctor Arce 37, 28002 Madrid, Spain

C. Frassoni, Istituto Nazionale C. Besta, Via Celoria 11, 20133 Milan, Italy

T.F. Freund, Institute of Experimental Medicine, Hungarian Academy of Sciences, Szigony u. 43, H-1083 Budapest, Hungary

L.M. Garcia-Segura, Instituto Cajal (CSIC), Avda. Doctor Arce 37, 28002 Madrid, Spain

M. Garzón, Departamento de Morfología, Facultad de Medicina, Universidad Autónoma de Madrid (UAM), Madrid, Spain

P.S. Goldman-Rakic, Department of Neurobiology, Yale University School of Medicine, 333 Cedar Street, New Haven, CT 06520-8001, USA

I. Gonzalez-Burgos, Laboratory of Psychobiology, CIBIMI, I.M.S.S., Morelia, Mich., Mexico

P.R. Hof, Department of Ophthalmology, Mount Sinai School of Medicine, One Gustave L. Levy Place, New York, NY 10029, USA

E.G. Jones, Center for Neuroscience, University of California, Davis, 1544 Newton Court, Davis, CA 95616, USA

N. Koibuchi, Department of Physiology, Gunma University School of Medicine, Maebashi, Gunma 371-8511, Japan

J.B. Levitt, Department of Biology, City College of the City University of New York, 138th Street and Convent Avenue, New York, NY 10031, USA

R.-W. Li, Department of Physiology and Neurobiology, 3107 Horsebarn Hill Road, U-4156, Storrs, CT 06269, USA

J.S. Lund, Department of Ophthalmology and Visual Science, Moran Eye Center, University of Utah, 50 North Medical Drive, Salt Lake City, UT 84132, USA

J.J. Mann, Department of Psychiatry, Columbia University College of Physicians and Surgeons, 1051 Riverside Drive, New York, NY 10032, USA

E. Mengual, Departmento de Anatomía, Facultad de Medicina, Universidad de Navarra, Irunlarrea 1, Pamplona 31008, Spain

C.P. Miralles, Department of Physiology and Neurobiology, 3107 Horsebarn Hill Road, U-4156, Storrs, CT 06269, USA

Z. Molnár, Department of Human Anatomy and Genetics, University of Oxford, South Parks Road, Oxford OX1 3QX, UK

J. Morante-Oria, Instituto de Neurociencias, Consejo Superior de Investigaciones Cientificas and Universidad Miguel Hernández, Campus de San Juan, Apartado 18, 03550 San Juan de Alicante, Spain

J.H. Morrison, Neurobiology of Aging Laboratories, Box 1639, Mount Sinai School of Medicine, One Gustave L. Levy Place, New York, NY 10029, USA

E. Mugnaini, Northwestern University Institute for Neuroscience, Searle Building 5-471, 320 E. Superior Street, Chicago, IL 60611, USA

R.M. Murillo, Instituto Cajal (CSIC), Avda. Doctor Arce 37, 28002 Madrid, Spain

B. Nadarajah, Department of Anatomy and Developmental Biology, University College London, London WC1E 6BT, UK

M. Nieto-Sampedro, Department of Neural Plasticity, Instituto Cajal de Neurobiología, CSIC, Avda. Doctor Arce 37, 28002 Madrid, Spain

J.G. Parnavelas, Department of Anatomy and Developmental Biology, University College London, London WC1E 6BT, UK

P. Pasik, Department of Neurology, Mount Sinai School of Medicine, New York, NY 10029, USA

T. Pasik, Department of Neurology, Mount Sinai School of Medicine, New York, NY 10029, USA

A. Peters, Department of Anatomy and Neurobiology, Boston University School of Medicine, 715 Albany Street, Boston, MA 02118-2526, USA

V.M. Pickel, Division of Neurobiology, Department of Neurology and Neuroscience, Weill Medical College of Cornell University, 411 East 69th Street, New York, NY 10021, USA

P. Rakic, Department of Neurobiology, Yale University School of Medicine, P.O. Box 208001, New Haven, CT 06520-8001, USA

C.E. Ribak, Department of Anatomy and Neurobiology, University of California at Irvine, College of Medicine, Irvine, CA 92697-1275, USA

R. Riquelme, Department of Physiology and Neurobiology, 3107 Horsebarn Hill Road, U-4156, Storrs, CT 06269, USA

P. Rudomin, Department of Physiology, Biophysics and Neurosciences, Centro de Investigación y Estudios Avanzados del Instituto Politécnico Nacional, 07000 Mexico D.F., Mexico

S. Sakakibara, Department of Histology and Neurobiology, Dokkyo University School of Medicine, Mibu, Tochigi 321-0293, Japan

G. Sáry, Department of Cell Biology, Vanderbilt University, Medical Center North C2310, Nashville, TN 37232-2175, USA

S.W. Schwarzacher, Institute of Anatomy, University of Goettingen, Kreuzbergring 36, D-37075 Goettingen, Germany

M. Segal, Department of Neurobiology, The Weizmann Institute, Rehovot 76100, Israel

C. Sotelo, INSERM U-106, Hôpital de la Salpétrière, 75013 Paris, France

K. Turlejski, Department of Neurophysiology, Nencki Institute of Experimental Biology, 3 Pasteur Street, 02-093 Warsaw, Poland

S. Ueda, Department of Histology and Neurobiology, Dokkyo University School of Medicine, Mibu, Tochigi 321-0293, Japan

M.D. Underwood, Department of Neuroscience and Department of Psychiatry, Columbia University College of Physicians and Surgeons, 1051 Riverside Drive, New York, NY 10032, USA

F. Valverde, Instituto Cajal (CSIC), Avda. Doctor Arce 37, 28002 Madrid, Spain

D.I. Vaney, Vision, Touch and Hearing Research Centre, School of Biomedical Sciences, The University of Queensland, Brisbane, Qld. 4072, Australia

E. Watanabe, Department of Histology and Neurobiology, Dokkyo University School of Medicine, Mibu, Tochigi 321-0293, Japan

P. Whitaker-Azmitia, Department of Psychology, State University of New York, Stony Brook, NY 11794-2500, USA

X. Xu, Department of Psychology, Vanderbilt University, Medical Center North C2310, Nashville, TN 37232-2175, USA

B.Y. Yang, Department of Physiology and Neurobiology, 3107 Horsebarn Hill Road, U-4156, Storrs, CT 06269, USA

K. Yoshimoto, Department of Legal Medicine, Kyoto Prefectural University of Medicine, Kawaramachi Hirokoji, Kamikyo-ku, Kyoto 602-0841, Japan

W. Yu, Department of Physiology and Neurobiology, 3107 Horsebarn Hill Road, U-4156, Storrs, CT 06269, USA

L. Zaborszky, Center for Molecular and Behavioral Neuroscience, Rutgers, The State University of New Jersey, 197 University Avenue, Newark, NJ 07102, USA

Contents

Section I. Neuronal changes during development and evolution

Section II. Inside the neuron: cytoskeleton, dendrites, and synapses

Section III. Character and function of specific neurons

Section VI. Functional circuits, mental diseases and brain aging

Neuronal changes during development and evolution

E.C. Azmitia, J. DeFelipe, E.G. Jones, P. Rakic and C.E. Ribak (Eds.)
Progress in Brain Research, Vol. 136

CHAPTER 1

Neuronal changes during development and evolution (an overview)

Facundo Valverde*

Instituto Cajal (CSIC), Avenida del Doctor Arce 37, 28002 Madrid, Spain

Abstract: This overview highlights the presentations made by several authors, with sidelights commentaries on the topics covered in this session. The Neurotropic hypothesis, formulated by Cajal more than one century ago, has been one of the fundamental tenets of modern Neuroscience. Research work is unveiling highly complex molecular mechanisms by means of which neuronal processes grow in the right direction leading to the formation of neural networks. Another interesting topic covered in this session pertains to the remarkably conserved similarity of most parts of the brain between reptiles, birds and mammals. The presence of the neocortex, which occurs in mammals, is discussed on the basis of different migratory behavior during development. The question of neuronal stability throughout the life cycle raises interesting aspects on the generation of new neurons. This is a particularly timely topic because recent evidence, denied by others, has shown the generation of new neocortical neurons in the adult. In another session, it was discussed the evidence showing that pyramidal cells and intrinsic cells of the neocortex have different developmental origins. Finally, several modern analyses show the role of different transcription factors in the formation of brain cortical maps before the arrival of their proper afferent connections.

The organization of the brain is an integral series of developmental processes which include cell birth, migration, differentiation, settling, and the establishment of connections. These were the topics covered in this session, and which I will present in the following lines. Through their presentations, all speakers agreed to give a tribute to Santiago Ramón y Cajal for his important contributions to, and also predictions on, each of these themes. Since several presentations in this session were more or less related to some studies carried out in my laboratory, I will take this opportunity to briefly include comments related to the general area of the topics covered in the session.

At a special evening lecture, Constantino Sotelo (INSERM, Hôpital de la Salpétrière, Paris) was awarded the Krieg Achievement Award by the Cajal Club, which he richly deserved in appreciation of his well-known scientific career. A good friend of mine since the early

sixties, when we were both postdoctoral fellows with Professor F. De Castro (the last living disciple of Santiago Ramón y Cajal), I was especially glad to be present at that moment. Constantino Sotelo reviewed the Neurotropic hypothesis formulated by Cajal in 1890. He recalled how Cajal observed and detailed for the first time the advancing tip of growing axons in the spinal cord of the chick embryo, in Cajal's words "... *that the silver chromate renders yellow-cinnamon*, (see Fig. 1A, arrows)". I can imagine what this might have represented for Cajal himself at a time in which he was gathering facts in favor of one of his basic tenets, the independence of nerve cells. Growing cones remained a simple curiosity for a long time, because nobody could imagine how growing axons, swimming in a tangle of cellular processes, could be able to reach their targets "... *without deviations and errors*". Two years later (1892) Cajal published his first concepts on the chemotactic hypothesis for explaining how certain 'chemical flows' guide growing axons to find their corresponding targets.

*Corresponding author: Tel.: 91 585 4707; Fax: 91 585 4754;
E-mail: fvalverde@cajal.csic.es

4

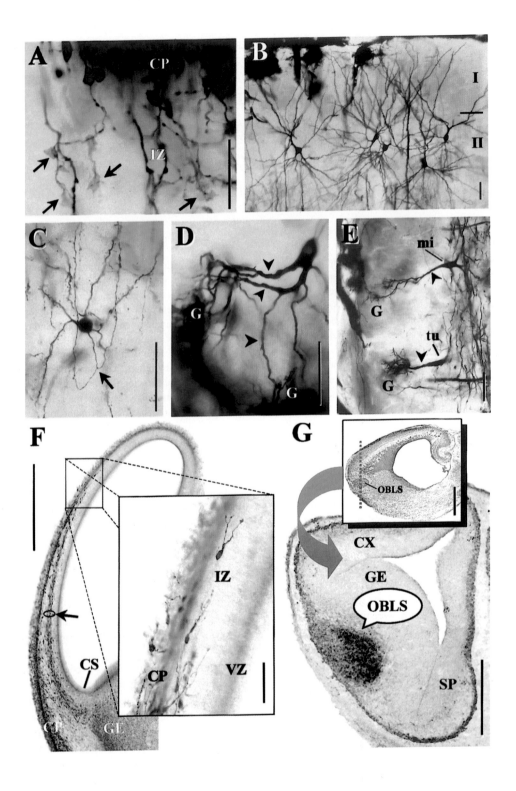

Sperry's (1963) formulation of the chemoaffinity hypothesis for the development of specific patterns of connections initiated a revival of Cajal's concepts on the chemotactic hypothesis, which still had to wait until recent years to provide direct evidence for a chemotropic guidance of growing axons. We now know that the guidance of axons depends on certain substances that can be attractive or repulsive (or both), secreted by intermediate targets and, not infrequently, thanks to the presence of specific cues or guide-post cells, developed along the pathways that the growing axons must follow. A family of these molecules has been identified, and even some of their genes have been cloned (e.g., Itoh et al., 1998; Brose et al., 1999). In his exposé, Constantino Sotelo reviewed his own work on the interpretations and functional correlates, as the ultimate challenge left to us by Cajal, in understanding the processes of axonal growth in development and regeneration. He addressed new scientific achievements in this field and his most recent work on long-range guidance molecules belonging to the family of semaphorins and Slits. He illustrated recent studies made with his collaborators (see references by De Castro and Nguyen-Ba-Charvet in his communication) on the complex interactions on mitral cell axons (lateral olfactory tract) exerted by different secreted semaphorins, and the response to different Slits by growing axons of the dorsal root ganglion neurons.

The lateral olfactory tract, which develops very early and is a phylogenetically old conserved tract, extends from the olfactory bulb to the olfactory cortex traveling in the lateral region of the basal telencephalon, away from the medial septum. One of the first indications that a chemorepulsive mechanism could play a role in target selection came from the studies made by Pini (1993) precisely in this fiber tract; when olfactory bulb and septum are cultured together, mitral cell axons emerged from the explant opposite to the side of the septum, indicating the existence of a diffusible chemorepellent. This repulsive factor was identified as the vertebrate homolog of the Slit protein, the ligand for Robo, by the group of Yi Rao (Li et al., 1999). Now, using an *in vitro* model, Sotelo showed that both Slit1 and Slit2 are implicated in the repulsive action on growing bulbar cells and that Sema 3B, released by the mesenchyme bordering the lateral olfactory tract, exerts an attractive influence on these axons. It is interesting to mention that these secreted chemorepellents and attractants appear conserved in the *Small Eye* mutant mice in which an, apparently normal, lateral olfactory tract arises from the olfactory bulb-like structure which develops ectopically in these mutants (López-Mascaraque et al., 1998; Jiménez et al., 2000).

Zoltán Molnár (University of Oxford, Oxford, UK) posed interesting questions for the study of homologies between diverse brain regions in different animals, to understand forebrain evolution. All of us who are familiar with his book (Molnár, 1998) know that he has been largely interested in the development and establishment of connections between the cortex and thalamus. During development, these connections travel through the cortico-striatal boundary which is delimited

Fig. 1A. Transverse section through the neocortex of a hedgehog embryo (*Erinaceus europaeus*) at a very early developmental stage, showing immature pyramidal cells of the cortical plate (CP) and their projecting axons entering the intermediate zone (IZ) below. The axons are tipped with delicate and faint growing cones (arrows) which appear as large triangular profiles, which Cajal, for images like this, liked to compare as the feet of web-footed animals. Golgi method. Scale bar = 50 μm. B. Transverse section through the somato-sensory cortex of an adult hedgehog *(Erinaceus europaeus)* showing a group of typical 'extraverted' pyramidal cells in layer II. These cells are characterized by their prominent dendritic ramifications extending into the thick layer I, where they receive a strong zonal input. Golgi method. Scale bar = 50 μm. C. Spiny stellate cell with recurving ascending axon (arrow) in sub-layer IVc of the primary visual cortex (area 17) of macaca (*Rhesus monkey*). The dendrites are moderately spinous; the axon bifurcates and turns into two ascending branches reaching the upper cortical layers. Golgi method. Scale bar = 50 μm. D. Mitral cell in the olfactory bulb of the mouse at embryonic day 20. Several dendrites (arrow-heads) approach distinct prospective glomeruli (G). Golgi method. Scale bar = 50 μm. E. Transverse section through the olfactory bulb of an adult hedgehog (*Erinaceus europaeus*). Mitral cells (mi) and tufted cells (tu) have single principal dendrites (arrow-heads) entering individual olfactory glomeruli (G). Golgi method. Scale bar = 50 μm. F. Transverse section through the telencephalic vesicle of the rat at embryonic day 15 showing GABA expression in cells in the marginal zone of the cortical plate (CP) and in cells of the prospective migratory stream (oval pointed by arrow), extending from the ganglionic eminence (GE) through the intermediate zone. The boxed area is amplified to denote the morphology of presumptive migratory cells in the intermediate zone (IZ). CP, cortical plate; CS, cortico-striatal sulcus; IZ, intermediate zone; VZ, ventricular zone. Large scale bar = 500 μm, scale bar in boxed area = 50 μm. G. Olfactory bulb like structure (OBLS) in homozygous Pax-6 mutant mouse at embryonic day 20 (see Jiménez et al., 2000). Box shows a Nissl-stained sagittal section in which the OBLS can be seen at the rostral tip of the telencephalic vesicle. Dotted line corresponds approximately to the level of the large transverse section. This section shows *Robo2* expression (purple) and calretinin immunolabeling (brown). Scale bar in the large transverse section = 500 μm, scale bar in box = 1 mm.

inside the lateral ventricle by the prominent cortico-striatal sulcus (see Fig. 1F, CS), and appears to be crucial not only for the traffic of fibers linking both cortex and thalamus, but also, as I shall discuss below (see also commentaries to John Parnavelas), for the passage of migrating cells entering the neocortex. Zoltán Molnár discussed relevant aspects of this particular boundary, which has been shown to present transient characteristics and gene expression patterns, in order to explain certain homologies between different animals. His hypothesis of field homology (in collaboration with Ann Butler) suggests that very specific gradients of pallial development at the cortico-striatal boundary represent a key issue in neocortical evolution, proposing that the anterior dorsal ventricular ridge of reptiles and birds (sauropsids), and the lateral neocortex and parts of the claustro-amygdaloid complex of mammals are homologous, representing elaborations of the deep part of the lateral cortex. This supports the hypothesis of a field homology of the anterior part of the dorsal ventricular ridge to these mammalian basal structures. Recent studies have shown the existence of a subdivision intercalated between the striatum and lateral pallium, whose derivatives, at least in the mouse, belong to the claustro-amygdaloid complex (Puelles et al., 2000), and that the *Pax6* gene, which controls the dorso-ventral regionalization of neocortex (Stoykova et al., 2000), may be in relation to the normal migratory pattern in the region of the cortico-striatal junction. Much in line with these observations, Zoltán Molnár has suggested that a mutation of the *Pax6* gene, or in any of the genes in its downstream cascade, in the ancestral amniote stock, might have been involved in the evolution of neocortex by changing the fate of cells in this crucial region.

It comes near at hand to consider, as the title of his presentation reads (Neuronal Changes During Evolution), something relative to neuronal morphology, that surely might have been accounted for during these evolutionary changes; thus, it seemed to me appropriate to discuss briefly some work in which I was engaged several years ago in relation to this interesting topic. The cortex appears not to be hardwired for specific elements, retaining during evolution the competence to adapt or modify its neuronal types to whatever is most convenient for its specific function. Comparative neuroanatomy reconstructs the process of evolution through the study of some living species that are thought to be almost exact replicas of those found in the fossil record. The insectivore

hedgehog (*Erinaceus*) has been considered a direct descendant of primitive eutherians and, therefore, the comparison of its brain organization offers a likely model for brain evolution in which several aspects of neuronal changes can be observed. The neocortex of the hedgehog contains, in layer II, large pyramidal cells with several dendrites arborizing profusely in layer I (Fig. 1B). These pyramidal cells, or 'extraverted neurons', as they were coined by the Sanides (Sanides, 1970; Sanides and Sanides, 1972), receive a strong input in the most superficial cortical layers and probably represent a stage of phylogenetic development, fully expressed at the amphibian level with the most accentuated dendritic extraversion and absence of basal dendrites. Thus, neocortical evolutionary differentiation might be related to changes in the laminar distribution of cortical afferents which may have shifted from layer I in primitive forms to predominate in the lower part of layer III and in layer IV, as seen in advanced mammals.

From my studies of the forms of cells with spinous dendrites in various mammals, I have always had the impression that they all may share a common phylogenetic origin, and that a continuum can be traced from lower forms to the primate brain. In the neocortex of the hedgehog, a complete series of intermediate forms, between the most 'extraverted' pyramidal cells and the typically developed pyramidal cells, can always be found (Valverde, 1986). At a later stage of development, some pyramidal cells lose their apical dendritic branches in layer I (which no longer maintains its primacy as the target for cortical input), retaining but a thin apical dendrite tapering at some distance from the cell body. This seems to be the case of the stellate or grain pyramids of the barrel field in the somatosensory and visual cortices of some rodents. In a final elimination of the remnant of their thin apical dendrites, these cells turn into typical spiny stellate cells (Fig. 1C), like those found in the visual cortices of the cat and monkey (Valverde, 1971a, 1985). These stages of pyramidal cell differentiation also involve variations in the axonal pattern, which changes from long projecting neurons (hedgehog, mouse, rat, cat) to intrinsic cells with strong recurving, ascending axons (Fig. 1C, arrow) that remain inside the cortex (primates). There is a long way, in evolutionary units (if I am allowed to use such a term), between the two examples presented in Fig. 1B and C, but they suggest to me that neocortical organization attained in higher mammals might have been accomplished by reshaping dendritic and axonal arbors of various categories of cortical cells, where differences can be minimal in closely related species, but are substantial when comparison is made between distant subjects.

Neuronal changes throughout the life cycle was another interesting topic covered by Kris Turlejski (Nencki Institute, Warsaw, Poland). Thus, we were given the opportunity to complete a general overview of neuronal changes, not only through the long course of evolution, as just commented on, but also through the short breadth of the life-span. Turlejski has been interested in several aspects of cell proliferation and cell death in the adult brain. For instance, he pointed out that cell migration occurs in the dentate gyrus and olfactory bulb, although in the former it stops in young adults, and that in the olfactory bulb in certain species it is seasonally modulated.

Developmental processes throughout the adult life of an animal include: proliferation and migration of neurons from stem cells (that now hits the headlines of almost every daily newspaper); programmed cell death (neurons collaborate in their own death by the synthesis of proteins that injure the cell, apoptosis); and reorganization of connections (including synapse formation and/or elimination), among other phenomena. Since the brain is a machine devised for continuous modification throughout the life cycle (think of the learning, behavior and memory processes), these phenomena provide the necessary basis for brain plasticity. In his hypothesis of brain function, Cajal already had the idea that axons and dendrites are continuously modified by the establishment of new connections, withdrawal of exuberant ramifications, and pruning of dendrites and axons, so that, in his own words, "...*the entire neuronal arborization, in visible traits, represents the history of the battles suffered during its embryonic life*" (Cajal, 1911). All of these are processes that explain the capacity to create new associations and modify the adaptative capacity of the human brain. But, as Kris Turlejski added, the remodeling of connections may also depend on extreme rearing environments, that reverts into pathological conditions, so that the importance of understanding the life cycle of neurons is enormous.

We know that many dendritic trees and their appendages (the dendritic spines), as well as axonal arborizations, are dynamic structures, and that the plasticity of these cell processes during development, or in response to experience and rearing in deprived

conditions, are well known. In this respect, I would like to recall my older studies on the reduction in the number of dendritic spines in pyramidal cells of the visual cortex in mice that were reared in complete darkness from birth (Valverde, 1967), and on the structural changes found in area striata of mice after enucleation (Valverde, 1968), all of them being performed in an epoch in which preliminary concepts and observations on brain plasticity were just beginning to appear. From these early experiments, we also learned that mice maintained in complete darkness for prolonged periods, never recover the normal number of dendritic spines when they were returned to normal conditions (Valverde, 1971b), confirming early studies by Wiesel and Hubel (1965) showing that part of the deficiency produced by sensory deprivation becomes irreversible. An example of dendritic remodeling is provided by some developing mitral cells of the olfactory bulb, a few of which have more than one principal dendrite for several olfactory glomeruli (Fig. 1D, arrowheads), in contrast to the adult pattern, in which only one principal dendrite of mitral/tufted cells reaching a single glomerulus appears to be the rule (Fig. 1E, arrowheads).

José María Frade (Instituto Cajal, CSIC, Madrid) reviewed some recent work concerning several aspects of the interkinetic nuclear movement (INM) and its implication in neurogenesis. INM is important for controlling cell density necessary to continuously produce a high number of neurons in G0, which are generated in an efficient way due to the definition of an apically located proneural cluster that contains equipotent precursors in the neurogenetic state.

The cerebral cortex contains two principal types of neurons: pyramidal cells projecting to distant targets, and intrinsic neurons with short axons that remain inside the cortex. John Parnavelas (University College, London, UK) reviewed recent evidence showing that these two neuronal types are generated in distinct proliferative zones. The cerebral cortex develops from the dorsal part of the telencephalic vesicle. Its precursor cells originate in the ventricular zone lining the walls of the third ventricle and slithering along radially oriented glial cells reach their final layer position following an inside-out gradient (Rakic, 1971, 1972). The ventral part of the telencephalic vesicle forms two major subdivisions known as the lateral and medial ganglionic eminences (LGE, MGE), components of the basal telencephalon, which will differentiate into the corpus striatum and pallidum of the adult. The germinative territories of both dorsal and ventral subdivisions of the telencephalic vesicle are separated by the prominent internal cortico-striatal sulcus, delimiting the cortico-striatal boundary, which was thought to restrict to their own domains the migration of precursor cells (Fishell, 1995). However, recent studies have shown that during development, many cells derived from both ganglionic eminences migrate tangentially, some of them transgressing the cortico-striatal limit, to enter the developing cortex (De Carlos et al., 1996; Anderson et al., 1997a; Tamamaki et al., 1997), while others migrate to distinct basal telencephalic structures (e.g., the olfactory bulb; Lois and Alvarez-Buylla, 1994). This is a particularly timely topic, because, in the short time elapsed since the first report from my laboratory of this new type of migration (De Carlos et al., 1996), a large number of studies have furthered interesting aspects of this migratory route and specified several characteristics of its cellular components (see review by Marín and Rubenstein, 2001). These cells express GABA (Anderson et al., 1997a; Tamamaki et al., 1997; Parnavelas, 2000), suggesting that a substantial number of cortical interneurons, known to express GABA, are derived from the ganglionic eminences. These cells appear reduced in number in Dlx-1 and Dlx-2 mutant mice (Anderson et al., 1997a, b), implicating both genes in this type of tangential migration. However, the molecular mechanisms guiding these migrating cells are still poorly understood. It has been shown that the ventricular zone of the ganglionic eminences secretes Slit which is repulsive for GABAergic neurons (Zhu et al., 1999). It has also been demonstrated that neuropilin receptors control the migration of interneurons from the ganglionic eminences (Marín et al., 2001), and recent studies in my laboratory show complementary patterns of expression of PSA-NCAM and Robo-2 which may be implicated in this migratory route.

It is still unclear whether these migrating cells originate from the MGE, the LGE or both ganglionic eminences. John Parnavelas and his collaborators (Lavdas et al., 1999) showed that the MGE is the source of a substantial number of cells: in the marginal zone, including some with features of Cajal-Retzius cells; in the subplate; and in the lower intermediate zone. Similar results were obtained by Wichterle et al. (1999) after grafting neuronal precursors taken from the MGE into the adult brain (see also Wichterle et al., 2001). Anderson et al. (2001) reported GABA-expressing cells migrating from the MGE into the cerebral cortex through the intermediate zone, while they found, at later stages, LGE-derived cells migrating via the subventricular zone. Thus, it appears that both the MGE and LGE are sources of different neurons following distinct migratory pathways.

Beginning at embryonic day 14 in the rat embryo, the flow of GABA-immunoreactive cells migrating in the intermediate zone is very impressive (Fig. 1F, arrow), and, at later embryonic stages, the migratory stream even reaches the medial side, approaching the primordium of the hippocampus. One can imagine these cells struggling to pass through a forest of perpendicularly arranged glial cells, ascending obliquely to reach their positions in the cerebral cortex. John Parnavelas described how these cells probably use tangential migratory paths within the intermediate and marginal zones to reach the developing cortex, possibly responding to certain positional cues and establishing communication with pyramidal cells before migrating to their destination. A key issue that came to my attention is the recent publication by Letinic and Rakic (2001), who have demonstrated that there are a substantial number of GABA-expressing cells migrating from the ganglionic eminences, in the human brain, into the dorsal thalamus. This type of migration, which appears to be unique to humans, can possibly be correlated with the evolution of the neocortex, and adds even more interest to the study of the significance of the ganglionic eminences, and the migration of their cells. I think it is now time to review Karten's (1991) theory of the dual developmental origin of the mammalian neocortex in the context of these new advances.

All of us interested in cortical development are familiar with Pasko Rakic's (Yale University, New Haven, USA) fundamental studies on cell lineage, origin, mode of migration and fate of cortical neurons (see Section IV). The cerebral cortex in the adult is parcelled into morphologically and functionally distinct cortical areas. The remarkable similarity of cortical topography across species is not the result of mere coincidence. Areas subserving the same function are located at comparable positions; e.g., the visual cortex is always located dorso-caudally, the somato-sensory cortex occupies a central position and is always placed behind the motor cortex, etc. Are areal identities already determined in the germinative epithelium of the ventricular zone? Or is their specification the result of interaction between uncommitted cell populations and their afferent fiber systems? An answer to the first question was derived from Pasko

Rakic's radial unit hypothesis (Rakic, 1988); the ventricular zone contains a number of proliferative units, constituting a *protomap* for the different cortical areas, which are expanded in the developing cerebral cortex thanks to the perfect alignment of radial glial fibers.

As an extension of the *protomap* hypothesis, Donoghue and Rakic (1999) have examined in embryonic material the expression of several transcription factors and the EphA receptor family, a group of cell surface-bound tyrosine kinases, which appear expressed in different prospective functional domains prior to the development of any afferent or efferent systems. An answer to the second question has also been derived from several experiments showing that factors extrinsic to the developing cortex (the arrival of thalamo-cortical fibers) control the specification of the different cortical areas (e.g., Schlaggar and O'Leary, 1991). Thus far, the evidence obtained from several studies using a variety of molecular and gene expression markers suggests that both of these mechanisms may be acting in sequence; thus, certain aspects of intrinsic cortical organization may already be present in the ventricular zone prior to the arrival of its extrinsic connections. At later stages, signals provided by thalamic input (and, eventually, any other afferent input) will refine and lead to the emergence of the proper structural specificity (Kennedy and Dehay, 1993). A special issue of *Cerebral Cortex,* devoted to the genetic control of cortical development, reviewed recent advances on these mechanisms (Rubenstein and Rakic, 1999).

The extension of the *protomap* hypothesis leads us to consider regional expression in other telencephalic structures in the absence of patterned afferent input. In this context, it has been generally accepted that the development and differentiation of the olfactory bulb depends on the arrival of olfactory receptor axons. Homozygous *small eye* mutant mice lack nasal structures, including the olfactory epithelium and, supposedly, the olfactory bulb. However, several studies carried out in my laboratory on these mutant mice (Jiménez et al., 2000), provide evidence that a prospective olfactory bulb, develops, albeit abnormally, in the absence of its proper afferent input (Fig. 1G, OBLS). This argues in favor of the existence of other similar compartmentalized functional domains in other brain regions, even when the establishment of their proper afferent connections are lacking.

We are still far from completing many aspects of brain development and evolution, but I am sure these will come in the near future; a solid background is at hand. Although we know many aspects and properties of guidance molecules that direct axons to their appropriate targets, our understanding of the more precise molecular mechanisms involved in specific inter-neuronal connectivity still remains limited; we only begin to understand how certain brain regions evolved from homologous parts of our ancestors, but ignore what evolutionary steps gave rise to the development of highly evolved structures, like the neocortex; not to mention our ignorance for the prevention and treatment of those neuronal processes that can lead to disordered clinical phenotypes. The key discoveries and brilliant insights left to us by Santiago Ramón y Cajal no doubt have contributed, and still will help to decipher, many of these important questions.

Acknowledgments

I would like to thank the organizers of this Cajal Club/Cajal Institute Joint Meeting for giving me the opportunity to act as chairman for this session and the helpful comments and discussion from all participants. I am especially indebted to Juan A. De Carlos, Harvey Karten, and M. Angela Nieto for valuable suggestions in the preparation of this commentary. Work in my lab is supported by Research Project PB96-0813 from the Ministerio de Ciencia y Tecnología (former Ministerio de Educación y Cultura of Spain).

References

Anderson, S.A., Eisenstat, D.D., Shi, L. and Rubenstein, J.L.R. (1997a) Interneuron migration from basal forebrain to neocortex: dependence on *Dlx* genes. *Science*, 278: 474–476.

Anderson, S.A., Qiu, M.-S., Bulfone, A., Eisenstat, D.D., Meneses, J., Pedersen, R. and Rubenstein, J.L.R. (1997b) Mutation of the homeobox genes *Dlx-1* and *Dlx-2* disrupt the striatal subventricular zone and differentiation of late-born striatal neurons. *Neuron*, 19: 27–37.

Anderson, S.A., Marín, O., Horn, C., Jennings, K. and Rubenstein, J.L.R. (2001) Distinct cortical migrations from the medial and lateral ganglionic eminences. *Development*, 128: 353–363.

Brose, K., Bland, K.S., Wang, K.-H., Arnott, D., Henzel, W., Goodman, C.S., Tessier-Lavigne, M. and Kidd, T. (1999) Slit proteins bind Robo receptors and have an evolutionary conserved role in repulsive axon guidance. *Cell*, 96: 795–806.

Cajal, S.R. (1890) A quelle époque apparaissent les expansions des cellules nerveuses de la moëlle épinière du poulet ? *Anat. Anz.*, 5: 609–613.

10

Cajal, S.R. (1892) La rétine des vertébrés. *La Cellule*, 9: 121–255.

Cajal, S.R. (1911) *Histologie du Système Nerveux de l'Homme et des Vertébrés.* Vols. 1 and 2, Maloine, Paris (Reimpress. Instituto Cajal, CSIC, 1952).

De Carlos, J.A., López-Mascaraque, L. and Valverde, F. (1996) Dynamics of cell migration from the lateral ganglionic eminence in the rat. *J. Neurosci.*, 16: 6146–6156.

Donoghue, M.J. and Rakic, P. (1999) Molecular evidence for the early specification of presumptive functional domains in the embryonic primate cerebral cortex. *J. Neurosci.*, 19: 5967–5979.

Fishell, G. (1995) Striatal precursors adopt cortical identities in response to local cues. *Development*, 121: 803–812.

Itoh, A., Miyabayashi, T., Ohno, M. and Sakano, S. (1998) Cloning and expression of three mammalian homologs of Drosophila Slit suggest possible roles for Slit in the formation and maintenance of the nervous system. *Mol. Brain. Res.*, 62: 175–186.

Jiménez, D., García, C., De Castro, F., Chédotal, A., Sotelo, C., De Carlos, J.A., Valverde, F. and López-Mascaraque, L. (2000) Evidence for intrinsic development of olfactory structures in *Pax-6* mutant mice. *J. Comp. Neurol.*, 428: 511–526.

Karten, H.J. (1991) Homology and evolutionary origins of the 'neocortex'. *Brain Behav. Evol.*, 38: 264–272.

Kennedy, H. and Dehay, C. (1993) Feature article: Cortical specification of mice and men. *Cerebral Cortex*, 3: 171–186.

Lavdas, A.A., Grigoriou, M., Pachnis, V. and Parnavelas, J.G. (1999) The medial ganglionic eminence gives rise to a population of early neurons in the developing cerebral cortex. *J. Neurosci.*, 19: 7881–7888.

Letinic, K. and Rakic, P. (2001) Telencephalic origin of human thalamic GABAergic neurons. *Nature Neurosci.*, 4: 931–936.

Li, H., Chen, J., Wu, W., Fagaly, T., Zhou, L., Yuan, W., Dupuis, S., Jiang, Z., Nash, W., Gick, C., Ornitz, D.M., Wu, J.Y., and Rao, Y. (1999) Vertebrate Slit, a secreted ligand for the transmembrane protein Roundabout, is a repellent for olfactory bulb axons. *Cell.*, 96: 807–818.

Lois, C. and Alvarez-Buylla, A. (1994) Long-distance neuronal migration in the adult mammalian brain. *Science*, 264: 1145–1148.

López-Mascaraque, L., García, C., Valverde, F. and De Carlos, J.A. (1998) Central olfactory structures in *Pax-6* mutant mice. *Ann. N. Y. Acad. Sci.*, 855: 83–94.

Marín, O. and Rubenstein, J.L.R. (2001) A long, remarkable journey: tangential migration in the telencephalon. *Nature Rev. Neurosci.*, 2: 1–11.

Marín, O., Yaron, A., Bagri, A., Tessier-Lavigne, M and Rubenstein, J.L.R. (2001) Sorting of striatal and cortical interneurons regulated by semaphorin-neuropilin interactions. *Science*, 293: 872–875.

Molnár, Z. (1998) *Development of Thalamocortical Connections*, Springer, Berlin.

Parnavelas, J. (2000) The origin and migration of cortical neurones: New vistas. *TINS*, 23: 126–131.

Pini, A. (1993) Chemorepulsion of axons in the developing mammalian central nervous system. *Science*, 261: 95–98.

Puelles, L., Kuwana, E., Puelles, E., Bulfone, A., Shimamura, K., Keleher, J., Smiga, S. and Rubenstein, J.L.R. (2000) Pallial and subpallial derivatives in the embryonic chick and mouse telencephalon, traced by the expression of the genes *Dlx-2, Emx-1, Nkx-2.1, Pax-6,* and *Tbr-1. J. Comp. Neurol.*, 424: 409–438.

Rakic, P. (1971) Guidance of neurons migrating to the fetal monkey neocortex. *Brain Res.*, 3: 471–476.

Rakic, P. (1972) Mode of cell migration to the superficial layers of fetal monkey. *J. Comp. Neurol.*, 145: 61–84.

Rakic, P. (1988) Specification of cerebral cortical areas. *Science*, 241: 170–176.

Rubenstein, J.L.R. and Rakic, P. (1999) Genetic control of cortical development. *Cerebral Cortex*, 9: 521–523.

Sanides, F. (1970) Functional architecture of motor and sensory cortices in primates in the light of a new concept of neocortex evolution. In: C.R. Noback and W. Montagna (Eds.), *The Primate Brain. Advances in Primatology*, Vol. 1, Appleton-Century-Crofts, New York, pp. 137–208.

Sanides, F. and Sanides, D. (1972) The "extraverted neurons" of the mammalian cerebral cortex. *Z. Anat. EntwGesch.*, 136: 272–293.

Schlaggar, B.L. and O'Leary, D.D.M. (1991) Potential of visual cortex to develop an array of functional units unique to somatosensory cortex. *Science*, 252: 1556–1560.

Sperry, R.W. (1963) Chemoaffinity in the orderly growth of nerve fiber patterns and connections. *Proc. Natl. Acad. Sci., USA*, 50: 703–710.

Stoykova, A., Treichel, D., Hallonet, M. and Gruss, P. (2000) *Pax6* Modulates the dorsoventral patterning of the mammalian telencephalon. *J. Neurosci.*, 20: 8042–8050.

Tamamaki, N., Fujimori, E., and Takauji, R. (1997) Origin and route of tangentially migrating neurons in the developing neocortical intermediate zone. *J. Neurosci.*, 17: 8313–8323.

Valverde, F. (1967) Apical dendritic spines of the visual cortex and light deprivation in the mouse. *Exp. Brain Res.*, 3: 337–352.

Valverde, F. (1968) Structural changes in the area striata of the mouse after enucleation. *Exp. Brain Res.*, 5: 274–292.

Valverde, F. (1971a) Short axon neuronal subsystems in the visual cortex of the monkey. *Int. J. Neurosci.*, 1: 181–197.

Valverde, F. (1971b) Rate and extent of recovery from dark rearing in the visual cortex of the mouse. *Brain Res.*, 33: 1–11.

Valverde, F. (1985) The organizing principles of the primary visual cortex in the monkey. In: A. Peters and E.G. Jones (Eds.), *Cerebral Cortex, Visual Cortex*, Vol. 3, Plenum Press, New York and London, pp. 207–257.

Valverde, F. (1986) Intrinsic neocortical organization: Some comparative aspects. *Neuroscience*, 18: 1–23.

Wichterle, H., García-Verdugo, J.M., Herrera, D.G. and Álvarez-Buylla, A. (1999) Young neurons from medial ganglionic eminence disperse in adult and embryonic brain. *Nat. Neurosci.*, 2: 461–466.

Wichterle, H., Turnbul, D.H., Nery, S., Fishell, G., and Alvarez-Buylla, A. (2001) In utero fate mapping reveals distinct migratory pathways and fates of neurons born in the mammalian basal forebrain. *Development*, 128: 3759–3771.

Wiesel, T.N. and Hubel, D.H. (1965) Extent of recovery from the effects of visual deprivation in kittens. *J. Neurophysiol.*, 28: 1060–1072.

Zhu, Y., Li, H.-S., Zhou, L., Wu, J.Y. and Rao, Y. (1999) Cellular and molecular guidance of GABAergic neuronal migration from an extracortical origin to the neocortex. *Neuron*, 23: 473–485.

E.C. Azmitia, J. DeFelipe, E.G. Jones, P. Rakic and C.E. Ribak (Eds.)
Progress in Brain Research, Vol. 136

CHAPTER 2

The chemotactic hypothesis of Cajal: a century behind

Constantino Sotelo*

*INSERM U-106, Hôpital de la Salpêtrière, 75013 Paris, France, and Cátedra de Neurobiología del Desarrollo
"Profesora Remedios Caro Almela", Instituto de Neurociencias, Universidad Miguel Hernandez,
03550 San Juan de Alicante, Spain*

Introduction

The precise birthdays of new scientific ideas are often difficult to determine. However, it is obvious for most neuroscientists that the present revolution we are living in our discipline, has its roots in Santiago Ramón y Cajal. During almost half a century (1887–1934) of patient work, he was able to show that the nervous system is made up of billions of independent, richly and precisely interconnected nerve cells, organized in detailed networks.

His studies on the architectural organization of the brain, and his prophetic predictions of its functions became the basis of neuroanatomy, neurophysiology, neuropathology, and what he named 'rational psychology'. This monumental work justifies his well-deserved title as founder of modern neuroscience.

Of course, despite the outstanding accomplishments of Cajal and his genius in unraveling the complexity of brain structure, the postulation and subsequent demonstration of the neuron doctrine was not solely the result of his own investigation. As it always happens in science, the contemporary knowledge in the field and the introduction of novel analytical and experimental methods greatly contributed to Cajal's achievements. During the second half of the 19th century, most investigators considered the nervous system as a huge syncitium within which protoplasmic processes emerging from cell bodies, after breaking up into thinner branches, dissolved

into a tight network that terminated by reconstituting the nerve fibers of the white matter. Investigators such as Wilhelm His in Germany and August Forel in Switzerland were the first to fight successfully the network, or reticularist, theory. Wilhelm His (1886, 1887), analyzing the early stage of nervous system development, was able to determine that embryonic axons were a continuation of the first process emerging from postmitotic nerve cells, and that they grew from the free distal end of this process. Forel (1887) based his conclusions on experiments showing that, after axonal avulsion of the motor cranial nerve roots, only those cells at the origin of the avulsed axons became atrophic. These observations inspired by Gudden, with whom he collaborated in Munich from 1875 to 1877, gave indirect proof of the reciprocal trophic dependency between axons and their cell bodies. There is no doubt, however, and despite some recent unfounded attacks, that Cajal was the sharp knife in solving the controversy about the way nerve cells communicate, and how their processes terminate. It was Cajal's technical skills in modifying Camillo Golgi's silver stain (*reazione nera*) and in developing new metallic impregnation methods, as well as his successful use of embryonic material and of degeneration approaches initiated by his predecessors, that provided the necessary tools for his discoveries.

Although research and technical advances contemporary with Cajal were instrumental in carrying out his work, it was his analytical power, particularly his genius for extracting patterns of nervous organization from collections of Golgi impregnated sections, and his brilliant

*Corresponding author: Tel.: 331 421 62671; Fax: 331 457 09990;
E-mail: sotelo@chups.jussieu.fr

interpretations and functional correlates that were solely responsible for his discoveries. We are indebted to him for opening up this new era in the history of neuroscience.

The morphology of the nervous system

After 10 years of work in the field of general histology (1877 to 1887), that could be considered as the period of cautious initiation to morphological research, Cajal started his important research on brain structure using the Golgi method (published by Golgi in 1873). This essential period of Cajal's work (1887–1903) corresponded to the most active and productive period of his own career. Thus, in his autobiography, 'Recollections of My Life', Cajal (1917, 1937) considered 1888 as '*my greater year, my year of fortune*'. The extraordinary large amount of new data obtained during this period is gathered in what is regarded to be Cajal's *Opus magnum*, the 'Textura del Sistema Nervioso del Hombre y de los Vertebrados' (1899 and 1904) (see its recent English translation by Pedro and Tauba Pasik, 1999, 2000).

When recently, I was asked to write a short note on 'Highlights in Twentieth Century Neuroscience' (Sotelo, 1999), I did not hesitate to select the French updated version of the 'Textura', published under the title 'Histologie du Système Nerveux de l'Homme et des Vertébrés' (Cajal, 1909, 1911). The book is so rich with ideas and drawings that finding a topic to focus on is as difficult as deciding what to buy in the shopping center, the only problem is to decide what you want to buy. Since this meeting was devoted to 'Changing views of Cajal's neuron', and since my own work is on axonal growth in development and regeneration, my current choice has been to discuss one of the most prophetic hypotheses put forward by Cajal, the hypothesis that took almost a century to be accepted. This hypothesis has become today one of the fastest expanding subjects in the field of axonal mechanisms underlying the building up of neuronal networks. Of course, I am talking about Cajal's concept of chemotactism or—as he named it—his 'neurotropic hypothesis' (Cajal, 1892).

Cajal and neuroembryology: the neurotropic theory

My tribute to Cajal's achievements will, therefore, concern the great importance of his work in the field of neuroembryology. He first started working on the developing nervous system, to collect evidence in favor of the neuron doctrine. But the embryonic nervous system captivated his interest, and he became devoted to its analysis which began with the study of the development of the spinal cord.

In 1890, Cajal made what he described as one of his most cherished discoveries: the axonal growth cone (Fig. 1a). The growth cone is one of the most sophisticated machines imaginable for steering the growing neural processes towards their terminal domains. Cajal, in his analysis of the development of dorsal commissural neurons and ventral motoneurons of the embryonic chick spinal cord, was impressed by the behavior of growing axons. At the end of E3, all the growth cones belonging to motoneuron axons had left the spinal cord through the ventral roots, whereas those belonging to commissural neurons were more dorsally located but already oriented toward the ventral midline (Fig. 1c). By E4, the growth cones of the commissural neurons had reached the ventral midline, and decussated through the floor plate (Fig. 1d). Quoting Cajal's own words, these axons "*will adopt pre-determined directions and establish connections with defined neural or extra neural elements… without deviations or errors, as if guided by an intelligent force*". A similar behavior was also reported for axons of mislaid neurons (even those fallen into the ventricular cavity) in the embryonic medulla oblongata. They re-entered the nervous parenchyma and re-oriented themselves to join the bundles of axons of their normally developed congeneric neurons (Fig. 1b). These fibers eventually reach their correct destinations. Cajal was, of course, immediately interested by the study of the forces that provide directionality to the growing axons. He proposed that target cells were able to secrete inducing or attracting substances, and that growth cones are provided with chemotactic sensitivity or chemically elicited ameboidism, formulating this way the 'neurotropic theory' (Cajal, 1892).

It is important to recall here that Cajal got his first position as Professor of Anatomy at the Medical School of the University of Valencia in 1884. A year later, owing to an epidemic of cholera that ravaged the town, Cajal was involved in bacteriological studies and was even tempted to abandon his morphological research and devote his career to microbiology. Indeed, his vocation pushed him toward bacteriology, but his final choice was determined by financial reasons: neuromorphological

Fig1a

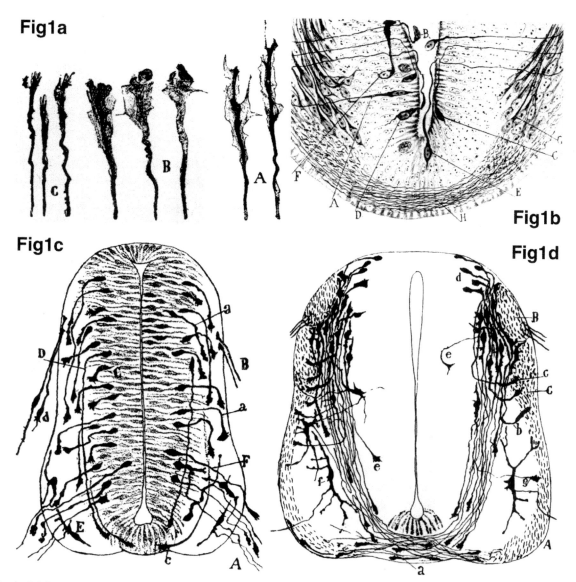

Fig1b

Fig1c

Fig1d

Fig. 1. Cajal's drawings illustrating his early discoveries in growth cone navigation. (**a**) Growth cones in the spinal cord of E4 chick embryos. Golgi impregnation. Note the diversity of shapes exhibited by the axonal growth cones: from relatively simple forms 'C' (growth cones traveling in the white matter) to much more complex forms, 'B' (cones within the ventral commissure) or 'A' (cones passing through the gray matter). This diversity corresponds to what we know today as the sensitivity of growth cones to cues in their micro-environment: the cones have simple shapes in straight paths, whereas in decision regions they adopt much more complex morphologies. (**b**) Young, immature neurons in the medulla oblongata of an E4 chick embryo. Reduced silver impregnation. Some of these neurons have erroneously fallen into the ventricular cavity 'B, C, E' and/or reentered the ventricular zone 'D'. These misplaced neurons have axons that came back to the bulbar parenchyma and, straight, reach the bundles of axons belonging to the normally developed congeneric neurons 'G'. These axons can, eventually, find their correct destinations. (**c**) Chick embryo spinal cord (E3). Golgi impregnation. Note that axons from motoneurons 'E, F' enter the ventral roots, whereas those belonging to commissural neurons 'D' grow in a ventral direction 'a' to reach the floor plate 'c'. (**d**) At E4, the commissural axons have crossed the floor plate and formed a ventral commissure 'a'. 'e' Growth cones lost in the ventricular zone; 'f' motoneurons.

research was much cheaper than bacteriology (Cajal, 1917). This short digression offered him the opportunity to follow the microbiological literature and to be aware of the important discoveries in the field, particularly work carried out by the Pasteur school in Paris during the decade 1882 to 1892 concerning the 'chemotactic ameboidism' of leukocytes (see in Elie Metchnikoff, 1892). For Cajal, the axonal growth cones have chemotactic sensibility, allowing them to identify substances produced by other neurons, epithelia or mesodermal cells. Thus, similar to leukocytes that are guided toward bacteria by diffusion gradients of bacterial toxins, growth cones are also oriented toward their target elements (muscle, neurons) by stimulating substances produced by the targets (neurotropic substances). The end product of this oriented, forward movement is the formation of specific and stable connections.

In his publication of 1892, Cajal envisaged that chemotaxic mechanisms could also be involved in the process of the migration of neuronal cell bodies, particularly those of the cerebellar granule cells and sensory ganglion cells. He admitted that, either a 'positive chemotaxis' (attraction) oriented towards the terminal domains of the migrating neurons, or a 'negative chemotaxis' (repulsion) for substances produced by their own axons might be possible in this case of neuronal migration. Over 100 years later, we published the first evidence that netrin-1 (see below) exerts a repulsive action on radially migrating granule cells in the postnatal cerebellum (Alcantara et al., 2000). However, this functional dichotomy soon disappeared, and in the *Textura* (Vol. 1, 1899) only attractive chemotropic influences were among the proposed mechanisms for axon guidance. Indeed, similar to his concept of interneuronal communication (synaptic transmission), that appeared to be always excitatory in all his functional considerations, especially in his 'law of dynamic polarization', axon guidance is not a binary process, and inhibitory or repulsive forces are excluded. He specifically wrote years later: "...*nothing indicated the intervention of negative neurotropic substances...*" (Cajal, 1913). Another important point is that the chemotactic forces are secreted or produced by the final targets: other neurons in the CNS and, in addition, muscle and peripheral target cells in the PNS (Cajal, 1909). Thus, although chemotropic molecules were supposed to be diffusible, the gradients envisaged by Cajal were much more extensive than those accepted today by modern embryology. In other terms,

the current concept of 'intermediate target' was missing in Cajal's considerations.

The problem with hypotheses, even the most appealing ones, is that they require validation by experimental data. Cajal soon abandoned the idea of getting the required evidence working with embryonic tissue. However, Cajal speculated on his neurotropic hypothesis in his monumental work on axonal regeneration, started on 1905 (Cajal, 1905). Some of these ideas are collected in his important monographic work devoted to 'Degeneration and Regeneration of the Nervous System' (Cajal, 1913, 1914). He wrote : "*Since we formulated in 1892 the hypothesis of chemotactism, that is, of amoeboidism of young axons brought about by an orienting stimulus from attracting or neurotropic substances many experiments have been undertaken with a view to supplying an objective basis for this conception... these experiments have dealt with nervous regeneration...(since) embryonic neurogenesis, is too difficult and delicate for experimental proof of the type wanted.*" In this book, Cajal gathered a large number of experiments that unequivocally demonstrated the constant behavior of regenerating peripheral axons: they emerged from the proximal stumps and, whatever the obstacles raised against their growth, they ended entering the distal stumps, as if the regenerating axons were strongly attracted by them. I am grateful to our colleagues Javier DeFelipe and Ted Jones who, in the cover page of the complete English translation of this important, but somewhat neglected work of Cajal (Cajal, 1991), have commemorated the chemotropic hypothesis by illustrating some of the key experiments (Fig. 2a). For instance, the importance of the distance between the proximal and distal stumps for the successful regeneration has been emphasized in the classical experiment in which a graft of a crushed and lacerated piece of sciatic nerve (Fig. 2a) was placed equidistantly from the two stumps. This experiment was completed by transplanting a piece of peripheral nerve treated with chloroform to kill all the Schwann cells (Fig. 2b). The growth of regenerating axons was oriented towards the grafted nerve only when living Schwann cells were present. These experiments clearly illustrate that the guidance of regenerative growth is not the result of mechanical or physical interactions. It is solely conditioned by the release of substances by living cells in the distal amputated or transplanted aneural nervous stumps, which are particularly rich in Schwann cells.

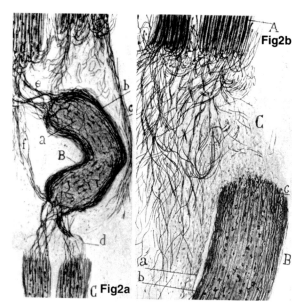

Fig2b

C

B

C Fig2a

Fig. 2. Illustrations of the peripheral grafts done by Cajal to show the neurotropic influences of Schwann cells in attracting regenerating nerve fibers from the proximal (up) to the distal stumps. (**a**) Graft of a crushed and lacerated piece of nerve in the wound of the sciatic nerve of an adult rabbit. The animal was killed 17 days after grafting. Distal stump 'C'; grafted segment 'B'. Axons regenerating from the proximal stump are attracted by the graft 'e' and, along the superficial region of the graft, enter 'd' the distal stump. (**b**) The main difference with the previous experiment is that here, the grafting was done with a piece of nerve killed by chloroform. Young cat killed 12 days after the operation. Central stump 'A'; dead graft 'B'; scar 'C'. Note that the regenerating axons emerging from the proximal stump do not enter the dead graft.

Experiments with peripheral nerve grafts in the central nervous system were started just at that time by Francisco Tello, the closest of Cajal's pupils (Tello, 1911). These experiments, cited by Cajal in his arguments in favor of the neurotropic hypothesis, also suggested the chemical nature of the guidance factors and the importance of Schwann cells in their elaboration. Two to five weeks after peripheral nerve grafting in the deep layers of the cerebral cortex, axon sprouts emerging from the lesioned white matter fibers behaved as peripheral axons: they grew exclusively within the sheaths of the aneural grafted peripheral nerve (Fig. 3a, b). Thus, peripheral nerve grafts not only provided a permissive environment for central axon regeneration, but also neurotropic attractive substances for its guidance. These classical experiments are currently of critical interest because it is possible that

the same chemotropic molecules (see below) that direct the outgrowth of developing axons could also be involved in the failure of adult central axons to regenerate and in the guidance of the few regenerating ones.

The decline and revival of neurotropism

Scientific disciplines are extremely influenced by fashion, and neuroscience is no exception. The lack of direct evidence to fully support the growth cone chemotaxis hypothesis, and the use of new tools—in this case *in vitro* studies, particularly by Ross Harrison (1910)—with new results and interpretations have marked the waning of Cajal's hypothesis. The latter was substituted by the idea that, since the growth cone cannot grow in a liquid medium but attached to specific substrates, what is important in axon guidance is the local environment of the growing axons, a hypothesis that years later was named 'contact guidance' (Paul Weiss, 1941). It is not surprising that Victor Hamburger (1988), in a review celebrating the 100 years of neuroembryology, wrote in relation to Cajal's chemotropism "*but while he asked the right question, his answer ... turned out to be incorrect*". However, this sentence was written five years after the publication of the seminal paper by Andrew Lumsden and Alan Davies (1986) who, with a new methodological approach (collagen gel co-cultures), showed that "*isolated virgin target tissue can elicit and orient primary neurite outgrowth from specific neurons*". These investigators used trigeminal sensory axons which, as in Cajal's hypothesis, were attracted by their final peripheral targets, the whisker pad epithelium. These results provided the first experimental evidence for natural chemoattractant activities during embryonic development. Moreover, Marc Tessier-Lavigne et al. (1988), using *in vitro* 'the dorsal region of the embryonic spinal cord' Cajal's favorite material, reported that commissural cell axons were attracted not by their final targets, but by intermediate targets, in this case the floor plate. Another milestone was the discovery by Adrian Pini (1993), also with collagen gel co-cultures—in this case of embryonic olfactory bulb and septal neurons (considered here an intermediate target)—that chemotropic influences were not only attractive but that they could also be inhibitory, meaning repulsive. Thus, it became clear that navigating growth cones during their pathfinding are guided, in addition to 'local contact influences' or short-range cues, by long

16

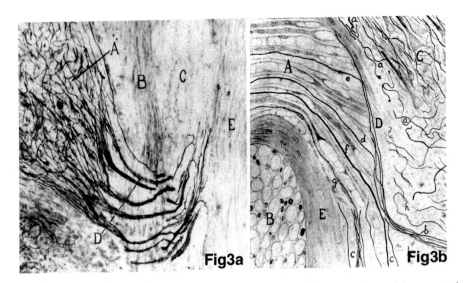

Fig. 3. Peripheral nerve grafts in the adult CNS done by Francisco Tello (1911) and used by Cajal in favor of the neurotropic hypothesis. (**a**) Retouched microphotograph. Aneural segments of sciatic nerves were grafted into the cerebral cortex of adult rabbits. Animals were sacrificed 14 days after the operation. White matter of the cortex 'A'; connective sheath of the nerve 'B'; bundles of cortical fibers, crossing the connective sheath, are oriented 'D' and enter the grafted segment. Reduced silver impregnation. (**b**) Drawing of a similar experiment. Longitudinal section of the grafted nerve 'A'; transverse section of the grafted nerve 'B'; deep region of the cerebral cortex 'C'. Note that white matter fibers 'd, e, f, g' have entered the graft, and are oriented by the bands of Büngner. These experiments not only suggest that central axons can regenerate but that they are attracted by Schwann cells as well.

range guidance cues, some attractive while others are repulsive. Moreover, attractive and/or repulsive cues are secreted by intermediate targets, distributed as landmarks all along the pathways that must be followed by the axons. Thus, it is accepted today that the coordination of four types of guidance cues (contact attraction, contact repulsion, chemoattraction and chemorepulsion) must be used by growing axons to navigate through the embryonic parenchyma of the brain during the formation of projection maps (Tessier-Lavigne and Goodman, 1996).

Marc Tessier-Lavigne succeeded in identifying the first molecules with chemotropic action in mammalian embryos. This was a major advance in favor of neurotropic axon guidance at a distance. These chemotactic molecules were named 'netrins' and were mainly produced by intermediate targets (Serafini et al., 1994). Other families of chemotropic molecules have been identified, such as secreted semaphorins, hepatocyte-growth factor/scatter factor, and Slits, that together with neurotrophins constitute the bulk of chemotactic molecules used by growth cones in their growth and elongation. Modern cellular and molecular studies have,

thus, elegantly revived the neurotropic hypothesis of Cajal in these last seven years.

Chemotactic cues in axonal guidance: the formation of the lateral olfactory tract

To illustrate the present status of the 'neurotropic hypothesis' in axonal guidance, I will present some of the work done in my laboratory by Alain Chédotal, Kim Nguyen-Ba-Charvet and Fernando de Castro. In particular, I will refer to the work on the development of olfactory connections. In agreement with Cajal's studies (Cajal, 1911), it is well established that axons from receptor neurons in the olfactory epithelium (OE) project ipsilaterally, through the olfactory nerve, to the olfactory bulb (OB), where they terminate in the glomeruli synapsing on the apical dendrites of mitral and tufted cells. The latter, particularly mitral cells, that are the earliest generated, project their axons, in the rat embryo from E15 onward, towards the anterior olfactory nucleus and higher olfactory centers, forming an axon bundle—the lateral olfactory tract (LOT)—located peripherally under the pial surface. Thus, mitral cell axons grow away from

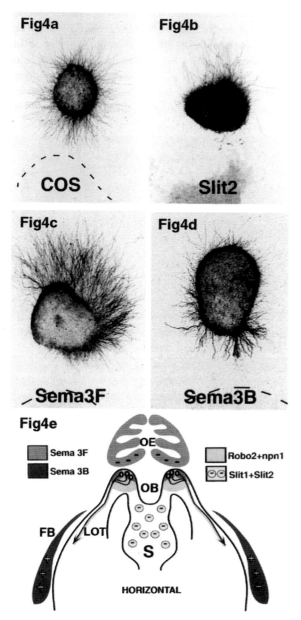

Fig4a
COS

Fig4b
Slit2

Fig4c
Sema3F

Fig4d
Sema3B

Fig4e

Sema 3F
Sema 3B
Robo2+npn1
Slit1+Slit2

OE

OB

FB LOT

S

HORIZONTAL

the OE, and leave the OB following a very specific location (equidistant from the neocortex, the ganglionic eminences and the septum) to reach their terminal domains.

The presumptive chemotropic actions of these molecules were tested *in vitro* using a slight modification of the method of Lumsden and Davies (1986). The explants of embryonic neurons were tested in collagen gel cultures without the presence of their presumptive intermediate targets. Instead, the explants were confronted with aggregates of epithelial (EBNA) or fibroblastic (COS) cell lines, transfected with cDNA coding for the chemotropic candidate molecule (Fig. 4). When E15 rat olfactory bulb explants were confronted to Slit-secreting cells (Slit1, Slit2), most of the emerging axons appeared in the distal quadrant of the explants, away from the Slit sources (compare Fig. 4a and b). Thus, Slits exert a repulsive action on growing mitral and tufted cell axons and, in addition, Slit2 exerts a powerful collapsing effect on the growth cone of these axons (Nguyen-Ba-Charvet et al., 1999). Since Slit1 and Slit2 are highly expressed in the developing septum, they appear to be the repulsive septal molecules anticipated by Pini (1993). Moreover, the study of the functional activity of class 3 semaphorins, revealed that Sema3F (Fig. 4c) had a strong repulsive action on mitral cell axons, whereas Sema3B (Fig. 4d) appeared to somewhat attract those axons. These observations indicate that a diffusible factor released by the olfactory epithelium could be Sema3F, where it is synthesized. Similarly, the mesenchyma bordering the lateral aspect of the forebrain, the only region close to the LOT expressing Sema3B, could exert an attractive influence on the growing mitral cell axons by releasing this semaphorin (de Castro et al., 1999). Thus, even the formation of a relatively simple projection pattern, like the mitral cells' projection, requires complex interactions of several chemotropic cues (Fig. 4e),

Fig. 4. Functional, confrontation assays in collagen gel cultures. E14–E15 rat olfactory bulb (OB) explants were co-cultured next to COS cell aggregates and stained with a neuronal marker, the anti-class III β-tubulin monoclonal antibody (Mab Tuj1). (**a**) The COS cells were transfected with *alkaline-phosphatase* (AP). The co-cultures were kept *in vitro* for 18 h. In these control assays, olfactory bulb axons confronted with AP-expressing cells have grown symmetrically. (**b**) In contrast, they grew away (in the distal quadrant) from hSlit2-expressing COS cells, even after only 18 h *in vitro*. When the OB explants were kept for 60 h next to aggregates of COS cells transfected with Sema3F, the axons grew almost exclusively in the distal quadrant (**c**), indicative of strong repulsion. Whereas, when the explants were co-cultured facing COS cells producing Sema3B, the axons grew in all quadrants, but they were significantly more numerous in the proximal quadrant (**d**), indicative of an attractive effect. (**e**) Schematic representation (horizontal plane) of the chemotactic cues expression patterns that influence the orientation of the forming lateral olfactory tract (LOT). Each nervous territory (olfactory epithelium : OE; septum : S; mesenchymal precursors of the frontal bone: FB) exhibits a different color, illustrating the expressed chemotactic molecule (Taken from de Castro et al., 1999 and Nguyen Ba-Charvet et al., 1999).

without considering the influence of their combination with a large variety of local cues.

Are contact and diffusible cues entirely different molecules?

I would like to finish this review, remembering that the rather simple dichotomies, short range/long range, attractant/repellent, that have led to the definition of the four classes of forces involved in axon guidance discussed above, are a real matter of debate. Indeed, neurotropic molecules—like netrins, semaphorins—are bifunctional (attractive and repulsive). Moreover, *in vitro*, the response of some growth cones to many chemotropic molecules depends on their activation state and can be switched after modulation of the intracytoplasmatic concentration of cyclic nucleotides, as discovered by Mu-Ming Poo (see Song and Poo, 1999). Finally, the extracellular domains of some membrane bound molecules (L1, axonin or Sema4D) can be proteolytically cleaved and released to the extracellular space, where they can provide long-range cues. On the contrary, most chemotropic molecules (class 3 semaphorins, netrins and Slits) are highly charged and tend to bind to the membrane of the cells that are secreting them, acting as short-range cues. Slit proteins are particularly interesting in this respect: they are proteolytically processed, thus diffusible but also membrane-associated, and can exert both positive and negative effects on developing axons (Nguyen Ba-Charvet et al., 2001a). *In vivo*, Slit2 is cleaved into 140 kD N-terminal (Slit2-N) and 55–60 kD C-terminal fragments, but uncleaved/full-length Slit2 can also be isolated from brain extracts. Because Slit2-N and full-length Slit2 bind tightly to cell membranes, we have studied the response of growing axons to substrate-bound Slit2 and fragments using the stripe assay. The experiments were performed on a different neuronal system, the NGF-sensitive dorsal root ganglion neurons. In the stripe assay (Nguyen Ba-Charvet et al., 2001b), the axons grow parallel to alternating stripes of two different proteins or protein combinations, making it possible to test the axons' preference for one substrate over the other (Fig. 5). In these assays, the DRG axons avoid the stripes coated with membranes of cells producing either Slit2, netrin1 or Sema3A, whereas they grow in stripes coated with control membranes. By using recombinant Slit2 protein and their fragments, the DRG axons avoided Slit2 fragments when coated as stripes on laminin. However,

when the Slit2 stripes were coated on fibronectin, the axons still avoided full-length Slit2 (Slit2-U; Fig. 5a) but grew preferentially on Slit2-N (Fig. 5b), contrary to the behavior of olfactory bulb axons that, when confronted with alternating lanes of Slit2-N and fibronectin, always preferred fibronectin (Nguyen-Ba-Charvet et al., 2001b). In addition, axon response to Slit2 fragments could be

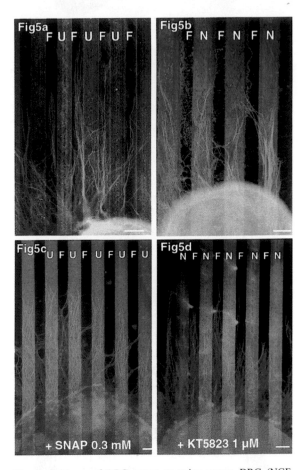

Fig. 5. Guidance of DRG axons on stripe assays. DRG (NGF-sensitive) explants, taken from E14–E15 rat embryos, were cultured on substrates patterned with alternating stripes of Slit2-U (U) or Slit2-N (N) and fibronectin (F), the Slit2-coated stripes were labeled with fluorescein-conjugated BSA. When the DRG axons were offered a choice between Slit2-U and fibronectin (**a**), they showed a preference for fibronectin. Whereas, when the choice was between Slit2-N and fibronectin (**b**), the axons grew on Slit2-N. These preferences were inverted by treating the cultures either by a PKG activator (SNAP), in the case of fibronectin over Slit2-U (**c**) preference, or a PKG inhibitor (KT5823) in the case of Slit2-N preference (**d**). These results testify in favor of a regulation by cyclic-GMP of the signaling of Slit proteins. (Taken from Nguyen Ba-Charvet et al., 2001b).

19

modulated by cGMP and by a laminin-1 peptide. We found that the preference for Slit2-N of DRG axon outgrowth in the context of fibronectin can be converted to a negative effect by lowering cGMP levels with KT5823, a PKG inhibitor (Fig. 5d). The treatment with a PKG activator (SNAP) changed the behavior of DRG axons in that they preferred to grow on Slit2-U lanes rather than on fibronectin (Fig. 5e). These results demonstrate a role for cyclic nucleotides in the signaling of Slit proteins. Thus, Slit2 and other diffusible factors (Sema3A, NT3) belong to group II, whose functions are regulated by cGMP levels (Nguyen Ba-Charvet et al., 2001b).

Our work reinforces the essential notions on the mechanisms for axon guidance. Like for most key processes taking place in the development of neuronal networks, there is: (i) phylogenetic preservation of the guiding mechanisms from worms and flies to human beings and (ii) redundancy of these mechanisms, since several diffusible molecules are implied in each axon guidance. In addition, the guidance cues are not only multiple—as I have already said—but each one can exert bifunctional actions (attraction and repulsion). Finally, our recent results show that, since extracellular matrix molecules can modulate the response of the growth cones, just by modulating cyclic nucleotide levels, the action of some of these molecules—Slit2 in particular—depends on the molecular context in which it is presented to the growth cone.

Now, at the beginning of the new millennium, Cajal's chemotaxis hypothesis has become one of the most promising fields to study late steps of neurodevelopment: those guiding afferent axons to their proper postsynaptic partners. We already know that the process of axon guidance is a highly complex molecular process, with molecular redundancy, and phylogenetic conservation. It is for the 21st century to understand this complexity, and to analyze the transduction pathways that allow axon growth cones to navigate within the embryonic CNS.

References

Alcantara, S., Ruiz, M., de Castro, F., Soriano, E. and Sotelo, C. (2000) Netrin-1 acts as an attractive or as a repulsive cue for distinct migrating neurons during the development of the cerebellar system. *Development*, 127: 1359–1372.

Cajal, S.R. (1890) A quelle époque apparaissent les expansions des cellules nerveuses de la moëlle épinière du poulet? *Anat. Anz.*, 5 (Nr. 21 and 22): 609–613, 631–639.

Cajal, S.R. (1892) La rétine des vertébrés. *La Cellule*, 9: 121–133.

Cajal, S.R. (1899, 1904) *Textura del Sistema Nervioso del Hombre y de los Vertebrados*. 2 vols. Moya, Madrid.

Cajal, S.R. (1905) Sobre la degeneración y regeneración de los nervios. Boletín del Instituto de Sueroterapia, Vacunación y Bacteriología de Alfonso XIII 1: 49–60, 113–119.

Cajal, S.R. (1909, 1911) *Histologie du Système Nerveux de l'Homme et des Vertébrés*. Translated by Léon Azoulay. Masson, Paris.

Cajal, S.R. (1913, 1914) *Estudios sobre la Degeneración y Regeneración del Sistema Nervioso*. 2 vols. Moya, Madrid.

Cajal, S.R. (1917) *Recuerdos de mi vida*. Vol 2. *Historia de mi Labor Científica*. Moya, Madrid.

Cajal, S.R. (1937) *Recollections of My Life*. Translated by E. H. Craigie *with the assistance of* J. Cano. American Philosophical Society: Philadelphia (Reprinted by MIT Press, Cambridge, MA; 1989).

Cajal, S.R. (1991) *Cajal's Degeneration & Regeneration of the Nervous System*. *Translated by* R. M. May. *Edited, with an Introduction & Additional Translations by* Javier De Felipe and Edward G. Jones. Oxford University Press, New York.

Cajal, S.R. (1999, 2000) *Texture of the Nervous System of Man and the Vertebrates*. *An Annotated and Edited Translation of the Original Spanish Text with the Additions of the French Version* by Pedro Pasik and Tauba Pasik. Springer, New York.

De Castro, F., Hu, L., Drabkin, H., Sotelo, C. and Chédotal, A. (1999) Chemoattraction and chemorepulsion of olfactory bulb axons by different secreted Semaphorins. *J. Neurosci.*, 19: 4428–4436.

Forel, A. (1887) Einige hirnanatomische Betrachtungen und Ergebnisse. *Arch. Psychiat. Nerv. Krankh.*, 18: 162–198.

Golgi, C. (1873) Sulla structura della sostanza grigia del cervello. *Gazz. Med. Ital.*, 6: 244–246.

Hamburger, V. (1988) Ontogeny of neuroembryology. *J. Neurosci.*, 8: 3535–3540.

Harrison, R.G. (1910) The outgrowth of the nerve fiber as a mode of protoplasmic movement. *J. Exp. Zool.*, 9: 787–846.

His, W. (1886) Zur Geschichte des menschlichen Rückenmarkes und der Nervenwurzeln. *Abhandl. Königl. Sächs. Ges. Wiss.* (*Math.-Phys. Kl*), 13: 479–514.

His, W. (1887) Die Entwicklung der ersten Nervenbahnen beim menschlichen Embryo. *Arch. Anat. Physiol. Leipzig* (*Anat. Abt.*), 368–378.

Lumsden, A.G.S. and Davies, A.M. (1986) Chemotropic effect of specific target epithelium in the development of the mammalian nervous system. *Nature*, 323: 538–539.

Metchnikoff, E. (1892) *Leçons sur la Pathologie Comparée de l'Inflamation* (*faites à l'Institut Pasteur en avril et mai 1891*) Masson, Paris.

Nguyen-Ba-Charvet, K.T., Brose, K., Wang, K., Marillat, V., Kidd, T., Goodman, C.S., Tessier-Lavigne, M., Sotelo, C. and Chédotal, A. (1999) Slit2-mediated chemorepulsion and collapse of developing forebrain axons. *Neuron*, 22: 463–473.

Nguyen-Ba-Charvet, K.T., Brose, K., Wang, K., Marillat, V., Ma, L., Sotelo, C., Tessier-Lavigne, M. and Chédotal, A. (2001a) Diversity ans specificity of actions of Slit2 proteolytic fragments in axon guidance. *J. Neurosci.*, 21: 4281–4289.

Nguyen-Ba-Charvet, K.T., Brose, K., Marillat, V., Sotelo, C., Tessier-Lavigne, M. and Chedotal, A. (2001b) Sensory axon response to substrate-bound slit2 is modulated by laminin and cyclic GMP. *Mol. Cell Neurosci.*, 17: 1048–1058.

Pini, A. (1993) Chemorepulsion of axons in the developing mammalian central nervous system. *Science*, 261: 95–98.

Serafini, T., Kennedy, T.E., Galko, M.J., Mirzayan, C., Jessell, T.M. and Tessier-Lavigne, M. (1994) The netrins define a family of axon outgrowth-promoting proteins homologous to *C. elegans* UNC-6. *Cell*, 78: 409–424.

Song, H.J. and Poo, M.M. (1999) Signal transduction underlying growth cone guidance by diffusible factors. *Opin. Curr Neurobiol.*, 9: 355–363.

Sotelo, C. (1999) From Cajal's chemotaxis to the molecular biology of axon guidance. *Brain Res. Bull.*, 50: 395–396.

Tello, F. (1911) La influencia del neurotropismo en la regeneración de los centros nerviosos. *Trab. Lab. Invest. Biol.*, Univ. Madrid 9: 123–159.

Tessier-Lavigne, M., Placzek, M., Lumsden, A.G., Dodd, J. and Jessell, T.M. (1988) Chemotropic guidance of developing axons in the mammalian central nervous system. *Nature*, 336: 775–778.

Tessier-Lavigne, M. and Goodman, C.S. (1996) The molecular biology of axon guidance. *Science*, 274: 1123–1133.

Weiss, P. (1941) Nerve patterns: the mechanisms of nerve growth. *Growth (Suppl.)*, 5: 163–203.

E.C. Azmitia, J. DeFelipe, E.G. Jones, P. Rakic and C.E. Ribak (Eds.)
Progress in Brain Research, Vol. 136

CHAPTER 3

Neuronal changes during forebrain evolution in amniotes: an evolutionary developmental perspective

Zoltán Molnár[a],* and Ann B. Butler[b]

[a]*Department of Human Anatomy and Genetics, University of Oxford, South Parks Road, Oxford OX1 3QX, UK*
[b]*Krasnow Institute for Advanced Study and Department of Psychology, George Mason University, Fairfax, VA 22030, USA*

Abstract: Embryology is the interface of genetic inheritance and phenotypic expression in adult forms, and as such is uniquely positioned to illuminate both. Embryonic cell migration pattern, transient connectivity, axonal growth kinetics and fasciculation patterns can clearly be substantially impacted at the striatocortical junction, which appears to be critical for telencephalic development. Similarly, the big questions concerning pallial evolution in amniotes all involve the pivotal region at the pallial-subpallial boundary, an area where complex developmental cross-currents may be involved in the specification of multiple structures that are thus related to each other. We review some of the positions based on recent genetic data and/or hodology, then suggest that comparative studies of intervening, embryological events may resolve some of the apparent conflicts and illuminate the evolutionary scenario. We propose a new hypothesis, the collopallial field hypothesis, which specifies that the anterior dorsal ventricular ridge of sauropsids and a set of structures in mammals—the lateral neocortex, basolateral amygdalar complex, and claustrum-endopiriform nucleus formation—are homologous to each other as derivatives of a common embryonic field. We propose that in mammals the laterally lying collopallium splits, or differentiates, into deep (claustroamygdalar) and superficial (neocortical) components, whereas in sauropsids, this split does not occur.

Introduction

Santiago Ramón y Cajal believed that "*Practitioners will only be able to claim that a valid explanation of a histological observation has been provided if three questions can be answered satisfactorily: what is the functional role of the arrangement in the animal; what mechanisms underlie this function; and what sequence of chemical and mechanical events during evolution and development gave rise to these mechanisms?*" The third point seems to be neglected nowadays, when most observations are made in a handful of laboratory animals ignoring the huge variety of vertebrates and the possible evolutionary relations. Before the turn of the previous century

*Corresponding author: Tel.: +44-1865-282664; Fax: +44-1865-272420; E-mail: zoltan.molnar@human-anatomy.oxford.ac.uk

evolutionary biology and developmental biology were very closely related, and studying homologies between parts of animals was considered a crucial way to understand anatomy. The comparative analysis of development is useful to all. Comparison of immature stages reveals features of evolution that are otherwise obstructed by the complexity of the mature brain. Reciprocally, to look at development by thinking in evolutionary terms helps to focus on the most biologically relevant mechanisms. Cajal provided the most complete and still the most reliable account of the morphological organization of virtually every part of the nervous system in all classes of vertebrates.

Most of the mammalian cerebral cortex comprises neocortex (isocortex), which has six cell and fiber layers (Fig. 1A). This part of the cortex has also been identified as dorsal pallium, in contrast to medial pallium

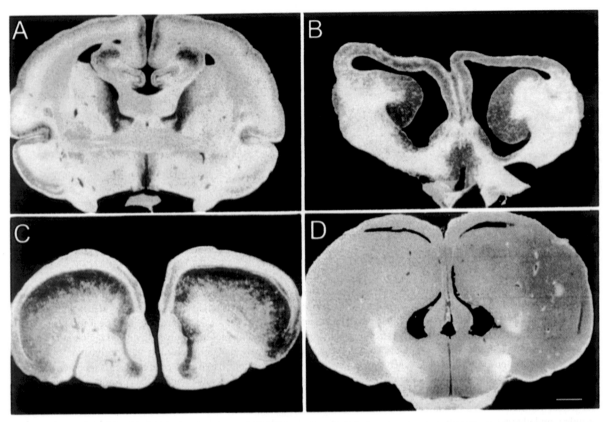

Fig. 1. Examples of fiber stained coronal sections of four different amniote brains viewed under dark field illumination to demonstrate the spectacular differences between forebrain organization in A: marsupial, Native Cat, *Dysaurus Hallucatus*, B: Turtle, *Pseudemus Scripta Elegans*, C: Iguana, *Iguana Iguana*, D: Crocodile (Australian). Note the thicker dorsal cortex in marsupial (A) and the huge ball-like structure in B–D protruding into the lateral ventricule. Scale bar: 1 mm.

(the three-layered hippocampal formation) and lateral pallium (which includes the three-layered olfactory-recipient cortex). The pallium of sauropsids—reptiles (Fig. 2A–C) and birds (Fig. 2E–G)—contains three major cortical regions, each with three cell and fiber layers: medial (hippocampal) pallium, dorsal pallium, or cortex—which includes the Wulst in birds—and lateral (olfactory) pallium, or cortex (see Butler and Hodos, 1996; Nieuwenhuys et al., 1998; Medina and Reiner, 2000). The sauropsid pallium also includes a large, bulging mass in its dorsolateral sector, the dorsal ventricular ridge (DVR), which has anterior (ADVR) and posterior (PDVR) portions (Figs. 1B–D, 2A–C).

In some reptiles (Fig. 2A, B) the DVR is of modest size and comprises a core nucleus bordered peripherally by a corticoid band of neurons; in other reptiles (Fig. 2C) the DVR is much larger and consists of multiple nuclear

groups (see Butler and Hodos, 1996). In birds, the DVR reaches its apogee, being of massive size and of numerous components (Karten and Hodos, 1967). The avian ADVR (Fig. 2E–G) contains regions mistakenly assumed to correspond to the mammalian striatum and so named, including the hyperstriatum accessorium (HA), hyperstriatum dorsale (HD), hyperstriatum ventrale (HV), and neostriatum (N). The latter consists of several areas including the ectostriatum (E). The PDVR contains a similarly named region, the archistriatum (A).

Of the many forebrain structures, some can be recognized unambiguously across amniotes. Others, including some dorsal thalamic nuclei and their telencephalic targets, have remained cryptic and are focuses of current controversy. Medial parts of neocortex, for example, appear to correspond to at least part of the reptilian dorsal cortex and its more elaborate, enlarged version in birds, the

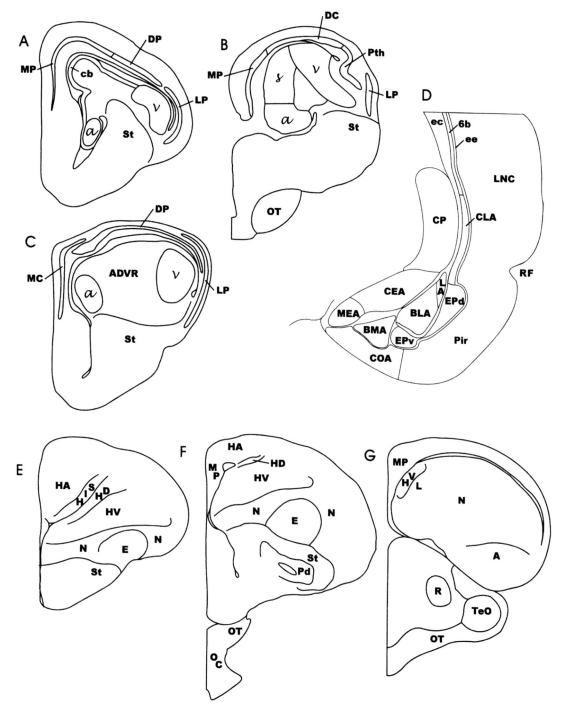

Fig. 2. The major components of the right telencephalon in reptiles (A: tuatara, B: turtle, C: iguana), the right forebrain in pigeon (E–G), and the lateral part of the telencephalon in rat (D). Tuatara (*Sphenodon*) redrawn from Reiner and Northcutt (2000); turtle from Ulinski (1983); iguana from Bruce and Butler (1984); rat from Swanson and Petrovich (1998); and pigeon from Karten and Hodos (1967). Drawings are not to the same scale.

Wulst. The homology of these structures, implying the presence of a similar, dorsal pallial component in the common ancestor, is relatively well established (Medina and Reiner, 2000). The visual parts of reptilian dorsal cortex and avian Wulst receive ascending projections from the dorsal lateral optic nucleus[1] in the dorsal thalamus, and this pathway is regarded as homologous to the dorsal lateral geniculate nucleus-striate cortex pathway in mammals (see Karten, 1969). Comparable somatosensory pathways exist as well (Wild, 1987). In contrast, lateral parts of neocortex—including auditory cortex and the multiple, extrastriate visual areas—are highly enigmatic as to their evolutionary origin and relationships to pallial structures in sauropsids. Identity of thalamic nuclei that project to these cortices in mammals and to possible counterparts in other amniotes is tied to the identity of their targets. Thus, circular arguments abound and frustrate attempts to solve the puzzle.

Part of the problem derives from hodology. Besides lateral neocortex, various ascending sensory pathways terminate in the amygdala, claustrum, and striatum (LeVay and Sherk, 1981; Jones, 1985; Doron and LeDoux, 1999). Immunohistochemical studies have definitively identified the subpallial striatum and pallidum across amniotes (see Medina and Reiner, 1995). In contrast, identifying sauropsid structures that may be homologous to the several pallial derivatives has proved to be labyrinthine. In discussing the amygdala, we adopted the nomenclature of Swanson and Petrovich (1998).

From genes to structures: conflicting interpretations

Genetic expression patterns support some interpretations of hodology and conflict with others. We first briefly review some of the positions based on recent genetic data and/or hodology. We then suggest that comparative studies of intervening, embryological events may resolve some of the apparent conflicts and illuminate the evolutionary scenario.

---

[1] The term dorsal lateral optic nucleus was introduced by Butler and Hodos (1996) to specify the major retinorecipient, dorsal thalamic nucleus that in turn projects to the telencephalic pallium (dorsal cortex, pallial thickening, Wulst) across all sauropsids. It is a homologue of the dorsal lateral geniculate nucleus of mammals and refers to variously named nuclei in sauropsids including nucleus intercalatus thalami of lizards, dorsal optic nucleus of turtles, and multiple components of the nucleus opticus principalis thalami complex of birds.

Gene expression patterns: shared patterns across amniotes

Gene expression during development reveals several clearly distinct subdivisions within the telencephalic pallium. Developmental expression of homeobox genes of the *Emx*, *Dlx*, and *Pax* families in embryonic forebrains of mouse, chick, turtle, and frog (Smith Fernández et al., 1998) demonstrated that the expression domains of *Emx1* in the pallium and *Dlx1* in the striatum are separated by a thin intermediate domain expressing neither gene. In sauropsids, this intermediate domain includes the ventral part of the ADVR but does not extend into its dorsal- and medial-most portions, which are *Emx1*-positive. In mouse, the intermediate domain appears to give rise to structures of the laterobasal telencephalic region, possibly including piriform (olfactory) cortex, amygdala, diagonal band, and medial septum. Thus, these data indicate homology of at least part of the ADVR to part of the mammalian amygdala, supporting the hypothesis of Bruce and Neary (1995), as discussed below. Since the intermediate domain in sauropsids has a protracted proliferation period in comparison to mammals, however, Smith Fernández et al. (1998) favored the hypothesis that the avian neostriatum and the major part of the DVR of turtles "have no developmental homolog" in the mouse. They argued that late-generated structures may not be homologous among taxa even if they are generated by homologous anlagen. These data nonetheless indicate a pivotal position for the intermediate domain in the developing pallium, which has strategic importance for comparisons across tetrapods.

From their analysis of gene expression patterns in chick and mouse embryos, Puelles et al. (2000) verified that the intermediate zone is pallial rather than striatal and proposed recognizing it as a new subdivision—the ventral pallium. They also proposed that lateral pallial derivatives include piriform cortex in both chick and mouse, the claustrum (dorsal claustrum, or claustrum proper) and basolateral amygdalar nucleus in mouse, and dorsal parts of the ADVR in chick, whereas ventral pallial derivatives comprise the endopiriform nucleus (ventral claustrum) and lateral amygdalar nucleus in mouse and more ventral parts of ADVR in chick. Puelles et al. (2000) noted that the implied homology of the murine claustrum with the avian hyperstriatum ventrale is consistent with exceptionally strong expression of kappa opioid receptor (Reiner et al., 1989) and neurotensin binding sites (Brauth et al., 1986) in both of these structures.

Hodology: adult phenotypic relationships

The PDVR is comparable to at least part of the mammalian amygdala (see Bruce and Neary, 1995)—particularly the accessory olfactory-recipient and autonomic components (Swanson and Petrovich, 1998)—and this hypothesis has achieved consensus. The ADVR was originally proposed by Källén (1962), based on embryological studies, to be homologous to various parts of neocortex. This hypothesis was supported by discovery of ascending sensory pathways to the ADVR in birds (see Karten, 1969, 1997; Karten and Shimizu, 1989) and similar pathways in reptiles (e.g., Hall and Ebner, 1970; Pritz, 1975; Bruce and Butler, 1984; and see Butler, 1994a,b). Karten (1969) proposed that homologous constituent neuronal populations are present in the pallium of all amniotes and that in sauropsids, these cell populations form 'cortical equivalent' circuits.

In birds, the ADVR visual pathway involves a relay via the midbrain tectum to nucleus rotundus in the dorsal thalamus and thence to ectostriatum (see Karten, 1969). This pathway has been compared to the mammalian pathway to extrastriate cortex via the superior colliculus and the lateralis posterior/pulvinar (LP/pul) (Mpodozis et al., 1996; Karten et al., 1997; Luksch et al., 1998). An auditory pathway comparable to the medial geniculate-auditory cortex pathway likewise appears to be present in sauropsids (see Karten, 1969), as is a visual/ somatosensory pathway (Korzeniewska and Güntürkün, 1990) comparable to the collicular-posterior nuclear group-somatosensory association cortices pathway in mammals (see Butler, 1994a,b).

Butler (1994b) generally supported Karten's hypothesis of ADVR evolution, but she did not assign a DVR per se to the common amniote ancestor, rather regarding it as an apomorphy (specialization) of the sauropsid line. She likewise considered lateral neocortex to be an apomorphy of the synapsid line that led to mammals. She assigned only the presence of various midbrain roof, dorsal thalamic-dorsolateral pallial sensory pathways to the common ancestor. Butler (1994a) recognized two fundamental divisions of the dorsal thalamus—the lemnothalamus and collothalamus—and she referred to the set of midbrain roof-relayed pathways to the ADVR in sauropsids and to lateral (temporal and parietal) neocortex in mammals as collothalamic pathways. The complementary set of lemnothalamic nuclei predominantly receive direct (lemniscal) sensory projections that do not synapse in the midbrain roof, and they project to dorsal cortex in reptiles, the Wulst in birds, and medial neocortical areas, such as striate and primary somatosensory cortices, in mammals.

Reiner (1993) independently recognized similar pallial divisions and sets of ascending pathways. Reiner (2000) recently proposed a 'common origin' hypothesis of temporal neocortex and [anterior] DVR, proposing that these structures each arose in their respective lines from an ancestral "proto-DVR [that did] not bulge into the ventricle" but did contain distinct and separate terminal fields similar to extrastriate (V2) and auditory cortices in mammals. Reiner (2000) contrasted this common origin hypothesis with the "temporal cortex *de novo* hypothesis," which generally summarizes various other viewpoints that support independent, homoplastic evolution of the sauropsid DVR (Northcutt and Kaas, 1995) and/or homologize it with part(s) of the mammalian amygdala and/or claustrum (Bruce and Neary, 1995; Striedter, 1997; Puelles et al., 2000). It asserts that the V2 and auditory cortices evolved *de novo* within the synapsid line to mammals.

Bruce and Neary (1995) proposed that the entire DVR is homologous to the amygdala of mammals. They have convincingly argued that the PDVR is homologous to central, medial, and basomedial parts of the amygdala and a portion of its basolateral part due to hodology. Their argument comparing the ADVR to part of the lateral amygdalar nucleus has been less persuasive, however, because necessary correspondences between respective afferent thalamic nuclei in sauropsids and mammals (Linke et al., 1999) are not widely accepted. Striedter (1997) agreed that the PDVR is homologous to parts of the amygdala, but he proposed on topo- logical grounds that the ADVR is homologous to the endopiriform nucleus and the pallial thickening (a lateral part of dorsal cortex present in turtles) to the claustrum proper. The claustrum and endopiriform nucleus receive projections from the intralaminar nuclei of the dorsal thalamus (LeVay and Sherk, 1981; Bayer and Altman, 1991).

Hodological comparisons are hazardous because in mammals multiple dorsolateral pallial structures receive dorsal thalamic projections. Collothalamic projections (Butler, 1994a,b) exhibit substantial overlap to lateral neocortical regions and to both the striatum (Beckstead, 1984; Lin et al., 1984; Takada et al., 1985) and the lateral part of the amygdala (Ryugo and Killackey, 1974; LeDoux et al., 1985; Namura et al., 1997; Doron and LeDoux, 1999; Linke et al., 1999). Interestingly, in the rat, even LP participates in the thalamoamygdalar projection system (Namura et al., 1997; Doron and LeDoux, 1999). Additionally, intralaminar nuclei (see Jones, 1985) have widespread projections not only to neocortex but also to claustrum and endopiriform nucleus (LeVay and Sherk, 1981; Bayer and Altman 1991).

The dorsolateral pallial sector is obviously the part of the telencephalon that is most resistant to evolutionary illumination. Two homologies are well established and generally accepted: homology of the lateral cortex in sauropsids with the lateral, piriform cortex of mammals and homology of the PDVR with the accessory olfactory-recipient and autonomic components (see Swanson and Petrovich, 1998) of the amygdala. Regarding the ADVR, the proposal of Bruce and Neary (1995) regarding an amygdalar homology cannot be falsified with current hodological data because possible correspondence of the collothalamic visual pathway in sauropsids with the tecto-suprageniculate-amygdalar pathways in mammals (Linke et al., 1999) has not been ruled out. The structures of the dorsolateral pallial sector in mammals that remain in serious contention for homology with part or all of the sauropsid ADVR thus emerge as the lateral neocortex, claustrum and endopiriform nucleus, and basolateral amygdalar complex [lateral anterior and basolateral anterior nuclei as discussed by Swanson and Petrovich (1998)].

From genes to structures: getting there is half the fun

A plethora of new information on gene expression patterns as well as on the intricate choreography of embryological processes offers tantalizing glimpses into the complexity and the logic of the developmental sequence. Events, such as early gene expression, cell migration, cell death and the development of early connectivity, when explored on a comparative basis, offer the best avenue of research for reconciling the disparate findings from studies of genetic expression patterns and hodology. Embryology is the interface of genetic inheritance and phenotypic expression in adult forms, and as such is uniquely positioned to illuminate both (Butler and Molnár, 1998).

Dual origin of the mammalian cerebral cortex cellular constituents

The principal neuronal types of the cerebral cortex are the excitatory pyramidal cells, which project to distant

targets, and the inhibitory nonpyramidal cells, which are the cortical interneurons. Pyramidal cells are generated in the cortical neuroepithelium and migrate radially to reside in the cortex in an inside first, outside last fashion (Rakic, 1995). Relatively few nonpyramidal cells are generated in the cortical ventricular zone (Mione et al., 1997; Parnavelas, 2000). The exact origin of the tangentially migrating GABAergic neurons in mammals has been controversial (De Carlos et al., 1996; Tamamaki et al., 1997; Anderson et al., 1997 and 1999; Meyer et al., 2000) and it has only relatively recently been discovered that the vast majority of these cells originate in the medial ganglionic eminence (MGE), the primordium of the globus pallidus of the ventral telencephalon (Lavdas et al., 1999; Parnavelas, 2000). Experiments in living whole forebrain slice cultures have shown that these neurons follow long tangential migratory routes to their positions in the developing cortex. These studies have also shown that the first wave of neurons to leave the medial ganglionic eminence are those destined for the marginal zone including the Cajal-Retzius cells. Neurons generated somewhat later reach the marginal zone as well as the lower intermediate zone and cortical plate (Gulisano et al., 1996; Frotscher, 1998; Mallamaci et al., 1998, 1999). In contrast with the pyramidal cells they seem to populate the cortex in an outside first-inside last fashion (Sadikot et al., 2000).

Possible tangential migration in reptiles

The discovery of tangential migration in mammals produced a renaissance of the idea of dual developmental and evolutionary origin of the neuronal constituents of mammalian neocortex (Karten, 1997). Initially it seemed very likely that the tangential component in embryonic mammals could be related to the reptilian-to-mammalian transition. In the light of more recent results, however, it seems that the origin of the tangentially migrating cells does not correspond to the sight postulated by Karten (1997). Furthermore, similar tangential migration may also exist in reptiles (Métin and Molnár unpublished observation). The cadré of GABA and calbindin immunopositive neurons progressively moves from ventral to dorsal during embryonic development in turtle, and these cells have a morphology that is characteristic for migrating neurons (Blanton and Kriegstein, 1991; Métin and Molnár unpublished observation). Carbocyanine dye labelling in embryonic turtle slice cultures (Stage 15–18) recently revealed that cells generated in the medial ganglionic eminence follow long tangential migratory routes to dorsal cortex (Métin and Molnár unpublished observation). This finding suggests that the tangential migration of GABAergic neurons might not be a unique feature of the mammalian pallium; rather, it seems that the combined radial and tangential migration patterns are both present in all amniotes and it might be a fundamental and highly conserved mechanism for the generation of the dorsal cortex. The mechanisms that guide tangentially migrating neurons from the ganglionic eminence to the cerebral cortex and the possible homology between the mammalian and reptilian population of these cells are presently not known.

Transient cell groups and their projections assist the development of thalamocortical projections

Thalamic axons have to travel through a considerable portion of the newly formed subdivisions of the embryonic forebrain at an early stage when most of the cells of the telencephalon are not even born and have not migrated into position (Figs. 3A,E,F and 4). Tracing studies have revealed the degree of order that thalamic fibers maintain and the cellular elements they encounter while they grow out from the diencephalon, through the internal capsule, and accumulate below the corresponding cortical region (Rakic, 1977;

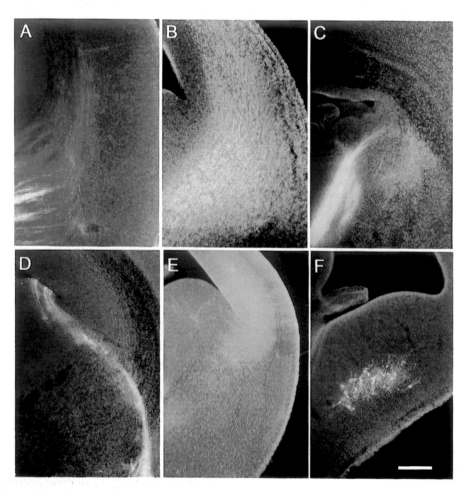

Fig. 3. Observations at the lateral corner of the lateral ventricle at the striatocortical junction during development. The panels indicate the path and fasciculation changes of the thalamocortical pathway in A: Normal, B: *reeler*, C: *L1* K.O. mice at P0, E18 and P1 (respectively), labeled with carbocyanine dye placements from the dorsal thalamus (see Molnár and Hannan, 2000 and Molnár et al., 1998a). D: radial glia labeled from carbocyanide dye crystal placement to the olfactory cortex, E: early corticofugal projections at E14 as their front lies up at the striatocortical junction. F: Cells of the internal capsule with early dorsal thalamic projections (through which they were labeled). Scale 500 μm.

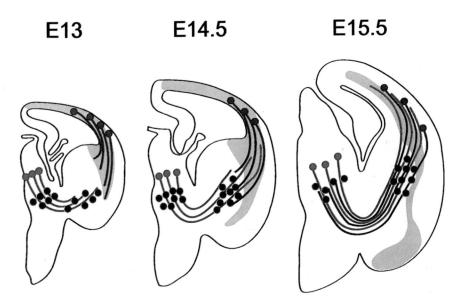

Fig. 4. The relationship between the developing reciprocal thalamocortical and corticofugal projections and early subdivisions of the embryonic mouse brain. Each diagram represent and imaginary coronal section through the left hemisphere, revealing the entire thalamocortical pathways. At E13, early thalamic (green) and corticofugal (blue) fibers synchronously approach the internal capsule. Red dots indicate cells which possess thalamic projections in the ventral thalamus and internal capsule, and the blue coloring mark the stripe of transient *Pax6* positive cells (Stoykova and Gruss, 1994; Smith Fernandez et al., 1998; Molnár et al., 2000) extending from the ventricular zone near the striatocortical junction towards the ventrolateral telencephalon. The growing corticofugal axons pause at the border of the *Pax6* compartment before they continue their journey towards the diencephalons and encounter the growing thalamic projections. Thalamic axons advance to the site of interactions among cells of the internal capsule which have already developed dorsal thalamic projections. The *Pax6* expression is gradually reduced, but continues to be present at the ventral telencephalon.

McConnell et al., 1989; Molnár, 1998). The interactions of the thalamocortical projections with the early generated, largely transient cells of the subplate, marginal zone, internal capsule and ventral thalamus are believed to play a crucial role in the organized deployment of thalamic projections through the subdivisions of the embryonic forebrain. It has been suggested that thalamic afferents reach the cortex by associating with pre-existing cells in the ventral thalamus and internal capsule and with preplate projections (De Carlos and O'Leary, 1992; Erzurumlu and Jhaveri, 1992; Métin and Godement, 1996; Molnár et al., 1998a,b,c).

Possible role of selective fasciculation in thalamic fiber deployment

The selective fasciculation of thalamic and preplate projections was proposed as a mechanism for the former to traverse the internal capsule and advance to the cortex through the striatocortical junction (Molnár and

Blakemore, 1995). The fiber ordering of the thalamic projections in *reeler* support this notion (Fig. 3B). In reeler mutant mice, the cortical plate develops below the early generated preplate cells and, therefore, separates the incoming thalamic fibers from their intermediate target cells in the 'superplate' (Caviness et al., 1988). The embryonic cortical plate is thought to be a nonpermissive environment for thalamic fiber ingrowth (Götz et al., 1992). The existence of privileged pathways for axon growth could explain how thalamic axons in *reeler* are able to penetrate the cortical plate and steer up to reach the equivalent cells in the superplate, while ignoring the hostile territory of cortical plate cells around them (Molnár et al., 1998b).

Cells of the embryonic internal capsule

Hodological analysis in mammalian embryonic brains reveals that thalamic reticular cells and some cells of the primitive internal capsule (perireticular cells) project to the dorsal thalamus from early embryonic ages (Mitrofanis and Guillery, 1993; Métin and Godement, 1996; Molnár et al., 1998a; Fig. 3F). The internal capsule cells with thalamic projections might be responsible for the early outgrowth of thalamic fibers and, perhaps, for the sorting of various corticofugal projections. This idea is supported by the observation that in Mash-1 knockout mice, which lack these cells, thalamic projections do not enter the internal capsule (Tuttle et al., 1999).

The intermediate zone

The corticostriatal junction is critical for the development of the thalamocortical connections. A puzzling behavior of thalamocortical and corticothalamic projections is observed at the stripe of cells located at the lateral end of the internal capsule (Molnár, 2000; Molnár and Hannan, 2000; Fig. 4). This transient stripe of cells is different from the cells of the internal capsule as revealed by their distinct gene-expression pattern and thalamic projections (Molnár and Cordery, 1999; Molnár, 2000). During early stages of forebrain development, thalamocortical and corticofugal projections pause before they cross this boundary. Cells within this stripe have been characterized by the expression of MAP2, calbindin and *Pax6* (Stoykova and Gruss, 1994; Smith Fernández et al., 1998; Molnár et al., 2000), of CAD11 (Simonneau and Thiery, 1998), and of semaphorin G (Skaliora et al., 1998). The role of this transient stripe of cells in the development of thalamocortical projections is presently unknown.

Comparative developmental examination of the transient stripe

Transient characters can be of key importance in tethering the alignment of developmental comparisons across taxa. Developmental events and gene expression patterns particularly when assessed in the context of topology, cytochemistry, adult homology, and other relevant characters, can inform our understanding of forebrain evolution. Early gene expression patterns in embryonic vertebrate brains, particularly the expression of *Emx1*, *Dlx1* and *Pax6* genes, helped to define regions in the embryonic pallium which started to produce some stable landmarks and useful reference points for further analysis (Smith Fernández et al., 1998; Puelles et al., 2000). There are numerous similar features in mammals, birds

and reptiles; nevertheless the defined regions change across species as if the cross-currents are affected in such a way that the proportions and relative positions come out differently. It appears that the corticostriatal junction is a rather puzzling area in this respect. The first observation is that the intermediate zone, defined by gene expression patterns *Pax6*-positive, but *Emx1*-negative and *Dlx1*-negative, appears much larger during development in birds and reptiles than mammals. Furthermore, the *Pax6*-positive cells remain dorsal in reptiles and birds while the same region acquires a ventrolateral position and is largely transient in dorsal regions in mammals. Hodological studies on the embryonic turtle by Cordery and Molnár (1999) support the significance of this genetically identified domain and demonstrate an algorithm similar to that of mammals. In mammals the population of internal capsule cells with thalamic projections is located medial to the region of the *Pax6*-positive intermediate territory defined by Smith Fernández et al. (1998) and does not extend into it (Molnár and Cordery, 1999). Similarly, the ADVR of turtles does not contain backlabelled cells after thalamic crystal placements (Cordery and Molnár, 1999). This result suggests that although the cortical intermediate zone in mammals and the ventral border of the DVR in reptiles are both close to the rostral portion of the backlabeled cells in the internal capsule, they are excluded from these structures.

Carbocyanine dye placements in the dorsal thalamus and other diencephalic sites in the embryonic turtle (Cordery and Molnár, 1999) revealed clear segregation of projections from nucleus rotundus to the dorsal ventricular ridge and projections of perirotundal nuclei (including the dorsal lateral optic nucleus) to the dorsal cortex. This specificity of innervation is apparent at early stages. Unfortunately it is not yet known whether the different thalamic nuclei have a different relationship to the *Pax6*-positive stripe in mammals.

Disturbed thalamocortical and corticofugal fiber growth at the striatocortical junction in various mutants

Hevner et al. (1998) and Kawano et al. (1999) described that in mice with mutations of transcription factor genes expressed in either cortex (*Tbr1*), dorsal thalamus (*Gbx2*), or both (*Pax6*), errors of corticothalamic and thalamocortical pathfinding occurred in the region of the internal capsule. Tracing experiments in these knock-out mice have shown that lack of early corticofugal projections is associated with abnormal development of thalamocortical projections. We do not yet understand what is responsible for the failure of both sets of fibers to cross the region in these mutants. The disturbed thalamocortical development in the above mentioned transgenic mice might be a very sensitive indicator of the disturbed early forebrain regionalization at the striatocortical junction.

There are several mutants (such as *Pax6*, *Tbr1*, *Gbx2*, *Emx2*) in which both thalamocortical and corticofugal pathfindings as well as tangential migration are arrested or altered at this particular site, suggesting that there might be a common mechanism orchestrating the processes. Both thalamocortical projections and tangentially migrating neurons have to traverse the corticostriatal junction (Fig. 4). The generative zone at the lateral corner of the telencephalic ventricle is clearly a crucial region. Cross-currents of influences intermix to produce complex and partially overlapping patterns. The developmental outcome of this region may be particularly vulnerable to shifts in timing and/or changes in genesis and wiring, such that any small alteration could have profound effects. Unfortunately, very little is known about this region even in mammals. There are several questions to be answered: What is the fate of the stripe? What is the origin of the cells constituting the stripe? Is it comprised of migrating cells? Is it a mixed population? What elements traverse the stripe? What is the relationship between the cells of the stripe and the tangentially migrating cells? When and why is it reduced during development, and what molecular changes occur at the region during normal development and in selected mutants with known defects of thalamocortical development and tangential migration? Many of these questions have direct relevance to questions of homology across vertebrates.

Collopallial field hypothesis

The common origin hypothesis and the *de novo* hypothesis (see Reiner, 2000) each have considerable merit. The various mammalian homologies proposed to date for the ADVR have all been on a 1:1 basis. None of these comparisons account, however, for evolution of all dorsolateral pallial components in mammals. The common origin hypothesis fails to specifically account for the basolateral amygdalar complex and claustrum and the *de novo* hypothesis for lateral neocortex. Only two possibilities appear to exist for evolution of lateral neocortex: a duplication of medial neocortex (see Puelles et al., 2000) or derivation from an embryonic field that in sauropsids includes the ADVR.

Four major structures in mammals—lateral neocortex, claustrum, endopiriform nucleus, and basolateral amygdalar complex—need to be accounted for. Among these structures, collothalamic afferents project to lateral neocortex and the lateral amygdalar nucleus (see Butler, 1994b; Doron and LeDoux, 1999). *Emx1* expression occurs during development in the lateral neocortex and in the dorsolateral part of the claustrum and basolateral amygdalar nucleus (Puelles et al., 2000). Swanson and Petrovich (1998) support the view that the basolateral amygdalar complex is a *"ventromedial extension of the claustrum"* and that this claustroamygdaloid formation constitutes the deepest layer of the overlying cortices. This view is consistent with that of Alheid et al. (1995) that the lateral, basolateral and basomedial nuclei of the amygdala are a *"functional extension of adjacent areas of the cortex,"* noting that the *"connections, cytology, ultra-structure, and histochemistry of these areas … in most instances … correspond to elements of the cortex"* and that *"several of these areas seem to possess cells whose morphology and connections are suggestive of a cortical-like processing scheme in the most general sense."*

Ramón y Cajal (1900) listed the claustrum as the eighth layer of the insular cortical region, lying deep to the extreme capsule as the seventh layer, but noted significant cellular differences between the claustrum and the cortex that he believed gainsaid its assignment as a true deep cortical layer. He contrasted the predominantly stellate cells of the claustrum with the somewhat smaller fusiform cells of the fifth and sixth layers of the insular cortex. On the other hand, Ramón y Cajal clearly recognized that the claustrum was not a part of the deeper basal ganglia. He concluded that the claustrum is a *"special formation different from the insular cortex and from the corpus striatum …"*

Of particular note is a set of non-GABAergic, pyramidal (and fusiform) neurons that express latexin, a carboxypeptidase A inhibitor, and are distributed within lateral neocortex, claustrum, and endopiriform nucleus (Arimatsu et al., 1994, 1998). These latexin-positive neurons span portions of the dorsal, lateral, and ventral pallia of Puelles et al. (2000). The distributions of *Emx1* expression, latexin expression, and collothalamic projections are thus not congruent, but instead are partially overlapping. This pattern suggests that the four major dorsolateral pallial components are developmentally related, i.e., derived from a single developmental field. The distribution of latexin-positive neurons in particular (Arimatsu et al., 1994) points to a unified developmental relationship for the claustrum, endopiriform nucleus, and lateral neocortex, while collothalamic projections unite the lateral neocortex with the lateral amygdalar nucleus.

Lateral neocortex has traditionally been considered a dorsal pallial derivative (see Butler, 1994b). The rhinal sulcus commonly has been perceived as a virtual River Styx between neocortex and piriform cortex but may in fact be a red herring. The sauropsid DVR has been regarded by some as a component of solely the lateral pallium (Holmgren, 1925; Northcutt, 1970; Striedter, 1997), and Northcutt (1974) noted a possible field homology of the amphibian lateral pallium with both piriform cortex and lateral neocortex in mammals and with both piriform cortex and DVR in sauropsids.

Butler (1994b) postulated that the DVR [ADVR] is an apomorphy for sauropsids, as is lateral neocortex in mammals, but maintained that both structures evolved from an expanded part of the pallial wall in ancestral amniotes that was in receipt of discrete collothalamic projections. We concur here with Northcutt's (1974) suggestion of lateral pallial derivation for both DVR and lateral neocortex as a general concept but prefer the term 'collopallium' to distinguish a nonolfactory, laterally lying, pallial entity. This moiety encompasses portions of the dorsal, lateral, and ventral pallia of Puelles et al. (2000). We have offered (Butler and Molnár, 2002; Molnár and Butler, 2002) a new, 'collopallial field hypothesis' (Fig. 5) that an expanded, nonolfactory pallial region was present in the common amniote ancestor, which in sauropsids gives rise to the ADVR, while in mammals it splits, or differentiates, to form lateral neocortex superficially as well as the deeper lying claustrum, endopiriform nucleus, and basolateral amygdalar complex. Thus, none of the latter structures have individual, 1:1 structural homologues in sauropsids. Instead, all of the superficial and deep components of the mammalian collopallial region are homologous to the ADVR only as a set of derivatives of a single embryonic field (Smith, 1967). In all amniotes, the olfactory-related

part of the lateral pallium splits to form piriform cortex superficially and its corresponding deep structures, the olfactory (and hypothalamic)-related parts of the amygdala/PDVR, which can thus be homologized respectively.

We thus generally concur that dorsoventral differentiation occurs as Puelles et al. (2000) describe, producing the respective derivatives of the *Emx1*-positive and -negative territories, but we also believe that a deep-to-superficial parcellation, or 'splitting,' occurs, which is normally expressed to a decreasing degree as one goes from lateral to medial and to a lesser extent in sauropsids than in mammals. The corollary of this hypothesis is that the medial part of the traditionally recognized "dorsal" pallium is evolutionarily and developmentally related to hippocampal pallium and gives rise only to the lemnopallium—medial neocortex and the dorsal cortex/ Wulst formation—again in agreement with Northcutt (1974) and also reconcilable with the findings and ideas of Martínez-García and Olucha (1988), Hoogland and Vermeulen-Van der Zee (1989), and Lohman and Smeets (1991). A bipartite (lateral versus medial) partitioning of the pallial mantle rather than a tripartite (lateral, dorsal, and medial) partitioning harks back to the ideas of Dart (1934) Abbie (1940), and Sanides (1970) regarding a dual origin of neocortex from hippocampal and piriform pallial regions. Despite contradictions to some aspects of that hypothesis (see Butler, 1994b), the basic idea of a medial and lateral pallial origin for two parts of neocortex appears robust.

In amphibians, Marín et al. (1998) clarified relationships of laterally-lying pallial structures and identified a region (LA) that lies ventral to the piriform area as homologous to the mammalian lateral amygdalar nucleus. The pallial topography in amphibians thus differs from that in amniotes (Fig. 5), in which the collopallial region, which includes the lateral amygdalar nucleus, lies dorsal to piriform cortex, as presumably also in the common amniote ancestor (CLP, Fig. 5). While this dorsoventral topographic relationship is not clearly apparent in most sauropsids, Reiner and Northcutt (2000) have recently described and confirmed it in the tuatara *Sphenodon*, in which the DVR has a very pronounced laminar (corticoid band) configuration: at rostral telencephalic levels the DVR lamina is continuous with the cellular lamina of dorsal cortex. Reiner and Northcutt (2000) convincingly argue that this DVR configuration was probably plesiomorphic for sauropsids.

32

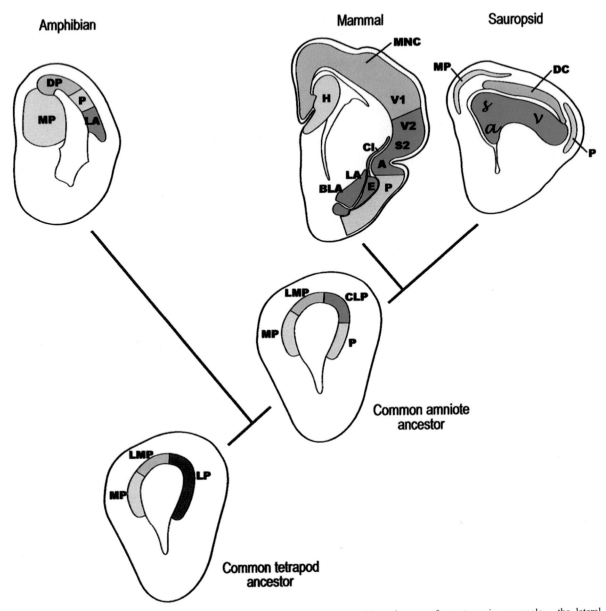

Fig. 5. Collopallial field hypothesis. Anterior dorsal ventricular ridge of sauropsids and a set of structures in mammals – the lateral neocortex, basolateral amygdalar complex, and claustrum – endopiriform nucleus formation – are homologous to each other as derivatives of a common embryonic field. In mammals the laterally lying collopallium splits, or differentiates, into deep (claustroamygdalar) and superficial (neocortical) components, whereas in sauropsids, this split does not occur. The common amniote ancestor is hypothesized to have had a unitary collopallial field, dorsal to piriform cortex. Extant amphibians exhibit a different topologic relationship of piriform cortex to their collopallial field, and thus a single, lateral collopallial/olfactory field may have been present in the common tetrapod ancestor that differentiated independently and differently in the amphibian and amniote lineages. Amphibian telencephalic hemisection redrawn from Northcutt and Kicliter (1980), ancestral and sauropsid hemisections from Butler (1994b), and lateral part of mammalian hemisection from Swanson and Petrovich (1998).

The differing pallial topography among extant tetrapods thus may result from independent derivation from a common, single, laterally lying pallial field in ancestral tetrapods.

Splitting of the pallial anlage in mammals

Rubenstein and Rakic (1999) have discussed factors involved in cortical regionalization, including cell position and cell capacity to respond to regulatory signals. We believe that 'splitting' of the pallial formation into deep and superficial components varies continuously along a lateromedial gradient that may be specified by such signals. The condition of least splitting, or parcellation (Ebbesson, 1980), is common to both sauropsids and mammals for the piriform (and vomeronasal) cortex and related parts of the amygdala (Swanson and Petrovich, 1998; Fig. 6). In sauropsids the collopallium remains a single, unparcellated structure—the ADVR—while in monotremes, both a small lateral neocortex and the basolateral component of the amygdala can be identified (Hines, 1929). In therian mammals, the split extends further dorsomedially, with an expanded region of lateral neocortex and the claustrum-endopiriform nucleus formation. The split is much less robust further medially but can be followed into medial neocortex with its deep component of layer 6b (see Swanson and Petrovich, 1998; Fig. 6). In the hippocampal pallium, only three cortical layers are present and no deep component can be perceived.

It is highly noteworthy for this scenario that monotremes lack a claustrum. Puelles (2000) suggested that if a prominent homologue of the claustrum is present in sauropsids, one might expect that a corresponding structure also would be *present and rather massive* in monotremes, in which the neocortex is *scarce and relatively primitive.* However, after careful searching, Divac et al. (1987) failed to find any trace of a claustrum in the echidna. Hines (1929) tentatively wondered about a small, ectopically located cell group (her Plate 68) in the platypus deep to temporal cortex, but no claustrum could be corroborated in the platypus (Paul Manger and Ann Butler, unpublished observations). The collopallial field hypothesis proposed here accounts for absence (or diminutive size) of a claustrum in monotremes: the ancestral lateral neocortical region was small and associated only with its most ventral deep component, the

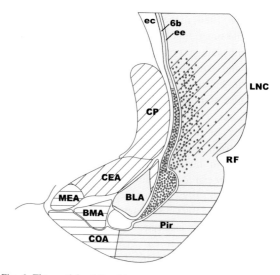

Fig. 6. The spatial relationships among components of the lateral part of the telencephalon of mammals, exemplified by the rat, redrawn after Swanson and Petrovich (1998) and including the distribution of markers (latexin-positive neurons as pink dots and *Emx1*-positive regions in light yellow) and hodology (collothalamic inputs indicated by diagonal lines and olfactory inputs by horizontal lines). The claustrum, filled with latexin-positive cells and *Emx1*-positive, is unlabeled here but corresponds to CLA of Fig. 2. Likewise the collothalamic-recipient LA is unlabeled and lies dorsolaterally adjacent to BLA, and the dorsal and ventral parts of the endopiriform nucleus are unlabeled and lie ventral to the claustrum as in Fig. 2. See text for references. An extreme capsule (ee), not present in rats, has been added to represent the more generalized mammalian condition.

basolateral amygdala. Later, dorsally directed expansion of the lateral neocortex by areal duplications (Kaas, 1995) in the ancestral therian line was linked to formation of additional deep components—a definitive endopiriform nucleus and claustrum.

Progressive splitting of the lateral pallial region over evolution is mirrored in the dorsal thalamus. During development in rats, a unitary dorsal pronucleus (Rose, 1942; Balmer et al., 1999) splits to form both the posterior nuclear group and LP. Neurons have fusiform profiles, indicating migration (Puelles et al., 1992) from the posterior nuclear group to LP (K.K. Cookson, C.W. Balmer, and A.B. Butler, unpublished observations). A field homology (Smith, 1967) of the nucleus rotundus-triangularis complex in sauropsids to both the posterior nuclear group and LP/pulvinar is thus also proposed here, in correlation with collopallial evolution. In support of this field homology, which is also an example of parcellation

34

(Ebbesson, 1980) in the mammalian line, cells within the superficial superior colliculus project to both LP and the suprageniculate part of the posterior group (Linke et al., 1999), and both LP and the posterior group nuclei project to the amygdala (Doron and LeDoux, 1999).

The idea of progressive splitting of the collopallium to produce the claustroamygdalar formation and lateral neocortex in therian mammals receives substantial support from genetic disorders that affect neuronal migration. In human females, mutation of the gene *doublecortin* can result in formation of a 'double cortex' (Gleeson et al., 1999), or subcortical laminar heterotopia (Palmini et al., 1993). An extensive layer of gray matter forms deep to the usual neocortical sheet but separated from it by a *"narrow but well-defined layer of white matter"* (Harding, 1996). In all three cases examined by Harding (1996) the heterotopic layer formed deep to most cortical areas, excepting only the striate, cingulate, and fusiform (occipitotemporal) gyri and the medial temporal areas—i.e., only the most medial cortical regions. The heterotopic band contains many pyramidal neurons, although of smaller size and in a more scattered array than in the overlying neocortex, and—of particular note—it incorporates the claustrum, as can be clearly seen in Fig. 6 of Harding (1996). It would thus appear that the heterotopic band produced by mutation of *doublecortin* represents a geographically elongated claustrum, formed by an abnormally extensive 'split' of the pallium that continues much farther medially than in the normal case.

Conclusions

The big questions concerning pallial evolution in amniotes all involve the pivotal region at the lateral corner of the lateral ventricle, an area where complex developmental cross-currents may be involved in the specification of multiple structures that are thus related to each other. Cell migrations, transient connectivity, axonal growth kinetics and patterns, and fasciculation behavior can clearly be substantially impacted in this region, which appears to be critical for thalamocortical development. We propose a new, collopallial field hypothesis, which specifies that the anterior dorsal ventricular ridge of sauropsids and a set of structures in mammals— the lateral neocortex, basolateral amygdalar complex, and claustrum-endopiriform nucleus formation—are

homologous to each other as derivatives of a common embryonic field. We propose that in mammals the laterally lying collopallium splits, or differentiates, into deep (claustroamygdalar) and superficial (neocortical) components, whereas in sauropsids, this split does not occur.

Acknowledgments

ABB expressly thanks John Allman for telling her about *doublecortin* and the double cortex syndrome. The sections for the pictures of Fig. 1 were kindly given to ZM by Jack Pettigrew, Paul Manger and Leah Krubitzer. This work was supported by Grants from The Royal Society, Swiss National Science Foundation (3100-56032.98), European Community (QLRT-1999-30158) and The Wellcome Trust to ZM and NSF Grant IBN-9728155 to ABB. We are thankful for the kind hospitality of the Senior Common Room of St John's College where some of these ideas were discussed by the authors.

Abbreviations used in figures

a	Collothalamic auditory area of ADVR
A	Archistriatum (Fig. 2); Auditory cortex (Fig. 5)
ADVR	Anterior dorsal ventricular ridge
BLA	Basolateral nucleus of the amygdala
BMA	Basomedial nucleus of the amygdala
cb	Corticoid band of the anterior dorsal ventricular ridge
CEA	Central nucleus of the amygdala
Cl	Claustrum (Fig. 5)
CLA	Claustrum (Fig. 2)
CLP	Collothalamic lateral pallium
COA	Cortical nucleus of the amygdala
CP	Caudate-putamen
DC	Dorsal cortex
DP	Dorsal pallium
E	Ectostriatum: collothalamic visual area of the ADVR (Fig. 2); Endopiriform nucleus (Fig. 5)
ec	External capsule
ee	Extreme capsule
EPd	Endopiriform nucleus, dorsal part
EPv	Endopiriform nucleus, ventral part
H	Hippocampus
HA	Hyperstriatum accessorium

HD	Hyperstriatum dorsale
HIS	Hyperstriatum intercalatus superior
HV	Hyperstriatum ventrale
L	Field L of Rose: collothalamic auditory area of ADVR
LA	Lateral nucleus of the amygdala
LMP	Lemnothalamic medial pallium
LNC	Lateral neocortex
LP	Lateral pallium
MEA	Medial nucleus of the amygdala
MNC	Medial neocortex
MP	Medial pallium
N	Neostriatum (part of the ADVR)
OC	Optic chiasm
OT	Optic tract
P	Piriform cortex (Fig. 5)
Pd	Dorsal pallidum (paleostriatum primitivum)
Pir	Piriform cortex (Figs. 2,6)
Pth	Pallial thickening
R	Nucleus rotundus
RF	Rhinal fissure
s	Collothalamic somatosensory area of ADVR
St	Dorsal striatum (paleostriatum augmentatum)
S2	Secondary somatosensory cortex
TeO	Optic tectum
v	Collothalamic visual area of ADVR
V1	Primary visual cortex
V2	Secondary visual cortex
6b	Layer 6b of neocortex

References

Abbie, A.A. (1940) Cortical lamination in the monotremata. J. Comp. Neurol., 72: 428–467.

Alheid, G.F., de Olmos, J.S. and Beltramino, C.A. (1995) Amygdala and extended amygdala. In: G. Paxinos, (Ed.), The Rat Nervous System, Academic Press, San Diego, pp. 495–578.

Anderson, S., Mione, M., Yun, K. and Rubenstein, J.L. (1999) Differential origins of neocortical projection and local circuit neurons: role of Dlx genes in neocortical interneuronogenesis. Cereb. Cortex, 9: 646–654.

Anderson, S.A., Eisenstat, D.D., Shi, L. and Rubenstein, J.L. (1997) Interneuron migration from basal forebrain to neocortex: dependence on Dlx genes. Science, 278: 474–476.

Arimatsu, Y., Kojima, M. and Ishida, M. (1998) Area- and lamina-specific organization of a neuronal subpopulation defined by expression of latexin in the rat cerebral cortex. J. Neurosci., 88: 93–105.

Arimatsu, Y., Nihonmatsu, I., Hirata, K. and Takiguchi-Hayashi, K. (1994) Cogeneration of neurons with a unique molecular phenotype in layers V and VI of widespread lateral neocortical areas in the rat. J. Neurosci., 14: 2020–2031.

Balmer, C.W., Cookson, K.K., Saini, H.S., Jones, M.J. and Butler, A.B. (1999) Dorsal thalamic differentiation in rats involves transient pronuclei consistent with the dual elaboration hypothesis of thalamic evolution. Soc. Neurosci. Abstr., 25: 103.

Bayer, S.A. and Altman, J. (1991) Development of the endopiriform nucleus and the claustrum in the rat brain. Neuroscience, 45: 391–412.

Beckstead, R.M. (1984). The thalamostriatal projection in the cat. J. Comp. Neurol., 223: 313–346.

Blanton, M.G. and Kriegstein, A.R. (1991) Morphological differentiation of distinct neuronal classes in embryonic turtle cerebral cortex. J. Comp. Neurol., 310: 558–570.

Brauth, S.E., Kitt, C.A., Reiner, A. and Quirion, R. (1986) Neurotensin binding sites in the forebrain and midbrain of the pigeon. J. Comp. Neurol., 253: 358–373.

Bruce, L.L. and Butler, A.B. (1984) Telencephalic connections in lizards. II. Projections to anterior dorsal ventricular ridge. J. Comp. Neurol., 229: 602–615.

Bruce, L.L. and Neary, T.J. (1995) The limbic system of tetrapods: a comparative analysis of cortical and amygdalar populations. Brain Behav. Evol., 46: 224–234.

Butler, A.B. (1994a) The evolution of the dorsal thalamus of jawed vertebrates, including mammals: cladistic analysis and a new hypothesis. Brain Res. Rev., 19: 29–65.

Butler, A.B. (1994b) The evolution of the dorsal pallium in the telencephalon of amniotes: cladistic analysis and a new hypothesis. Brain Res. Rev., 19: 66–101.

Butler, A.B. and Hodos, W. (1996) Comparative Vertebrate Neuroanatomy: Evolution and Adaptation. Wiley-Liss, New York.

Butler, A.B. and Molnár, Z. (1998) Development and evolution in nervous systems: development and evolution of ideas. Meeting report. Trends Neurosci., 21: 177–178.

Butler, A.B. and Molnár, Z. (2002) Development and Evolution of the Collopallium in Amniotes: a New Hypothesis of Field Homology. Brain Res. Bull., in press.

Cajal, S.R. (1900) Studies on the human cerebral cortex III: Structure of the acoustic cortex. Rev. Trimest. Microgr., 5: 129–183. Translated and reprinted in: J. DeFelipe and E.G. Jones (Eds.), Cajal on the Cerebral Cortex: An Annotated Translation of the Complete Writings. Oxford University Press, New York, 1988, pp. 251–288.

Caviness, V.S., Jr., Crandall, J.E. and Edwards, M.A. (1988). The reeler malformation, implications for neuronal histogenesis. In: E.G. Jones, and A. Peters, (Eds.), Cerebral Cortex, Development and Maturation of Cerebral Cortex, Vol. 7, Plenum Press, New York-London, pp. 59–89.

Cordery, P. and Molnár, Z. (1999) Embryonic development of connections in turtle pallium. J. comp. Neurol., 413: 26–54.

Dart, R.A. (1934) The dual structure of the neopallium: its history and significance. J. Anat., 69: 3–19.

De Carlos, J.A. and O'Leary, D.D.M. (1992) Growth and targeting of subplate axons and establishment of major cortical pathways. J. Neurosci., 12: 1194–1211.

De Carlos, J.A., Lopez-Mascaraque, L. and Valverde, F. (1996) Dynamics of cell migration from the lateral ganglionic eminence in the rat. J. Neurosci., 16: 6146–6156.

Divac, I., Holst, M.C., Nelson, J. and McKenzie, J.S. (1987) Afferents of the frontal cortex in the echidna (Tachyglossus aculeatus). Brain Behav. Evol., 30: 303–320.

Doron, N.N. and LeDoux, J.E. (1999) Organization of projections to the lateral amygdala from auditory and visual areas of the thalamus in the rat. *J. Comp. Neurol.*, 412: 383–409.

Ebbesson, S.O.E. (1980) The parcellation theory and its relation to interspecific variability in brain organization, evolutionary and ontogenetic development and neuronal plasticity. *Cell Tissue Res.*, 213: 179–212.

Erzurumlu, R.S. and Jhaveri, S. (1992) Emergence of connectivity in the embryonic rat parietal cortex. *Cereb. Cortex*, 2: 336–352.

Frotscher, M. (1998) Cajal-Retzius cells, Reelin, and the formation of layers. *Curr. Opin. Neurobiol.*, 8: 570–575.

Gleeson, J.G., Minnerath, S.R., Fox, J.W., Allen, K.M., Luo, R.F., Hong, S.E., Berg, M.J., Kuzniecky, R., Reitnauer, P.J., Borgatti, R., Mira, A.P., Guerrini, R., Holmes, G.L., Rooney, C.M., Berkovic, S., Scheffer, I., Cooper, E.C., Ricci, S., Cusmai, R., Crawford, T.O., Leroy, R., Andermann, E., Wheless, J.W., Dobyns, W.B., Ross, M.E. and Walsh, C.A. (1999) Characterization of mutations in the gene doublecortin in patients with double cortex syndrome. *Ann. Neurol.*, 45: 146–153.

Götz, M., Novak, N., Bastmayer, M. and Bolz, J. (1992) Membrane-bound molecules in rat cerebral cortex regulate thalamic innervation. *Develop.*, 116: 507–519.

Gulisano, M., Broccoli, V., Pardini, C. and Boncinelli, E. (1996) *Emx1* and *Emx2* show different patterns of expression during proliferation and differentiation of the developing cerebral cortex in the mouse. *Eur. J. Neurosci.*, 8: 1037–1050.

Hall, W.C. and Ebner, F.F. (1970) Thalamotelencephalic projections in the turtle (*Pseudemys scripta*). *J. Comp. Neurol.*, 140: 101–122.

Harding, B. (1996) Gray matter heterotopia. In: R. Guerrini, R. Canapicchi, B. Zifkin, F. Andermann, J. Roger, and P. Pfanner (Eds.), *Dysplasias of Cerebral Cortex and Epilepsy*, Lippincott-Raven, Philadelphia, pp. 81–88.

Hevner, R.F., Miyashita, E., Martin, G. and Rubenstein, J.L.R. (1998) Lack of thalamocortical connections in mutants affecting cortical (*TBR-1*) or thalamic (*GBX-2*) gene expression. *Soc. Neurosci. Abstr.*, 24: 58.

Hines, M., IV. (1929) The brain of *Ornithorhynchus Anatinus*. *Phil. Trans. Roy. Soc. Lond. B*, 217: 155–287 and plates.

Holmgren, N. (1925) Points of view concerning forebrain morphology in higher vertebrates. *Acta Zool. Stockh.*, 6: 413–477.

Hoogland, P.V. and Vermeulen-Van der Zee, E. (1989) Efferent connections of the dorsal cortex of the lizard *Gekko gecko* studied with *Phaseolus vulgaris*-leucoagglutinin. *J. Comp. Neurol.*, 285: 289–303.

Jones, E.G. (1985) The Thalamus. Plenum Press, New York.

Kaas, J.H. (1995) The evolution of isocortex. *Brain Behav. Evol.*, 46: 187–196.

Källén, B. (1962) Embryogenesis of brain nuclei in the chick telencephalon. *Ergeb Anat Entwicklungsgesch*, 36: 62–82.

Karten, H.J. (1969) The organization of the avian telencephalon and some speculations on the phylogeny of the amniote telencephalon. *Ann NY Acad. Sci.*, 167: 146–179.

Karten, H.J. (1997) Evolutionary developmental biology meets the brain: the origins of mammalian cortex. *Proc. Natl. Acad. Sci. USA*, 94: 2800–2804.

Karten, H.J. and Hodos, W. (1967) *A Stereotaxic Atlas of the Brain of the Pigeon (Columba livia)*, The Johns Hopkins Press, Baltimore.

Karten, H.J. and Shimizu, T. (1989) The origins of neocortex: connections and lamination as distinct events in evolution. *J. Cognitive Neurosci.*, 1: 291–301.

Karten, H.J., Cox, K. and Mpodozis, J. (1997) Two distinct populations of tectal neurons have unique connections within the retinotectorotundal pathway of the pigeon (*Columba livia*). *J. Comp. Neurol.*, 387: 449–465.

Kawano, H., Fukuda, T., Kubo, K., Horie, M., Uyemura, K., Takeuchi, K., Osumi, N., Eto, K. and Kawamura, K. (1999) *Pax6* is required for thalamocortical pathway formation in fetal rats. *J. Comp. Neurol.*, 408: 147–160.

Korzeniewska, E. and Güntürkün, O. (1990) Sensory properties and afferents of the n. dorsolateralis posterior thalami of the pigeon. *J. Comp. Neurol.*, 292: 457–479.

Lavdas, A.A., Grigoriou, M., Pachnis, V. and Parnavelas, J.G. (1999) The medial ganglionic eminence gives rise to a population of early neurons in the developing cerebral cortex. *J. Neurosci.*, 19: 7881–7888.

LeDoux, J.E., Ruggiero, D.A. and Reis, D.J. (1985) Projections to the subcortical forebrain from anatomically defined regions of the medial geniculate body in the rat. *J. Comp. Neurol.*, 242: 182–213.

LeVay, S. and Sherk, H. (1981) The visual claustrum of the cat. I. Structure and connections. *J. Neurosci.*, 1: 956–980.

Lin, C.-S., May, P.J. and Hall, W.C. (1984) Nonintralaminar thalamostriatal projections in the gray squirrel (*Sciurus carolinensis*) and tree shrew (*Tupaia glis*). *J. Comp. Neurol.*, 230: 33–46.

Linke, R., De Lima, A.D., Schwegler, H. and Pape, H.-C. (1999) Direct synaptic connections of axons from superior colliculus with identified thalamo-amygdaloid projection neurons in the rat: possible substrates of a subcortical visual pathway to the amygdala. *J. Comp. Neurol.*, 403: 158–170.

Lohman, A.H.M. and Smeets, W.J.A.J. (1991) The dorsal ventricular ridge and cortex of reptiles in historical and phylogenetic perspective. In: B.L. Finlay, G. Innocenti and H. Scheich (Eds.), *The Neocortex: Ontogeny and Phylogeny*, Plenum, New York, pp. 59–74.

Luksch, H., Cox, K. and Karten, H.J. (1998) Bottlebrush dendritic endings and large dendritic fields: motion-detecting neurons in the tectofugal pathway. *J. Comp. Neurol.*, 396: 399–414.

Mallamaci, A., Iannone, R., Briata, P., Pintonello, L., Mercurio, S., Boncinelli, E. and Corte, G. (1998) EMX2 protein in the developing mouse brain and olfactory area. *Mech. Dev.*, 77: 165–172.

Mallamaci, A., Muzio, L., Chan, C.-H., Parnavelas, J. and Boncinelli, E. (1999) Area identity shifts in the early cerebral cortex of *Emx2*–/– mutant mice. *Nat. Neurosci.*, 679–686.

Marín, O., Smeets, W.J.A.J. and González, A. (1998) Basal ganglia organization in amphibians: chemoarchitecture. *J. Comp. Neurol.*, 392: 285–312.

Martínez-García, F. and Olucha, F.E. (1988) Afferent projections to the Timm-positive areas of the telencephalon of lizards. In: W.K. Schwerdtfeger, and W.J.A.J. Smeets, (Eds.), *The Forebrain of Reptiles: Current Concepts of Structure and Function*. Basel, Karger, pp. 30–40.

McConnell, S.K., Ghosh, A., and Shatz, C.J. (1989) Subplate neurons pioneer the first axon pathway from the cerebral cortex. *Science*, 245: 978–982.

Medina, L. and Reiner, A. (1995) Neurotransmitter organization and connectivity of the basal ganglia in vertebrates: implications for the evolution of basal ganglia. *Brain Behav. Evol.*, 46: 235–258.

Medina, L. and Reiner, A. (2000) Do birds possess homologues of mammalian primary visual, somatosensory and motor cortices? *Trends Neurosci.*, 23: 1–12.

Métin, C. and Godement, P. (1996) The ganglionic eminence may be an intermediate target for corticofugal and thalamocortical axons. *J. Neurosci.*, 16: 3219–3235.

Meyer, G., Castro, R., Soria, J.M. and Fairen, A. (2000) The subpial granular layer in the developing cerebral cortex of rodents. *Results Probl. Cell. Differ.*, 30: 277–91.

Mione, M.C., Cavanagh, J.F.R., Harris, B. and Parnavelas, J.G. (1997) Cell specification and symmetrical/asymmetrical divisions in the developing cerebral cortex. *J. Neurosci.*, 2018–2029.

Mitrofanis, J. and Guillery, R.W. (1993) New views of the thalamic reticular nucleus in the adult and developing brain. *Trends in Neurosci.*, 16: 240–245.

Molnár, Z. (1998) Development of Thalamocortical Connections. Berlin. Springer-Verlag; and Georgetown, TX. R.G. Landes Company.

Molnár, Z. (2000) Conserved developmental algorithms during thalamocortical circuit formation in mammals and reptiles. In: G.R. Bock and G. Cardew (Eds.), *Evolutionary Developmental Biology of the Cerebral Cortex. Novartis Found Symp 223.* Chichester, pp. 148–172.

Molnár, Z. and Blakemore, C. (1995) How do thalamic axons find their way to the cortex? *Trends in Neurosci.*, 18: 389–397.

Molnár, Z. and Butler, A.B. (2002) The corticostriatal junction: a crucial region for forebrain development and evolution. *Bioessays*, in press.

Molnár, Z. and Cordery, P.M. (1999) Connections between cells of the internal capsule, thalamus and cerebral cortex in embryonic rat. *J. Comp. Neurol.*, 413: 1–25.

Molnár, Z. and Hannan, A. (2000) Development of thalamocortical projections in normal and mutant mice. In: A. Goffinet and P. Rakic (Eds.), *Mouse Brain Development*, Springer-Verlag, Heidelberg, pp. 293–332.

Molnár, Z., Adams, R. and Blakemore, C. (1998a) Mechanisms underlying the establishment of topographically ordered early thalamocortical connections in the rat. *J. Neurosci.*, 18: 5723–5745.

Molnár, Z., Adams, R., Goffinet, A.M. and Blakemore, C. (1998b) The role of the first postmitotic cells in the development of thalamocortical fiber ordering in the reeler mouse. *J. Neurosci.*, 18: 5746–5785.

Molnár, Z., Knott, G.W., Blakemore, C. and Saunders, N.R. (1998c) Development of thalamocortical projections in the south American grey short-tailed Opossum (*Monodelphis Domestica*). *J. Comp. Neurol.*, 398: 491–514.

Molnár, Z., Mather, N.K., Katznelson, A., Voelker, C., Bronchti, G., Welker, E. and Taylor, J.S.H. (1999) Disturbed fasciculation, but ordered cortical termination of thalamocortical projections in L1 knock-out mice. *Soc. For Neurosci. Abstr.*, 25: 1305.

Molnár, Z., Modoux, D., Gruss, P. and Stoykova, A. (2000) Development of thalamocortical and corticofugal projections in the *Pax6-LacZ* mice. *Soc. For Neurosci. Abstr.*, 26: 290.

Mpodozis, J., Cox, K., Shimizu, T., Bischof, H.-J., Woodson, W. and Karten, H.J. (1996) GABAergic inputs to the nucleus rotundus (pulvinar inferior) of the pigeon (*Columba livia*). *J. Comp. Neurol.*, 374: 204–222.

Namura, S., Takada, M., Kikuchi, H. and Mizuno, N. (1997) Collateral projections of single neurons in the posterior thalamic region to both the temporal cortex and the amygdala: a fluorescent retrograde double-labeling study in the rat. *J. Comp. Neurol.*, 384: 59–70.

Nieuwenhuys, R., ten Donkelaar, H.J. and Nicholson, C. (1998) *The Central Nervous System of Vertebrates*, Springer, Berlin.

Northcutt, R.G. (1970) The telencephalon of the western painted turtle (*Chrysemys picta belli*), University of Illinois Press, Urbana, Illinois.

Northcutt, R.G. (1974) Some histochemical observations on the telencephalon of the bullfrog, *Rana catesbeiana* Shaw. *J. Comp. Neurol.*, 157: 379–390.

Northcutt, R.G. and Kaas, J.H. (1995) The emergence and evolution of mammalian neocortex. *Trends Neurosci.*, 18: 373–379.

Northcutt, R.G. and Kicliter, E. (1980) Organization of the amphibian telencephalon. In: S.O.E. Ebbesson (Ed.), *Comparative Neurology of the Telencephalon*, Plenum Press, New York, pp. 203–255.

Palmini, A., Andermann, F., de Grissac, H., Tampieri, D., Robitaille, Y., Langevin, P., Desbiens, R. and Andermann, E. (1993) Stages and patterns of centrifugal arrest of diffuse neuronal migration disorders. *Devel. Med. Child Neurol.*, 35: 331–339.

Parnavelas, J.G. (2000) The origin and migration of cortical neurons: new vistas. *Trends Neurosci.*, 23: 126–131.

Pritz, M.B. (1975) Anatomical identification of a telencephalic visual area in crocodiles: ascending connections of nucleus rotundus in *Caiman crocodilus. J. Comp. Neurol.*, 164: 323–338.

Puelles, L. (2000) In Discussion after Krubitzer LA. How does evolution build a complex brain? In: G.R. Bock and G. Cardew, (Eds.), *Evolutionary Developmental Biology of the Cerebral Cortex*. John Wiley & Sons, Ltd., Chichester, p. 226.

Puelles, L., Kuwana, E., Puelles, E., Bulfone, A., Shimamura, K., Keleher, J., Smiga, S. and Rubenstein, J.L.R. (2000) Pallial and subpallial derivatives in the embryonic chick and mouse telencephalon, traced by the expression of the genes *Dlx-2, Emx-1, Nkx-2.1, Pax-6*, and *Tbr-1. J. Comp. Neurol.*, 424: 409–438.

Puelles, L., Sanchez, M.P., Spreafico, R. and Fairen, A. (1992) Prenatal development of calbindin immunoreactivity in the dorsal thalamus of the rat. *Neurosci.*, 46: 135–147.

Rakic, P. (1977) Prenatal development of the visual system in the rhesus monkey. *Phil. Trans. Roy. Soc. Lond. B Biol. Sci.*, 278: 245–260.

Rakic, P. (1995) Radial versus tangential migration of neuronal clones in the developing cerebral cortex. *Proc. Natl. Acad. Sci. USA*, 92: 11323–11327.

Reiner, A. (1993) Neurotransmitter organization and connections of turtle cortex: implications for the evolution of mammalian isocortex. *Comp. Biochem. Physiol. A Comp. Physiol.*, 104: 735–748.

Reiner, A. (2000) A hypothesis as to the organization of cerebral cortex in the common amniote ancestor of modern reptiles and mammals. In: G.R. Bock, and G. Cardew (Eds.), *Evolutionary Developmental Biology of the Cerebral Cortex, Novartis Foundation Symposium 228*, John Wiley & Sons Ltd., Chichester, pp. 83–108.

Reiner, A., Brauth, S.E., Kitt, C.A. and Quirion, R. (1989) Distribution of *mu*, *delta*, and *kappa* opiate receptor types in the forebrain and midbrain of pigeons. *J. Comp. Neurol.*, 280: 359–382.

Reiner, A. and Northcutt, R.G. (2000) Succinic dehydrogenase histochemistry reveals the location of the putative primary visual and auditory areas within the dorsal ventricular ridge of *Sphenodon punctatus*. *Brain Behav. Evol.*, 55: 26–36.

Rubenstein, J.L.R. and Rakic, P. (1999) Genetic control of cortical development. *Cerebral Cortex*, 9: 521–654.

Rose, J.E. (1942) The ontogenetic development of the rabbit's diencephalon. *J. Comp. Neurol.*, 77: 61–129.

Ryugo, D.K. and Killackey, H.P. (1974) Differential telencephalic projections of the medial and ventral divisions of the medial geniculate body of the rat. *Brain Res.*, 82: 173–177.

Sadikot, A.F., Rymar, V., Muttal, S. and Luk, K. (2000) Neurogenesis of calretinin- and parvalbumin-immunoreactive GABAergic interneurons in the mammalian cerebral cortex. *Soc. Neurosci. Abstr.*, 26: 1857.

Sanides, F. (1970) Functional architecture of motor and sensory cortices in primates in the light of a new concept of neocortical evolution. In: C.R. Noback and W. Montagna (Eds.), *The Primate Brain: Advances in Primatology*, Vol. 1. Appleton-Century-Crofts, New York, pp. 137–208.

Simonneau, L. and Thiery, J.P. (1998) The mesenchimal cadherin-11 is expressed in restricted sites during the ontogeny of the rat brain in modes suggesting novel functions. *Cell Adhesion Commun.*, 6: 431–450.

Skaliora, I., Singer, W., Betz, H. and Püschel, A.W. (1998) Differential patterns of semaphoring expression in the developing rat brain. *Eur. J. Neurosci.*, 10: 1215–1229.

Smith, H.M. (1967) Biological similarities and homologies. *Syst. Zool.*, 16:101–102.

Smith Fernández, A., Pieau, C., Repérant, J., Boncinelli and Wassef, M. (1998) Expression of the *Emx-1* and *Dlx-1* homeobox genes define three molecularly distinct domains in the telencephalon of mouse, chick, turtle and frog embryos: implications for the evolution of telencephalic subdivisions in amniotes. *Develop.*, 125: 2099–2111.

Stoykova, A. and Gruss, P. (1994) Roles of Pax-genes in developing and adult brain as suggested by expression patterns. *J. Neurosci.*, 14: 1395–1412.

Striedter, G.F. (1997) The telencephalon of tetrapods in evolution. *Brain Behav. Evol.*, 49: 179–213.

Striedter, G.F. and Northcutt, R.G. (1991) Biological hierarchies and the concept of homology. *Brain Behav. Evol.*, 38: 177–189.

Swanson, L.W. and Petrovich, G.D. (1998) What is the amygdala? *Trends Neurosci.*, 21: 323–331.

Takada, M., Itoh, K., Sugimoto, T. and Mizuno, N. (1985) Topographical projections from the thalamus to the putamen in the cat. *Neurosci. Lett.*, 54: 207–212.

Tamamaki, N., Fujimori, K.E. and Takauji, R. (1997) Origin and route of tangentially migrating neurons in the developing neocortical intermediate zone. *J. Neurosci.*, 17: 8313–23.

Tuttle, R., Nakagawa, Y., Johnson, J.E. and O'Leary, D.D. (1999) Defects in thalamocortical axon pathfinding correlate with altered cell domains in Mash-1-deficient mice. *Develop.*, 126: 1903–1916.

Ulinski, P.S. (1983) *Dorsal Ventricular Ridge: A Treatise on Forebrain Organization in Reptiles and Birds*, John Wiley & Sons, New York.

Wild, J.M. (1987) The avian somatosensory system: connections of regions of body representation in the forebrain of the pigeon. *Brain Res.*, 412: 205–223.

E.C. Azmitia, J. DeFelipe, E.G. Jones, P. Rakic and C.E. Ribak (Eds.)
Progress in Brain Research, Vol. 136

CHAPTER 4

Life-long stability of neurons: a century of research on neurogenesis, neuronal death and neuron quantification in adult CNS

Kris Turlejski* and Ruzanna Djavadian

Department of Neurophysiology, Nencki Institute of Experimental Biology, 3 Pasteur Street, 02-093 Warsaw, Poland

Abstract: In this chapter we provide an extensive review of 100 years of research on the stability of neurons in the mammalian brain, with special emphasis on humans. Although Cajal formulated the Neuronal Doctrine, he was wrong in his beliefs that adult neurogenesis did not occur and adult neurons are dying throughout life. These two beliefs became accepted "common knowledge" and have shaped much of neuroscience research and provided much of the basis for clinical treatment of age-related brain diseases. In this review, we consider adult neurogenesis from a historical and evolutionary perspective. It is concluded, that while adult neurogenesis is a factor in the dynamics of the dentate gyrus and olfactory bulb, it is probably not a major factor during the life-span in most brain areas. Likewise, the acceptance of neuronal death as an explanation for normal age-related senility is challenged with evidence collected over the last fifty years. Much of the problem in changing this common belief of dying neurons was the inadequacies of neuronal counting methods. In this review we discuss in detail implications of recent improvements in neuronal quantification. We conclude: First, age-related neuronal atrophy is the major factor in functional deterioration of existing neurons and could be slowed down, or even reversed by various pharmacological interventions. Second, in most cases neuronal degeneration during aging is a pathology that in principle may be avoided. Third, loss of myelin and of the white matter is more frequent and important than the limited neuronal death in normal aging.

Introduction

One of the greatest achievements of Don Santiago Ramón y Cajal was proving the neuronal theory first formulated by His (1890). Many neuroanatomists like Paladino (1893), Sedgwick (1894) or Held (1907), supported the opposing syncytial (reticular, catenary) theory. Cajal mastered and further developed the Golgi (1886) technique, and this allowed him to prove that the CNS is built of separate cells. Cajal strongly adhered to the theory that in the mammalian CNS cell divisions stop in the prenatal period (Cajal, 1913, 1928). Therefore,

he believed that the mammalian brain reaches its maximal number of neurons prenatally. Another popular theory held that adult neurons gradually die out, and therefore their numbers decrease with age. This gradual depletion of the neuronal pool seemed to account for the functional deterioration during normal aging. Although both those premises were periodically contested, controversies concerning both of them remained, and therefore the question of stability of neuronal population throughout life is still open.

In this chapter we review the history of attempts to determine the number of neurons in various structures of the adult mammalian CNS and the evidence of adult proliferation and cell death. Two problems within the scope of this debate will be left out. First, we will not

*Corresponding author: Tel.: 48 22 659 8571 ext. 326;
Fax: 48 22 822 5342; E-mail: krist@nencki.gov.pl

discuss the period of early postnatal development in mammals. The main reason of this exclusion is, that there are enormous differences in the developmental stage at the time of birth among various species of mammals, from marsupials at one extreme, to ungulates and cetaceans at another. Processes of developmental proliferation of neurons in the postnatal period (Farel and McIlwain, 2000) and of the developmental cell death (Hamburger and Oppenheim, 1982; Cowan et al., 1984, Gould et al., 1991; Thomaidou et al., 1997) are well documented by now, and in this respect theories prevailing for half a century were completely rejected. Attempts at scaling of the developmental stages (Economos, 1982; Dreher and Robinson, 1988; Robinson and Dreher, 1990), although very important, are as yet few and limited. Second, we are not going to discuss the relation of age to neuronal depletion due to disease. Although originally dementia was considered to be a natural consequence of senility, at present it has clearly moved into the sphere of pathology, which is out of scope of this review.

Are new neurons added to the CNS of adult mammals?

History of the controversy

Many of Cajal's meticulous observations were done on the developing CNS (Cajal, 1899–1904, 1913). In parallel to such prominent neuroanatomists as Kolliker (1882, 1905) and His (1890, 1904), Cajal described proliferations of cells in the subependymal zone of the neural tube, migration of neuroblasts and then growth of neurons that start to extend axons and spread their dendritic trees. He concluded, that neurons are generated exclusively during the prenatal phase of development and this theory survived for over a century.

However, from the very beginning there were facts and ideas contradicting this theory. Some neuroanatomists, like Schaper (1897) and Levi (1898) claimed, that in the CNS of vertebrates, form fish to human, there is a pool of undifferentiated cells (medulloblasts – Kershman, 1938) that might proliferate and differentiate into new neurons. Hamilton (1901) found mitotic figures in the CNS of the four-day-old rats. Allen (1912) observed dividing cells in the brain of the 120-day-old rats. Later, Sugita (1918) reported that the number of neurons in the rat's cortex continued to increase during first 20 postnatal days.

However, such evidence was firmly rejected by the majority of prominent scientists like His (1904) and Cajal (1913, 1928). It was almost impossible to trace the fate of those scarce dividing cells and prove that the newly-born cells are neurons and not glia (Cajal, 1913). Besides, those observations were in conflict with another generalization about the mechanisms of development of the nervous system, namely that the newborn neurons generated in the subependymal zone of ventricles and central canal move out of that zone and into their proper places along the radial glia (Boll, 1873–1874; Kolliker, 1882; His, 1890; Lenhossek, 1890). As there is no radial glia in the adult brain, there would be no way of incorporating these newly created neurons into the functioning nervous system. In spite of repeating contests (Kershman, 1938), the dogma of "no new neurons after birth" lasted until a new method of labeling dividing cells with [^{3}H]-thymidine was developed (Leblond et al., 1959).

The [^{3}H] thymidine is incorporated into newly formed DNA during the S-phase of the cell cycle and may be detected with autoradiography (Sidman et al., 1959). Smart (1961) was the first to show that some neurons are born in the adult mouse brain. He found proliferations proceed in the subependymal layer and afterwards these newborn cells migrate and differentiated into neurons or glia. Altman (1962, 1963, 1966, 1969; Altman and Das, 1965) showed that those new neurons are added to only two structures of the adult rat's brain, the hippocampal dentate gyrus and the olfactory bulb (see Korr, 1982). Recently, another marker of the S-phase, a synthetic thymidine analogue, bromodeoxyuridine (BrdU) has been introduced (Gratzner, 1982; Morstyn et al., 1983; Miller and Nowakowski, 1988), which allowed for stereological determination of the total number of newly created cells. Another breakthrough was isolation of the stem cells from adult brains *in vitro* (Reynolds and Weiss, 1992; Moorshead et al., 1997).

Dentate gyrus

Postnatal cell proliferation within the hippocampal dentate gyrus is seen in various rodents: mouse (Kempermann et al., 1997; Rietze, 2000), rat (Altman, 1962, 1963, Altman and Das, 1965, 1966; Schlessinger et al., 1975; Kaplan and Hinds, 1977; Bayer, 1982; Cameron et al., 1993; Cameron and McKay, 1999, 2001), golden hamster (Huang et al., 1998); guinea pig (Altman and Das, 1967); gerbil (Dawirs et al., 2000); vole (Galea and McEwen, 1999); grey squirrel (Lavenex et al., 2000a,b) and primates: human (Eriksson et al., 1998); macaque (Rakic and Nowakowski, 1981; Eckenhoff and Rakic, 1988; Gould et al., 1999a; Kornack and Rakic, 1999; see however Rakic 1985); marmoset (Gould et al., 1998). It was also confirmed in the macroscelid tree shrew (Gould et al., 1997), lagomorph rabbit (Gueneau et al., 1982) and carnivores, cat (Altman, 1963; Wyss and Srinipanidkulchai, 1985) and dog (Blakemore and Jolly, 1972). It was also found in the brain of the marsupial brush-tailed possum (Sanderson and Wilson, 1997). However, the investigated carnivores were very young, still in the period of development. Members of other large mammalian orders, such as insectivores or bats, were not tested yet. Bialoskorska et al. (2001) reported preliminary data on the hippocampal proliferation in the adult shrews (Insectivora, see below).

Cameron and McKay (2001) who labeled dividing cells with BrdU, calculated that approximately 9000 new cells are generated in the adult rat dentate gyrus each day and 50% of them differentiate into neurons. If most of these neurons survive for four weeks then they constitute 6% of the total number of hippocampal granule cells (West et al., 1991), and about 70% in a year. There are reports of postnatal increases of the numbers of neurons in the rat's dentate gyri (Bayer, 1982; Bayer et al., 1982, Crespo et al., 1986). However, these increases were lower than it would be predicted from the rate of neurogeneration and other investigators did not report significant life-long increases (e.g. Boss et al., 1985). Therefore, there is a turnover of neurons in this structure, with some neurons dying out and being replaced by the new ones (Biebl et al., 2000). An interplay of cell divisions and cell death was first postulated for adult neurogenesis by Sturrock (1979).

The rate of neurogenesis in the mouse dentate gyrus is different in various strains of mice (Yanai, 1979; Wimer et al., 1976, 1978, 1980, 1988; Wimer and Wimer 1982; Symons et al. 1988; Barkats et al. 1996; Kempermann et al., 1997) and rat (Perfilieva et al. 2001). The rate of divisions in the dentate gyrus is also sensitive to many epigenetic factors. Stress and the increased level of adrenal steroids inhibit the rate of proliferation in the dentate gyrus (Gould et al., 1997, 1998, see however Sousa et al. 1998). Interestingly, reactivity to novelty is correlated with a diminished rate of proliferation in the dentate gyrus (Lemaire et al., 1999). On the other hand, absence of the adrenal steroids results in necrosis of the dentate gyrus (Maehlen and Torvik, 1990) and chronic injections of cortisol without evoking stress did not change the number of hippocampal neurons in the monkey (Leverenz et al., 1999).

Neurogenesis in the dentate gyrus also depends on the level of male and female hormones (Madeira et al., 1988; Tanapat et al., 1999). This sexual dimorphism was abolished in the hypothyroid rats (Madeira et al., 1988). Dietary restrictions increased the number of newly generated neurons in the dentate gyrus. The rate of survival of those neurons also depends on various factors. Performing a hippocampus-dependent learning tasks (Gould et al., 1999a) and the complexity of environment (Kempermann et al., 1997, 1998) decrease the proportion of neurons that die shortly after generation, while stress increases the rate of cell death (Lucassen, 2001).

In some mammals, seasonal differences in the rate of hippocampal proliferation were found. In the golden hamster (Huang et al., 1998) there is an autumnal increase, and in the meadow vole the non-breeding females had higher rates of proliferation in the hippocampus than the breeding ones and males (Galea and McEwen, 1999). Voles transferred from the short to long photoperiod show a non-significant 7.8% change in total brain DNA content (Dark et al., 1990). Such modulation may play an important role in the ecology of those species, as it is the case with various species of birds (Kirn and Nottebohm, 1993; Barnea and Nottebohm, 1994; Clayton, 1998; Scharff, 2000). However, the rate of hippocampal proliferations did not change in the grey squirrels that seasonally cache food (Lavenex et al., 2000a,b). Therefore, influence of seasonal factors on the rate of neurogeneration in the dentate gyrus of adult mammals may be species-specific.

Those newly generated neurons may be important for functioning of the dentate gyrus. It was postulated, that neurogeneration in the dentate gyrus is necessary for acquisition of the hippocampal-dependent memory (Gould et al., 1999c; Shors et al., 2001). However, the rate of neurogeneration, though high in early life, decreases markedly in the adult mice, that are still learning the hippocampus-dependent tasks (Kempermann et al., 1997, 1998). The same was found in the rat, where the rate of generation in the 12th month of life is markedly reduced in comparison to the 6th month (Kuhn et al., 1996). Our research on two insectivoran species of *Sorex* shrews

(Bialoskorska et al., 2001) showed high frequency of proliferations in the dentate gyrus of young, newly weaned animals, but the rate of proliferation drastically decreased in the autumn and winter, to stop almost completely in the spring, when these shrews are attaining sexual maturity. For the rest of their life, (about 6 months) proliferations in the dentate gyrus were barely detectable or absent. As the life-long pattern of neurogeneration in the dentate gyrus is species-dependent, its function still needs to be fully explained.

Subventricular zone of the lateral ventricles and olfactory bulbs

Proliferation in the subventricular zone originally drew little attention, but at present it is investigated intensively. Early papers of Altman (1963) and Bayer (1983) carefully documented its existence and extent in the rat and cat. Neurogenesis in the subventricular zone of lateral ventricles was described in the adult humans (Eriksson et al., 1998; Kukekov et al., 1999). Many cells in that zone of human brain show the characteristics of young, migrating neuroblasts (Bernier et al., 2000; Weickert et al., 2000). Proliferation in the subventricular zone and newly born neurons differentiating in the olfactory bulb were also observed in the macaque and cynomolgus monkeys (Lewis, 1968; Kaplan, 1983; McDermott and Lantos, 1991; Gould et al., 1999b; Kornack and Rakic, 2001; Pencea et al., 2001) and in the new-world monkey (McDermott and Lantos, 1990). In the dog, Blakemore and Jolly (1972) found neurons of the olfactory bulb that incorporated ^{3}H-thymidine. Several papers investigated this pool of proliferating cells in the adult mice (Luskin, 1994; Lois and Alvarez-Buylla, 1994; Lois et al., 1996; Doetsch et al., 1997; Goldman and Luskin, 1998; Temple and Alvarez-Buylla, 1999; Chazal et al., 2000), rat (Betarbet et al., 1996) and vole (Smith et al., 2001). Bialoskorska et al. (2001) investigated proliferation of cells in the brains of shrews (Insectivora) and found, that two days after injection of BrdU labeled nuclei were found in the periventricular zone of lateral ventricles and the rostral migration stream, while 14 days after injections they were located in the olfactory bulb.

These newly created neurons differentiate into granular and periglomerular neurons of the olfactory bulb (Corotto et al., 1993; Luskin, 1994; Lois and Alvarez-Buylla, 1994; Doetsch and Alvarez-Buylla, 1996;

Kato et al., 2000; Kornack and Rakic, 2001). They are predominantly GABA-ergic (Betarbet et al., 1996; Gheusi et al., 2000), but also dopaminergic (Betarbet et al., 1996) and many of them are calretinin-immunoreactive (Kato et al., 2001). In all investigated mammalian species proliferations around the lateral ventricles were more vigorous than in the dentate gyrus and seemed to continue throughout life, although decreasing with age (Pencea et al., 2001a). As the size of the olfactory bulb does not change in adults, a precise balance appears to exist between incorporation of new neurons and cell death. Investigations of Kato et al. (2000, 2001) showed that in the rat this pool of interneurons is rapidly exchanged: about 70% of them are replaced in the period of 6 weeks. Accordingly, in the NCAM-deficient mice, where migration of neuroblasts to the olfactory bulb is impaired, the granule and periglomerular layers are 40% thinner than in the control mice (Gheusi et al., 2000). These mice show impaired discrimination between odors, but unaltered thresholds of odor perception and short-term memory of odors. Proliferations in the subventricular zone and rostral migrations of the new neurons continued even after removal of the olfactory bulb (Kirschenbaum et al., 1999). In female voles, the rate of proliferation increased during estrus (Smith et al., 2001), and unilateral odor deprivation resulted in unilaterally decreased rate of generation in the periventricular zone and decreased survival of the new granule cells in the olfactory bulb (Corotto et al., 1994). This unexpected result indicates feedback signaling, through which the level of activity of the peripheral receptors influences the rate of cell generation in the subventricular zone. Mason et al. (2001) investigated *in vitro* mechanisms regulating migration of neuroblasts in that zone.

Other structures of the CNS

Gould et al. (1999b) found that new neurons may be added to some areas of the association, but not the sensory cortex of the adult monkey. The precursor cells appeared to come from cells dividing in the subventricular zone of lateral ventricles that usually generate new interneurons of the olfactory bulb. Rietze et al. (2000) found that in the mouse new neurons are generated and incorporated not only in the dentate gyrus, but also in other hippocampal areas, although at a much slower rate. Farel and McIlwain (2000) reviewed evidence for continuing neurogenesis in the spinal cord of juvenile mammals, and concluded that the majority of newly generated cells were glia (Horner et al., 2000). Nevertheless, stem cells seem to be present in the spinal cord (Weiss et al. 1996).

Proliferative potential of the mammalian CNS and its significance.

Discovery of the adult neurogenesis was a great achievement of neurobiology. It had a great impact on our thinking about brain and aging (O'Leary, 1993; van der Kooy and Weiss, 2000). However, a very old dogma of the exclusively foetal neurogenesis had to die in order to accept this knowledge (Gross, 2000). Clearly, the very limited neurogenesis in adult mammals is not typical, and is an exception in the animal world of both invertebrates and vertebrates (for review see Hastings et al., 2000). From the evolutionary point of view, reptiles' olfactory bulb and their equivalent of the dentate gyrus already are showing vigorous proliferations, and some new neurons are added to a variety of other structures (Perez-Canelas and Garcia-Verdugo, 1996; Perez-Canelas et al., 1997). However, such proliferations can be activated in various parts of the mammalian brain, including cortex, after e.g. ischemic damage to the nervous system (Liu et al., 2000; Magavi et al., 2000; Jin et al., 2001; Kee et al., 2001; Zhang et al., 2001). It is possible, that the neural stem cells in the subventricular zone of mammals (Gage, 2000) are activated by some factors released by the trauma or during healing. These stem cells may generate both neurons and glia (Nait-Oumesmar et al., 1999, Dutton and Bartlett, 2000; Kuhn et al., 2001; Pencea et al., 2001b). Alternatively, those new neurons may be produced either in the subventricular zone, or locally from those astrocytes that are derived from the transformed radial glia (Alvarez-Buylla and Lois, 1995; Doetsch et al., 1999; Noctor et al., 2001).

In conclusion, it is now firmly established that in mammals new granular neurons are being constantly incorporated into two brain structures, the dentate gyrus and olfactory bulb, while older neurons in these structures are in the same time removed. Although several external factors may change the balance of those two processes, in most cases they were found to be at equilibrium, and therefore neuronal populations in those two structures seemed to be numericaly constant,

although some investigations of the dentate gyrus suggested an age-dependent increasing trend. Existence of such dynamic equilibria in the mammalian brain has not been ever predicted or suggested until recently. This fact raises interesting questions about the purpose of the exchange in those two areas and about mechanisms of such precise regulation of neuronal numbers.

Do neurons in the CNS of adult mammals die out during normal progress of aging?

History of the claim

The nineteenth century pathologists noted that the weight of human brain slightly decreases with age (Broca, 1878). This was attributed to a reduction of the volume of gray matter. Reduction of the white matter was not taken into account, though, as we now know it accounts for a substantial part of the loss (Corselis, 1976; Peters et al., 2000). The acceptance of the neuronal theory prompted the question how many neurons are there in the brain. In 1894 Hodge published the first paper with an estimate of changes in the number of neurons with age. He reported his observations on the density of neurons in sections of brains of men and honeybees of various ages. Hodge found lower nuclear volume and lower density of neurons in old individuals of both species. He calculated that the number of neurons in the ganglia of old honeybees is reduced almost three times in comparison to the young ones. This decrease of the number of neurons supposedly explained the reduction of the volume of grey matter. Hodge concluded that during normal, healthy progress of life of all animals, including human, neurons are gradually dying out, until their numbers are too low to support functioning of the organism, and this is the main cause of the age-dependent functional deterioration.

The first estimate of the total number of neurons in a mammalian central nervous structure was published by Donaldson (1895), who used data collected by Meynert and calculated that there is 1.2 billion of neurons in the human neocortex. However, a much higher number of the human neocortical neurons (9.3 billion) was published shortly after by Thompson (1899), who used Hammarberg's data, and in 1925 von Economo and Koskinas published an even higher number (14.0 billions). These numerical discrepancies precluded investigations of the gradual changes of numbers of neocortical neurons.

44

Aghdur (1941) made corrections for double-counting of neurons and estimated that the number of neurons in human neocortex is 5.0 billions. Shariff (1953) using the Abercrombie's correction (1946) published a similar estimate: 6.9 billions. For the next thirty years the numbers of 5–7 billions neocortical neurons and about 10–12 billions of neurons in the whole human brain were generally accepted as satisfying approximations (Kappers et al., 1936–1965; Noback, 1967). These numbers had to be revised when new, unbiased techniques of counting (Sterio, 1984; Gundersen et al., 1988) were introduced. In 1985 Haug et al., applied the technique of disector and found that cortical neurons are twice more numerous (13.9 billions). Then Pakkenberg found the number of neocortical neurons should be almost doubled again, closer to 25 billions (from 22.8—Pakkenberg and Gundersen, 1997 to 27.4—Pakkenberg et al., 1989). Revisions of the total number of neurons in the human brain were even more substantial. It is now estimated that it contains 150–200 billions of neurons, and its largest population is that of the cerebellar granule cells, that alone count about 100 billions (Andersen et al., 1992). Earlier estimates for granule and Purkinje cells were two orders of magnitude lower (Harvey and Napper, 1988). This was the greatest revision resulting from the new stereological methods.

The first evidence of the age-related decrease of the absolute numbers of mammalian neurons (Ellis, 1919, 1920) concluded that about 25% of Purkinje neurons in the human cerebellum die out in the course of life. Corbin and Gardner (1937) and Gardner (1940) reported similar decreases of the number of neurons in sensory ganglia of middle-aged humans. Then Kuhlenbeck (1944) reported an age-related loss of neurons in the neocortical layers 2/3 of very old rats and Riese (1946) found the same in old humans. Brody (1955, 1970) established a substantial reduction of the number of neurons in the normal progress of life in the human cerebral cortex. He found that reduction of the numbers of cortical neurons between 18 and 95 years varies from 50% in the superior temporal cortex, to none in the inferior temporal. The overall reduction was estimated to be in the range of 30%. Other authors confirmed an age-related loss of neurons in the CNS of various mammalian species (Colon, 1971, 1972; Brizzee, 1973; Ordy et al., 1978; Brizzee and Ordy, 1979; Brizzee et al., 1980; Henderson et al., 1980).

The first experimental paper reporting no age-related decrease of neuronal numbers in the CNS was published by Inukai (1928), who found stable numbers of cerebellar Purkinje cells in the rat. Similarly, Delorenzi (1931) did not find any decrease of the numbers of Purkinje cells in humans. Their findings were in clear opposition to those of Ellis (1919, 1920), who investigated density of the same neuronal population. Investigations of the number of neurons in the peripheral ganglia, though technically much simpler, also brought variable results: Maleci (1934), Corbin and Gardner (1937) and Gardner (1940) found an age-related decrease of the number of neurons in the human sensory ganglia, while Van Buskirk (1945) found a stable population of those neurons. Brizzee et al. (1968) reported stable density of neocortical neurons in the rat. Brody himself (Monagle and Brody, 1974) found no change in the inferior olive and Cragg (1975) none in the frontal and temporal cortex of humans. Konigsmark and Murphy (1970) put in doubt the very idea of the age-related cell loss, when they critically analyzed Brody's data and found that his evidence of the neuronal loss was inconclusive. Hanley (1974) after an extensive review concluded that there is no good evidence for the process of progressive loss of neurons. Later, Brody noted differences in the rate of neuronal loss dependent on the species, area and time (Brody, 1980). In the later review, Flood and Coleman (1988) summarized that comparative data are still scarce and conflicting. In spite of this, the still prevailing layman belief is that "*while getting old we are losing our neurons and that's the main problem with aging*".

Olfactory bulb

Hinds and McNelly (1977) found that numbers of mitral cells in rats' olfactory bulbs were stable until the age of 24 months and then sharply decreased in the next three months. Interneurons of the granule and periglomerular layers of the olfactory bulb are constantly added to this structure throughout life (see above). However, numbers of those neurons do not seem to increase throughout life, as they are being constantly replaced.

Retina

The numbers of human retinal ganglion cells decrease with age (Gao and Hollyfield, 1992; Curcio and Drucker, 1993; Harman et al., 2000). Counts of the numbers of fibers in the optic nerves gave the same results

(Dolman et al., 1980; Balazsi et al., 1984; Johnson et al., 1987; Mikelberg et al., 1989; Jonas et al., 1990; see however Repka and Quigley, 1989, who found no change). Up to 25% of the human ganglion cells could have been lost throughout life, but the individual variance of neuronal numbers was high (Curcio and Drucker, 1993). There was no age-related decrease of the population of human foveal cones, while the numbers of parafoveal rods decreased by 30% over adulthood (Curcio, 2001). Kim et al. (1996) did not observe any decrease of the total number of ganglion cells in the retinas of old rhesus monkeys, in agreement with the counts of axons in their optic nerves (Morrison et al., 1990). Contrary to that, Sandell and Peters (2001) found that the numbers of fibers in the optic nerves of old monkeys were reduced by over 40%. Numbers of both retinal ganglion cells (Katz and Robinson, 1986) and optic nerve fibers (Weisse, 1995) were reduced in the aging rats. Age did not influence the numbers of ganglion cells in mice (Williams et al., 1996), and neither in the quokka wallaby (Fleming et al., 1996; Harman and Moore, 1999). In mice there were substantial strain differences in the average number of ganglion cells (from 32 to 87 thousands).

Neocortex

Neocortical neurons are the second largest population of neurons in the human brain. At present their number is estimated to be from 10 to 20 billions (Haug, 1985), or 19.3 billions in females and 22.8 billions in males, but varying from less than 15 billions to more than 30 billions, and therefore differing by the factor of two in the healthy adults individuals (Braendegaard et al., 1990; Pakkenberg and Gundersen, 1997). Numbers of neurons in area 17 of various species were compared by Colonnier and O'Kusky (1981).

The age-related loss of cortical neurons in primates was discussed by Peters (1993) and Peters et al. (1996, 1998). Many earlier studies of the numbers of neurons in various human neocortical areas indicated that this structure loses substantial or moderate numbers of those neurons with age (Brody, 1955, 1970; Shefer, 1973; Devaney and Johnson, 1980; Henderson et al., 1980; Anderson et al., 1983). However, results of other authors working with similar methods (Cragg, 1975; Curcio and Coleman, 1982; Haug, 1985, 1987; Terry et al., 1987; Leuba and Kraftsik, 1994a,b) questioned that

conclusion, as they did not find any age-related change of the number of cortical neurons. The majority of authors using stereological methods of estimation of the number of neurons found no change. Gomez-Isla et al. (1997) did not observe any decrease in the association cortex of the superior temporal sulcus. Many studies focused on those human neocortical areas that are most damaged by the Alzheimer disease: the entorhinal (Heinsen et al., 1994; Gomez-Isla et al., 1996; Gazzaley et al., 1997; West and Slomianka, 1998; Merrill et al., 2000; Price et al., 2001) and frontal cortex (Peters et al., 1994). All those authors used stereological methods and found stable numbers of neurons in healthy individuals. The only exceptions were Pakkenberg and Gundersen (1997) who found a 10% life-long decrease of the number of neocortical neurons in healthy old people and Heinsen et al. (1994), who found a continuous age-dependent decrease of neuronal numbers in the entorhinal cortex. A postulate of postnatal increase of the number of cortical neurons was published by Shankle, who analyzed data of J.L. Conel consisting of four millions measurements. Shankle concluded, that the number of neurons in the human neocortex increases postnatally, so at the age of six years this number is twice that at birth (Shankle et al., 1998a,b; Landing et al., 1998; Shankle et al., 1999). These estimations were criticized by Korr and Schmitz (1999).

In the macaque monkey, investigators using non-stereological methods showed an age-related decrease of neuronal numbers in the prefrontal cortex (Brizzee et al., 1980; Coleman and Flood, 1987), but an investigation using stereological methods showed no loss of neurons in area 46 (Peters et al., 1994). Data for somatosensory cortex are also contradictory, as Brizzee (1973) found a decrease of the number of neurons with age, while Tigges et al. (1990) observed no age-associated loss of neurons in that area. O'Kusky and Colonnier (1982) and Vincent et al. (1989) found no overall reduction of the number of neurons in the monkey's area 17. Investigators using unbiased stereological procedures confirmed this result (Kim et al., 1997; Peters et al., 1997; Nielsen and Peters, 2000). Neither was there any loss of the specialized neurons of area 17: the Meynert and layer IVB cells (Peters and Sethares, 1993; Hof et al., 2000). The entorhinal cortex of monkey did not show any loss of its layer II neurons either (Gazzaley et al., 1997).

In the rat, numerically stable populations of cortical neurons were reported by Brizzee (1973) and Peng and

Lee (1979) and area 17 did not show any neuronal decrease (Peters et al., 1983). The same was true in the frontal lobe of aging rats (Peinado et al. 1993). Mulders et al. (1997) calculated absolute numbers of neurons in the adult rat's presubiculum, parasubiculum and the entorhinal cortex. In the mouse, numbers of neurons in the barrel cortex, a part of the primary somatosensory area, were stable from the 4th till 33rd months of life (Curcio and Coleman, 1982). This result is especially reliable because of clear demarcation of the anatomical borders of that structure. Heuman and Leuba (1983) estimated numbers of neocortical neurons across the whole life span of the mouse (up to 720 days) and found a decrease in the layers II–IV of the aged animals. They also found a massive decrease of the numbers of cortical neurons during early postnatal development.

Hippocampus

West and Gundersen (1990) found 60 million neurons in human hippocampus and a significant age-dependent decrease only in the area CA1. Similar results were reported by Simic et al. (1997). However, in his next paper West (1993) found that the age-related loss was visible only in the subiculum (52%) and hilus of the dentate gyrus, and in the following paper (West et al., 1994) reported no loss in the area CA1 during normal aging. Other investigators (Peters et al., 1996) found no age-related changes in the hippocampus. Harding et al. (1998) recently reported that the number of neurons in the human area CA1 is more closely correlated with the volume of cerebrum than with age. The age-related reduction of hippocampal neurons is at best small. Taking into account the very substantial and easily detectable neuronal loss in the area CA1 due to the Alzheimer disease, the age-related loss is probably functionally insignificant. None of the investigators reported an age-related increase of the number of neurons in the dentate gyrus, and as new granular cells are generated there (Eriksson et al., 1998), there must be a constant turnover of those neurons.

In the monkey, an earlier investigation by Brizzee et al. (1980) showed a decrease of the number of neurons in the area CA1 of aging monkeys. However, two recent reports using stereological estimates did not confirm this (Rosene, 1993; Amaral, 1993).

In the rat, Brizzee and Ordy (1979) and Landfield et al. (1981) showed a substantial loss of hippocampal neurons

in the process of aging. Counts of the numbers of hippocampal neurons in the Wistar and Sprague-Dawley rats (Boss et al., 1985, 1987) showed substantial strain differences, with Wistars having on average 25–35% neurons less in all hippocampal areas. In the Sprague-Dawley rats numbers of neurons in the areas CA1 and CA3 (420 and 330 thousands respectively) was not significantly changed from the second postnatal day till adulthood (Boss et al., 1987). The number of neurons in the dentate gyrus in Sprague-Dawleys was constant from the first till the 12th month of life (about one million – Boss et al., 1987) while in Wistars it increased from 0.7 in the first to 1.0 million in the 4th month, and then it decreased again to 0.8 millions in the 12th month (Boss et al., 1985). Two authors investigating numbers of hippocampal neurons in the Wistar rats with stereological methods (Rasmussen et al., 1996; Rapp and Gallagher, 1996) concluded that in the old rats there was no loss of neurons in any of the hippocampal fields. Even the behaviorally impaired old animals had normal numbers of neurons in all hippocampal areas (Rasmussen et al., 1996). Kadar et al. (1994) studied different strains of rats and concluded that loss of neurons from the area CA3 showed the best correlation with the impairment of memory.

Research conducted on mice gave parallel results. Absolute numbers of neurons in the murine hippocampus are highly dependent on the strain (Wimer et al., 1976, 1978, 1980; Wimer and Wimer, 1982; Abusaad et al., 1999). Various inbred strains of mice could have as little as 230 thousands or as much as 430 thousands granular neurons in the dentate gyrus, with 86% of the variability determined by the genetic component and 11% by environmental factors (Abusaad et al., 1999). In mice there was no age-dependent loss of hippocampal neurons (Calhoun et al., 1998; Jucker et al., 2000). Even in the aged beta-amyloid precursor protein-null mice with impaired spatial learning there was no decrease of the number of hippocampal and basal cholinergic neurons (Phinney et al., 1999).

Basal ganglia

Oorschot (1996) studied the rat and found 2.79 millions of neostriatal neurons, 49.2 thousands of other neurons of the globus pallidus, 13.6 thousands in the subthalamic nucleus, 7.2 in the substantia nigra pars compacta and 26.3 thousands in substantia nigra pars reticularis.

Changes in the substantia nigra pars compacta indicate a reduction of dopaminergic cells, which is the most significant pathological finding in the Parkinson's disease (Foix, 1921; Pakkenberg and Brody, 1965; Fearnley and Lees, 1990; Pakkenberg et al., 1991). In humans population of the pigmented neurons of substantia nigra pars compacta are reduced during normal aging: almost 1% per year (Ma et al., 1999b), and the number of neurons expressing the dopamine transporter decreased at a comparative rate (Ma et al., 1999a). This is one of the greatest "natural" reductions indicating that this neuronal population of the human brain is vulnerable to degeneration.

There seems to be no overall age-related reduction of the volume of substantia nigra in the rhesus monkey (Siddiqui and Peters, 1999; Matochik et al., 2000) and the total number of nigral neurons in this species (Pakkenberg et al., 1995; Peters et al., 1996). However, the number of neurons immunoreactive for tyrosine hydroxylase (presumably dopaminergic) decreased dramatically—by 50% over the monkey's life span (i.e. for about 2% per year). The degree of reduction of this neuronal population correlated with the extent of motor impairment of the animals (Emborg et al., 1998). In the rat and mouse, there was no age-related loss of the nigrostriatal dopaminergic neurons (Emerich et al. 1993; McNeil and Koek, 1990).

There is less consensus on the age-related reduction of the number of cholinergic neurons in the basal forebrain, even though this is a postulated mechanism of mental deterioration in old age. In the human nucleus basalis of Meynert (NBM), there are reports of no correlation of age with the number of cholinergic neurons (Chui et al., 1984; Mesulam et al., 1987), or a modest reduction (up to 25%, starting after the 60th years of life—Bigl et al., 1987; 23% at the age of 90, in comparison to newborns—Lowes-Hummel et al., 1989). Others reported severe loss (about 50%, heavier in the rostral part of the nucleus, between the 30th and 90th years of life—de Lacalle et al., 1991 or significant decrease of the neuronal numbers and gliosis—Szenborn, 1993).

Stroessner-Johnson et al. (1992) found no change in the numbers of cholinergic septal neurons and a 19.3% age-related reduction in the rhesus monkeys' NBM. The neuronal loss was different than that seen in humans: the most substantial reduction (41%) was found in the caudal part of this nuclear complex, while its rostral part was normal. Voytko et al. (1995) found age-related neuronal loss only in the middle part of monkeys' NBM, and the extent of this depletion correlated with the degree of deterioration of spatial memory. The stereological study of Smith et al. (1999) showed that the number of neurons in the intermediate part of area Ch4 of the rhesus monkey did not differ in the adult and aged groups (60 vs 57 thousands). However, in the aged monkeys the number of cholinergic neurons was reduced by 43%. Treatment of the old monkeys with NGF increased the number of the labeled neurons to the adult level. Therefore, in this structure aging resulted in neuronal atrophy and functional loss, but not the cell death.

Neurons were evenly reduced (average 26%) in all cholinergic structures of the aged Wistar rats (Altavista et al., 1990). Similar (30%) reduction of neurons stained with cholinergic markers in the rat's NBM was observed by Smith and Booze (1995) and an even greater reduction (40%) was found in the rats showing impairment of spatial memory (Martinez-Serrano et al., 1995). However, in these studies cells were not counted on the Nissl stained sections, and therefore discrimination between atrophy (loss of label) and cell death was not possible. In the murine NBM numbers of those neurons did not seem to decrease with age (Hornberger et al., 1985; Phinney et al., 1999; Jucker et al., 2000). The DBA/2 strain has 20–32% more cholinergic neurons (depending on the nucleus) than the C57B strain. McNeil and Koek (1990) found that in the latter strain numbers of cholinergic neurons in the striatum significantly decreased with age. Largest loss (up to 38%) was found in the rostral part of the nucleus. There was also a decrease in the number of striatal nitric oxide synthase-immunoreactive neurons in the rat (Cha et al., 2000). Two reviews of the question of natural age-related loss of cholinergic neurons (Decker, 1987; Wenk and Willard, 1998) differ in their conclusions.

Navarro and Gonzalo (1991) found a substantial loss of neurons (36–47%, depending on nucleus) in the amygdala of aged humans. There was no change in the numbers of small neurons of human putamen (Pesce and Reale, 1987) and in the whole population of neostriatal neurons in aged rats (Zoli et al., 1993) and mice (Sturrock, 1986). In two other papers Sturrock (1991c, 1993) reported that there was no age-related neuronal loss in the murine posterolateral nucleus of stria terminalis, while reductions in the posteromedial nucleus of stria terminalis and bed nucleus of the anterior commissure were significant.

48

Diencephalon

There was no significant age-related loss of neurons in the lateral geniculate nucleus of monkey (Ahmad and Spear, 1993). These authors estimated that there is about 1,267 thousands of neurons in the parvicellular and 148 thousands in the magnocellular layers of monkey LGNd, with a 1.9-fold difference in those numbers among different brains. Satorre et al. (1985) showed stable numbers of the LGNd neurons in the aged rats. However, Diaz et al. (1999) found that in the rat's LGNd numbers of neurons decreased with age. In the rat's, thalamic reticular nucleus, density of neurons decreased between the 3rd and 24th month and then it increased between the 24th and 30th month (Ramos et al., 1995). In the mice, stable numbers of neurons were observed in the anterodorsal thalamic nucleus during their adult age and senility (Sturrock, 1989c).

Most counts of neurons in hypothalamic nuclei show no age-related change in neuronal numbers. In the human mammillary nucleus there were 32 thousands of neurons in young humans and these numbers did not significantly change throughout life (Begega et al., 1999). There were about 520 thousands neurons in the infundibular nucleus of both young and old women (Abel and Rance, 2000). In the rat hypothalamus, stable numbers were found (Peng and Hsu, 1982; Sartin and Lamperti, 1985; Flood and Coleman, 1993; Madeira et al., 1995; Leal et al., 1998). The only reported age-related decrease was found in three hypothalamic nuclei (out of seven investigated) of the female rats (Hsu and Peng, 1978). No age-related changes of the neuronal numbers were observed in three hypothalamic nuclei of the mouse (Sturrock, 1989c, 1991a).

Cerebellum

Andersen et al. (1992) estimated the number of cerebellar granule cells in the adult humans with stereological methods and found, that it may be in the range of 100 billions, while there is only about 30 millions of Purkinje cells. By comparison, there is about 2.2 billions of granule cells and 1.2–1.3 millions of Purkinje cells in the cat's cerebellum (Palkovits et al., 1971a,b). In the cerebellum of the adult rat there is 265 millions of granule cells (Korbo et al., 1993). There are still big differences in the estimates of the number of the Purkinje

cells. Their absolute numbers were given as being in the range of 610 thousands (Korbo et al., 1993), 230 thousands (Dlugos and Pentney, 1994) or 410 thousands (Larsen et al., 2000) in the normal, adult rats. It is possible that strain differences may be at least partially responsible for those discrepancies.

There are no reports of the age-related changes in the numbers of cerebellar granule neurons in humans. Population of the granule cells was unchanged in 20 year-old monkeys (Nandy, 1981). Druge et al. (1986), Quackenbush et al. (1990), Dlugos and Pentney (1994) found no change in the numbers of the cerebellar granular cells in the aging rats. Sturrock (1989d) reported the same in the mouse.

The age-related decline of the number of Purkinje neurons in humans is still controversial. Hall et al. (1975) found a 25% decrease of their numbers over a lifetime, and Torvik et al. (1986) confirmed a decrease. However, Torvik's data showed that individual variations in the absolute numbers of Purkinje cells were large, and that half of the people over 80 years had Purkinje cell densities similar to those of 60-year-old people. Investigators who used stereological methods (Nairin et al., 1989; Mayhew et al., 1990; Andersen et al., 1992) showed half the numbers of the Purkinje cells in a group of elders (76–93 years) in comparison to young adults. Decrease of the numbers of Purkinje neurons was also reported by (Sjobeck et al., 1999). However, estimations done by Karhunen et al. (1994) did not show any age-related decrease in humans of the age range 35–69 years. In the 20-year-old cynomolgus monkey the number of Purkinje cells was reduced in comparison to a four-year-old individual (Nandy, 1981).

Decrease of the numbers of Purkinje cells in senescent rats is also questionable. While Rogers et al. (1984) found a significant 15% age-related reduction of the numbers of Purkinje cells, Bakalian et al. (1991) found a non-significant 10% reduction in the extremely old Wistar rats. No changes were reported by Druge et al. (1986), Quackenbush et al. (1990) and Dlugos and Pentney (1994). In a recent research on the Sprague-Dawley rats, Larsen et al. (2000) showed a small (11%, significant) decrease of the number of Purkinje cells between the 5th and 23rd months of life. Moreover, in the same experiments, aged rats that were physically exercised throughout their life did not show any decrease in the numbers of Purkinje cells (Larsen et al., 2000). Therefore both strain and epigenetic factors could have influenced results of various authors. Sturrock (1989d,e,f, 1990b,d) reported that in the mouse cerebellum numbers of the granule, Golgi II and pale neurons did not decline with age (between the 6th and 31st months), whereas there was a substantial (30%) loss of the Purkinje, stellate and basket cells. The decrease of the number of Purkinje cells occurred mainly between the 15th and 31st months (Sturrock, 1989f). This author found an even greater age-related loss of neurons in the cerebellar nuclei of the mouse (about 40%, Sturrock, 1989e).

Brainstem nuclei

Many studies of neuronal changes were done in the nucleus locus coeruleus. Earlier investigations showed a pronounced decrease of the number of neurons in the locus coeruleus of aged humans (Vijayashankar and Brody, 1979; Wree et al., 1980; Lohr and Jeste, 1988). However, Marcyniuk et al. (1989) found only a modest, diffuse cell loss in that nucleus of mentally normal old people. Two unbiased estimations of the numbers of neurons in that nucleus (Mouton et al., 1994, Ohm et al., 1997) did not show any decrease with age. There were marked individual differences: from 12 to 25 thousands of neurons unilaterally (Ohm et al., 1997). On the other hand, Manaye et al. (1995) found a similar absolute numbers of coerulean neurons in young people (average —21 thousands), and a large reduction (about 50%) throughout life. This loss was significantly greater in the rostral part of the nucleus, which projects to the forebrain. In the rat, Goldman and Coleman (1981) found no age-related changes. Sturrock and Rao (1985) showed a large reduction in the old mice. Young mice had on the average 1.5 thousands of neurons in this nucleus, with a large interindividual and within strain variance.

A significant reduction was found in the human vestibular nucleus (Lopez et al., 1997; Alvarez et al., 1998, 2000). In the rat, loss of neurons was found in the medial nucleus of trapezoid body, but not in the olivary nucleus (Casey, 1990). In the mouse, numbers of neurons decreased with age in the vestibular (Sturrock, 1989b) and dorsal, but not posteroventral cochlear nucleus (Idrizbegovic et al., 2001). Counts of neurons in the posteroventral cochlear nucleus of gerbils did not show any age-related decrease (Czibulka and Schwartz, 1991).

Our knowledge about age-related changes of neuronal numbers is scarce in other brainstem structures. Sjobeck et al. (1999) found that numbers of neurons in the human inferior olivary nucleus were non-significantly reduced with age. Manaye et al. (1999) found no change in the number of the cholinergic neurons in the human pedunculopontine and laterodorsal tegmental nuclei. Kloppel et al. (2001) found no difference in the percentage of neurons synthesizing serotonin in raphe nuclei between the young and old humans. However, Kemper et al. (1997) found decreases in serotonergic neurons and interneurons of the nucleus centralis superior in the old rhesus monkeys. Counts of myelinated axons in the human vagus nerve (Lu et al., 2001) showed no age-related changes in their numbers. In the mouse, there were no age-related changes in the red nucleus (Sturrock, 1990a), parabigeminal nucleus (Sturrock, 1989a) and motor nucleus of the trigeminal nerve (Sturrock, 1987), while in other brainstem structures such as the mesencephalic nucleus (Sturrock, 1987), tegmental nuclei of Gudden (Sturrock, 1991b) and pontine nuclei (Sturrock, 1990c) the numbers of neurons decrease with age.

Spinal cord and neurons of sensory ganglia

The numbers of human motoneurons decrease with age either in the cervical segments (Zhang et al., 1996; Yuan et al., 2000) or on the segment L4 (Terao et al., 1996), or in all segments of the spinal cord (Cruz-Sanchez et al., 1998). The small neurons of the intermediate zone were lost, while the medium-sized and large motoneurons were stable. In the rat, the number of motoneurons of the segments L4/L5 decreases with age (Jacob, 1998). In the peripheral cholinergic system, neuronal population of the human ciliary ganglion was stable till the age of 60 and then it was reduced by 20% until 90 years (Bigl et al., 1987).

The counts of primary sensory ganglia are widely divergent and estimates of the age-related changes inconsistent (for review, see Coleman and Flood, 1987). Counts of neurons performed on exactly the same material with various methods, resulted in large differences (Smolen et al., 1983, Popken and Farel, 1997). Recent attempts at estimation of the number of neurons in the rat's dorsal root ganglia with stereological methods showed a 19% increase of the numbers between the 11th and 80th postnatal days (Popken and Farel, 1997) and then a very modest (12%) decrease (Bergman and Ulfhake, 1998). This was consistent with an earlier estimation of a 14% loss (Keithley and Feldmann, 1979). These volume decreases do not explain the old-age-related perceptual loss. In agreement, stable numbers were also found between the 3rd and 24th month in the lumbosacral ganglions of the rat (Mohammed and Santer, 2001). Human spiral ganglia did not show an age-related loss of neurons (Hinojosa et al., 1985), while the vestibular ganglion showed a 19% reduction between the 30th and 60th years of life (Park et al., 2001).

What did we learn since the times of Cajal?

In the century that passed since the Cajal's neuronal theory, investigations of generation and death of neurons continued to be an important part of neurophysiology. An important advance in the pursuit of these questions has been methodological.

Progress in the technique of counting and comparing neuronal populations

An important part of the progress that has been made in the last century is the methods of counting neurons. First attempts were simple: the number of the nuclei or cell bodies was taken as the number of those elements in the thickness of section. It took half a century before the first corrections excluding counts of the nuclei with their centers placed outside of the thickness of sections were developed (Aghdur, 1941; Abercrombie, 1946). These corrections resulted in an underestimation of the number of objects. This was corrected by Coupland (1968), but the correction demanded a computer program to be executed (Banks et al., 1977). The new methods changed the accepted numbers of neurons in a given structure (see the chapter on neocortex). The problem of the bias in our assumptions about the shape and size of neurons and in the method of sampling of their populations was removed when new, stereological methods were introduced (Gundersen et al., 1988). Applying of these techniques resulted in dramatic revisions of the estimates of the total number of neurons, especially in the cerebellum and neocortex. The technique of disector that was introduced by Gundersen, is still the most reliable when the absolute numbers of neurons have to be counted. It was since then modified and new methods were

developed (for a recent review see West, 1999). The most troublesome problem remaining is the enormous heterogeneity of the nervous system, which was underestimated in the original stereological formulas. When comparing structures that differ in neuronal size between groups and where the changes of neuronal numbers are modest, a small methodological error may result in the error of count that would be twice as high as the real difference (Smolen et al., 1983).

Other permanent problems are independent of the method of counting yet equally troubling, especially for those who work with human brains. First of all, these are problems with collecting comparable groups of brains. Therefore, in many cases the numbers of brains in each group must be markedly increased. The problem of differential, age dependent shrinkage (Haug et al., 1984) is especially relevant when comparing brains of animals of different ages. Once discovered, this factor may be relatively easily eliminated.

Several methods of estimation of the total cell number that were alternative to the counting were tried. They are based either on estimation of the content of DNA in the investigated structure (Peng and Lee, 1979), or on the cell dispersion and hemacytometer counting (Devaney and Johnson, 1980, 1984). They both suffer from the problems of separating neurons and glia, but seem to be worth developing for specific purposes.

Changed views on the stability of neuronal populations

Cajal's ideas heavily influenced development of neuroscience. His neuronal theory has been accepted. He believed mammalian neurons are born during an early, prenatal phase of development and gradually die producing functional impairments, senility and death. Both these hypotheses concerning the life cycle of neurons were revised or rejected. At present, the scientific theory on the life-long dynamics of neuronal populations is very different from that a century ago. Neurons may be created not only during early development, but also in principle throughout life; the main period of cell death occurs during early development and not throughout life.

Probably the biggest impact on our thinking about neuronal populations was the acceptance, that under physiological conditions in the majority of brain structures neuronal populations are constant throughout life, even during aging. Some important exceptions are addressed below. The general conclusion that emerged after years of investigations has a great impact on our thinking about the ways of treatment of functional impairments in the old age. In general, it gives us hope for restoration of the brain functions in old age through pharmacological interventions that would revive impaired neurons and their function.

Contrary to the original idea, large-scale cell death in the CNS occurs mainly during early development. It is particularly active and robust shortly after cell divisions are completed (Thomaidou et al., 1997). This idea was ignored, as it did not fit the widely accepted paradigm, claiming that during development neurons proliferate and do not immediately die. However, current research emphasizes that apoptotic cell death plays an extremely important developmental role. Disruption of apoptotic pathways during early neurogenesis leads to either death of the fetus or severe malformations (Haydar et al., 1999). Overexpression of the *bcl2* gene, that inhibits developmental apoptosis, brings mice that have brains 1.5 larger than the wild ones (Martinou et al., 1994). Interestingly, visual system of those mice does not show any higher-than-normal acuity (Gianfranceschi et al., 1999). Therefore, there seems to be no functional advantage in reducing developmental cell death.

Adult neurogenesis had a relatively small impact on the answer to the question of stability of neuronal populations. It has changed our views on the physiology of two CNS structures: the dentate gyrus and olfactory bulb. Here a dynamic stability is based on a constant turnover of neurons. Such a dynamic system would be almost unthinkable a century ago. Recently it was postulated, that besides memory (Gould et al., 1999), adult neurogenesis might serve important psychological functions (Jacobs et al., 2000). However, the events in those two structures appear to be exceptions from the general rule. Adult neurogenesis in other structures of adult mammalian brain for the purpose of addition or replacement of neurons is either extremely rare or controversial.

Widespread pools of stem cells appear to exist in the adult mammalian brain (Weiss et al., 1996; Morshead et al., 1997; Johansson et al., 1999). The newly created neurons may migrate far away from the place of cell division and extend their axons within the tissue of the adult, organized brain (Lois and Alvarez-Buylla, 1994; Stanfield and Trice, 1988). This observation, if true, introduces new possibilities of treatment of degenerative diseases of the CNS. It may help explain the source of vigorous neurogenesis taking place in some structures after cerebral ischemia (Zhang et al., 2001). Unfortunately, this post-ischemic neurogenesis may not be sufficient for a satisfactory replacement of the lost neurons.

Neurons in some structures seem to decrease during presumably healthy ageing. The case is best documented for the substantia nigra and motoneurons. There are also some indications that the number of cerebellar Purkinje cells may decrease with age without any clear pathological influences. These three neuronal populations are involved in regulation and execution of movements, therefore impaired ability of movement execution in the old age may be especially difficult to compensate. A different strategy for replacement of motor loss is needed than for memory or mental impairments.

On the other hand, aging rats exercising throughout life did not loose their Purkinje cells (Larsen et al., 2000). "Normal" epigenetic factors may be deleterious not only for functioning, but also for the integrity of the nervous system. These epigenetic factors can act prenatally (Jonson et al., 1976) or in neonates (Ibanez, 1998), targeting the vulnerable neuronal populations (Brody 1980). Aside from the three populations named above, increased vulnerability occurs in the basal forebrain cholinergic system and entorhinal cortex. Hippocampal area CA1 is especially vulnerable to hypoxia (Liu et al., 2000). Neurons in the cerebral cortex seem to be selectively susceptible to DNA damage (Mandavilli and Rao, 1996). Accidental deleterious events may cause great interindividual differences in impairment of adult and senile groups (Kadar et al., 1994). This selective vulnerability of neuronal populations to various avoidable epigenetic factors and its causes should be investigated further (Azmitia, this volume and Sapolsky, 1987, 1991).

However, the genetic factor has a great influence on the fate of neurons. Initial numbers of neurons and their rate of decrease during the process of aging heavily depend on the investigated species (Flood and Coleman, 1988; Austad, 1997), strain (Wimer and Wimer, 1982; Ingram and Jucker, 1999, Shimada, 1999) and individual (Collier and Coleman, 1991; Rapp et al., 1996). For example, analysis of variance of neuronal numbers in the dentate gyrus of two strains of mice and their hybrids (Wimer and Wimer, 1982) showed, that an overwhelming part of the variance could be attributed to the genetic factors. This may also explain big (frequently twofold) differences in the total numbers of neurons among adult individuals of the same species. The staggerer mutation in mice results in reduction of the Purkinje cells by 25% between the age of 15 and 24 months, while in the younger mice their numbers were stable (Doulazmi et al., 1999; Vogel et al., 2000). Therefore, genetic factors may interact with the process of aging.

Is neuronal loss correlated with impairment of function?

Parkinson's disease is an exemplary case. Correlation between the loss of dopaminergic neurons of the substantia nigra pars compacta and the impairment of function is very high (Pakkenberg et al., 1991). However, this population of neurons seems to be vulnerable to various factors and to decrease during normal aging (Ma et al., 1999b).

In Alzheimer's disease, functional impairment is highly correlated with the depletion of neurons in human entorhinal cortex (Gomez-Isla et al., 1996; Morrison and Hof, 1997) and the area CA1 of the hippocampus (West et al., 1994, 2000). Similar depletion in the hippocampus may be the result of heavy alcoholism (Jensen and Pakkenberg, 1993) or hypoxia (Liu et al., 2000). The cerebellar Purkinje cells seem to be highly vulnerable to various deleterious factors, like the Parkinson's disease (Sjobeck and Englund, 2001) or alcoholism (Baker et al., 1999), while animal studies showed that the numbers of cerebellar granule cells did not decrease in the aged, ethanol fed rats (Tabbaa et al., 1999). In these structures, the numbers of neurons in healthy old people seem to be either stable, or their reduction is marginal. Neuronal loss in these areas is clearly a sign of a pathology and not the normal process of aging. The neuronal loss due to apoptosis in the cerebral cortex of Alzheimer's patients is low and compatible with the slow pace of this disease (Jellinger and Stadelmann, 2000).

Correlation between neuronal depletion and functional impairment is frequently absent (see above). Functional impairment may proceed without neuronal loss, or function may be preserved in spite of severe neuronal loss. Normal numbers of neurons were found in the mediodorsal thalamic nucleus of schizophrenics (Thune et al., 2001) or the forebrain of hydrocephalic rats (Tinsley et al., 2001). Neocortical neurons, particularly the large ones, are heavily destroyed in the progress of AIDS, while the patients are becoming progressively demented. Yet, there seems to be no correlation between the extent of functional and structural loss (Weis et al., 1993; Fischer et al., 1999). In Alzheimer's disease, correlation between symptoms of the disease and neuronal loss in human association cortex is poor, with profound depletion occurring long before the appearance of symptoms of functional deterioration (Gomez-Isla et al., 1997). On the other hand, the age-related neuronal loss in that cortex is minimal even when the functions of the cortex are impaired in old age (see above). Even in chronic alcoholics, some investigators found no loss of neocortical neurons or of the volume of neocortex (Jensen and Pakkenberg, 1993). Therefore, neocortex has a vast compensatory capacity that allows it to function with substantial losses. The functioning of neocortex may be impaired by factors other than neuronal death, like impairment of connectivity and destruction of myelin (Jensen and Pakkenberg, 1993; Peters, this Volume).

Finally, neuronal changes in adult life and aging suggest three causes of functional impairment in old age. First, age-related neuronal atrophy seems to be the major factor in functional deterioration of existing neurons (Long et al., 1999), this could possibly be slowed down, or even reversed by various pharmacological interventions (Azmitia and Whitaker-Azmitia, 1997). Second, neuronal degeneration during aging is pathology, and raises the question of its epidemiology (Jellinger and Stadelmann, 2000). Discovery of adult neurogenesis raised hopes for finding a way of restoration of the lost neuronal populations, possibly by manipulating the levels of neurotrophins (Pencea et al., 2001). Third, destruction of myelin and of the white matter seems to be more frequent and important than the limited neuronal death in normal aging. The age-related impairment of the myelin sheaths of neurons would cause serious difficulties in long-distance communication (Peters et al., 2000). Again, replacement of the lost oligodendrocytes is an idea worth investigating.

Ten questions

Although a century of research on the neuronal populations of the mammalian brain brought new information and some breakthroughs in our thinking, several old and new questions are still waiting to be answered:

(1) What are the molecular mechanisms of inter-species differences in the rate of aging? Why do neurons in

the 3-year-old rats show severe senile changes, while in the dogs of the same age the neurons are typical for a mature animal, and in the humans are still growing? Differences of size or metabolism of the species do not fully explain this problem.

(2) Which genetic and epigenetic factors influence inter-individual differences of neuronal numbers? At what stage of life do the numbers diverge? How significant are those differences?

(3) In humans, why do some structures performing very important and complex functions have modest numbers of neurons (like the entorhinal cortex and hippocampus), while others have enormous neuronal populations (like cerebellum)? The numbers of neurons in those structures in small mammals do not have this spread.

(4) What is "normal" for the old age? Is it possible to live a natural life span without loss of neurons? If not, then do individual genetic differences in neuronal vulnerability play a dominant role?

(5) Why are some neuronal populations more vulnerable than others? This particularly refers to human entorhinal area, which seems to succumb to various pathological processes much easier, than e.g. visual cortex. Answers to this question may differ for each neuronal population and species.

(6) What is the maximum percentage of neuronal loss that each of those populations might bear without showing detectable dysfunctions?

(7) Why should the potential for neuronal proliferation be so severely restricted in the CNS of adult mammals (and birds) in comparison to lower vertebrates, including reptiles? What are the mechanisms of this restriction?

(8) Why do neuronal proliferations in mammalian dentate gyrus and the anterior part of subventricular zone occur and what is their function? Already in reptiles proliferation in these structures is higher than in others active in the adult animal. If they serve reworking of the spatial memory in the dentate gyrus, then what is the function of such exchange in the olfactory bulb?

(9) Why are the majority of new interneurons of the olfactory bulb produced in the proliferation zone placed outside of the olfactory bulb? Why was it necessary and advantageous to develop a special mechanism of tangential migration in that part of the subventricular zone?

(10) How is the dynamic balance between proliferation and cell death in the dentate gyrus and olfactory bulb achieved?

We have listed 10, but many more questions concerning the numbers and stability of neuronal populations are still worth answering. Most of these questions could not even have been asked in the time of Cajal, as he was unaware of many facts that have been discovered since then that have expanded our knowledge about neurons across the life cycle. Although much has changed, the more we know the more we continue to ask.

Acknowledgments

The authors express their thanks and gratitude to Dr Efrain C. Azmitia and Dr Charles E. Ribak for improving the manuscript of this review. Supported by the grant of the Polish State Committee for Scientific Research to the Nencki Institute for statutable research, and the Nencki Institute internal grant to Dr R. Djavadian.

References

Abel, T.W. and Rance, N.E. (2000) Stereologic study of the hypothalamic infundibular nucleus in young and older women. J. Comp. Neurol., 424: 679–688.

Abercrombie, M. (1946) Estimation of nuclear population from microtome sections. Anat. Rec., 94: 239–247.

Abusaad, I., MacKay, D., Zhao, J., Stanford, P., Collier, D.A. and Everall, I.P. (1999) Stereological estimation of the total number of neurons in the murine hippocampus using the optical disector. J. Comp. Neurol., 408: 560–566.

Agduhr, E. (1941) A contribution to the technique of determining the number of nerve cells per unit volume of tissue. Anat. Rec., 80: 191–202.

Ahmad, A. and Spear, P.D. (1993) Effects of aging on the size, density, and number of rhesus monkey lateral geniculate neurons. J. Comp. Neurol., 334: 631–643.

Allen, E. (1912) The cessation of mitosis in the central nervous system of the albino rat. J. Comp. Neurol., 19: 547–568.

Altavista, M.C., Rossi, P., Bentivoglio, A.R., Crociani, P. and Albanese, A. (1990) Aging is associated with a diffuse impairment of forebrain cholinergic neurons. Brain Res., 508: 51–59.

Altman, J. (1962) Are new neurons formed in the brains of adult mammals? Science, 135: 1127–1128.

Altman, J. (1963) Autoradiographic investigation of cell proliferation in the brains of rats and cats. Postnatal growth and differentiation of the mammalian brain, with implications for a morphological theory of memory. Anat. Rec., 145: 573–591.

Altman, J. (1966) Autoradiographic and histological studies of postnatal neurogenesis. II. A longitudinal investigation of the kinetics,

54

migration and transformation of cells incorporating tritiated thymidine in infant rats, with special reference to postnatal neurogenesis in some brain regions. *J. Comp. Neurol.*, 128: 431–474.

Altman, J. (1969) Autoradiographic and histological studies of postnatal neurogenesis. IV. Cell proliferation and migration in the anterior forebrain, with special reference to persisting neurogenesis in the olfactory bulb. *J. Comp. Neurol.*, 137: 433–458.

Altman, J. and Das, G.D. (1965) Autoradiographic and histological evidence of postnatal hippocampal neurogenesis in rats. *J. Comp. Neurol.*, 124: 319–335.

Altman, J. and Das, G.D. (1966) Autoradiographic and histological studies of postnatal neurogenesis. I. A longitudinal investigation of the kinetics, migration and transformation of cells incorporating tritiated thymidine in neonate rats, with special reference to postnatal neurogenesis in some brain regions. *J. Comp. Neurol.*, 126: 337–390.

Altman, J. and Das, G.D. (1967) Postnatal neurogenesis in the guinea-pig. *Nature*, 214: 1098–1101.

Alvarez, J.C., Diaz, C., Suarez, C., Fernandez, J.A., Gonzalez del Rey, C., Navarro, A. and Tolivia, J. (1998) Neuronal loss in human medial vestibular nucleus. *Anat. Rec.*, 251: 431–438.

Alvarez, J.C., Diaz, C., Suarez, C., Fernandez, J.A., Gonzalez del Rey, C., Navarro, A. and Tolivia, J. (2000) Aging and the human vestibular nuclei: morphometric analysis. *Mech. Ageing Dev.*, 114: 149–172.

Alvarez-Buylla A. and Lois, C. (1995) Neuronal stem cells in the brain of adult vertebrates. *Stem Cells*, 13: 263–272.

Amaral, D.G. (1993) Morphological analyses of the brains of behaviorally characterized aged nonhuman primates. *Neurobiol. Aging*, 14: 671–672.

Anderson, J.M., Hubbard, B.M., Coghill, G.R. and Slidders, W. (1983) Neuropsychological changes in healthy adults across the age range. *Neurobiol. Aging*, 14: 623–625.

Andersen, B.B., Korbo, L. and Pakkenberg, B. (1992) A quantitative study of the human cerebellum with unbiased stereological techniques. *J. Comp. Neurol.*, 326: 549–560.

Austad, S.N. (1997) Comparative aging and life histories in mammals. *Exp. Gerontol.*, 32: 23–38.

Azmitia, E.C. and Whitaker-Azmitia, P.M. (1997) Development and Neuroplasticity of Central Serotonergic Neurons. In: H.G. Baumgarten and M. Gothert (Eds.), *Handbook Of Experimental Pharmacology: Serotonergic Neurons and 5-HT Receptors in the CNS*. Chpt. 1, pp. 1–39.

Bakalian, A., Corman, B., Delhaye-Bouchaud, N. and Mariani, J. (1991) Quantitative analysis of the Purkinje cell population during extreme ageing in the cerebellum of the Wistar/Louvain rat. *Neurobiol Aging*, 12: 425–430.

Baker, K.G., Harding, A.J., Halliday, G.M., Kril, J.J. and Harper, C.G. (1999) Neuronal loss in functional zones of the cerebellum of chronic alcoholics with and without Wernicke's encephalopathy. *Neuroscience*, 91: 429–438.

Balazsi, A.G., Rootman, J., Drance, S.M., Schulzer, M. and Douglas, G.R. (1984) The effect of age on the nerve fiber population of the human optic nerve. *Am. J. Ophtalmol.*, 97: 760–766. Banks,

Banks, B.E.C., Hendry, I.A. and Khan, A.A. (1977) A program to compute the sizes and numbers of spherical bodies from observations made on tissue sections. *J. Neurocytol.*, 5: 231–239.

Barkats, M., Bertholet, J.Y. and Cohen-Salmon, C. (1996) age-related morphological changes in the hippocampus in two mouse strains. *Mech. Ageing Dev.*, 87: 155–164.

Barnea, A. and Nottebohm, F. (1994) seasonal recruitment of hippocampal neurons in adult free ranging black-capped chickadees. *Proc. Natl. Acad. Sci. USA*, 91: 11217–11221.

Bayer, S.A. (1982) Changes in the total number of dentate gyrus cells in juvenile and adult rats: a correlated volumetric and ^{3}H-thymidine autoradiographic study. *Exp. Brain Res.* 46: 315–323.

Bayer, S.A. (1983) 3H-thymidine-radioautographic studies of neurogenesis in the rat olfactory bulb. *Exp. Brain Res.*, 50: 329–340.

Bayer, S.A., Yackel, J.W. and Puri, P.S. (1982) Neurons in the rat dentate gyrus granular layer substantially increase during juvenile and adult life. *Science*, 216: 890–892.

Begega, A., Cuesta, M., Santin, L.J., Rubio, S., Astudillo, A. and Arias, J.L. (1999) Unbiased estimation of the total number of nervous cells and volume of medial mammillary nucleus in humans. *Exp. Gerontol.*, 34: 771–782.

Bergman, E. and Ulfhake, B. (1998) Loss of primary sensory neurons in the very old rat: neuron number estimates using the disector method and confocal optical sectioning. *J. Comp. Neurol.*, 396: 211–222.

Bernier P.J., Vinet, J., Cossette, M. and Parent, A. (2000) Characterization of the subventricular zone of the adult human brain: evidence for the involvement of Bcl-2. *Neurosci Res.*, 37: 67–78.

Betarbet, R., Zigova, T., Bakay, R.A. and Luskin, M.B. (1996) Dopaminergic and GABAergic interneurons of the olfactory bulb are derived from the neonatal subventricular zone. *Int. J. Dev. Neurosci.*, 14: 921–930.

Bialoskorska, K., Taylor, J., Djavadian, R. and Turlejski, K. (2001) Changes in the rate of generation of the brain cells in the life cycle of shrews (Insectivora). *Abstracts of the conference "Changing views of Cajal's Neuron"*, Madrid 2001. p. A2.

Biebl, M., Cooper, C.M., Winkler, J. and Kuhn, H.G. (2000) Analysis of neurogenesis and programmed cell death reveals a self-renewing capacity in the adult rat brain. *Neurosci. Lett.*, 8: 17–20.

Bigl, V., Arendt, T., Fischer, S., Fischer, S., Werner, M. and Arendt, A. (1987) The cholinergic system in aging. *Gerontology*, 33: 172–180.

Blakemore, W.F. and Jolly, R.D. (1972) The subependymal plate and associated ependyma in the dog. An ultrastructural study. *J. Neurocytol.*, 1: 69–84.

Boll, F. (1873–1874) Histologie und Histogenese der nervosen Centralorgane. *Arch f. Psychiatr.*, Berl., 4: 1–138.

Boss, B.D., Peterson, G.M. and Cowan, W.M. (1985) On the number of neurons in the dentate gyrus of the rat. *Brain Res.*, 338: 144–150.

Boss, B.D., Turlejski, K., Stanfield, B.B. and Cowan, W.M. (1987) On the numbers of neurons in fields CA1 and CA3 of the hippocampus of Sprague-Dawley and Wistar rats. *Brain Res.*, 406: 280–287.

Braendegaard, H., Evans, S.M., Howard, C.V. and Gundersen, H.J.G. (1990) The total number of neurons in the human neocortex unbiasedly estimayed using optical disectors. *J. Microsc.*, 257: 285–304.

Brizzee, K.R. (1973) Quantitative histological studies on aging changes in cerebral cortex of Rhesus monkey and albino rat with notes on effects of prolonged low-dose ionizing irradiation in the rat. *Prog. Brain Res.*, 40: 141–160.

Brizzee, K.R. and Ordy, J.M.(1979) Age pigments, cell loss and hippocampal function. *Mech. Ageing Dev.*, 9: 143–162.

Brizzee, K.R., Ordy, J.M. and Bartus, R.T. (1980) Localization of cellular changes within multimodal sensory regions in aged monkey brain: possible implications for age-related cognitive loss. *Neurobiol. Aging*, 1: 45–52.

Brizzee, K.R., Sherwood, N. and Timiras, P.S. (1968) A comparison of cell populations at various depth levels in cerebral cortex of young adult and aged Long-Evans rats. *J. Gerontol.*, 23: 289–297.

Broca, P. (1878) Anatomie comparee des circonvolutions cerebrales. Le grand lobe limbique dans la serie des mammiferes. *Revue d'anthropologie.*, 384–498.

Brody, H. (1955) Organization of the cerebral cortex, Part 3 (A study of aging in cerebral cortex). *J. Comp. Neurol.*, 102: 511–556.

Brody, H. (1970) Structural changes in the aging nervous system. *Interdisciplinary Top. Gerontol.*, 7: 9–21.

Brody, H. (1980) The nervous system and aging. *Adv. Pathobiol.*, 7: 200–209.

Cajal, S.R. (1913) Degeneration and Regeneration of the Nervous System (trans. Day, R.M., from the 1913 Spanish edn) (Oxford University Press, London, 1928).

Cajal, S.R. (1899–1904) Texture of the Nervous System of Man and the Vertebrates (trans. Pasik, P. and Pasik, T., from the 1899–1904 Spanish edn) (Springer, Vienna, 1999).

Cajal, S.R. (1928) *Degeneration and Regeneration of the Nervous System.* Oxford University Press, London.

Calhoun, M.E., Kurth, D., Phinney, A.L., Long, J.M., Hengemihle, J., Mouton, P.R., Ingram, D.K. and Jucker, M. (1998) Hippocampal neuron and synaptophysin-positive bouton number in aging C57BL/6 mice. *Neurobiol. Aging*, 19: 599–606.

Cameron, H.A. and McKay, R.D.G. (1999) Restoring production of hippocampal neurons in old age. *Nature Neuroscie.*, 2: 894–897.

Cameron, H.A. and McKay, R.D.G. (2001) Adult neurogenesis produces a large pool of new granule cells in the dentate gyrus. *J. Comp. Neurol.*, 435: 406–417.

Cameron, H.A., Woolley, C.S., McEwen, B.S. and Gould, E. (1993) Diferentiation of newly born neurons and glia in the dentate gyrus of the adult rat. *Neuroscience*, 56: 337–344.

Casey, M.A. (1990) The effects of aging on neuron number in the rat superior olivary complex. *Neurobiol. Aging*, 11: 391–394.

Cha, C.I., Sohn, S.G., Chung, Y.H., Shih, C. and Baik, S.H. (2000) Region-specific changes of NOS-IR cells in the basal ganglia of the aged rat. *Brain Res.*, 854: 239–244.

Chazal, G., Durbec, P., Jankovski, A., Rougon, G. and Cremer, H. (2000) Consequences of neural cell adhesion molecule deficiency on cell migration in the rostral migratory stream of the mouse. *J. Neurosci.*, 20: 1446–1457.

Chui, H.C., Bondareff, W., Zarow, C. and Slager, U. (1984) Stability of neuronal number in the human nucleus basalis of Meynert with age. *Neurobiol. Aging*, 5: 83–88.

Clayton, N.S. (1998) Memory and the hippocampus in food-storing birds: a comparative approach. *Neuropharmacology*, 37: 441–452.

Coleman, P.D., and Flood, D.G. (1987) Neuron numbers and dendritic extent in normal aging and Alzheimer's disease. *Neurobiol. Aging*, 8: 521–545.

Collier, T.J., and Coleman, P.D. (1991) Divergence of biological and chronological aging: evidence from rodent studies. *Neurobiol. Aging*, 12: 685–693.

Colon, E.J. (1971) Quantitative cytoarchitectonics of the human cerebral cortex. *Psychiatr. Neurol. Neurochir.*, 74: 291–302.

Colon, E.J. (1972) The elderly brain. A quantitative analysis in the cerebral cortex of two cases. *Psychiatr. Neurol. Neurochir.*, 75: 261–270.

Colonnier, M. and O'Kusky, J. (1981) Number of neurons and synapses in the visual cortex of diferent species. (In French). *Rev. Can. Biol.*, 40: 91–99.

Corbin, K.B. and Gardner, E.D. (1937) Decrease in the number of myelinated fibers in human spinal roots with age. *Anat. Rec.*, 68: 529–536.

Corsellis, J.A.N. (1976) Some observations on the Purkinje cell population and on brain volume in human aging. In: R.D. Terry and S. Gershon (Eds.) *Neurobiology of Aging.* Raven Press, New York.

Corotto, F.S., Henegar, J.A. and Maruniak, J.A. (1993) Neurogenesis persists in the subependymal layer of the adult mouse brain. *Neurosci. Lett.*, 149:111–114.

Corotto, F.S., Henegar, J.R. and Maruniak, J.A. (1994) Odor deprivation leads to reduced neurogenesis and reduced neuronal survival in the olfactory bulb of the adult mouse. *Neuroscience*, 61: 739–744.

Coupland, R.E. (1968) Determining sizes of spherical bodies such as chromaffin granules in tissue sections. *Nature*, 217: 384–388.

Cowan, W.M., Fawcett, J.W., O'Leary D.D.M. and Stanfield, B.B. (1984) Regressive events in neurogenesis. *Science*, 225: 1258–1265.

Cragg, B.G. (1975) The density of synapses and neurones in normal, mentally defective and ageing human brains. *Brain*, 98: 81–90.

Crespo, D., Stanfield, B.B. and Cowan, W.M. (1986) Evidence that late-generated granule cells do not simply replace earlier formed neurons in the rat dentate gyrus. *Exp. Brain Res.*, 62: 541–548.

Cruz-Sanchez, F.F., Moral, A., Tolosa, E., de Belleroche, J. and Rossi, M.L. (1998) Evaluation of neuronal loss, astrocytosis and abnormalities of cytoskeletal components of large motor neurons in the human anterior horn in aging. *J. Neural. Transm.*, 105: 689–701.

Curcio, C.A. (2001) Photoreceptor topography in aging and age-related maculopathy. *Eye*, 15: 376–383.

Curcio, C.A. and Coleman, P.D. (1982) Stability of neuron number in cortical barrels of aging mice. *J. Comp. Neurol.*, 212: 158–172.

Curcio, C.A. and Drucker, D.N. (1993) Retinal ganglion cells in Alzheimer's disease and aging. *Ann. Neurol.*, 33: 248–257.

Czibulka, A. and Schwartz, I.R. (1991) Neuronal populations in the gerbil PVCN: effects of age, hearing status and microcysts. *Hear Res.*, 52: 43–57.

Dark, J., Spears, N., Whaling, C.S., Wade, G.N., Meyer, J.S. and Zucker, I. (1990) Long day lengths promote brain growth in meadow voles. *Dev. Brain Res.*, 53: 264–269.

Dawirs, R.R., Teuchert-Noodt, G., Hildebrandt, K. and Fei, F. (2000) Granule cell proliferation and axon terminal degradation in the dentate gyrus of gerbils (Meriones unguiculatus) during maturation, adulthood and aging. *J. Neural. Transm.*, 107: 639–647.

Decker, M.W. (1987) The effects of aging on hippocampal and cortical projections of the forebrain cholinergic system. *Brain Res.*, 434: 423–438.

Delorenzi, E. (1931) Costanza numerica delle cellule di Purkinje del cerveletto dell'uomo in individui di varia eta. *Z. Zellforsch. Mikrosk. Anat.*, 14: 310–316.

Devaney, K.O. and Johnson, H.A. (1980) Neuron loss in the aging visual cortex of man. *J. Gerontol.*, 35: 836–841.

Devaney, K.O. and Johnson, H.A. (1984) Changes in cell density within the human hippocampal formation as a function of age. *Gerontology*, 30: 100–109.

Diaz, F., Villena, A., Gonzalez, P., Requena, V., Rius, F., Perez De Vargas, I. (1999) Stereological age-related changes in neurons of the rat dorsal lateral geniculate nucleus. *Anat. Rec.*, 255: 396–400.

Dlugos, C.A. and Pentney, R.J. (1994) Morphometric analysis of Purkinje and granular cells in aging F344 rats. *Neurobiol. Aging*, 15: 435–440.

Doetsch, F. and Alvarez-Buylla, A. (1996) Network of tangential pathways for neuronal migration in adult mammalian brain. *Proc. Natl. Acad. Sci. U S A.*, 93: 14895–14900.

Doetsch, F., Caille, I., Lim, D.A., Garcia-Verdugo, J.M. and Alvarez-Buylla, A. (1999) Subventricular zone astrocytes are neural stem cells in the adult mammalian brain. *Cell*, 97: 703–716.

Doetsch, F., Garcia-Verdugo, J.M. and Alvarez-Buylla, A. (1997) Cellular composition and three-dimensional organization of the subventricular germinal zone in the adult mammalian brain. *J. Neurosci.*, 17: 5046–5061.

Dolman, C.L., McCormick, A.Q. and Drance, S.M. (1980) Aging of the optic nerve. *Arch. Ophthalmol.*, 98: 2053–2058.

Donaldson, H.H. (1895) *The Growth of the Brain*. Chicago.

Doulazmi, M., Frederic, F., Lemaigre-Dubreuil, Y., Hadj-Sahraoui, N., Delhaye-Bouchaud, N. and Mariani, J. (1999) Cerebellar Purkinje cell loss during life span of the heterozygous staggerer mouse (Rora(+)/Rora(sg)) is gender-related. *J. Comp. Neurol.*, 411: 267–273.

Dreher, B. and Robinson, S.R. (1988) Development of the retinofugal pathway in birds and mammals: evidence for a common 'timetable'. Review: *Brain Behav. Evol.*, 31: 369–90.

Druge, H., Heinsen, H. and Heinsen, Y.L. (1986) Quantitative studies in ageing Chbb: THOM (Wistar) rats. II. Neuron numbers in lobules I, VIb + c and X. *Bibl. Anat.*, 28: 121–137.

Dutton, R. and Bartlett, P.F. (2000) Precursor cells in the subventricular zone of the adult mouse are actively inhibited from diferentiating into neurons. *Devel. Neurosci.*, 22: 96–105.

Eckenhoff, M.F. and Rakic, P. (1988) Nature and fate of proliferative cells in the hippocampal dentate gyrus during the life span of the rhesus monkey. *J. Neurosci.*, 8: 2729–2747.

Economo, C. von and Koskinas, G.N. (1925) Die Cytoarchitektonik der Hirnrinde des erwachsenen Menschen. Berlin.

Economos, A.C. (1982) Mammalian design and rate of living. *Exp. Gerontol.*, 17: 145–152.

Ellis, R.S. (1919) A preliminary quantitative study of the Purkinje cell in normal, subnormal and senescent human cerebella, with some notes on functional localization. *J. Comp. Neurol.*, 30: 229–252.

Ellis, R.S. (1920) Norms for some structural changes in the human cerebellum from birth to old age. *J. Comp. Neurol.*, 32: 1–33.

Emborg, M.E., Ma, S.Y., Mufson, E.J., Levey, A.I., Taylor, M.D., Brown, W.D., Holden, J.E. and Kordower, J.H. (1998) Age-related declines in nigral neuronal function correlate with motor impairments in rhesus monkeys. *J. Comp. Neurol.*, 401: 253–265.

Emerich, D.F., McDermott, P., Krueger P., Banks, M., Zhao, J., Marszalkowski, J., Frydel, B., Winn, S.R. and Sanberg, P.R. (1993) Locomotion of aged rats: relationship to neurochemical but not morphological changes in nigrostriatal dopaminergic neurons. *Brain Res. Bull.*, 32: 477–486.

Eriksson, P.S., Perfilieva, E., Bjork-Eriksson, T., Alborn, A.-M., Nordborg, C., Peterson, D.A. and Gage, F.H. (1998) Neurogenesis in the adult human hippocampus. *Nature Medicine*, 4: 1313–1317.

Farel, P.B. and McIlwain, D.L. (2000) Neuronal addition and enlargment in juvenile and adult animals. *Brain Res. Bull.*, 53: 537–546.

Fearnley, J.M. and Lees, A.J. (1990) Striatonigral degeneration. A clinicopathological study. *Brain*, 113: 1823–1842.

Fischer, C.P., Jorgen, G., Gundersen, H. and Pakkenberg, B. (1999) Preferential loss of large neocortical neurons during HIV infection: a study of the size distribution of neocortical neurons in the human brain. *Brain Res.*, 828: 119–126.

Fleming, P.A., Harman, A.M. and Beazley, L.D. (1996) Development and aging of the RPE in a marsupial, the quokka. *Exp. Eye Res.*, 62: 457–470.

Flood, D.G. and Coleman, P.D. (1988) Neuron numbers and sizes in aging brain: comparison of human, monkey and rodent data. *Neurobiol. Aging*, 9: 453–463.

Flood, D.G. and Coleman, P.D. (1993) Dendritic regression dissociated from neuronal death but associated with partial deafferentation in aging rat supraoptic nucleus. *Neurobiol. Aging*, 14: 575–587.

Foix, M.C. (1921) Les Lesions anatomiques de la Maladie de Parkinson. *Rev. Neurol.*, 38: 593–600.

Gage, F.H. (2000) Mammalian neural stem cells. *Science*, 287: 1433–1438.

Galea, L.A. and McEwen, B.S. (1999) Sex and seasonal differences in the rate of cell proliferation in the dentate gyrus of adult wild meadow voles. *Neuroscience*, 89: 955–964.

Gao, H. and Hollyfield, J.G. (1992) Aging of the human retina. *Invest. Ophthalmol. Vis. Sci.*, 33: 1–17.

Gardner, E.D. (1940) Decrease in human neurones with old age. *Anat. Rec.*, 77: 529–536.

Gazzaley, A.H., Thakker, M.M., Hof, P.R. and Morrison, J.H. (1997) Preserved number of entorhinal cortex layer II neurons in aged macaque monkeys. *Neurobiol. Aging*, 18: 549–553.

Gheusi, C., Cremer, H., McLean, H., Chazal, G., Vincent, J.D. and Lledo, P.M. (2000) Importance of newly generated neurons in the adult olfactory bulb for odor discrimination. *Proc. Natl. Acad. Sci. USA*, 97: 1823–1828.

Gianfranceschi, L., Fiorentini, A. and Maffei, L. (1999) Behavioral visual acuity of wild type and *bcl2* transgenic mouse. *Vision Res.*, 39: 569–574.

Goldman, G. and Coleman, P.D. (1981) Neuron numbers in locus coeruleus do not change with age in Fisher 344 rat. *Neurobiol. Aging*, 2: 33–36.

Goldman, S.A. and Luskin, M.B. (1998) Strategies utilized by migrating neurons of the postnatal vertebrate forebrain. *Trends Neurosci.*, 21:107–114.

Golgi, C. (1886) Sulla fina anatomia degli organi centrali del sistema nervoso. U. Hoepli, Milano.

Gomez-Isla, T., Hollister, R., West, H., Mu, S., Growdon, J.H., Petersen, R.C., Parisi, J.E. and Hyman, B.T. (1997) Neuronal loss correlates with but exceeds neurofibrillary tangles in Alzheimer's disease. *Ann. Neurol.*, 41: 17–24.

Gomez-Isla, T., Price, J.L., McKeel jr., D.W., Morris, J.C., Growdon, J.H. and Hyman, B.T. (1996) Profound loss of layer II entorhinal cortex neurons occurs in very mild Alzheimer's disease. *J. Neurosci.*, 16: 4491–4500.

Gould, E., Beylin, A., Tanapat, P., Reeves, A. and Shors, T.J. (1999a) Learning enhances adult neurogenesis in the hippocampal formation. *Nat. Neurosci.*, 2: 260–265.

Gould, E., McEwen, B.S., Tanapat, P., Galea, L.A. and Fuchs, E. (1997) Neurogenesis in the dentate gyrus of the adult tree shrew is regulated by psychosocial stress and NMDA receptor activation. *J. Neurosci.*, 17: 2492–2498.

Gould, E., Reeves, A.J., Graziano, M.S. and Gross, C.G. (1999b) Neurogenesis in the neocortex of adult primates. *Science*, 286: 548–552.

Gould, E., Tanapat, P., Hastings, N.B. and Shors, T.J. (1999c) Neurogenesis in adulthood: a possible role in learning. *Trends in Cognitive Sci.*, 3: 186–192.

Gould, E., Tanapat, P., McEwen, B.S., Flugge, G. and Fuchs, E. (1998) Proliferation of granule cell precursors in the dentate gyrus of adult monkeys is diminished by stress. *Proc. Natl. Acad. Sci. USA*, 95: 3168–3171.

Gould, B., Woley, C.S. and McEwen, B. (1991) Naturally occuring cell death in the developing dentate gyrus of the rat. *J. Comp. Neurol.*, 304: 408–418.

Gratzner, H.G. (1982) Monoclonal antibody to 5-bromo- and 5-iododeoxyuridine: a new reagent for detection of DNA replication. *Science*, 218: 474–475.

Gross, C.G. (2000) Neurogenesis in the adult brain: death of a dogma. *Nature Reviews*, 1: 67–73.

Gueneau, G., Privat, A., Drouet, J. and Court, L. (1982) Subgranular zone of the dentate gyrus of young rabbits as a secondary matrix. A high-resolution autoradiographic study. *Dev Neurosci.*, 5: 345–358.

Gundersen, H.J.G., Bendtsen, T.F., Korbo, L., Marcussen, N., Moller, A., Nielsen, K., Nyengard, J.R., Pakkenberg, B., Sorensen, F.B., Vesterby, A. and West, M.J. (1988) Some new, simple and efficient stereological methods and their use in pathological research and diagnosis. Review article., *APMIS*, 96: 379–394.

Hall, T.C., Miller, A.K.H. and Corselis, J.A.N. (1975) Variations in the human Purkinje cell population according to age and sex. *Neuropathol. Appl. Neurobiol.*, 1: 267–292.

Hamburger, V. and Oppenheim, R.W. (1982) Naturally occuring neuronal death in vertebrates. *Neurosci. Comm.*, 1: 39–55.

Hamilton, A. (1901) The division of differentiated cells in the central nervous system of the white rat. *J. Comp. Neurol.*, 11: 297–320.

Hanley, T. (1974) Neuronal fall-out in the aging brain: A critical review of the quantitative data. *Age Aging*, 3: 133–151.

Harding, A.J., Halliday, G.M. and Kril, J.J. (1998) Variation in hippocampal neuron number with age and brain volume. *Cereb. Cortex*, 8: 710–718.

Harman, A., Abrahams, B., Moore, S. and Hoskins, R. (2000) Neuronal density in the human retinal ganglion cell layer from 16–77 years. *Anat. Rec.*, 260: 124–131.

Harman, A.M. and Moore, S. (1999) Number of neurons in the retinal ganglion cell layer of the quokka wallaby do not change throughout life. *Anat. Rec.*, 256: 78–83.

Harvey, R.J. and Napper, R.M. (1988) Quantitative study of granule and Purkinje cells in the cerebellar cortex of the rat. *J. Comp. Neurol.*, 274: 151–157.

Hastings, N.B., Tanapat, P. and Gould, E. (2000) Comparative views of adult neurogenesis. *Neuroscientist*, 6: 315–325.

Haug, H. (1985) Are neurons of the human cerebral cortex really lost during aging? A morphometric evaluation. In: J. Traber and W.H., Gispen, (Eds.) *Senile dementia of the Alzheimer type*, Springer, Berlin, pp. 150–163.

Haug, H. (1987) Brain sizes, surfaces, and neuronal sizes of the cortex cerebri: a stereological investigation of man and his variability and a comparison with some mammals (primates, whales, marsupials, insectivores, and one elephant). *Am. J. Anat.*, 180: 126–142.

Haug, H., Kuhl, S., Mecke, E., Sass, N.L. and Wasner, K. (1984) The significance of morphometric procedures in the investigation of age changes in cytoarchitectonic structures of human brain. *J. Hirnforsch.*, 25: 354–374.

Haydar, T.F., Kuan, C.-Y., Flavell, R.A. and Rakic, P. (1999) The role of cell death in regulating the size and shape of the mammalian forebrain. *Cereb. Cortex*, 9: 621–626.

Heinsen, H., Henn, R., Eisenmenger, W., Gotz, M., Bohl, J., Bethke, B., Lockemann, U. and Puschel, K. (1994) Quantitative investigations on the human entorhinal area: left-right asymmetry and age-related changes. *Anat. Embryol. (Berl).*, 190: 181–194.

Held, H. (1907) Kritische Bemarkungenzu der Verteidigung der Neuroblasten und der Neuronentheorie durch R. Cajal. *Anat. Anz.*, 30: 369–391.

Henderson, G., Tomlinson, B.E. and Gibson, P.H. (1980) Cell counts in human cerebral cortex in normal adults throughout life using an image analysing computer. *J. Neurol. Sci.*, 46: 113–136.

Heumann, D. and Leuba, G. (1983) Neuronal death in the development and aging of the cerebral cortex of mouse. *Neuropathol. Appl. Neurobiol.*, 9: 297–311.

Hinojosa, R., Seligshorn, R. and Lerner S.A. (1985) Ganglion cell counts in the cochleae of patients with normal audiograms. *Acta Otolaryngol.*, 99: 8–13.

Hinds, J.W. and McNelly, N.A. (1977) Aging of the rat olfactory bulb: growth and atrophy of constituent layers and changes in size and number of mitral cells. *J. Comp. Neurol.*, 72: 345–367.

His, W. (1890) Histogenese und Zusammmenhang der Nervenelemente. *Arch. f. Anat. u. Physiol. Leipz., Anat. Abth.*, supp., 95–119.

58

His, W. (1904) Die Entwickelung des menschlichen Gehirns (Hirzel, Leipzig).

Hodge, C.F. (1894) Changes in ganglion cells from birth to senile death. Observations on man and honey-bee. *J. Physiol.*, 17: 129–134.

Hof, P.R., Nimchinsky, E.A., Young, W.G. and Morrison, J.H. (2000) Numbers of meynert and layer IVB cells in area V1: a stereologic analysis in young and aged macaque monkeys. *J. Comp. Neurol.*, 420: 113–126.

Hornberger, J.C., Buell, S.J., Flood, D.G., McNeill, T.H. and Coleman, P.D. (1985) Stability of numbers but not size of mouse forebrain cholinergic neurons to 53 months. *Neurobiol. Aging*, 6: 269–275.

Horner, P.J., Power, A.E., Kempermann, G., Kuhn, H.G., Palmer, T.D., Winkler, J., Thal, L.J. and Gage, F.H. (2000) Proliferation and diferentiation of progenitor cells throughout the intact adult rat spinal cord. *J. Neurosci.*, 20: 2218–2228.

Hsu, H.K. and Peng, M.T. (1978) Hypothalamic neuron number of old female rats. *Gerontology*, 24: 434–440.

Huang, L., DeVries, G.J. and Bittman, E.L. (1998) Photoperiod regulates neuronal bromodeoxyuridine labeling in the brain of seasonally breeding mammal. *J. Neurobiol.*, 36: 410–420.

Ibanez, C.F. (1998) Emerging themes in structural biology of neurotrophic factors. *Trends Neurosci.*, 21: 438–444.

Idrizbegovic, E., Canlon, B., Bross, L.S., Willott, J.F. and Bogdanovic, N. (2001) The total number of neurons and calcium binding protein positive neurons during aging in the cochlear nucleus of CBA/CaJ mice: a quantitative study. *Hear Res.*, 158: 102–115.

Inukai, T. (1928) On the loss of Purkinje cells with advancing age from the cerebral cortex of the albino rat. *J. Comp. Neurol.*, 45: 1–31.

Ingram, D.K. and Jucker, M. (1999) Developing mouse models of aging: a consideration of strain differences in age-related behavioral and neural parameters. *Neurobiol. Aging*, 20: 137–145.

Jacob, J.M. (1998) Lumbar motor neuron size and number is affected by age in male F344 rats. *Mech. Ageing Dev.*, 106: 205–216.

Jacobs, B.L., Praag, H. and Gage, F.H. (2000) Adult brain neurogenesis and psychiatry: a novel theory of depression. *Mol. Psychiatry*, 5: 262–269.

Jellinger, K.A. and Stadelmann, C.H. (2000) The enigma of cell death in neurodegenerative disorders. *J. Neural Transm. Suppl.*, 60: 21–36.

Jensen, G.B. and Pakkenberg, B. (1993) Do alcoholics drink their neurons away? *Lancet*, 342: 1201–1204.

Jin, K., Minami, M., Lan, J.Q., Mao, X.O., Batteur, S., Simon, R.P. and Greenberg, D.A. (2001) Neurogenesis in dentate subgranular zone and rostralsubventricular zone after cerebral ischemia in the rat. *Proc. Natl. Acad. Sci. USA*, 98: 4710–4715.

Johansson, C.B., Momma, S., Clarke, D.L., Risling, M., Lendahl, U., and Frisen, J. (1999) Identification of a neural stem cell in the adult mammalian central nervous system. *Cell*, 96: 25–34.

Johnson, B.M., Miao, M. and Sadun A.A. (1987) Age related decline of human optic nerve axon populations. *Age*, 10: 5–9.

Jonas, J.B., Muller-Bergh, J.A., Schlotzer-Schrehardt, U.M. and Naumann, G.O.H. (1990) Human optic nerve fibre count and optic disc size. *Invest. Ophthalmol. Vis. Sci.*, 33: 2012–2018.

Jonson, K.M., Lyle, J.G., Edwards, M.J. and Penny, R.H. (1976) Effects of prenatal heat stress on brain growth and serial discrimination reversal learning in the guinea pig. *Brain Res. Bull.*, 1: 133–150.

Jucker, M., Bondolfi, L., Calhoun, M.E., Long, J.M. and Ingram, D.K. (2000) Structural brain aging in inbred mice: potential for genetic linkage. *Exp. Gerontol.*, 35: 1383–1388.

Kadar, T., Arbel, I., Silbermann, M. and Levy, A. (1994) Morphological hippocampal changes during normal aging and their relation to cognitive deterioration. *J. Neural Transm. Suppl.*, 44: 133–143.

Kaplan, M.S. (1983) Proliferation of subependymal cells in the adult primate CNS: differential uptake of DNA labelled precursors. *J. Hirnforsch.*, 24: 23–33.

Kaplan, M.S. and Hinds, J.W. (1977) Neurogenesis in the adult rat: electron microscopic analysis of light autoradiographs. *Science*, 197:1092–1094.

Kappers, A., Huber, G.C. and Crosby, E.C. (1936–1965) *The Comparative Anatomy of the Nervous System of Vertebrates, including man.* Vol. I, II, III, Hafner, New York.

Karhunen, P.J., Erkinjuntti, T. and Laippala, P. (1994) Moderate alcohol consumption and loss of cerebellar Purkinje cells. *B.M.J.*, 308: 1663–1667.

Kato, L., Yokouchi, K., Kawagishi, K., Fukushima, N., Miwa, T. and Moriizumi, T. (2000) Fate of newly formed periglomerular cells in the olfactory bulb. *Acta Oto-laryngologica*, 120: 876–879.

Kato, L., Yokouchi, K., Fukushima, N. Kawagishi, K., Li, Z.Y. and Moriizumi, T. (2001) Continual replacement of newly-generated olfactory neurons in adult rats. *Neurosci. Lett*, 307: 17–20.

Katz, M.L. and Robinson, W.G. (1986) Evidence of cell loss from the rat retina during senescence. *Exp. Eye Res.*, 42: 293–304.

Kee, N.J., Preston, E. and Wojtowicz, J.M. (2001) Enhanced neurogenesis after transient global ischemia in the dentate gyrus of the rat. *Exp. Brain Res.*, 136: 313–320.

Keithley, E.M. and Feldman M.L. (1979) Spiral ganglion cell count in an age-graded series of rat cochleas. *J. Comp. Neurol.*, 1: 429–442.

Kemper, T.L., Moss, M.B., Rosene, D.L. and Killiany, R.J. (1997) Age-related neuronal loss in the nucleus centralis superior of the rhesus monkey. *Acta Neuropathol. (Berl).*, 94: 124–130.

Kempermann, G., Kuhn, H.G. and Gage, F.H. (1997) More hippocampal neurons in adult mice living in an enriched environment. *Nature*, 386: 493–495.

Kempermann, G., Kuhn, H.G. and Gage, F.H. (1998) Experience-induced neurogenesis in the senescent dentate gyrus. *J. Neurosci.*, 18: 3206–3212.

Kershman, J. (1938) The medulloblast and the medulloblastoma. *Arch. Neurol. Psychiat.*, 40: 937–967.

Kim, C.B., Pier, L.P. and Spear, P.D. (1997) Effects of aging on numbers and sizes of neurons in histochemically defined subregions of monkey striate cortex. *Anat. Rec.*, 247: 119–128.

Kim, C.B., Tom, B.W. and Spear, P.D. (1996) Effects of aging on the densities, numbers, and sizes of retinal ganglion cells in rhesus monkey. *Neurobiol. Aging*, 17: 431–438.

Kirn, J.R. and Nottebohm, F. (1993) Direct evidence for loss and replacement of projection neurons in adult canary brain. *J. Neurosci.*, 13: 1654–1663.

Kirschenbaum, B., Doetsch, F., Lois, C. and Alvarez-Buylla, A. (1999) Adult subventricular zone neuronal precursors continue to proliferate and migrate in the absence of the olfactory bulb. *J. Neurosci.*, 19: 2171–280.

Kloppel, S., Kovacs, G.G., Voigtlander, T., Wanschitz, J., Flicker, H., Hainfellner, J.A., Guentchev, M. and Budka, H. (2001) Serotonergic nuclei of the raphe are not affected in human ageing. *Neuroreport*, 12: 669–671.

Kolliker v., A. (1882) Embryologie; ou, Traite complet du developpement de l'homme et des animaux superieurs. Tr. By A. Schneider. Reinwand, Paris.

Kolliker v., A. (1905) Die Entwicklung der Elemente des Nervensystems. *Ztschr. f. wissensch. Zool.*, 82: 1–38.

Konigsmark, B.W. and Murphy, E.A. (1970) Neuronal populations in human brain. *Nature*, 228: 1335–1336.

Korbo, L., Andersen, B.B., Ladefoged, O. and Moller, A. (1993) Total numbers of various cell types in rat cerebellar cortex estimated using an unbiased stereological method. *Brain Res.*, 609: 262–268.

Kornack, D.R. and Rakic, P. (1999) Continuation of neurogenesis in the hippocampus of the adult macaque monkey. *Proc. Natl. Acad. Sci. U S A*, 96: 5768–5773.

Kornack, D.R. and Rakic, P.R. (2001) The generation and differentiation of olfactory neurons in the adult primate brain. *Proc. Natl. Acad. Sci. USA*, 98: 4752–4757.

Korr, H. (1982) Proliferation of different cell types in the brain of senile mice. Autoradiographic studies with ^{3}H- and ^{14}C-Thymidine. In: Hoyer S. (Ed.) *The Aging Brain*. Spriger, Berlin, Heidelberg, New York, pp. 51–57.

Korr, H. and Schmitz, C. (1999) Facts and fictions regarding post-natal neurogenesis in the developing human cerebral cortex. *J. Theor. Biol.*, 7: 291–197.

Kuhlenbeck, H. (1944) Senile changes in the brain of Wistar Institute rats. *Anat. Rec.*, 88: 441.

Kuhn, H.G., Dickinson-Anson, H. and Gage, F.H. (1996) Neurogenesis in the dentate gyrus of the adult rat: age-related decrease of neuronal progenitor proliferation. *J. Neurosci.*, 16: 2027–2033.

Kuhn, H.G., Palmer, T.D. and Fuchs, E. (2001) Adult neurogenesis: a compensatory mechanism for neural damage. *Eur. Arch. Psychiatry Clin. Neurosci.*, 251: 152–158.

Kukekov, V.G., Laywell, E.D., Suslov, O., Davies, K., Scheffler, B., Thomas, L.B., O'Brien, T.F., Kusakabe, M. and Steindler, D.A. (1999) Multipotent stem/progenitor cells with similar properties arise from two neurogenic regions of adult human brain. *Exp. Neurol.*, 156: 333–344.

Lacalle, de, S., Iraizoz, I., Gonzalo L.M. (1991) Differential changes in cell size and number in topographic subdivisions of human basal nucleus in normal aging. *Neuroscience*, 43: 445–456.

Landfield, P.W., Braun, L.D., Pitler, T.A., Lindsey, J.D. and Lynch, G. (1981) Hippocampal aging inrats: a morphometric study of multiple variables in semithin sections. *Neurobiol. Aging*, 2: 265–275.

Landing, B.H., Shankle, W.R. and Hara, J. (1998) Constructing the human cerebral cortex during infabcy and childhood: types and numbers of cortical columns and numbers of neurons in such columns at different age points. *Acta Paediatr. Jpn.*, 40: 530–543.

Larsen, J.O., Skalicky, M. and Viidik, A. (2000) Does long-term physical exercise counteract age-related Purkinje cell loss? A stereological study of rat cerebellum. *J. Comp. Neurol.*, 428: 213–222.

Lavenex, P., Steele, M.A. and Jacobs, L.F. (2000a) The seasonal pattern of cell proliferation and neuron number in the dentate gyrus of wild adult eastern grey squirrels. *Eur. J. Neurosci.*, 12: 643–648.

Lavenex, P., Steele, M.A. and Jacobs, L.F. (2000b) Sex differences, but no seasonal variations in the hippocampus of food-caching squirrels: a stereological study. *J. Comp. Neurol.*, 425: 152–166.

Leal, S., Andrade, J.P., Paula-Barbosa, M.M. and Madeira, M.D. (1998) Arcuate nucleus of the hypothalamus: effects of age and sex. *J. Comp. Neurol.*, 401: 65–88.

Leblond, C.P., Mesier, B. and Kopriwa, B. (1959) Thymidine-H3 as a tool for the investigation of the renewal of cell populations. *Lab. Invest.*, 8: 276–306.

Lemaire, V., Aurousseau, C., Le Moal, M. and Abrous, D.N. (1999) Behavioural trait of reactivity to novelty is related to hippocampal neurogenesis. *Eur. J. Neurosci.* 11: 4006–4014.

Lenhossek, V.M. (1890) Uber Nervenfasern in den hinteren Wurzeln, welche aus dem Vorderhorn entspringen. *Anat. Anz.*, 5: 360–362.

Leuba, G. and Kraftsik, R. (1994a) Changes in volume, surface estimate, three-dimensional shape and total number of neurons of the human primary visual cortex from midgestation until old age. *Anat. Embryol. (Berl).*, 190: 351–366.

Leuba, G. and Kraftsik, R. (1994b) Visual cortex in Alzheimer's disease: occurrence of neuronal death and glial proliferation, and correlation with pathological hallmarks. *Neurobiol. Aging*, 15: 29–43.

Leverenz, J.B., Wilkinson, C.W., Wamble, M., Corbin, S., Grabber, J.E., Raskind, M.A. and Peskind, E.R. (1999) Effect of chronic high-dose exogenous cortisol on hippocampal neuronal number in aged nonhuman primates. *J. Neurosci.*, 19:2356–2361.

Levi, G. (1898) Sulla carcinogenesi delle cellule nervose. *Riv. Patol. Nerv. Ment.*, 3: 97–113.

Lewis, P.D. (1968) Mitotic activity in the primate subependymal layer and the genesis of gliomas. *Nature*, 217: 974–975.

Liu, J., Bernabeu, R., Lu, A. and Sharp, F.R. (2000) Neurogenesis and gliogenesis in the postischemic brain. *Neuroscientist*, 6: 362–370.

Lohr, J.B. and Jeste, D.V. (1988) Locus ceruleus morphometry in aging and schizophrenia. *Acta Psychiatr. Scand.*, 77: 689–697.

Lois, C. and Alvarez-Buylla, A. (1994) Long-distance neuronal migration in the adult mammalian brain. *Science*, 264: 1145–1148.

Lois, C., Garcia-Verdugo, J.M. and Alvarez-Buylla, A. (1996) Chain migration of neuronal precursors. *Science*, 271: 978–981.

Long, J.M., Mouton, P.R., Jucker, M. and Ingram, D.K. (1999) What counts in brain aging? Design-based stereological analysis of cell number. *J. Gerontol. A Biol. Sci. Med. Sci.*, 54: B407–B417.

Lopez, I., Honrubia, V. and Baloh, R.W. (1997) Aging and the human vestibular nucleus. *J. Vestib. Res.*, 7: 77–85.

Lowes-Hummel, P., Gertz, H.J., Ferszt, R. and Cervos-Navarro, J. (1989) The basal nucleus of Meynert revised: the nerve

60

cell number decreases with age. *Arch. Gerontol. Geriatr.*, 8: 21–27.

Lu, S., Goto, N., Goto, J., Tajima, N. and Ishikawa, H. (2001) Morphometric analysis of myelinated axons in the human vagus nerve. *Okajimas Folia Anat.*, 78: 1–5.

Lucassen, P.J., Vollmann-Honsdorf, G.K., Gleisberg, M., Boldizsar, C., De Kloet, E.R. and Fuchs, E. (2001) Chronic psychosocial stress differentially affects apoptosis in hippocampal subregions and cortex of the adult tree shrew. *Eur. J. Neurosci.*, 14: 161–166.

Luskin, M.B. (1994) Neuronal cell lineage in the vertebrate central nervous system. *FASEB J.*, 8:722–730.

Ma, S.Y., Ciliax, B.J., Stebbins, G., Jaffar, S., Joyce, J.N., Cochran, E.J., Kordower, J.H., Mash D.C., Levey, A.I. and Mufson E.J. (1999 a) Dopamine transporter-inmunoreactive neurons decrease with age in the human substantia nigra. *J. Comp. Neurol.*, 409: 25–37.

Ma, S.Y., Roytt, M., Collan, Y. and Rinne, J.O. (1999 b) Unbiased morphometrical measurements show loss of pigmented nigral neurones with ageing. *Neuropathol. Appl. Neurobiol.*, 25: 394–399.

Madeira, M.D., Paula-Barbosa, M.M., Cadette-Leite, A. and Tavares, M.A. (1988) Unbiased estimate of hippocampal granule cell numbers in hypothyroid and sex-age-matched control rats. *J. Hirnforsch.*, 29: 643–650.

Madeira, M.D., Sousa, N., Santer, R.M., Paula-Barbosa, M.M. and Gundersen, H.J. (1995) Age and sex do not affect the volume, cell numbers, or cell size of the suprachiasmatic nucleus of the rat: an unbiased stereological study. *J. Comp. Neurol.*, 361: 585–601.

Maehlen, J. and Torvik, A. (1990) Necrosis of granule cells of hippocampus in adrenocortical failure. *Acta Neuropathol. (Berl.)*, 80: 85–87.

Magavi, S.S., Leavitt, B.R. and Macklis, J.D. (2000) Induction of neurogenesis in the neocortex of adult mice. *Nature*, 405: 892–893.

Maleci, O. (1934) Contributo all conoscenza delle variazioni quantitative delle cellule nervose nelle senescenza. *Arch. Ital. Anat. Estilog. Patolog.*, 33: 883–901.

Manaye, K.F., McIntire, D.D., Mann, D.M. and German, D.C. (1995) Locus coeruleus cell loss in the aging human brain: a non-random process. *J. Comp. Neurol.*, 358: 79–87.

Manaye, K.F., Zweig, R., Wu, D., Hersh, L.B., De Lacalle, S., Saper, C.B. and German, D.C. (1999) Quantification of cholinergic and select non-cholinergic mesopontine neuronal populations in the human brain. *Neuroscience*, 89: 759–770.

Mandavilli, B.S. and Rao, K.S. (1996) Neurons in the cerebral cortex are most susceptible to DNA damage in aging rat brain. *Biochem. Mol. Biol. Int.*, 40: 507–14.

Marcyniuk, B., Mann, D.M. and Yates, P.O. (1989) The topography of nerve cell loss from the locus caeruleus in elderly persons. *Neurobiol. Aging*, 10: 5–9.

Martinez-Serrano, A, Fisher, W. and Bjorklund, A. (1995) Reversal of age-dependent cognitive impairments and cholinergic neuron atrophy by NGF-secreting neural progenitors grafted to the basal forebrain. *Neuron*, 15: 473–484.

Martinou, J.C., Dubois-Dauphin, M., Staple, J.K., Rodriguez, I., Frankowski, H., Missotten, M., Albertini, P., Talbot, D., Catsicas, S., Pietra, C. and Huarte, J. (1994) Overexpression of Bcl-2 in transgenic mice protects neurons from naturally occurring cell death and experimental ischemia. *Neuron*, 13: 1017–1030.

Mason, H.A., Ito, S. and Corfas, G. (2001) Exstracellular signals that regulate the tangential migration of olfactory bulb neuronal precursors: inducers, inhibitors and repellents. *J. Neuroscience*, 21: 7654–7663.

Matochik, J.A., Chefer, S.I., Lane, M.A., Woolf, R.I., Morris, E.D., Ingram, D.K., Roth, G.S. and London, E.D. (2000) Age-related decline in striatal volume in monkeys as measured by magnetic resonance imaging. *Neurobiol. Aging*, 21: 591–598.

Mayhew, T.M., MacLaren, R. and Henery, C.C. (1990) Fractionator studies on Purkinje cells in the human cerebellum: numbers in right and left halves of male and female brains. *J. Anat.*, 169: 63–70.

McDermott, K.W. and Lantos, P.L. (1990) Cell proliferation in the subependymal layer of the postnatal marmoset, Callithrix jacchus. *Dev. Brain Res.*, 57: 269–277.

McDermott, K.W. and Lantos, P.L. (1991) Distribution and fine structural analysis of undifferentiated cells in the primate subependymal layer. *J. Anat.*, 178: 45–63.

McNeill, T.H. and Koek, L.L. (1990) Differential effects of advancing age on neurotransmitter cell loss in the substantia nigra and striatum of C57BL/6N mice. *Brain Res.*, 521: 107–117.

Merrill, D.A., Roberts, J.A. and Tuszynski, M.H. (2000) Conservation of neuron number and size in entorhinal cortex layers II, III, and V/VI of aged primates. *J. Comp. Neurol.*, 422: 396–401.

Mesulam, M.M., Mufson, E.J. and Rogers, J. (1987) Age-related shrinkage of cortically projecting cholinergic neurons: a selective effect. *Ann. Neurol.*, 22: 31–36.

Mikelberg, F.S., Drance, S.M., Schulzer, M., Yidegiligne, H.M. and Weis M.M. (1989) The normal human optic nerve. *Ophthalmology*, 96: 1325–1328.

Miller, M.W. and Nowakowski, R.S. (1988) Use of bromo-deoxyuridine-immunohistochemistry to examine the proliferation, migration and time of origin of cells in the central nervous system. *Brain Res.*, 457: 44–52.

Mohammed, H.A. and Santer, R.M. (2001) Total neuronal numbers of rat lumbosacral primary afferent neurons do not change with age. *Neurosci. Lett.*, 304: 149–152.

Monagle, R.D. and Brody, H. (1974) The effects of age upon the main nucleus of the inferior olive in the human. *J. Comp. Neurol.*, 155: 51–66.

Moorshead, C., van der Kooy, D. and Weiss, S. (1997) Do multilineage potential neural stem cells really exist in the brain of adult mammals? *TINS* 20: 203–204.

Morrison, J.C., Cork, L.C., Dunkelberg, G.R., Brown, A. and Quigley H.A. (1990) Aging changes of the rhesus monkey optic nerve. *Invest. Ophthalmol. Vis. Sci.*, 31: 1623–1627.

Morrison, J. H. and Hof, P.R. (1997) Life and death of neurons in the aging brain. *Science*, 278: 412–419.

Morstyn, G., Hsu, S.M., Kinsella, T., Gratzner, H., Russo, A. and Mitchell, J.B. (1983) Bromodeoxyuridine in tumors and chromosomes detected with a monoclonal antibody. *J. Clin. Invest.*, 72: 1844–1850.

Mouton, P.R., Pakkenberg, B., Gundersen, H.J. and Price, D.L. (1994) Absolute number and size of pigmented locus coeruleus neurons in young and aged individuals. *J. Chem. Neuroanat.*, 7: 185–190.

Mulders, W.H., West, M.J. and Slomianka, L. (1997) Neuron numbers in the presubiculum, parasubiculum, and entorhinal area of the rat. *J. Comp. Neurol.*, 385: 83–94.

Nairn, J.G., Bedi, K.S, Mayhew, T.M. and Campbell, L.F. (1989) On the number of Purkinje cells in the human cerebellum: unbiased estimates obtained by using the "fractionator". *J. Comp. Neurol.*, 290: 527–532.

Nait-Oumesmar, B., Decker, L., Lachapelle, F., Avelana-Adalid, V., Bachelin, C. and Baron-Van Evercooren, A. (1999) Progenitor cells of the dult mouse subventricular zone proliferate, migrate and differentiate into oligodendrocytes after demyelination. *Eur. J. Neurosci.*, 11: 4357–4366.

Nandy, K. (1981) Morphological changes in the cerebellar cortex of aging Macaca nemestrina. *Neurobiol. Aging*, 2: 61–64.

Navarro, C. and Gonzalo, L.M. (1991) Changes in the human amygdaloid complex due to age. *Rev. Med. Univ. Navarra*, 35: 7–12.

Nielsen, K. and Peters, A. (2000) The effects of aging on the frequency of nerve fibers in rhesus monkey striate cortex. *Neurobiol. Aging*, 21: 621–628.

Noback, C.R. (1967) *The Human Nervous System*. McGraw Hill, New York.

Noctor, S.C., Flint, A.C., Weissman, T.A., Dammerman, R.S. and Kriegstein A.R. (2001) Neurons derived from radial glial cells establish radial units in neocortex. *Nature*, 409: 714–720.

Ohm, T.G., Busch, C. and Bohl, J. (1997) Unbiased estimation of neuronal numbers in the human nucleus coeruleus during aging. *Neurobiol. Aging*, 18: 393–399.

O'Kusky, J. and Colonnier, M. (1982) Postnatal changes in the number of neurons and synapses in the visual cortex (area 17) of the macaque monkey: a stereological analysis in normal and monocularly deprived animals. *J. Comp. Neurol.*, 210: 291–306.

O'Leary, D.D.M. (1993) Adding neurons to the adult mammalian brain. *Proc. Natl. Acad. Sci. USA*, 90: 2101–2102.

Oorschot, D.E. (1996) Total number of neurons in the neostriatal, pallidal, subthalamic, and substantia nigral nuclei of the rat basal ganglia: a stereological study using the Cavalieri and optical disector methods. *J. Comp. Neurol.*, 366: 580–599.

Ordy, J.M., Brizzee, K.R., Kaack, B. and Hansche, J. (1978) Age differences in short-term memory and cell loss in the cortex of the rat. *Gerontology*, 24: 276–285.

Pakkenberg, H., Andersen, B.B., Burns, R.S. and Pakkenberg, B. (1995) A stereological study of substantia nigra in young and old rhesus monkeys. *Brain Res.*, 693: 201–206.

Pakkenberg, H. and Brody, H. (1965) The number of nerve cells in the substantia nigra in paralysis agitans. *Acta Neuropathol. (Berl).*, 5: 320–324.

Pakkenberg, H., Evans, S.M., Moller, A., Braendegaard, H. and Gundersen, H.J.G. (1989) Total number of neurons in human neocortex related to age and sex estimated by way of optical disector. *Acta Stereol.*, 8: 251–256.

Pakkenberg, B. and Gundersen, H.J. (1997) Neocortical neuron number in humans: effect of sex and age. *J. Comp. Neurol.*, 384: 312–320.

Pakkenberg, B., Moller, A., Gundersen, H.J., Mouritzen Dam A. and Pakkenberg, H. (1991) The absolute number of nerve cells in substantia nigra in normal subjects and in patients with Parkinson's disease estimated with an unbiased stereological method. *J. Neurol. Neurosurg. Psychiatry*, 54: 30–33.

Paladino, G. (1893) De la continuation de la nevroglie dans le squelette myelinique des fibres nerveuses et de la constitution pluricellulaire du cylinderaxe. *Arch. Ital. de Biol.*, 19: 26–32.

Palkovits. M., Magyar, P. and Szentagothai, J. (1971a) Quantitative histological analysis of the cerebellar cortex in the cat. I. Number and arrangement in space of the Purkinje cells. *Brain Res.*, 32: 1–13.

Palkovits, M., Magyar, P. and Szentagothai, J. (1971b) Quantitative histological analysis of the cerebellar cortex in the cat. II. Cell numbers and densities in the granular layer. *Brain Res.*, 32: 15–30.

Park, J.J., Tang, Y., Lopez, I. and Ishiyama, A. (2001) Age-related change in the number of neurons in the human vestibular ganglion. *J. Comp. Neurol.*, 431: 437–443.

Peinado, M.A., Martinez, M., Pedrosa, J.A., Quesada, A. and Peinado, J.M. (1993) Quantitative morphological changes in neurons and glia in the frontal lobe of the aging rat. *Anat. Rec.*, 237: 104–108.

Pencea, V., Bingaman, K.D., Freedman, L.J. and Luskin, M.B. (2001a) Neurogenesis in the subventricular zone and rostral migratory stream of the neonatal and adult primate forebrain. *Exp. Neurol.*, 172: 1–16.

Pencea, V., Bingaman K.D., Wiegand, S.J. and Luskin, M.B. (2001b) Infusion of brain-derived neurotrophic factor into the lateral ventricle of the adult rat leads to new neurons in the parenchyma of the striatum, septum, thalamus and hypothalamus. *J. Neuroscience*, 21: 6706–6717.

Peng, M.T. and Hsu, H.K. (1982) No neuron loss from hypothalamic nuclei of old male rats. *Gerontology*, 28: 19–22.

Peng, M.T. and Lee, L.R. (1979) Regional differences of neuron loss of rat brain in old age. *Gerontology*, 25: 205–211.

Perez-Canellas, M.M., Font, E. and Garcia-Verdugo, J.M. (1997) Postnatal neurogenesis in the telencephalon of turtles; evidence for nonradial migration of new neurons from distant proliferative ventricular zones to the olfactory bulb. *Dev. Brain Res.*, 18: 101: 125–137.

Perez-Canellas, M.M. and Garcia-Verdugo, J.M. (1996) Adult neurogenesis in the telencephalon of a lizard: a [3H] thymidine autoradiographic and bromodeoxyuridine immunocytochemical study.. *Dev. Brain Res.*, 18: 93: 49–61.

Perfilieva, E., Risedal, A., Nyberg, J., Johansson, B.B. and Eriksson P.S. (2001) Gender and strain influence on neurogenesis in dentate gyrus of young rats. *J. Cerb. Blood Flow Metab.*, 21: 211–217.

Pesce, C. and Reale, A. (1987) Aging and the nerve cell population of the putamen: a morphometric study. *Clin. Neuropathol.*, 6: 16–18.

Peters, A. (1993) The absence of significant neuronal loss from cerebral cortex with age. *Neurobiol. Aging*, 14: 657–658.

Peters, A., Feldman, M.L. and Vaughan, D.W. (1983) The effect of aging on the neuronal population within area 17 of adult rat cerebral cortex. *Neurobiol Aging*, 4: 273–282.

Peters, A., Leahu, D., Moss, M.B. and McNally, K.J. (1994) The effects of aging on area 46 of the frontal cortex of the rhesus monkey. *Cereb. Cortex*, 4: 621–635.

Peters, A., Morrison, J.H., Rosene, D.L. and Hyman B.T. (1998) Are neurons lost from the primate cerebral cortex during normal aging? *Cereb. Cortex*, 8: 295–300.

Peters, A., Moss, M.B. and Sethares C. (2000) Effects of aging on myelinated nerve fibers in monkey primary visual cortex. *J. Comp. Neurol.*, 419: 364–376.

Peters, A., Nigro, N.J. and McNally, K.J. (1997) A further evaluation of the effect of age on striate cortex of the rhesus monkey. *Neurobiol. Aging*, 18: 29–36.

Peters, A., Rosene, D.L., Moss, M.B., Kemper T.L., Abraham, C.R., Tigges, J. and Albert, M.S. (1996) Neurobiological bases of age-related cognitive decline in the rhesus monkey. *J. Neurophathol. Exp. Neurol.*, 55: 861–874.

Peters, A. and Sethares, C. (1993) Aging and the Meynert cells in rhesus monkey primary visual cortex. *Anat Rec.*, 236: 721–729.

Phinney, A.L., Calhoun, M.E., Wolfer, D.P., Lipp, H.P., Zheng, H. and Jucker, M. (1999) No hippocampal neuron or synaptic bouton loss in learning-impaired aged beta-amyloid precursor protein-null mice. *Neuroscience*, 90: 1207–1216.

Popken, G.J. and Farel, P.B. (1997) Sensory neuron number in neonatal and adult rats estimated by means of stereologic and profile-based methods. *J. Comp. Neurol.*, 386: 8–15.

Price, J.L., Ko, A.I., Wade, M.J., Tsou, S.K., McKeel, D.W. and Morris, J.C. (2001) Neuron number in the entorhinal cortex and CA1 in preclinical Alzheimer disease. *Arch. Neurol.*, 58: 1395–1402.

Quackenbush, L.J., Ngo, H. and Pentney, R.J. (1990) Evidence for nonrandom regression of dendrites of Purkinje neurons during aging. *Neurobiol. Aging*, 11: 111–115.

Rakic, P. (1985) Limits of neurogenesis in primates. *Science*, 227: 1054–1056.

Rakic, P. and Nowakowski, R.S. (1981) The time of origin of neurons in the hippocampal region of the rhesus monkey. *J. Comp. Neurol.*, 196: 99–128.

Ramos, R., Requena, V., Diaz, F., Villena, A., Perez de Vargas, I (1995) Evolution of neuronal density in the ageing thalamic reticular nucleus. *Mech Aging Dev.*, 83: 21–29.

Rapp, P.R., Burwell, R.D. and West, M.J. (1996) Individual differences in aging: implications for stereological studies of neuron loss. *Neurobiol. Aging*, 17: 495–496.

Rapp, P.R. and Gallagher, M. (1996) Preserved neuron number in the hippocampus of aged rats with spatial learning deficits. *Proc. Natl. Acad. Sci. USA*, 93: 9926–9930.

Rasmussen, T., Schliemann, T., Sorensen, J.C., Zimmer, J. and West, M.J. (1996) Memory impaired aged rats: no loss of principal hippocampal and subicular neurons. *Neurobiol. Aging*, 17: 143–147.

Repka, M.X. and Quigley, H.A. (1989) The effect of age on normal human optic nerve fiber number and diameter. *Ophthalmology*, 96: 26–32.

Reynolds., B.A. and Weiss S. (1992) Generation of neurons and astrocytes from isolated cells of the adult mammalian central nervous system. *Science*, 255: 1707–1712.

Riese, W. (1946) The cerebral cortex in the very old human brain. *J. Neuropath. Exp. Neurol.*, 5: 160–164.

Rietze, R., Poulin, P. and Weiss, S. (2000) Mitotically active cells that generate neurons and astrocytes are present in multiple regions of the adult mouse hippocampus. *J. Comp. Neurol.*, 424: 397–408.

Robinson, S.R. and Dreher, B. (1990) The visual pathways of eutherian mammals and marsupials develop according to a common timetable. *Brain Behav Evol.*, 36: 177–195.

Rogers, J., Zornetzer, S.F., Bloom, F.E. and Mervis, R.E. (1984) Senescent microstructural changes in rat cerebellum. *Brain Res.*, 292: 23–32.

Rosene, D.L. (1993) Comparing age-related changes in the basal forebrain and hippocampus of the rhesus monkey. *Neurobiol. Aging*, 14: 669–670.

Sandel, J.H. and Peters, A. (2001) Effects of age on nerve fibers in the rhesus monkey optic nerve. *J. Comp. Neurol.*, 429: 541–553.

Sanderson, K.J. and Wilson, P.M. (1997) Neurogenesis in septum, amygdala and hippocampus in the marsupial brushtailed possum (*Trichosurus vulpecula*). *Rev. Bras. Biol.*, 57: 323–325.

Sapolsky, R.M. (1987) Second generation questions about senescent neuron loss. *Neurobiol. Aging*, 8: 547–548.

Sapolsky, R.M. (1991) Energetics and neuronal death: hibernating bears or starving refugees? *Neurobiol. Aging*, 12: 317–324.

Sartin, J.L. and Lamperti, A.A. (1985) Neuron numbers in hypothalamic nuclei of young, middle-aged and aged male rats. *Experientia*, 41: 109–111.

Satorre, J., Cano, J. and Reinoso-suarez, F. (1985) Stability of the neuronal population of the dorsal lateral geniculate nucleus (LGNd) of aged rats. *Brain Res.*, 339: 375–377.

Schaper, A. (1897) Die fruhesten differenzierungsvorgange im centralnervensystems. *Arch. f. Entw.-Mech. Organ.*, 5: 81–132.

Scharff, C. (2000) Chasing fate and function of new neurons in adult brains. *Curr. Opin. Neurobiol.*, 10: 774–783.

Schlessinger A.R., Cowan, W.M. and Cottlieb, D.I. (1975) An autoradiographic study of the time of origin and the pattern of granule cell migration in the dentate gyrus of the rat. *J. Comp. Neurol.*, 159: 159–176.

Sedgwick, A. (1894) On the inadequacy of the cellular theory of development, and on the early development of nerves, particularly of the third nerve and of the sympathetic in Elasmobranchii. *Quart. J. Micr. Sc., Lond.*, 37: 87–101.

Shankle, W.R., Landing, B.H., Rafii, M.S., Schiano, A., Chen, J.M. and Hara, J. (1998a) Evidence for a postnatal doubling of neuron number in the developing human cerebral cortex between 15 months and 6 years. *J. Theor. Biol.*, 191: 115–140.

Shankle, W.R., Romney, A.K., Landing, B.H. and Hara, J. (1998b) Developmental patterns in the cytoarchitecture of the human cerebral cortex from birth to 6 years examined by correspondence analysis. *Proc. Natl. Acad. Sci. USA*, 95: 4023–4028.

Shankle, W.R., Rafii, M.S., Landing, B.H. and Fallon J.H. (1999) Approximate doubling of numbers of neurons in postnatal human cerebral cortex and in 35 specific cytoarchitectural areas from birth to 72 months. *Pediatr. Dev. Pathol.*, 2: 244–259.

Shariff, G.A. (1953) Cell counts in the primate cerebral cortex. *J. Comp. Neurol.*, 98: 381–400.

Shefer, V.F. (1973) Absolute number of neurons and thickness of the cerebral cortex during aging, senile and vascular dementia, and Pick's and Alzheimer's diseases. *Neurosci. Behav. Physiol.* 6: 319–324.

Shimada, A. (1999) Age-dependent cerebral atrophy and cognitive dysfunction in SAMP10 mice. *Neurobiol. Aging*, 20:125–136.

Shors, T.J., Miesegaes, G., Beylin, A., Zhao, M., Rydel, T. and Gould E. (2001) Neurogenesis in the adult is involved in the formation of trace memories. *Nature*, 410: 372–375.

Sidman, R.L., Miale, I.L. and Feder, N. (1959) Cell proliferation and migration in the primitive ependymal zone; an autoradiographic study of histogenesis in the nervous system. *Exp. Neurol.*, 1: 322–333.

Siddiqi, Z.A. and Peters, A. (1999) The effect of aging on pars compacta of the substantia nigra in rhesus monkey. *J. Neuropathol. Exp. Neurol.*, 58: 903–920.

Sjobeck, M., Dahlen, S. and Englund, E. (1999) Neuronal loss in the brainstem and cerebellum—part of the normal aging process? A morphometric study of the vermis cerebelli and inferior olivary nucleus. *J. Gerontol. A Biol. Sci. Med. Sci.*, 54: B363–368.

Sjobeck, M. and Englund, E. (2001) Alzheimer's disease and the cerebellum: a morphologic study on neuronal and glial changes. *Dement. Geriatr. Cogn. Disord.*, 12: 211–218.

Simic, G., Kostovic, I., Winblad, B. and Bogdanovic, N. (1997) Volume and number of neurons of the human hippocampal formation in normal aging and Alzheimer's disease. *J. Comp. Neurol.*, 379: 482–494.

Smart, I. (1961) The subependymal layer of the mouse brain and its cell production as shown by autography after $[H^3]$-thymidine injection. *J. Comp. Neurol.*, 116: 325–347.

Smith, D.E., Roberts, J., Gage, F.H. and Tuszynski, M.H. (1999) Age-associated neuronal atrophy occurs in the primate brain and is reversible by growth factor gene therapy. *Proc. Natl. Acad. Sci. USA*, 96: 10893–10896.

Smith, M.L. and Booze, R.M. (1995) Cholinergic and GABAergic neurons in the nucleus basalis region of young and aged rats. *Neuroscience*, 67: 679–688.

Smith, M.T., Pencea, V., Wang, Z., Luskin, M.B. and Insel, T.R. (2001) Increased number of BrdU-labeled neurons in the rostral migratory stream of the estrous prairie vole. *Horm. Behav.*, 39: 11–21.

Smolen, A.J., Wright L.L. and Cunningham, T.J. (1983) Neuron numbers in the superior cervical sympathetic ganglion of the rat: a critical comparison of methods for cell counting. *J. Neurocyt.*, 12: 739–750.

Sousa N., Almeida, O.F., Holsboer, F., Paula-Barbosa M.M. and Madeira M.D. (1998) Maintenance of hipocampal cell numbers in young and aged rats submitted to chronic unpredictable stress. Comparison with the effects of corticosterone treatment. *Stress*, 2: 237–249.

Stanfield, B.B. and Trice, J.E. (1988) Evidence, that granule cells generated in the dentate gyrus of adult rats extend axonal projections. *Exp. Brain Res.*, 72: 399–406.

Sterio, D.C. (1984) The unbiased estimation of number and sizes of arbitrary particles using the disector. *J. Microsc.*, 134: 127–136.

Stroessner-Johnson, H.M., Rapp, P.R. and Amaral, D.G. (1992) Cholinergic cell loss and hypertrophy in the medial septal nucleus of the behaviorally characterized aged rhesus monkey. *J. Neurosci.*, 12: 1936–1944.

Sturrock, R.R. (1979) A quantitative lifespan study of changes in cell number, cell division and cell death in various regions of the mouse forebrain. *Neuropath. Appl. Neurobiol.*, 5: 433–456.

Sturrock, R.R. (1986) A quantitative histological study of the indusium griseum and neostriatum of elderly mice. *J. Anat.*, 149: 195–203.

Sturrock, R.R. (1987) Changes in the number of neurons in the mesencephalic and motor nuclei of the trigeminal nerve in the ageing mouse brain. *J. Anat.*, 151: 15–25.

Sturrock, R.R. (1989a) Stability of neuron and glial number in the parabigeminal nucleus of the ageing mouse. *Acta Anat. (Basel).*, 134: 322–326.

Sturrock, R.R. (1989b) Age related changes in neuron number in the mouse lateral vestibular nucleus. *J. Anat.*, 166: 227–232.

Sturrock, R.R. (1989c) A quantitative histological study of the anterodorsal thalamic nucleus and the lateral mammillary nucleus of ageing mouse. *J. Hirnforsch.*, 30: 191–195.

Sturrock, R.R. (1989d) Changes in neuron number in the cerebellar cortex of the ageing mouse. *J. Hirnforsch.*, 30: 499–503.

Sturrock, R.R. (1989e) Loss of neurons from the intracerebellar nuclei of the ageing mouse. *J. Hirnforsch.*, 30: 517–519.

Sturrock, R.R. (1989f) Age related changes in Purkinje cell number in the cerebellar nodulus of the mouse. *J. Hirnforsch.*, 30: 757–760.

Sturrock, R.R. (1990a) Age related changes in neuron number in the mouse red nucleus. *J. Hirnforsch.*, 31: 399–403.

Sturrock, R.R. (1990b) A comparison of quantitative histological changes in different regions of the ageing mouse cerebellum. *J. Hirnforsch.*, 31: 481–486.

Sturrock, R.R.(1990c) Age related changes in neuron number in the combined ventral and lateral pontine nuclei of the mouse. *J. Hirnforsch.*, 31: 811–815.

Sturrock, R.R. (1990d) A quantitative histological study of Golgi II neurons and pale cells in different cerebellar regions of the adult and ageing mouse brain. *Z Mikrosk. Anat. Forsch.*, 104: 705–714.

Sturrock, R.R. (1991a) Stability of neuron number in the subthalamic and entopeduncular nuclei of the ageing mouse brain. *J. Anat.*, 179: 67–73.

Sturrock, R.R. (1991b) Age related changes in neuron number in the tegmental nuclei of Gudden of the mouse. *J. Hirnforsch.*, 32: 89–92.

Sturrock, R.R. (1991c) Variation with age in neuron number in the bed nucleus of the mouse anterior comissure. *J. Hirnforsch.*, 32: 775–777.

Sturrock, R.R. (1993) The effect of ageing on the posterior medial and posterior lateral subnuclei of the bed nucleus of the stria terminalis in the mouse. *Anat. Anz.*, 175: 189–193.

Sturrock, R.R. and Rao, K.A. (1985) A quantitative histological study of neuronal loss from the locus coeruleus of ageing mice. *Neuropathol. Appl. Neurobiol.*, 11: 55–60.

Sugita, N. (1918) Comparative studies on the growth of the cerebral cortex. *J. Comp. Neurol.*, 29: 61–117.

Symons, J.P., Davis, R.E. and Marriott, J.G. (1988) Water-maze learning and effects of cholinergic drugs in mouse strains with high and low hippocampal pyramidal cell counts. *Life Sci.* 42: 375–383.

Szenborn, M. (1993) Neuropathological study on the nucleus basalis of Meynert in mature and old age. *Patol. Pol.*, 44: 211–216.

Tabbaa, S., Dlugos, C. and Pentney, R. (1999) The number of granule cells and spine density on Purkinje cells in aged, ethanol-fed rats. *Alcohol*, 17: 253–260.

Tanapat, P., Hastings, N.B., Reeves, A.J. and Gould, E. (1999) Estrogen stimulates a transient increase in the number of new neurons in the dentate gyrus of the adult female rat. *J. Neurosci.*, 19: 5792–5801.

Temple, S. and Alvarez-Buylla, A.(1999) Stem cells in the adult mammalian central nervous system. *Curr. Opin. Neurobiol.*, 9: 135–141.

Terao, S., Sobue, G., Hashizume, Y., Li, M., Inagaki, T. and Mitsuma, T. (1996) Age-related changes in human spinal ventral horn cells with special reference to the loss of small neurons in the intermediate zone: a quantitative analysis. *Acta Neuropathol. (Berl).*, 92: 109–114.

Terry, R.D., DeTeresa, R. and Hansen, L.A. (1987) Neocortical cell counts in normal human adult aging. *Ann. Neurol.*, 21: 530–539.

Thomaidou, D., Mione, M.C., Cavanagh, J.F.R., and Parnavelas, J.G. (1997) Apoptosis and its relation to the cell cycle in the developing cerebral cortex. *J. Neuroscience*, 17: 1075–1085.

Thompson, H. (1899) The total number of functional nerve cells in the cerebral cortex of man. *J. Comp. Neurol.*, 9: 113–140.

Thune, J.J., Uylings, H.B. and Pakkenberg, B. (2001) No deficit in total number of neurons in the prefrontal cortex in schizophrenics. *J. Psychiatr. Res.*, 35: 15–21.

Tigges, J., Herndon, J.G. and Peters, A. (1990) Neuronal population of area 4 during the life span of the rhesus monkey. *Neurobiol. Aging*, 11: 201–208.

Tinsley, C.J., Bennett, G.W., Mayhew, T.M. and Parker, T.L. (2001) Stereological analysis of regional brain volumes and neuron numbers in rats displaying a spontaneous hydrocephalic condition. *Exp. Neurol.*, 168: 88–95.

Torvik, A., Torp, S. and Lindboe, C.F. (1986) Atrophy of the cerebellar vermis in ageing. A morphometric and histologic study. *J. Neurol. Sci.*, 76: 283–294.

Yuan, H., Goto, N., Akita, H., Shiraishi, N. and He, H.J. (2000) Morphometric analysis of the human cervical motoneurons in the aging process. *Okajimas Folia Anat. Jpn.*, 77: 1–4.

Van Buskirk, C. (1945) The seventh nerve complex. *J. Comp. Neurol.*, 82: 303–333.

Van der Kooy, D. and Weiss, S. (2000) Why stem cells? *Science*, 287: 1439–1441.

Vijayashankar, N. and Brody, H. (1979) A quantitative study of the pigmented neurons in the nuclei locus coeruleus and subcoeruleus in man as related to aging. *J. Neuropathol. Exp. Neurol.*, 38: 490–497.

Vincent, S.L., Peters, A. and Tigges, J. (1989) Effects of aging on the neurons within area 17 of rhesus monkey cerebral cortex. *Anat. Rec.*, 223: 329–341.

Vogel, M.W., Sinclair, M., Qiu, D. and fan, H. (2000) Purkinje cell fate in straggerer mutants: agenesis versus cell death. *J. Neurobiol.*, 42: 323–337.

Voytko, M.L., Sukhov, R.R., Walker, L.C., Breckler, S.J., Price, D.L. and Koliatsos, V.E. (1995) Neuronal number and size are preserved in the nucleus basalis of aged rhesus monkeys. *Dementia*, 6: 131–141.

Weickert, C.S., Webster, M.J., Colvin, S.M., Herman, M.M., Hyde, T.M., Weinberger, D.R. and Kleinman, J.E. (2000) Localization of epidermal growth factor receptors and putative neuroblasts in human subependymal zone. *J. Comp. Neurol.* 423: 359–372.

Weisse, I. (1995) Changes in the aging rat retina. *Ophthal. Res.*, 27: 54–163.

Weis, S., Haug, H. and Budka, H. (1993) Neuronal damage in the cerebral cortex of AIDS brains: a morphometric study. *Acta Neuropathol. (Berl)*, 85: 185–189.

Weiss, S., Dunne, C., Hewson, J., Wohl, C., Wheatley, M., Peterson, A.C. and Reynolds, B.A. (1996) Multipotent CNS stem cells are present in the adult mammalian spinal cord and ventricular neuraxis. *J. Neurosci.* 16: 7599–7609.

Wenk, G.L. and Willard, L.B. (1998) The neural mechanisms underlying cholinergic cell death within the basal forebrain. Int. *J. Dev. Neurosci.*, 16: 729–735.

West, M.J. (1993) Regionally specific loss of neurons in the aging human hippocampus. *Neurobiol. Aging*, 14: 287–293.

West, M.J. (1999) Stereological methods for estimating the total number of neurons and synapses: issues of precision and bias. *Trends Neurosci.* 22: 51–61.

West, M.J., Coleman, P.D., Flood, D.G. and Troncoso, J.C. (1994) Differences in the pattern of hippocampal neuronal loss in normal aging and Alzheimer's disease. *Lancet*, 344: 769–772.

West, M.J. and Gundersen, H.J. (1990) Unbiased stereological estimation of the number of neurons in the human hippocampus. *J. Comp. Neurol.*, 296: 1–22.

West, M.J., Kawas, C.H., Martin, L.J. and Troncoso, J.C. (2000) The CA1 region of the human hipocampus is a hot spot in Alzheimer's disease. *Ann. N.Y. Acad. Sci.*, 908: 255–259.

West, M.J. and Slomianka, L. (1998) Total number of neurons in the layers of the human entorhinal cortex. *Hippocampus*, 8: 69–82.

West, M.J., Slomianka, L. and Gundersen, H.J. (1991) Unbiased stereological estimation of the number of neurons in the subdivision of the hippocampus using the optical fractionator. *Anat. Rec.*, 231: 482–497.

Williams, R.W., Strom, R.C., Rice, D.S. and Goldowitz, D. (1996) Genetic and enviromental control of variation in retinal ganglion cell number in mice. *J. Neurosci.*, 16: 7193–7205.

Wimer, R.E. and Wimer, C.C. (1982) A biometrical-genetic analysis of granule cell number in the area dentata of house mice. *Devel. Brain Res.*, 2: 129–140.

Wimer, R.E., Wimer, C.C. and Alameddine, L. (1988) On the development of strain and sex differences in granule cell number in the area dentata of house mice. *Dev. Brain Res.*, 42: 191–197.

Wimer, R.E., Wimer, C.C., Chernow, C.R. and Balvanz, B.A. (1980) The genetic organization of neuron number in the pyramidal cell layer of hippocampal regio superior in house mice. *Brain Res.*, 196: 59–77.

Wimer, R.E, Wimer, C.C., Vaughn, J.E., Barber, R.P., Balvanz, B.A. and Chernow, C.R. (1976) The genetic organization of neuron number in Ammon's horns of house mice. *Brain Res.*, 118: 219–243.

Wimer, R.E., Wimer, C.C., Vaughn, J.E., Barber, R.P., Balvanz, B.A. and Chernow, C.R. (1978) The genetic organization of neuron number in the granule cell layer of the area dentata in house mice. *Brain Res.*, 157: 105–122.

Wree, A., Braak, H., Schleicher, A. and Zilles, K. (1980) Biomathematical analysis of the neuronal loss in the aging human brain of both sexes, demonstrated in pigment preparations of the pars cerebellaris loci coerulei. *Anat. Embryol (Berl)*, 160: 105–119.

Wyss, J.M. and Srinipanidkulchai, B. (1985) The development of Ammon's horn and the fascia dentata in the cat: a [³H] thymidine analysis. *Brain Res.*, 350: 185–198.

Yanai, J. (1979) Strain and sex differences in the adult brain. *Acta Anat.*, 103: 150–158.

Yuan, H., Goto, N., Akita, H. Shiraishi, N. and He, H.J. (2000) Morphometric analysis of the human cervical motoneurons in the aging process. *Okajimas Folia Anat. Jpn.*, 77: 1–4.

Zhang, C., Goto, N., Suzuki, M. and Ke, M. (1996) Age-related reductions in number and size of anterior horn cells at C6 level of the human spinal cord. *Okajimas Folia Anat. Jpn.*, 73: 171–177.

Zhang, R.L., Zhang, Z.G., Zhang, L. and Chopp, M. (2001) Proliferation and differentiation of progenitor cells in the cortex and subventricular zone in the adult rat after focal cerebral ischemia. *Neuroscience*, 105: 33–41.

Zoli, M., Ferraguti, F., Toffano, G., Fuxe K. and Agnati, L.F. (1993) Neurochemical alterations but not nerve cell loss in aged rat neostriatum. *J. Chem. Neuroanat.*, 6: 131–145.

E.C. Azmitia, J. DeFelipe, E.G. Jones, P. Rakic and C.E. Ribak (Eds.)
Progress in Brain Research, Vol. 136

CHAPTER 5

Interkinetic nuclear movement in the vertebrate neuroepithelium: encounters with an old acquaintance

José María Frade*

Instituto Cajal (CSIC), Avenida del Doctor Arce 37, 28002 Madrid, Spain

Abstract: The vertebrate neuroepithelium is a highly efficient structure with respect to the process of neurogenesis. The orthogonal arrangement of the nuclei with respect to the surface of the epithelium facilitates the dramatic increase in cell density necessary to produce a high number of neurons. Moreover, the spatial organization of the neuroepithelium reflects the segregation of cells that are transiently embarked upon distinct functions, thereby avoiding any interference between these populations in terms of their physiological activities. Two main regions can be distinguished: an apical *neurogenetic zone*, where lateral inhibitory signals and neurogenic gene expression can be observed, and a basally located *pre-neurogenetic zone*, which contains cells replicating their DNA and able to receive the signals that will modify their fate.

Introduction

The vertebrate neuroepithelium initially appears to be a pseudostratified tissue wherein the interphase nuclei are scattered across virtuallly its whole thickness and mitotic figures are restricted to the region that lines the lumen. During the working life of Santiago Ramón y Cajal, it was difficult to correctly interpret this structure since the only approaches available to study the neuroepithelium were based on microscopic techniques. Thus, the conclusions drawn by Cajal from his studies using the Golgi method, essentially agreed with the initial descriptions made by Wilhelm His (Cajal, 1909). Both considered neuroepithelial cells to be of one of two types. Either they were mitotically active germinal cells, neuronal precursors that are located close to the lumen of the neural tube, or they were spongioblasts whose processes span the whole thickness of the neuroepithelium and that can be considered to be glial precursors (His, 1889). According to His, germinal cells divide repeatedly,

*Corresponding author: Tel.: +34 91 585 4740; Fax: +34 91 585 4754; E-mail: frade@cajal.csic.es

giving rise to one daughter cell that remains close to the lumen and re-enters the mitotic cycle, and another daughter cell that becomes a neuroblast. The first morphologist to realize that both cell types might represent alternative stages in the mitotic cycle of the same cell was Alfred Schaper, who suggested that germinal cells might be spongioblasts that have moved closer to the lumen during mitosis (Schaper, 1897). Unfortunately, his work was ignored for some decades until F. C. Sauer again proposed the existence of interkinetic nuclear movement (also referred to as intermitotic nuclear migration; INM) in the vertebrate neuroepithelium (Sauer, 1935). Sauer based his argument on the correlation between the size and histological appearance of the nuclei in the neural tube of pig and chick embryos in relation to their distance from the lumen. This was only circumstantial evidence for the existence of INM, and unequivocal evidence took over two decades to arrive. In 1956, Watterson and collaborators, used colchicine to inhibit mitosis in the chick neural tube and observed an increase in the number of cells that were arrested in metaphase close to the lumen (Watterson et al., 1956). These observations were later confirmed by

Källén (1962), and by Langman et al. (1966), who used vincristine sulphate to inhibit mitosis. These experiments clearly showed that all cells at any level in the neural epithelium could undergo mitosis once they had displaced their nuclei to the luminal surface. Finally, two independent experimental approaches provided unequivocal proof of the existence of INM. On the one hand, cytophotometric measurements were made of the DNA content of nuclei located at different positions in the neuroepithelium (Sauer and Chittenden, 1959). Meanwhile, the second approach involved the labelling of nuclei with ^{3}[H]-thymidine and determining their position in the neuroepithelium at distinct time points after labelling (Sauer and Walker, 1959).

The confirmation that INM occurs raises a number of questions as those concerning the mechanisms and the significance of this to-and-fro movement of the nuclei. In the following sections, we will summarize some recent work revealing novel aspects of this particular nuclear behavior.

Molecular mechanism of the INM

As in other columnar epithelia, neuroepithelial cells are known to attach to each other at their apical domain by means of classical adherens junctions (Chen et al., 1998). This fact was observed by Sauer (Sauer, 1935), who described the existence of terminal "bars" at the free surface of the neuroepithelial cells that constitute the neural plate. He suggested that "the migration of the inter-kinetic nucleus to the lumen is associated with the facts that the cells acquire a rounded shape in mitosis, and that they are attached to each other at the lumen by terminal bars. A cell that is to change from a columnar to a rounded form, and at the same time to maintain its attachment to the terminal bar net, must obviously move the mass of its cytoplasm, together with the nucleus, to the region of the lumen". This interpretation still can be considered correct in light of our current knowledge regarding the cellular and molecular basis of INM.

Adherens junctions are anchored to a scaffold of microtubules that are involved in the nuclear migration by means of an apical ring of actin microfilaments (Messier, 1978; Chen et al., 1998). This ring has been shown to be crucial for the process of INM as cytochalasin B, a drug that disrupts contractile microfilaments, blocks nuclear migration (Karfunkel, 1972; Messier and

Auclair, 1974; Webster and Langman, 1978). Once the nucleus reaches the apical surface, the cell rounds up in preparation for mitosis. At this point, microtubules lose their apico-basal orientation and the apical microfilament ring relaxes to allow a broadening of the luminal surface (Nagele and Lee, 1979).

These cytological observations of the change from a fusiform to a round shape in neuroepithelial cells entering mitosis have been further adorned with information regarding the molecular changes that occur. Neuroepithelial cells have been shown to acquire a round shape in the presence of lysophosphatidic acid (LPA; Fukushima et al., 2000). LPA is a phospholipid that mediates diverse cellular responses, including the formation of stress fibers and cell rounding through mechanisms involving Rho and Rho-associated kinase. The action of LPA is mediated by the receptor named lpA1, previously isolated as a novel G-protein-coupled receptor that is highly expressed by neuroepithelial cells at the ventricular zone (Chun and Jaenisch, 1996; Hecht et al., 1996). Interestingly, LPA is predominantly produced by postmitotic neurons. Thus, it is possible that the signals that initiate the changes in shape of neuroepithelial cells could well emanate from these postmitotic neurons located beneath the basal membrane of the neuroepithelium (Fig. 1).

Functional implications of the INM

Not much is known about the reasons why vertebrates have adopted such a high energy-consuming way of organizing their neuroepithelia based on the to-and-fro nuclear movement. Some authors have speculated that INM might help to facilitate the invagination of the neural plate during neurulation. They argue that INM results in the accumulation of nuclei at the basal zone of the neuroepithelium and that this could help to generate the force involved in the bending of the neural plate (Langman et al., 1966; Messier, 1978).

INM and neurogenesis

INM might also represent the vertebrate solution to the problem of increasing the density of precursor cells whilst maintaining adherens junctions during mitosis (see above). Having such a large number of precursors probably facilitates the high rate of neuronal production that is crucial to build up a vertebrate brain within which the

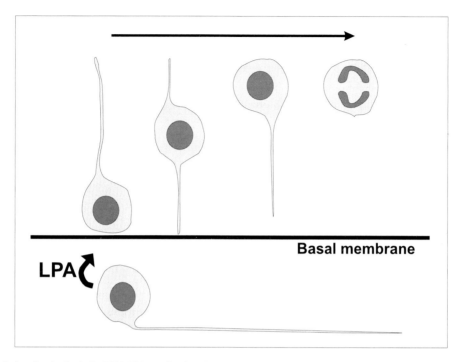

Fig. 1. Hypothetical molecular basis for INM. LPA, predominantly produced by post-mitotic neurons, is able to interact with its receptor LpA1, located on the surface of the neuroepithelial cells. Once activated, this receptor is able to transduce signals that result in the changes in precursor morphology, whereby the precursor adopts a round shape in preparation for mitosis. Modified from Fukushima et al. (2000).

cells are unable to proliferate once they have left the neuroepithelium. In accordance with this idea, some areas of the vertebrate neuroepithelium with limited neurogenic capacity present a low proliferation rate and absence of INM. This is the case at the boundaries between the rhombomeres in the chick embryo where INM has been shown to be reduced or absent (Guthrie et al., 1991).

Recently, it has been pointed out that the capacity of neuronal precursors to respond to environmental signals changes as they progress through the cell cycle. Thus, neural precursors can modify their fate in response to the signals in older developmental environments if grafted, or cultured, during S-phase, but not during G2/M/G1 (McConnell and Kaznowski, 1991; Belliveau and Cepko, 1999). Indeed, neurogenic genes such as *Notch1* and *Delta1*, and proneural determination genes such as *Ngn2* start to be expressed more intensely when chick neuroepithelial cells enter G2/M (Murciano et al., 2001), an observation that may explain the loss of plasticity observed in these stages of the mitotic cycle.

As a consequence of INM, the cyclic changes that neuroepithelial cells undergo are reflected in the segregation of the neuroepithelium into discrete specialized regions (Fig. 2). Thus, for instance, Notch1 expression is particularly enhanced in the apical zone, thus restricting the influence of lateral inhibitory signals to this area (Murciano et al., 2001). This emphasizes the importance of the three-dimensional structure of the neuroepithelium with respect to efficient neuronal production. As such, in the absence of INM, one would expect a higher degree of interaction between cells with the capacity to express proneural and neurogenic genes with those lacking such a property. The resulting decrease in lateral inhibition would lead to an increase of neurogenesis and the depletion of neuroepithelial cells, finally resulting in a decrease in neuronal production (Murciano et al., 2001).

Another consequence of their segregation into specific regions within the neuroepithelium is that precursors in S-phase with the capacity to sense environmental signals (McConnell and Kaznowski, 1991; Belliveau and Cepko, 1999) concentrate in the basal region of the neuroepithelium (Fig. 2). In this region, they would have complete access to instructive signals released by differentiating neurons located adjacent to the neuroepithelium. This is

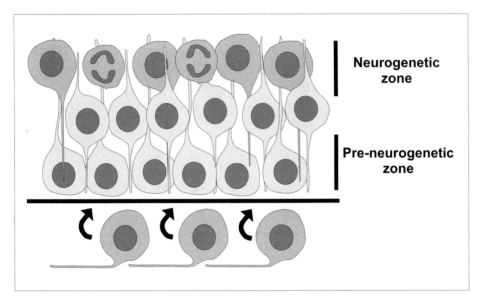

Fig. 2. Scheme representing the functional organization of the neuroepithelium in terms of neurogenesis. The orthogonal arrangement of the oscillating nuclei is translated into the segregation of two zones each made up of precursors that are transiently involved in distinct functions. In the apical region (neurogenic zone), proliferating cells express proneural and neurogenic genes (dark grey), are subjected to lateral inhibition, and are refractive to environmental signals able to alter their potential cell fate. In the basal region (Pre-neurogenic zone), precursors are undergoing DNA synthesis while they are receptive to environmental signals, likely to be released from post-mitotic neurons (arrows), that can modulate their cell fate, perhaps by selecting a new combination of proneural genes as they enter G2.

probably the case in the retina of the chick embryo, where mature retinal ganglion cells can release factors that inhibit their own production (González-Hoyuela et al., 2001; Zhang and Yang, 2001).

INM and the local synchronization of precursors

Across the animal kingdom, neurogenesis has frequently been shown to be associated with synchronized waves of cell cycle progression, the reasons for this remaining obscure. Thus, in the Drosophila embryo, the process of singling out of neuroblasts is preceded by a block in the cell cycle at G2 (Hartenstein et al., 1994). In anamniotes, primary neurons that withdraw from the mitotic cycle before the pseudostratified neuroepithelium is fully differentiated (Hartenstein, 1989, 1993) are born during a wave of mitosis that sweeps over the neural plate in a lateral to medial direction (Hartenstein, 1989). These strategies are characterized by the existence of long periods in which neurons are not born, which in the case of Drosophila is counterbalanced by the proliferative

capacity of the neuroblasts. One singularity of employing INM in the vertebrate neuroepithelium is that the continuous production of neurons can be maintained whilst ensuring that precursors embark upon the differentiation pathway only in G2/mitosis, a prerequisite that seems to be a constant in the neuronal production across the animal kingdom. This has surely led to a greater efficiency in terms of neurogenesis.

Acknowledgments

The author is grateful to Mark Sefton for grammatical corrections of the manuscript.

References

Belliveau, M.J. and Cepko, C.L. (1999) Extrinsic and intrinsic factors control the genesis of amacrine and cone cells in the rat retina. *Development*, 126: 555–566.

Cajal, S.R. (1909) *Histologie du système nerveux de l'homme et des vertebrés*. Reprinted by Consejo Superior de Investigaciones Científicas, Instituto Ramón y Cajal, 1952–1955.

Chen, A., Zhang, Y.A., Chang, B.T. and McConnell, S.K. (1998) Intrinsic polarity of mammalian neuroepithelial cells. *Mol. Cell Neurosci.*, 11: 183–193.

Chun, J. and Jaenish, R. (1996) Clonal cell lines produced by infection of neocortical neuroblasts using multiple oncogenes transduced by retroviruses. *Mol. Cell. Neurosci.*, 7, 304–321.

Fukushima, N., Weiner, J.A. and Chun, J. (2000) Lysophosphatidic acid (LPA) is a novel extracellular regulator of cortical neuroblast morphology. *Dev. Biol.*, 228: 6–18.

González-Hoyuela, M., Barbas, J.A. and Rodríguez-Tébar, A. (2001) The autoregulation of retinal ganglion cell number. *Development*, 128: 117–124.

Guthrie, S., Butcher, M. and Lumsden, A. (1991) Patterns of cell division and interkinetic nuclear migration in the chick embryo hindbrain. *J. Neurobiol.*, 22: 742–754.

Hartenstein, V. (1989) Early neurogenesis in Xenopus : the spatio-temporal pattern of proliferation and cell lineages in the embryonic spinal cord. *Neuron*, 3: 399–411.

Hartenstein, V. (1993) Early pattern of neuronal differentiation in the Xenopus embryonic brainstem and spinal cord. *J. Comp. Neurol.*, 328: 213–231.

Hartenstein, V., Yonoussi-Hartenstein, A. and Lekven, A. (1994) Delamination and division in the Drosophila neurectoderm: spatiotemporal pattern, cytoskeletal dynamics, and common control by neurogenic and segment polarity genes. *Dev. Biol.*, 165: 480–499.

Hecht, J.H., Weiner, J.A., Post, S.R. and Chun, J. (1996) Ventricular zone gene-1 (vzg-1) encodes a lysophosphatidic acid receptor expressed in neurogenic regions of the developing cerebral cortex. *J. Cell. Biol.*, 135: 1071–1083.

His, W (1889) Die Neuroblasten und deren Entstehung im embryonalen Mark. *Abh. d. Math.-physisc. Klasse d. k., Sächs. Ges. d. Wissen.*, 15: 313–372.

Källén, B. (1962) Mitotic patterning in the central nervous system of chick embryos studied by a colchicine method. *Z. Anat. Entwicklungsgeschichte.*, 123: 309–319.

Karfunkel, P. (1972) The activity of microtubules and microfilaments in neurulation in the chick. *J. Exp. Zool.*, 181: 289–302.

Langman, J., Guerrant, R.L. and Freeman B.G. (1966) Behaviour of neuroepithelial cells during closure of the neural tube. *J. Comp. Neurol.*, 127: 399–410.

Messier P.-E. and Auclair C. (1974) Effect of cytochalasin B on interkinetic nuclear migration in the chick embryo. *Dev. Biol.*, 36: 218–223.

McConnell, S.K. and Kaznowski, C.E. (1991) Cell cycle dependence of laminar determination in developing neocortex. *Science*, 254: 282–285.

Messier, P.-E. (1978) Microtubules, interkinetic nuclear migration and neurulation. *Experientia*, 34: 289–296.

Murciano, A., Zamora, J., López-Sánchez, J. and Frade, J.M. (2001) Interkinetic nuclear movement provides spatial clues for the regulation of neurogenesis. *Int. J. Dev. Biol.*, 45 (Suppl. 1): S172.

Nagele, R.G. and Lee H.Y. (1979) Ultrastructural changes in cells associated with interkinetic nuclear migration in the developing chick epithelium. *J. Exp. Zool.*, 210: 89–106.

Sauer, F.C. (1935) Mitosis in the neural tube. *J. Comp. Neurol.*, 62: 377–405.

Sauer, M.E. and Chittenden, A.C. (1959) Deoxyribonucleic acid content of cell nuclei in the neural tube of the chick embryo: evidence for intermitotic migration of nuclei. *Exp. Cell Res.*, 16: 1–6.

Sauer, M.E. and Walker, B.E. (1959) Radioautographic study of interkinetic nuclear migration in the neural tube. *Proc. Soc. Exp. Biol. Med.*, 101: 557–560.

Schaper, A. (1897) The earliest differentiation in the central nervous system of the vertebrates. *Science*, 5: 430–431.

Watterson, R.L., Veneziano, P. and Bartha, A. (1956) Absence of a true germinal zone in neural tubes of young chick embryos as demonstrated by the colchicine technique. *Anat. Rec.*, 124: 379.

Webster, W. and Langman, J. (1978) The effect of cytochalasin B on the neuroepithelial cells of the mouse embryo. *Am. J. Anat.*, 152: 209–221.

Zhang, X.M. and Yang, X.J. (2001) Regulation of retinal ganglion cell production by Sonic hedgehog. *Development*, 128: 943–957.

E.C. Azmitia, J. DeFelipe, E.G. Jones, P. Rakic and C.E. Ribak (Eds.)
Progress in Brain Research, Vol. 136

CHAPTER 6

The origin and migration of cortical neurons

John G. Parnavelas*, Pavlos Alifragis and Bagirathy Nadarajah

Department of Anatomy and Developmental Biology, University College London, London WC1E 6BT, UK

Introduction

The structure of the mammalian cerebral cortex captured the interest of Santiago Cajal more than any other part of the brain (Cajal, 1911). Cajal also devoted considerable effort in the study of the histogenesis of the cortex and in the growth and differentiation of its cellular elements (Cajal, 1960). The cerebral cortex develops from the rostral dorsal part of the neural tube named the telencephalic pallium. The wall of the pallium is at first formed of neuroepithelial germinal cells whose continued proliferation causes the outward bulging of the pallial walls to form the cerebral vesicles. The radial alignment of the neuroepithelial cells imposes a radial pattern on histogenesis of the pallium. This early radial organization is progressively distorted by the generation and growth of neurons and glial cells and by the formation of the afferent and efferent connections that impose a horizontal lamination on the radial pattern. The conventional scheme of cortical formation depicted in Fig. 1 (Boulder Committee, 1970; Uylings et al., 1990), shows that early postmitotic neurons migrate away from the germinal ventricular zone (VZ) towards the surface of the cerebral vesicles to form the primordial plexiform layer or preplate (PP). The later-generated neurons migrate to form a layer within the PP, the so-called cortical plate (CP), thus splitting it into a superficial marginal zone (MZ; layer I) and a deep subplate (SP). The neurons of the CP assemble into

---
*Corresponding author: Tel.: +44 20 7679-3366;
Fax: +44 20 7679-7349; E-mail: j.parnavelas@ucl.ac.uk

layers II–VI in an 'inside-out' sequence and show regional differences of time of origin. Both the MZ and SP contain the earliest generated neurons of the cerebral cortex. Those in layer I differentiate as Cajal-Retzius cells and other types of neurons that have not yet been fully characterized (Bradford et al., 1977; Meyer et al., 1999). The SP is separated from the VZ by the intermediate zone (IZ), a layer that will eventually contain the afferent and efferent axonal tracts of the cortex (future white matter). As the CP emerges, another layer of proliferating cells appears between the VZ and IZ, the so-called subventricular zone (SVZ). This germinal zone contains cells, produced in the VZ, that mainly give rise to glia. The SVZ expands greatly in late gestation and in early postnatal life as the VZ disappears.

Development of neuronal lineages

All areas of the cortex contain two broad classes of neurons, the pyramidal and nonpyramidal cells, in approximately the same proportions (Rockel et al., 1980). These neurons show characteristic morphological (Szentágothai, 1973), neurochemical (Parnavelas et al., 1989) and functional (Gilbert, 1983) properties. The pyramidal cells, which are defined by the shape of their cell bodies and by the strict pattern of their dendritic arborization, are the projection neurons of the cortex which use the excitatory amino acid, glutamate, as a neurotransmitter. Nonpyramidal cells, the cortical interneurons, are a much more diverse group of cells that display a range of morphologies and molecular identities

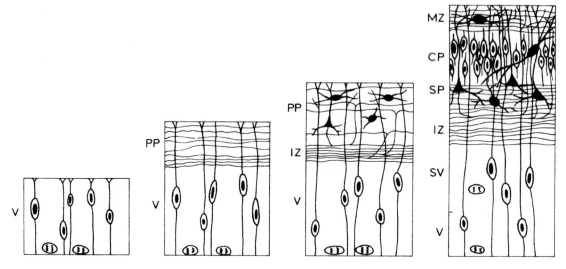

Fig.1. Four panels illustrate the layers of the cerebral wall at different stages of development. VZ, ventricular zone; PP, preplate; IZ, intermediate zone; MZ, marginal zone; CP, cortical plate; SP, subplate; SV, subventricular zone.

(Fairén et al., 1984; Naegele and Barnstable, 1989). They all contain the inhibitory neurotransmitter GABA, and also one or more neuropeptides (Parnavelas et al., 1989).

At what point do undifferentiated cells in the VZ commit themselves to become pyramidal or nonpyramidal in form? Such knowledge would facilitate our efforts to understand the mechanisms that control the development of these neuronal cell classes, as is possible for individual cells in simpler systems. The study of cell lineages in the cerebral cortex has become possible with the use of recombinant retroviruses (Sanes et al., 1986; Price et al., 1987). The advantage of this technique is that by infecting single progenitor cells with virus, a marker gene is introduced into them that can be inherited undiluted by all their progeny. Therefore, the expression of the marker gene provides a histochemically detectable label of infected clones. One example is the *lacZ* gene that encodes for β-galactosidase, a bacterial enzyme that acts on 5-bromo-4-chloro-3-indolyl-β-D-galactopyranoside (X-gal) to produce a blue color in the cell. More recently, alkaline phosphatase has been used as a histochemical marker (Reid et al., 1995).

Earlier lineage studies, using predominantly the BAG retrovirus, observed single labeled cells or discrete clusters of two or more neurons in the cerebral cortex following intraventricular injections at any day of gestation during cortical neurogenesis in rats and mice (Luskin et al., 1988; Price and Thurlow, 1988). The clones of two or more cells contained for the most part either neurons or glial cells, a finding that was confirmed in dissociated cell cultures (Luskin et al., 1988; Price et al., 1992). When neuronal clones were examined further with electron microscopy or immunohistochemistry, it was found that they were nearly all homogeneous, composed of all pyramidal or all nonpyramidal cells (Parnavelas et al., 1991; Luskin et al., 1993; Mione et al., 1994). These early observations suggested that the VZ, the germinal layer of the embryonic cortex, may be viewed as a mosaic of progenitor cells each with a different restricted potential.

Further examination of clonally related neurons from brains injected with retrovirus at different stages of corticogenesis revealed remarkable differences in the number and laminar distribution of pyramidal and nonpyramidal neurons injected with retrovirus. Nonpyramidal cells appeared either as single cells or as clones of two neurons present in the same or in adjacent layers. Clones of pyramidal neurons were larger, and they were either dispersed in one layer or in several layers following earlier injections. Their size and laminar distribution was progressively reduced following later injections (Luskin et al., 1993). This finding suggested the existence of different mechanisms that generate the two main neuronal types of the cerebral cortex. More recent lineage analyses have utilized libraries of retroviral vectors carrying a large number of DNA tags, each of which can be distinguished by the polymerase chain reaction (Walsh and Cepko, 1992). These studies have shown that not all clonally related cells maintain the spatial relationship that they had before migration (Walsh and Cepko, 1993), but it is noteworthy that those that do invariably show the same phenotype (Reid et al., 1995).

The more recent use of a retroviral marker in combination with bromodeoxyuridine (BrdU) has shown that only pyramidal neurons maintain a close spatial relationship with their clonal relatives in the developing cortex, which can be achieved through radial migration (Mione et al., 1997). In contrast, labeled nonpyramidal cells were found, in agreement with earlier lineage analyses, as isolated cells or pairs of clonally related neurons. Their low content of BrdU indicated that these cells were part of larger clones, and suggested that their isolation was the result of non-radial (tangential) migration. These findings pose two alternative interpretations: either clonally related cells, instructed to develop a particular phenotype, are also endowed with the ability to use a specific migratory pathway, or cues encountered during radial and tangential migration are responsible for the pyramidal and nonpyramidal phenotypes. Experiments by Tan et al. (1998) have provided evidence for the former possibility with regard to the generation and migration of pyramidal neurons. Using highly unbalanced mouse embryonic stem cell chimeras, these authors found that radially dispersed neurons contained glutamate, the marker of pyramidal neurons, whereas tangentially dispersed cells were predominantly GABAergic. Their study has also demonstrated that specification of the pyramidal lineage occurs at the level of the progenitor, before the onset of neurogenesis.

Our understanding of the origin and development of nonpyramidal cell lineages is not as clear. The studies of Mione et al. (1997) have suggested that nonpyramidal cells, scattered in the cortex as isolated neurons or pairs of clonally related cells, were part of larger clones. This raised the question of whether there exist in the cortical VZ progenitors committed to producing only nonpyramidal cells. The analysis of chimeric mice by Tan and colleagues (1998) raised the same question, and concluded that whether these neurons are generated from progenitors with single or mixed potential, they have the tendency to be diffusely scattered in the cortex. We suggest that the dispersed sibling cells described in the lineage studies of Walsh and Cepko (1993) were indeed nonpyramidal types, as were the neurons found to

migrate tangentially in the developing cortex after they were labeled with a fluorescent marker in the VZ (O'Rourke et al., 1995). The presence in the cortex of a relatively small number of nonpyramidal neurons compared with the often very large pyramidal clones suggests that there are other potential sources of nonpyramidal neurons.

Radial migration of pyramidal neurons

Neuronal migration begins when the first cohort of postmitotic neurons leaves the VZ to form the PP at the margin of the cerebral wall. How do cortical neurons migrate to their destinations? The migration of young neurons to their positions in many regions of the developing brain is largely dependent on radial glia. Serial-section electron microscopy of fetal monkey neocortex has shown that migrating neurons are closely apposed to radial glial fibers, suggesting that these specialized glia provide the substrate for their migration (Rakic 1972, 1974). It should be mentioned that the geometric arrangement of radial glial cells had prompted Cajal to imply long before that these cells serve as scaffolding in the rapidly changing embryonic nervous system and direct neurons during their migration. A number of adhesive molecules and receptors have been implicated in glia-directed migration of cortical neurons. These include the neuronal proteins astrotactin, neuregulin (Anton et al., 1997) and its receptor erB4 (Rio et al., 1997), as well as components of the extracellular matrix such as tenascin (for review, see Hatten, 1999).

Prior to the demonstration of glial-aided neuronal migration, Morest (1970) using Golgi stained fetal opossum tissue, described 'perikaryal translocation' as the mode by which young cortical neurons migrate to their destinations. In support of Morest's observations, a recent study has identified early neuronal populations in the developing rodent cortex with morphological features that closely resemble cells undergoing perikaryal or somal translocation (Brittis et al., 1995). However, it was real-time imaging experiments in acute cortical slices which demonstrated that somal translocation and glial-guided locomotion are indeed two distinct modes of radial neuronal migration in the developing rodent cortex (Nadarajah et al., 2001). Translocating cells typically have distinct morphological features with long radially oriented processes terminating at the pial surface and a short transient trailing process. Time-lapse imaging has demonstrated that as the soma translocates towards the pial surface, the leading process becomes thicker and progressively shorter, while its terminal remains attached to the pial surface. A distinct feature of cells undergoing somal translocation is their continuous advancement, resulting in faster average speeds of movement (60 µm/h). By contrast, glial-guided locomoting cells have a freely motile leading process that maintains a relatively constant length as the cell migrates forward. Further, these cells show a characteristic saltatory pattern of migration—short bursts of forward movements interspersed with stationary phases, resulting in slower average speeds (35 µm/h). Since long-range translocation is prevalent during early corticogenesis, it has been suggested that at this stage, when the cortical anlage is thin, neurons might use somal translocation to reach their final positions. Interestingly, glial-guided cells have been shown to switch to translocation in the terminal phase of their movement once their leading process reaches the MZ. These observations indicate that somal translocation is temporally regulated, and that neurons generated in the cortical VZ may utilize both somal translocation and glial guidance in their radial ascent towards the developing CP.

Studies of mutant mice with migration defects have led to the discovery of molecules that are involved in controling the developmental events that occur at the end of migration. Best-known of these mutants is reeler (Caviness and Rakic, 1978). In these animals, cell proliferation and the early phase of cell migration are normal, but the PP does not split into the MZ and the SP as the migration of the CP neurons is impeded. Neurons of the CP accumulate beneath the undivided PP, which has been termed 'superplate' in these mutants. Also, the layers of the CP are formed in the opposite order to normal, with superficial layers being generated first and the deep parts later. The *reeler* gene has recently been identified. It encodes a large extracellular matrix-like protein, called reelin, that is secreted by the Cajal-Retzius cells of the PP (Ogawa et al., 1995; Curran and D'Arcangelo, 1998). Through reelin, Cajal-Retzius cells positioned strategically in the MZ are believed to control cell–cell interactions and cell positioning in the developing cortex (D'Arcangelo et al., 1995; Curran and D'Arcangelo, 1998). Recent studies (Trommsdorff et al., 1999) have suggested that cell-surface receptors, known as very-low-density-lipoprotein receptor and

apolipoprotein-E receptror 2, together with members of cadherin-related neuronal receptor family (Senzaki et al., 1999) have been identified as likely receptors for reelin. They are essential components of a signaling pathway that mediates the transmission of the reelin signal across the plasma membrane to intracellular kinases that regulate neuronal migration.

Following the discovery of reelin, considerable progress has been made in identifying the downstream signaling components. One member of the reelin signaling pathway is *mDabl* (Gonzalez et al., 1997; Howell et al., 1997; Sheldon et al., 1997). *mDabl* encodes a cytoplasmic protein in CP neurons that is likely to function as an adapter molecule by binding to non-receptor tyrosine kinases, including Abl and Fyn. Defects in cortical lamination have also been identified in mutant mice that lack the cyclin-dependent kinase 5 (Cdk5; Gilmore et al., 1998), a brain-specific kinase, and its neuronal specific activator p35 (Chae et al., 1997). It remains to be shown whether Cdk5 /p35 are involved in the reelin signaling cascade, although more recent studies have indicated a possible interaction of these proteins with cell adhesion molecules (Kwon et al., 2000). Other genes that have been associated with the directed migration of neurons from the VZ, and known to cause migrational anomalies in humans, are *filamin 1* (*FLN*1; Fox et al., 1998), *doublecortin* (*DCX*; Gleeson et al., 1999) and *LIS1* (Hirotsune et al., 1998). It seems that while the molecular mechanisms underlying the glia-guided migration are currently being unraveled, the molecular events associated with somal translocation are largely unknown. Interestingly, a feature consistently noted in all mutant mice with cortical malformations is the normal development of the PP, whereas the subsequent layers are aberrantly formed. A plausible interpretation would be that during early corticogenesis, when the cortical anlage is thin, neurons may move by long-range somal translocation, a mode of migration that might be independent of reelin and associated downstream signaling cascades.

Nonpyramidal neurons: origin and tangential migration

Sources of neurons destined for the cerebral cortex have been discovered in the ganglionic eminence, the primordium of the basal ganglia in the ventral telencephalon or subpallium. Porteus et al. (1994) first reported that cells expressing *Dlx2* appear to migrate from the ventral telencephalon to the neocortex. Subsequently, De Carlos et al. (1996) and Tamamaki et al. (1997) provided unequivocal evidence that cells in the lateral ganglionic eminence (LGE), the primordium of the striatum, migrate into the developing neocortex, and are distributed predominantly in the IZ. More recently, a number of tracing studies (Anderson et al., 1997; Lavdas et al., 1999; Wichterle et al., 1999) have shown that the cells that migrate from the ventral telencephalon to the cortex are indeed GABAergic. Three different streams of neurons originating in the ventral telencephalon were observed to round the corticostriatal notch and follow tangentially oriented paths to enter the cortex. An early cohort (E12 in mouse; E14 in rat), originating in the medial ganglionic eminence (MGE), invades mainly the PP. These cells are tangentially oriented and show features typical of Cajal-Retzius cells. A second and more prominent cohort, composed also of MGE cells, has been observed to migrate predominantly through the IZ slightly later in development (E13-15 mouse; E15-17 rat). At the late stages of corticogenesis, cells originating in the LGE and MGE appear in the lower IZ and SVZ (Anderson et al., 2001). Genetic manipulations have provided further evidence for the origin of the cortical GABAergic interneurons in the subpallium. Thus, mice lacking transcription factors that regulate regionalization (*Nkx2.1*) or differentiation (*Dlx1/2*, *Mash1*) in the ventral telencephalon have significantly reduced numbers of GABAergic neurons in the cortex (Anderson et al., 1997; Casarosa et al., 1999; Sussel et al., 1999). Specifically, *Nkx2.1* mutants that lack a functional MGE show approximately a 50% reduction in GABA-containing neurons in the cortex, but the olfactory bulbs of these mutants contain nearly a normal number of GABAergic cells. Further, tracing studies in slice cultures of these mutants showed a significantly reduced migration of labeled cells in the cortex from the LGE or from the abnormal 'MGE'. In contrast, the *Dlx1/2* mutants that lack migration of cells out of the LGE and MGE in slice cultures, have about a 75% reduction of GABA cells in the cortex and virtually no GABAergic cells in the olfactory bulb. These observations suggest that the MGE is the main source of interneurons to the cerebral cortex, while the LGE provides some cells to the cortex and many to the olfactory bulb. This is supported by the finding that dissociated MGE cells injected into the lateral ventricle tend to migrate to the striatum, pallidum and neocortex, while LGE cells migrate predominantly into the striatum and olfactory bulb (Wichterle at al., 1999). In a more recent study, Stühmer et al. (2002) have shown that all cortical GABAergic neurons in the adult mouse brain are derived from cells that express the *Dlx* genes. This finding suggests that the vast majority, if not all, GABA-containing neurons in the mammalian cortex are derived from progenitors in the ventral telencephalon.

Neurons of the ganglionic eminence destined for the developing cerebral cortex express the LIM homeobox gene *Lhx6* (Grigoriou et al., 1998; Lavdas et al., 1999). In the later stages of corticogenesis and in postnatal life, *Lhx6* has been found to be expressed in cells scattered throughout the cortical thickness. Although double-labeling experiments have not yet been conducted, the distribution of these cells resembles that of the GABA-containing neurons (our unpublished observations), suggesting that cortical interneurons express *Lhx6* during corticogenesis and in later life. LIM homeodomain transcription factors have been previously implicated in neurotransmitter expression (Thor and Thomas, 1997), and it may be that the expression of GABA in cortical interneurons is under the control of *Lhx6*.

The molecular mechanisms that guide the migration of interneurons from the ganglionic eminence, around the corticostriatal notch and into the neocortex are unknown. What signals trigger the migration of these neurons? A number of factors have been shown to stimulate motogenic activity in neural and non-neural tissue. One of these molecules, hepatocyte growth factor/scatter factor (HGF/SF) and its receptor MET have recently been shown to be important in the migration of cortical interneurons. Disruption of the normal expression of HGF/SF appears to result in undirected scattering of cells from the ganglionic eminence and in a significant reduction of interneurons in the cortex at the time of birth (Powell et al., 2001). Little is known about the substrates used by interneurons to reach the cortex, but their tangential migration appears largely independent of interactions with radial glia. However, a close association has been observed between tangentially oriented cells and corticofugal axons, predominantly in the IZ and MZ of the developing cortex (Métin and Godement, 1996), suggesting that interneurons may use this axonal system as a scaffold for their migration into the cortex. Recent studies (Denaxa et al., 2001) have provided evidence that

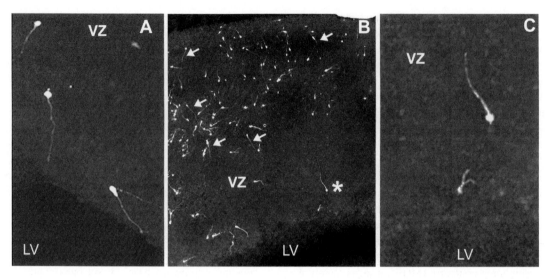

Fig. 2. Cells migrate into the neocortex following placement of the fluorescent marker CMTMR in the ventral telencephalon of brain slices of rat embryos. Dye-labeled cells appeared in the ventricular zone (VZ) after 2 days in culture following placement of CMTMR in the ganglionic eminence of an E16 rat brain slice (A), or in the cortical plate (CP) and intermediate zone (IZ) (arrows, B). Labeled cells with leading processes oriented towards the pial surface were also observed in the VZ (asterisk in B and higher magnification in C). LV, lateral ventricle.

the neural adhesion molecule TAG-1, a member of the immunoglobulin superfamily present on corticofugal fibers, serves as a substrate upon which GABAergic interneurons migrate. Blocking TAG-1 function in cortical slices with anti-TAG-1 antibodies or soluble TAG-1 protein results in marked reduction of migrating GABAergic interneurons (Denaxa et al., 2001).

If tangentially migrating neurons use the corticofugal system to enter the neocortex, how do they become distributed as GABAergic interneurons at all levels of the developing cortex? Using time-lapse imaging of cortical slices, Nadarajah et al. (2002) have shown that interneurons leave the IZ to migrate towards the cortical VZ (Fig. 2). After a pause in this proliferative zone, they migrate radially in the direction of the pial surface to take up positions in the developing CP. Earlier birthdating studies have demonstrated that both pyramidal and non-pyramidal neurons are disposed in an 'inside-out' pattern within the CP (Miller, 1985). How is it that two neuronal types generated in two distinct regions of the developing brain, the pallium and subpallium, and shown to follow different migratory paths assemble in the cortex in a way that they are linked temporally and spatially? Nadarajah and colleagues (2002) have proposed that cortical interneurons follow ventricle-directed migration actively seeking the VZ in order to obtain the type of positional

information that the pyramidal cells acquire prior to becoming postmitotic. These cues may be obtained from the local environment or from the pyramidal cells themselves through neural–neural interactions. The mechanism that guides interneurons to the VZ before they move

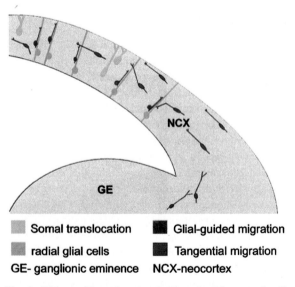

Fig. 3. Diagram illustrating the three modes of neuronal cell movement in the developing cerebral cortex: glia-guided radial migration, somal translocation, and tangential migration.

to the positions in the developing cortex are not known, but a combination of chemoattractant (e.g. semaphorins) and chemorepellent (e.g. Slit) molecules may be involved. The finding of ventricle-directed migration together with the recent demonstration of two modes of radial migration, locomotion and somal translocation, suggest that young neurons use different modes of cell movement to reach their positions in the developing cortex (Fig. 3).

References

Anderson, S.A., Eisenstat, D.D., Shi, L. and Rubenstein, J.L.R. (1997) Inreneuron migration from the basal forebrain to neocortex: dependence on Dlx genes. *Science*, 278: 474–476.

Anderson, S.A., Marin, O., Horn, C., Jennings, K. and Rubenstein, J.L.R. (2001) Distinct cortical migrations from the medial and lateral ganglionic eminences. *Development*, 128: 353–363.

Anton, E.S., Marchionni, M.A., Lee, K.F. and Rakic, P. (1997) Role of GGF/neuregulin signaling in interactions between migrating neurons and radial glia in the developing cerebral cortex. *Development*, 124: 3501–3510.

Boulder Committee (1970) Embryonic vertebrate central nervous system: revised terminology. *Anat. Rec.*, 166: 257–262.

Bradford, R., Parnavelas, J.G. and Lieberman, A.R. (1977) Neurons in layer I of the developing occipital cortex of the rat. *J. Comp. Neurol.*, 176: 121–132.

Brittis, P.A., Meiri, K., Dent, E. and Silver, J. (1995) The earliest patterns of neuronal differentiation and migration in the mammalian central nervous system. *Exp. Neurol.*, 134: 1–12.

Cajal, S.R. (1911) *Histologie du Système nerveux de l'Homme et des Vertébrés*, Vol. 2, Paris: Maloine.

Cajal, S.R. (1960) *Studies on Vertebrate Neurogenesis*, Translated by Lloyd Guth, Springfield, IL: Thomas.

Casarosa, S., Fode, C. and Guillemot, F. (1999) Mash1 regulates neurogenesis in the ventral telencephalon. *Development*, 126: 525–534.

Caviness, V.S. Jr. and Rakic, P. (1978) Mechanisms of cortical development: a view from mutations of mice. *Ann. Rev. Neurosci.*, 1: 297–326.

Chae, T., Kwon, Y.T., Bronson, R., Dikkes, P., Li, E. and Tsai, L.H. (1997) Mice lacking p35, a neuronal specific activator of Cdk5, display cortical lamination defects, seizures, and adult lethality. *Neuron*, 18: 29–42.

Curran, T. and D'Arcangelo, G. (1998) Role of reelin in the control of brain development. *Brain Res. Rev.*, 26: 285–294.

D'Arcangelo, G., Miao, G.G., Chen, S.-C., Soares, H.D., Morgan, J.I. and Curran, T. (1995) A protein related to exracellular matrix proteins deleted in the mouse mutant reeler. *Nature*, 374: 719–723.

De Carlos, J.A., Lopez-Mascaraque, L. and Valverde, F. (1996) Dynamics of cell migration from the lateral ganglionic eminence in the rat. *J. Neurosci.*, 16: 6146–6156.

Denaxa, M., Chan, C.-H., Schachner, M., Parnavelas, J.G. and Karagogeos, D. (2001) The adhesion molecule TAG-1 mediates the migration of cortical interneurons from the ganglionic eminence along the corticofugal fiber system. *Development*, 128: 4635–4644.

Fairén, A., De Felipe, J. and Regidor, J. (1984) Nonpyramidal neurons: general account. In: A. Peters and E.G. Jones (Eds.), *Cerebral Cortex, Cellular Components of the Cerebral Cortex*, Vol. 1, Plenum, New York, pp. 201–253.

Fox, J.W., Lamperti, E.D., Eksioglu, Y.Z., Hong, S.E., Feng, Y., Graham, D.A., Scheffer, I.E., Dobyns, W.B., Hirsch, B.A., Radtke, R.A., Berkovic, S.F., Huttenlocher, P.R. and Walsh, C.A. (1998) Mutations in filamin 1 prevent migration of cerebral cortical neurons in human periventricular heterotopia. *Neuron*, 21: 1315–1325.

Gilbert, C.D. (1983) Microcircuitry of the visual cortex. *Ann. Rev. Neurosci.*, 6: 217–247.

Gilmore, E.C., Ohshima, T., Goffinet, A.M., Kulkarni, A.B. and Herrup, K. (1998) Cyclin-dependent kinase 5-deficient mice demonstrate novel developmental arrest in cerebral cortex. *J. Neurosci.*, 18: 6370–6377.

Gleeson, J.G., Lin, P. T., Flanagan, L.A. and Walsh, C.A. (1999) Doublecortin is a microtubule-associated protein and is expressed widely by migrating neurons. *Neuron*, 23: 257–271.

Gonzalez, J.L., Russo, C.J., Goldowitz, D., Sweet, H.O., Davisson, M.T. and Walsh, C.A. (1997) Birthdate and cell marker analysis of scrambler: a novel mutation affecting cortical development with a reeler-like phenotype. *J. Neurosci.*, 17: 9204–9211.

Grigoriou, M., Tucker, A.S., Sharpe, P.T. and Pachnis, V. (1998) Expression and regulation of Lhx6 and Lhx7, a novel subfamily of LIM homeodomain encoding genes, suggests a role in mammalian head development. *Development*, 125: 2063–2074.

Hatten, M.E. (1999) Central nervous system neuronal migration. *Ann. Rev. Neurosci.*, 22: 511–539.

Hirotsune, S., Fleck, M.W., Gambello, M.J., Bix, G.J., Chen, A., Clark, G.D., Ledbetter, D.H., McBain, C.J. and Wynshaw-Boris, A. (1998) Graded reduction of Pafah1b1 (Lis1) activity results in neuronal migration defects and early embryonic lethality. *Nat. Genet.*, 19: 333–339.

Howell, B.W., Hawkes, R., Soriano, P. and Cooper, J.A. (1997) Neuronal position in the developing brain is regulated by mouse disabled-1. *Nature*, 389: 733–737.

Kwon, Y.T., Gupta, A., Zhou, Y., Nikolic, M. and Tsai, L.H. (2000) Regulation of N-cadherin-mediated adhesion by the p35-Cdk5 kinase. *Curr. Biol.*, 10: 363–372.

Lavdas, A.A., Grigoriou, M., Pachnis, V. and Parnavelas, J.G. (1999) The medial ganglionic eminence gives rise to a population of early neurons in the developing cerebral cortex. *J. Neurosci.*, 19: 7881–7888.

Luskin, M.B., Pearlman, A.L. and Sanes, J.R. (1988) Cell lineage in the cerebral cortex of the mouse studied *in vivo* and *in vitro* with a recombinant retrovirus. *Neuron*, 1: 635–647.

Luskin, M.B., Parnavelas, J.G. and Barfield, J.A. (1993) Neurons, astrocytes, and oligodendrocytes of the rat cerebral cortex originate from separate progenitor cells: an ultrastructural analysis of clonally related cells. *J. Neurosci.*, 13: 1730–1750.

Mètin, C. and Godement, P. (1996) The ganglionic eminence may be an intermediate target for corticofugal and thalamocortical axons. *J. Neurosci.*, 16: 3219–3235.

Meyer, G., Goffinet, A.M. and Fairén, A. (1999) What is a Cajal-Retzius cell? A reassessment of a classical cell type based on

80

recent observations in the developing cortex. *Cereb. Cortex*, 9: 765–775.

Miller, M.W. (1985) Cogeneration of retrogradely labeled cortico-cortical projection and GABA-immunoreactive local circuit neurons in cerebral cortex. *Dev. Brain Res.*, 23: 187–192.

Mione, M.C., Danevic, C., Boardman, P., Harris, B. and Parnavelas, J.G. (1994) Lineage analysis reveals neurotransmitter (GABA and glutamate) but not calcium-binding protein homogeneity in clonally related cortical neurons. *J. Neurosci.*, 14: 107–123.

Mione, M.C., Cavanagh, J.F.R., Harris, B. and Parnavelas, J.G. (1997) Cell fate specification and symmetrical/asymmetrical divisions in the developing cerebral cortex. *J. Neurosci.*, 17: 2018–2029.

Morest, D.K. (1970) A study of neurogenesis in the forebrain of opossum pouch young. *Z. Anat. Entwicklungsgesch.*, 130: 265–305.

Nadarajah, B., Brunstrom, J.E., Grutzendler, J., Wong, R.O. and Pearlman, A.L. (2001) Two modes of radial migration in early development of the cerebral cortex. *Nat. Neurosci.*, 4: 143–150.

Nadarajah, B., Alifragis, P., Wong, R. and Parnavelas, J.G. (2002) Ventricle-directed migration in the developing cerebral cortex. *Nat. Neurosci.*, in press.

Naegele, J. and Barnstable, C.J. (1989) Molecular determinants of GABAergic local-circuit neurons in the visual cortex. *Trends Neurosci.*, 12: 28–34.

Ogawa, M., Miyata, T., Nakajima, K., Yagyu, K., Seike, M., Ikenaka, K., Yamamoto, H. and Mikoshiba, K. (1995) The reeler gene-associated antigen on Cajal-Retzius neurons is a crucial molecule for laminar organization of cortical neurons. *Neuron*, 14: 899–912.

O'Rourke, N.A., Sullivan, D.P., Kaznowski, C.E., Jacobs, A.A. and McConnell, S.K. (1995) Tangential migration of neurons in the developing cerebral cortex. *Development*, 121: 2165–2176.

Parnavelas, J.G., Dinopoulos, A. and Davies, S.W. (1989) The central visual pathways. In: A. Björklund, T. Hökfelt and S.W. Swanson (Eds.), *Handbook of Chemical Neuroanatomy, Integrated Systems of the CNS*, Vol. 7: Part II, Elsevier, Amsterdam, pp. 1–164.

Parnavelas, J.G., Barfield, J.A., Franke, E. and Luskin, M.B. (1991) Separate progenitor cells give rise to pyramidal and nonpyramidal neurons in the rat telencephalon. *Cereb. Cortex*, 1: 463–468.

Porteus, M.H., Bulfone, A., Liu, J.K., Puelles, L., Lo, L.C. and Rubenstein, J.L.R. (1994) DLX-2, MASH-1, and MAP-2 expression and bromodeoxyuridine incorporation define molecularly distinct cell populations in the embryonic mouse forebrain. *J. Neurosci.*, 14: 6370–6383.

Powell, E.M., Mars, W.M. and Levitt, P. (2001) Hepatocyte growth factor/scatter factor is a motogen for interneurons migrating from the ventral to the dorsal telencephalon. *Neuron*, 30: 79–89.

Price, J. and Thurlow, L. (1988) Cell lineage in the rat cerebral cortex: a study using retroviral-mediated gene transfer. *Development*, 104: 473–482.

Price, J., Turner, D. and Cepko, C. (1987) Lineage analysis in the vertebrate nervous system by retrovirus-mediated gene transfer. *Proc. Natl. Acad. Sci. USA*, 84: 156–160.

Price, J., Williams, B. and Grove, E. (1992) The generation of cellular diversity in the cerebral cortex. *Brain Path.*, 2: 23–29.

Rakic, P. (1972) Mode of cell migration to the superficial layers of fetal monkey neocortex. *J. Comp. Neurol.*, 145: 61–83.

Rakic, P., Stensas, L.J., Sayre, E., and Sidman, R.L. (1974) Computer-aided three-dimensional reconstruction and quantitative analysis of cells from serial electron microscopic montages of foetal monkey brain. *Nature*, 250: 31–34.

Reid, C.B., Liang, I. and Walsh, C. (1995) Systematic widespread clonal organization in cerebral cortex. *Neuron*, 15: 299–310.

Rio, C., Rieff, H.I., Qi, P., Khurana, T.S. and Corfas, G. (1997) Neuregulin and erbB receptors play a critical role in neuronal migration. *Neuron*, 19: 39–50.

Rockel, A.J., Hiorns, R.W. and Powell, T.P.S. (1980) The basic uniformity in structure of the neocortex. *Brain*, 103: 221–244.

Sanes, J.R., Rubenstein, J.L.R. and Nicolas, J.-F. (1986) Use of recombinant retrovirus to study post-implantation cell lineage in mouse embryos. *EMBO J.*, 5: 3133–3142.

Senzaki, K., Ogawa, M. and Yagi, T. (1999) Proteins of the CNR family are multiple receptors for Reelin. *Cell*, 99: 635–647.

Sheldon, M., Rice, D.S., D'Arcangelo, G., Yoneshima, H., Nakajima, K., Mikoshiba, K., Howell, B.W., Cooper, J.A., Goldowitz, D. and Curran, T. (1997) Scrambler and yotari disrupt the disabled gene and produce a reeler-like phenotype in mice. *Nature*, 389: 730–733.

Stühmer, T., Puelles, L., Ekker, M. and Rubenstein, J.L.R. (2002) Expression from a Dlx gene enhancer marks adult mouse cortical GABAergic neurons. *Cereb. Cortex*, 12: 75–85.

Sussel, L., Marin, O., Kimura, S. and Rubenstein, J.L.R. (1999) Loss of Nkx2.1 homeobox gene function results in a ventral to dorsal molecular respecification within the basal telencephalon: evidence for a transformation of the pallidum into the striatum. *Development*, 126: 3359–3370.

Szentágothai, J. (1973) Synaptology of the visual cortex. In: R. Jung (Ed.), *Handbook of Sensory Physiology*, Vol. VII/3, Part B, Springer-Verlag, Berlin, pp. 269–324.

Tamamaki, N., Fugimori, K.E. and Takauji, R. (1997) Origin and route of tangentially migrating neurons in the developing neocortical intermediate zone. *J. Neurosci.*, 17: 8313–8323.

Tan, S.S., Kalloniatis, M., Sturm, K., Tam, P.P.L., Reese, B.E. and Faulkner-Jones, B. (1998) Separate progenitors for radial and tangential cell dispersion during development of the cerebral cortex. *Neuron*, 21: 295–304.

Thor, S. and Thomas, J.B. (1997) The Drosophila islet gene governs axon pathfinding and neurotransmitter identity. *Neuron*, 18: 397–409.

Trommsdorff, M., Gotthardt, M., Hiesberger, T., Shelton, J., Stockinger, W., Nimpf, J., Hammer, R.E., Richardson, J.A. and Herz, J. (1999) Reeler/Disabled-like disruption of neuronal migration in knockout mice lacking the VLDL receptor and ApoE receptor 2. *Cell*, 97: 689–701.

Uylings, H.B.M., Van Eden, C.G., Parnavelas, J.G. and Kalsbeek, A. (1990) The prenatal and postnatal development of rat cerebral cortex. In: B. Kolb and R.C. Tees (Eds.), *The Cerebral Cortex of the Rat*, MIT Press, Cambridge, MA, pp. 35–76.

Walsh, C. and Cepko, C.L. (1992) Widespread dispersion of neuronal clones across functional regions of the cerebral cortex. *Science*, 255: 434–440.

Walsh, C. and Cepko, C.L. (1993) Clonal dispersion in proliferative layers of developing cerebral cortex. *Nature*, 362: 632–635.

Wichterle, H., Garcia-Verdugo, J.M., Herrera, D.G. and Alvarez-Buylla, A. (1999) Young neurons from medial ganglionic eminence disperse in adult and embryonic brain. *Nat. Neurosci.*, 2: 461–466.

Inside the neuron: cytoskeleton, dendrites, and synapses

E.C. Azmitia, J. DeFelipe, E.G. Jones, P. Rakic and C.E. Ribak (Eds.)
Progress in Brain Research, Vol. 136

CHAPTER 7

Inside the neuron: cytoskeleton, dendrites, and synapses (an overview)

Enrico Mugnaini*

Northwestern University Institute for Neuroscience, Searle Bldg. 5-471, 320 E. Superior Street, Chicago, IL 60611, USA

The birth of modern neuroscience is commonly traced to the work of Camillo Golgi, Santiago Ramón y Cajal, Charles Sherrington, and their contemporaries around the turn of the previous century. Cajal certainly towered among all neuroanatomists. His scientific output was so extensive, masterfully illustrated, incisively written, and uniquely visionary, that his contributions remain vivid nearly seventy years after his death. The Cajal Club meetings celebrate the memory of the great master and, at the same time, help new generations of neuroscientists throughout the world to develop a historical perspective on the patterns of discovery. In this section, the reader will find six stimulating chapters which illuminate evolving views on several of Cajal's favored topics, including the neuronal cytoskeleton and the effects of glial factors on its plasticity (by E. C. Azmitia), the dendritic spines (by G. N. Elston and J. DeFelipe, A. Feria-Velasco and coworkers, and M. Segal), the interactions among processes of special types of nerve cells (by V. M. Pickel and coworkers), and the make-up of interneuronal contacts (by S. B. Christie and coworkers, presented by A. L. de Blas).

Perhaps, a flew reflections are in order as a thread through these papers. Cajal was both a man of his time and in most respects a visionary neuroscientist, who used his data to derive both specific functional explanations and general principles of organization of the nervous system. He had an admirable acumen in sensing the true

*Corresponding author: Tel.: 312 503 4300; Fax: 312 503 7345; E-mail: e-mugnaini@northwestern.edu

limitations of the methods he used. He left few brain centers and cell types untouched, and made few mistakes. Moreover, Cajal was a bold thinker and did not shy from speculative ideas. (Incidentally, he also largely published without peer-review!) Even today, his ideas offer the ground to 'benevolent exegesis'; a host of modern discoveries trace back to him or link his work of historical proportion to the most novel findings.

Thus, one may recognize the theme of 'Cajal the visionary' in all the chapters. Azmitia highlights Cajal's studies on regenerating axons, linking the great master's 'neurobiones' to microtubules and the 'Schwann cell trophic factor' to S-100β, a protein extruded by peripheral and central glia. Azmitia proposes a neuronal-glial-neuronal interplay mediated by serotonin, S-100β, and microtubule associated proteins that involves the neuronal cytoskeleton and is part of the many complex interactions between transmitters, trophic, and tropic factors that regulate birth, growth, life, and death of the neuron.

As Sherrington wrote (quoted by Cowan and Kandel, 2001), "*A trait very noticeable in [Cajal] was that in describing what the microscope showed he spoke habitually as though it were a living scene.*" Such living scenes are observable today by video microscopy and laser-scanning confocal microscopy of cells transfected with cytoskeletal protein/green fluorescent protein constructs. Intermediate filament subunits associate as microscopic particles and squiggles, possibly related to the neurobiones, that move along microtubule tracks with kinesin- and/or actin-dependent mechanisms

(Prahlad et al., 1998, 2000; Chou and Goldman, 2001; Shah et al., 2000; Wang et al., 2000). Spines also appear to be dynamic structures.

Discovery of the dendritic spine is one of the most conspicuous examples of Cajal's superior power of observation. Many would agree with Feria-Velasco and coworkers that the spine pattern probably represents a more powerful means to establish 'neuronal typology' than patterns of dendritic branching, targets of axonal projections, and expression of particular gene products. It is intriguing to realize that Camillo Golgi, the discoverer of the '*reazione nera*', must have seen thousands of neurons provided with spines, and yet he left the spine in the shadow. One may pardon Golgi this grand oversight, for the notion of impregnation artifacts loomed large and a misinterpretation would have retarded acceptance of his new method by the scientific community (Szenthágothai, 1975). [The interested reader will find a cogent analysis of Golgi's advances, preoccupations, and career in a thoughtful biography (Mazzarello, 1999)]. Cajal, however, immediately grasped how far the Golgi method could be trusted, and provided further evidence for the existence of spines with the methylene blue stain. A few years after identification of the synaptic junctions as specialized, asymmetric forms of intercellular contact (Palay, 1956), the reality of both the spines and the encrustation-like 'excrescences' was ultimately demonstrated by electron microscopy, and these dendritic evaginations were shown to bear chemical synapses (Gray, 1959a,b; Blackstad and Kjaerheim, 1961).

Elston and DeFelipe review data from the literature and from their own extensive investigations emphasizing dendritic plasticity and topographic and interspecies differences in spine densities in cortical pyramidal neurons. They conclude that both cell-intrinsic and epigenetic factors determine spine distribution, and argue that back-propagation of action potentials is the most probable activity-dependent mechanism. Correlations between quantitative measures of back-propagation and spine density would be helpful in strengthening their argument. However, back-propagation seems unlikely as a universal principle, because Purkinje cells have negligible back-propagation and possess the highest density of spines in brain.

Feria-Velasco and co-workers analyze the complex effect of a tryptophan restricted diet on hippocampal CAI pyramidal neurons and uncover spine changes that may be transynaptically linked to understimulation of serotonin receptors. Segal reviews the history of our knowledge on spines, their involvement with calcium-dependent processes, their apparent regulation by changes in synaptic activity of the neural network, and the question of their motility. His exciting studies on the visualization of spines in living neurons, together with several investigations published during the current year on signal transduction and protein–protein interaction in spines, favor a highly dynamic view of this organelle (Cowan et al., 2001). As molecules that affect spine shape and size are being discovered (Pak et al., 2001; Sala et al., 2001), it is apparent that several of these molecules are linked to actin, a cytoskeletal component that represents a major actor in development, function, and plasticity, but actin was unknown to Cajal. The chemical make-up of spines on different portions of the somatodendritic compartment may differ even within an individual neuron. Morando et al. (2001) recently highlighted the complexity of dendritic plasticity involving spines of a single type of neuron. They showed that the proximal dendrites of mature Purkinje cells relinquish their contacts with the climbing fibers in the absence of activity and become covered with new spines that establish new synapses mainly with parallel fibers. Thus, afferent systems competing for the same target neurons do not follow uniform rules, and activity may differentially affect not only different types of neurons but also different types of axo-spinous contacts. We are barely beginning to understand why data on spines obtained from studying different types of neurons, *in vitro*, *ex vivo*, or *in situ*, differ. It will take a number of years before we reach down to the spine by combinations of *quantitative* molecular, cellular, and electrophysiological methods and fully appreciate common and differential properties of spines under varying developmental and functional conditions.

The chapters of Pickel and de Blas and their coworkers demonstrate the power of immunoelectron microscopy to elucidate synaptic and extrasynaptic neurotransmitter based interactions between dendritic and axonal domains utilizing antibodies to plasma membrane transporters, vesicular transporters, and receptors. The existence of dendrodendritic interactions, which could more easily be related to the work of Golgi than to that of Cajal, is now well proven, although the mechanisms regulating their operations are still debated. Pickel and coworkers emphasize the role of dendritic tubulovesicular organelles provided with vesicular transporters, which they observed in monoaminergic and cholinergic neurons, but which might extend to neurons utilizing other neurotransmitters. Obviously we need to know more about the functions of these organelles and how they differ from the better known axonal vesicular and endocytic elements (De Camilli et al., 2001).

Finally, Christie and coworkers review molecular and immunocytochemical advances on GABAergic synapses and the distribution and targeting of postsynaptic and extrasynaptic GABA receptors in specific neuronal systems. Although, Cajal is widely praised for having provided many accurate wiring diagrams of what we now know are inhibitory neuronal connections, such as those in the hippocampus and cerebellum, he did not envision the role of inhibition in central processes (Cowan and Kandel, 2001). [Putative inhibitory interneurons, however, were envisioned by Cajal's pupil, Rafael Lorente de Nó (reviewed by Fairén, 1993) to explain the mechanism of nystagmus and the circuitry of the entorhinal cortex (Lorente de Nó, 1933a,b; 1938)]. Christie and coworkers emphasize the discovery of the type 1 and type 2 synapses by Gray (1959a,b; 1961a), that introduced the notion of a morphological dichotomy among synapses. This dichotomy was soon linked to excitation and inhibition (Blackstad and Flood, 1963; Uchizono, 1965). In retrospect, the string of papers published by George Gray in the late 1950s and the early 1960s on the ultrastructure of the nervous system equaled in acumen the early contributions of Cajal (for an early description of gap junctions/light junctions in brain, see Gray, 1961b). With clarification of the sequence and membrane topology of excitatory and inhibitory neurotransmitters and discovery of PSD-95, gephyrin, GABARAP, and other postsynaptic proteins, the basis for the morphological differences between excitatory and inhibitory synapses is beginning to emerge (Sheng, 2001). The role of local synthesis of postsynaptic proteins in synaptic diversity (Kiebler and Degroseillers, 2000; Pierce et al., 2001) is also receiving renewed interest. Advances on targeting mechanisms, molecular motors, cargos, and adaptors of glutamate receptors (Miki et al., 2001; Wong et al., 2001), suggest that specific adaptors also exist for the subunits of inhibitory neurotransmitter receptors. However, possible differences in the components of the presynaptic membranes and the synaptic cleft materials of type 1 and type 2 synapses remain largely unknown. Some evidence suggests that the prion protein might be part of the presynaptic GABAergic machinery (Collinge et al., 1994; Ferrer et al., 2000; but see the more general distribution of prion protein proposed by Lainé et al., 2001).

Neuronal diversity will continue to engender many challenges for anatomical, biochemical, and electrophysiological studies. Although neurons share a fundamental machinery that regulates neurotransmitter secretion and postsynaptic receptor organization, it is likely that this machinery is differentially regulated—and may even vary in some of its elements—in types and subsets of neurons. Synapses with features intermediate between the type 1 and type 2 categories exist in many brain regions. Moreover, synapses between GABAergic boutons and spines with thick postsynaptic densities and wide synaptic clefts, like those of type 1 synapses, although not ubiquitous, are far from rare. Do these GABAergic type 1 synapses contain special combinations of $GABA_A$ receptor subunits and postsynaptic spine proteins, or do they represent developmental errors and repair processes? We do not know, but further investigations of the complex make-up of inhibitory and excitatory synapses in general and of synapses of specific networks in particular is expected to resolve many open issues.

In conclusion, while the chapters in this session express an aspect of Cajal's remembrance, they also represent the evolutionary nature of scientific discovery. They emphasize combinations of modern molecular and anatomical approaches that pick up the story where Cajal left it at the end of his long and extraordinarily productive life and advance it towards new vistas. Far from the "structura obscura, obscuriores morbi, functiones obscurissimae" of the pre-Golgi/Cajal era (Szentágothai, 1975), bright lights now illuminate the new pathways.

References

Blackstad, T.W. and Flood, P.R. (1963) Ultrastructure of hippocampal axo-somatic synapses. Nature, 198: 542–543.

Blackstad, T.W. and Kjaerheim, A. (1961) Special axo-dendritic synapses in the hippocampal cortex: electron and light microscopic studies on the layer of mossy fibers. J. Comp. Neurol., 117: 133–159.

Chou, Y.-H. and Goldman, R.D. (2001) Intermediate filaments on the move. J. Cell Biol., 150: F101–F105

Collinge, J., Whittington, M.A., Sidle, K.C.L., Smith, J., Palmer, M.S., Clarke, A.R. and Jeffreys, J.G.R. (1994) Prion protein is necessary for normal synaptic function. Nature, 370: 295–297.

Cowan, W.M. and Kandel E.R. (2001) A brief history of synapses and synaptic transmission. In: W.M. Cowan, T.C. Sudhof, C.F. Stevens, (Eds.), Synapses. Johns Hopkins University Press, Baltimore, pp. 1–87.

Cowan, W.M., Südhof, T.C. and Stevens, C.F. (2001) *Synapses*. Johns Hopkins University Press, Baltimore.

DeCamilli P., Slepnev, V.I., Shupliakov, O. and Brodin, L. (2001) Synaptic vesicle endocytosis. In: W.M. Cowan, T.C. Südhof and C.F. Stevens, (Eds.) *Synapses*. Johns Hopkins University Press, Baltimore, pp. 217–274.

Fairén, A. (1993). Axonal patterns of interneurons in the cerebral cortex: in memory of Rafael Lorente de Nó. In: M.A. Merchán, J.M. Juiz, D.A. Godfrey, E. Mugnaini, (Eds.). *The Mammalian Cochlear Nuclei: Organization and Function*. NATO ASI Series A; *Life Sciences*, Vol. 239. Plenum Press, New York, pp. 467–473.

Ferrer, I., Puig, B., Blanco, R. and E. Martí (2000) Prion protein deposition and abnormal synaptic protein expression in the cerebellum of Creutzfeldt-Jakob disease. *Neuroscience*, 97: 715–726.

Gray, E.G. (1959a) Electron microscopy of synaptic contacts on spines of dendrites of the cerebral cortex. *Nature*, 183: 1592–1593.

Gray, E.G. (1959b) Axo-somatic and axo-dendritic synapses of the cerebral cortex: an electron microscope study. *J. Anat.*, 93: 420–433.

Gray, E.G. (1961a) The granule cells, mossy synapses and Purkinje spine synapses of the cerebellum: light and electron microscope observations. *J. Anat.* 95: 345–356.

Gray, E.G. (1961b) Ultrastructure of synapses of the cerebral cortex and of certain specialisations of neuroglial membranes. In: J.D. Boyd, Johnson, F.R., Lever, J.D (Eds.) *Electron Microscopy in Anatomy*. Edwards Arnold, London, pp. 54–73.

Kiebler, M.A., Desgroseillers, L. (2000) Molecular insights into mRNA transport and local translation in the mammalian nervous system. *Neuron*, 25: 19–28.

Lainé, J., Marc, M.E., Sy, M.S., Axelrad, H. (2001) Cellular and subcellular morphological localization of normal prion protein in rodent cerebellum. *Eur. J. Neurosci.*, 14: 47–56.

Lorente De Nó, R. (1933a) Vestibulo-ocular reflex arc. *Arch. Neurol. Psychiat.*, 30: 245–291.

Lorente De Nó, R. (1933b) Studies on the structure of the cerebral cortex. I. The area enthorinalis. *J. Psychol. Neurol. (Lpz.)*, 45: 381–438.

Lorente De Nó, R. (1938) Analysis of the activity of the chains of internuncial neurons. *J. Neurophysiol.*, 1: 207–244.

Mazzarello, P. (1999) *The Hidden Structure: A Scientific Biography of Camillo Golgi*. Oxford University Press, Oxford.

Miki, H., Setou, M., Kaneshiro, K. and Hirokawa, N. (2001) All kinesin superfamily protein, KIF, genes in mouse and human. *Proc. Natl. Acad. Sci. USA*, 98: 7004–7011.

Morando, L., Cesa, R., Rasetti, R., Harvey and R., Strata, P. (2001) Role of glutamate delta-2 receptors in activity-dependent competition between heterologous afferent fibers. *Proc. Natl. Acad. Sci. USA* 98: 9954–9959.

Pak, D.T., Yang, S., Rudolph-Correia, S., Kim, E. and Sheng, M. (2001) Regulation of dendritic spine morphology by SPAR, a PSD-95-associated RapGAP. *Neuron*, 31: 289–303.

Palay, S.L. (1956) Synapses in the central nervous system. *J. Biophys. Biochem. Cytol.* 2 (suppl.): 193–202.

Pierce, J.P., Mayer, T. and McCarthy. J.B. (2001) Evidence for a satellite secretory pathway in neuronal dendritic spines. *Curr. Biol.*, 11: 351–355

Prahlad, V., Yoon, M., Moir, R.D., Vale, R.D. and Goldman, R.D. (1998) Rapid movement of vimentin on microtubule tracks: kinesin-dependent assembly of intermediate filament networks. *J. Cell Biol.*, 143: 159–170.

Prahlad, V., Helfand, B.T., Langford, G.M., Vale, R.D. and Goldman, R.D. (1998) Fast transport of neurofilament protein along microtubules in squid axoplasm. *J. Cell Sci.*, 113: 3939–3946.

Sala, C., Piech, V., Wilson, N.R., Passafaro, M., Liu, G. and Sheng, M. (2001) Regulation of dendritic spine morphology and synaptic function by Shank and Homer. *Neuron*, 31: 115–130.

Shah, J.V., Flanagan, L.A., Janmey, P.A. and Leterrier, J.-F. (2000) Bidirectional translocation of neurofilaments along microtubules mediated in part by dynein/dynactin. *Mol. Biol. Cell.*, 11: 3495–3508.

Sheng, M., H.-T. (2001) The postsynaptic specialization. In: W.M. Cowan, T.C. Südhof and C.F. Stevens (Eds.), *Synapses*. Johns Hopkins University Press, Baltimore, pp. 315–355.

Szentágothai, J. (1975) What the "reazione near" has given to us. In: M. Santini (Ed.), *Golgi Centennial Symposium: Perspectives in Neurobiology*. Raven Press, New York, pp. 1–12.

Uchizono, K. (1965) Characteristics of excitatory and inhibitory synapses of the central nervous system. *Nature*, 207: 642–643.

Wang, L., Ho, C.-L., Sun, D.-M., Liem, R.K.H. and Brown, A. (2000) Rapid movement of axonal neurofilaments interrupted by prolonged pauses. *Nature Cell Biol.*, 2: 137–141.

Wong, R.W., Setou, M. and Hirokawa, N. (2001) Turning the current up on AMPA receptor trafficking. *Trends Cell Biol.*, 11: 320.

E.C. Azmitia, J. DeFelipe, E.G. Jones, P. Rakic and C.E. Ribak (Eds.)
Progress in Brain Research, Vol. 136
© 2002 Elsevier Science B.V. All rights reserved

CHAPTER 8

Cajal's hypotheses on neurobiones and neurotropic factor match properties of microtubules and S-100β

Efrain C. Azmitia*

Departments of Biology and Psychiatry, Center for Neural Science, New York University, 100 Washington Square East, New York, NY 10003, USA

Abstract: Cajal described both the morphology and plasticity of neurons. He summarized the structure of neurons as composed of membrane, protoplasm, Golgi apparatus, nucleus, spongioplasm and neurofibrils (cytoskeleton). He initially considered the cytoskeleton as absorbing excitation energy and forming a "*conductive pathway in the protoplasm*" within the neuron. Later, he viewed the neurofibrillary threads as independent, living entities and called them neurobiones. Cajal recognized neuroplasticity in development, memory, sleep, injury and dementia, as well as after exposure to cold and starvation. He noted cytoskeletal changes during these events. However, he did not causatively connect the plastic changes in neurons with the changes in cytoskeleton. Finally, Cajal proposed a theory of chemoaffinity in 1892, and modified his neurotropic theory over the next 40 years. Today we accept that changes in the cytoskeleton produce changes in neuronal morphology. The properties of the cytoskeleton and neurobione as described by Cajal are similar to those of microtubules. These long intraneuronal neurofibrils are polymers of the protein tubulin and, whilst not being living entities, are highly dynamic, sensitive to environmental stimuli, and stabilized by microtubule associated proteins (MAPs). Furthermore, Cajal was very specific in his characterization of the neurotropic factor derived from Schwann cells. Initially, he thought the chemicals attracted the axonal fibers, but later he wrote that the factor was not attractant but rather was involved in assimilation, growth and ramifications. The neurotropic hypothesis described by Cajal in *Degeneration and Regeneration in the Nervous System* is more similar to a neurite extension factor (NEF) than to a neurotrophic growth factor or specific chemoaffinity (attractant) molecule. S-100β is the major NEF found in PNS Schwann cells and CNS astroglial cells. In summary, the views of Cajal on neuroplasticity, its frequency and function, agree with the modern hypothesis of neuronal instability. This concept states that MAPs regulate microtubule stability by a S-100β sensitive phosphorylation processes. Serotonin, by acting on the astroglial 5-HT1A receptor, releases S-100β and regulates neuronal morphology and apoptosis. This neuronal-glial connection provides a fresh view for linking neuroplasticity, mental illness, and memory with changes in the cytoskeleton.

Introduction

The brain contains thousands of billions of neurons which have been classified by their function and location, as well as by their chronological and maturation age, chemical content, genotype and phenotype. Before

---

*Corresponding author: Tel.: 212-998-8235; Fax: 212-995-4015;
Email: efrain.azmitia@nyu.edu

the Golgi stain was discovered, neuroanatomists had classified neurons into three principal classes: motoneurons, sensory neurons and interneurons. The shapes of neurons are typically described as oval, spindle, unipolar or multipolar. However this simple classification does not fully convey the vast array of shapes assumed by neurons in the nervous system. The dendritic tree of a Purkinje neuron is very different from that of a motoneuron (Fig. 1). Amacrine and horizontal neurons in the retina may lack an axon, while pyramidal and spinal ganglion neurons have

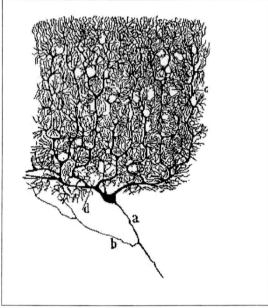

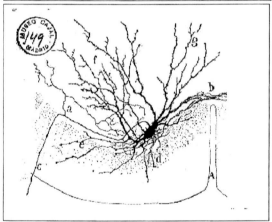

Fig. 1. Using Golgi stained material, Cajal was able to draw single neurons with all their dendritic and axonal processes. Top picture [Fig. 9] Purkinje cell of human cerebellum. Bottom picture [Fig. 11] Motor cell of the spinal cord. Cat fetus. (Copied with permission from Cajal, 1899).

extensive axons. The axons of the reticular formation, especially those which contain monoamines such as serotonin, dopamine or norepinephrine, have millions of branches projecting throughout the neuroaxis from a single cell body. In contrast, the axons from a thalamic sensory neuron or from a spinal cord motoneuron may project to a select target neuron or muscle fiber, respectively. All these distinct morphologies are modified by the environment of the cell throughout the life of the organism.

For a long time neuroscientists knew of the electrical properties of neurons and most of the brain pathways. They viewed the brain as a static organ and Descartes (1662) even advanced the idea of the brain as a machine, with predictable pathways and functions. This idea of a static organ was the basis of phrenology which held that skull morphology reflected the genetically inherent structure and function of the underlying brain. Even today, in some respects, the view of fixed and static categories of neurons prompts the search for specific genes which determine specific brain structures, organizations, functions and diseases.

The various classifications of neurons in the fixed nervous system obscures one important principle, that every neuron is individual, unique and influenced by external factors. This is clearly reflected in Cajal's early views of a dynamic and plastic nervous system. He writes "*Morphology of the nerve cell does not obey an imminent and fatal tendency, maintained by hereditary, as certain authors have defended, but it depends entirely on the physical and chemical circumstances present in the environment*" (p. 55, Cajal, 1917). This idea fits more with the current findings of stem cells and neuronal instability in the adult brain, than it did with Cajal's later views of a CNS having "*proliferation inability and irreversibility of intraprotoplasmic differentiation.*" Cajal, in his final years described the neurons as "*impotent*" with respect to their ability to regenerate, but he paradoxically recognized their ability to change shape.

Cytoskeleton

What determines the shape of cells? Today it is clear that it is the cytoskeleton. The fibrillar texture in the protoplasm of nerve cells was first noticed by Remark in 1893. However, Cajal's view of the cytoskeleton was primitive and underwent various transformations during his career. Using a reduced silver nitrate method, Cajal became aware of the cytoskeleton of neurons (Fig. 2). The neurofibrillary processes ran throughout the soma, dendrites and axons. Although he did not indicate that the fibrils formed the foundation of cell structure, he accurately described their appearance and organization in all parts of the neuron, even in the smallest dendrites. "*Thus, the packets of neurofibrils becomes progressively thinner, until only one, very slender, pale, with no varicosities, remains within the core of a dendritic branchlet*" (p. 147, Cajal, 1899).

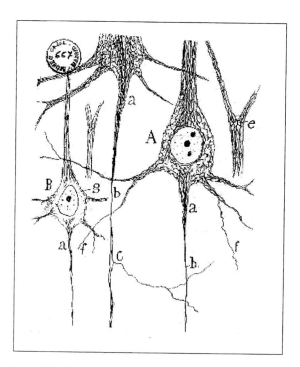

Fig. 2. [Fig. 60] Giant Pyramidal cell: ten-day dog. The neuronal cytoskeleton as drawn by Cajal using reduced silver nitrate method. Note that single neurofibrils are depicted in the smallest neurites (f). The neurofibrils are seen in all areas of the neuron (cell body (A), dendrites (e,f) and axon (a,b). In the dendrites, certain neurofibrils are seen stretching between two branches. (Copied with permissionn from Cajal, 1899).

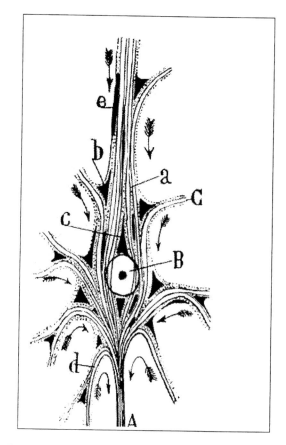

Fig. 3. [Fig. 51] Schematic drawing by Cajal showing the assumed passage of neuronal impluse using the cytoskeleton as a pathway (a and d) from the dendrites [C] through the cell body (B) and into the axon (A). Arrows indicate the direction of impluses (Copied with permission from Cajal 1899).

A function for these neurofibrils was proposed before they were even discovered. Cajal initially thought that the *"clear space between Nissl bodies must contain a system for the conduction of the nerve impulse"* and later felt that the discovery of the neurofibrillary framework justified his idea. *"These neurofibrils, which are the sole conductors of neural excitation, form bundles in axons and dendrites"* (142, Cajal, 1899) (see Fig. 3) Cajal's adherence to an electrical function for the cytoskeleton may have prevented him from appreciating the morphological consequences of the plasticity of the cytoskeleton.

Cajal knew about neuroplasticity. After various forms of damage produced by rabies or lesions to the nervous system, Cajal observed the retraction of dendritic processes. (Fig. 4). As can be seen in the figures, the dendritic tree is shown to be absorbed into the cell body of this cortical pyramidal neuron. This retraction of dendrites was also seen in rabbits exposed to cold temperature for 8 h. In this study, the neurofibrils can

again be seen to condense and retract into the soma. A similar phenomenon was seen in the lizard, where increased temperature, cold and fasting all resulted in a disruption of the cytoskeleton. Finally, in hibernating lizards, Cajal observed that not only was the neuron reduced in size and branching, but there was also a corresponding loss of connections (Fig. 5).

Neuroplasticity occurs during normal brain functions and may be the cause of mental illness. Cajal appears to accept neurite retraction during sleep. *"According to this scholar [Duvall, 1895] nerve cell processes have amoeboid movement and contacts between terminal axonal branches and the soma and dendrites could loosen by protoplasmic retraction. In this way, dissociation would take place with the consequent functional rest of the*

90

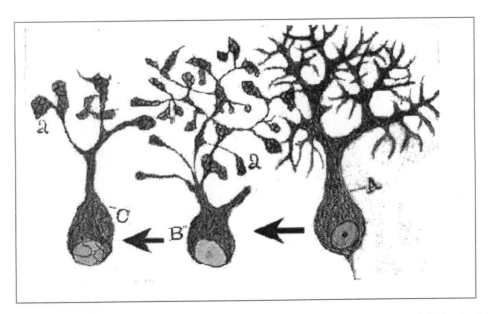

Fig. 4. [Fig. 40]. Purkinjee cells of cat of twenty-five, sacraficed two days after the traumatic lesion. A Normal, B, C cells which retracted dendrites terminate in reticulated clubs. (Copied with permission from Cajal, 1933).

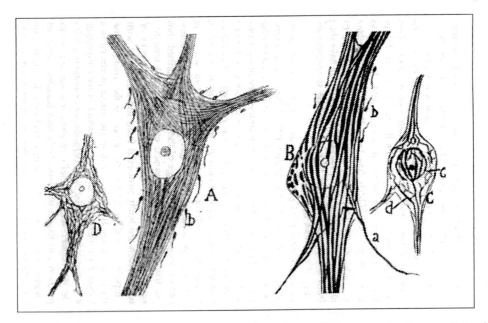

Fig. 5. [Fig. 72] Cells of lizard spinal cord; illustration demonstrates the changes in neurofibillar net according to season. Reduced silver nitrate method. A, D, cells of a lizard kept in warm in an incubator for some hours. B,C, cells of a lizard in a state of hibernation in hibernating lizards, Cajal observed that not only was the neuron reduced in size and branching, but there was also a corresponding los of connections (Copied with permission, Cajal 1899).

cells. Thus during sleep, dendrites of pyramidal cells would shrink and cease excitation arriving from the sense organs" (p. 189, Cajal, 1899). Cajal writes that according to Lupine (1894), "… in certain pathological states, particularly in motor and sensory paralyses of hysteric females, articulations established among neurons could become looser so that the passage of impulses could be partially or totally arrested" (p. 189, Cajal, 1899). Cajal writes "… reabsorption of spines, atrophy and deformation of dendritic appendages and even dendritic trunks are noted in the cerebral cortex of patients affected with progressive paralysis of the insane … and in other mental disorders … epileptic dementias and other hallucinatory states … epilepsy … rabid patients … alcoholism … [and] diphtheria" (p. 197, Cajal, 1899). For Cajal, "The filamentous framework of the nerve cell is not an immutable structure… [but] subjected to the physico-chemical variations in the neuronal environment." (p. 198, Cajal, 1899)

The amazing thing is that Cajal did not associate the changes in cytoskeleton with the corresponding changes in dendritic shape and their connections. He was certainly aware at this time (1906) that morphogenesis was a functionally important process with regard to nervous function, and might even be the structural basis of memory, but he failed to understand the subcellular (molecular) basis of this form of neuroplasticity.

Neurobiones

The years of 1905 and 1906 are coincident with the zenith of Cajal's scientific career. As Cajal devoted more attention to the neuronal doctrine, he became increasingly interested in the intraprotoplasmic neurofibrils. At this time, he described four new observations on the initial events of regeneration, which were summarized in his *Recuerdos de mi Vida*, but not translated into English by Craigie (39–40, Cajal, 1917).

1. *"That the first sprouts of the central stump sprout preferentially at the level of the axonal thickenings adjacent to the junctional disc (medullatred axons). [*At the node of Ranvier.]*

2. *"That the axons of the peripheral stump do not die instantly when they are suddenly cut off from their tropic centers, rather, they pass, especially in the vicinity of the scar, through a certain agonal process, during which they attempt to form growth cones, boutons and ramifications [which are] ephermeral and*

frustrated productions because they are not influenced by the lifegiving ferments emanating from the trophic center (the neuron with its nucleus).

3. *"That when the axon dies suddenly, as in crushing or other traumatic injuries, the necrotic protoplasm, with a pale and granular appearance, is frequently invaded by isolated fibers of recurrent formation, which ends by means of rings, handles and other [structures] (see in Fig. 123, a,c,d) (Fig. 6), the curious intra-axonal sproutings of the neurofibrils engendered in the living portion of the axon). Such phenomena take place also in the peripheral stumps of the cut nerves (Fig. 122,a).*

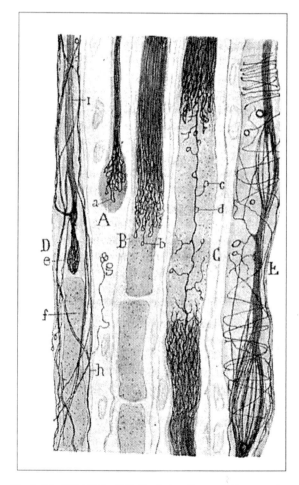

Fig. 6. [Fig. 109 A] [Fig. 122]. Crushed portion–necrotic segment—of a nerve compressed by a forcept. Cat killed 52 hours (or 48 h) after the operation. Note in the zone near the wound phenomena of survival and regnewration of neuroibrils (C, D). (Cat, 48 h [after] the operation.) (Copied with permission from Cajal, 1913–14) (see also Cajal 1917).

92

4. *"Finally, that these and other vegetative acts of isolated neurofibrils, as well as the above mentioned phenomena of metamorphosis of the neurofibrillar skeleton of the neuronal soma (rabies, action of cold, etc.) imply that the threads of the axon [that are] stainable with silver are composed of infinitesimal living entities, the neurobiones; [these are] capable of growing and multiplying with relative autonomy in the bosom of the neuroplasm, and capable of being arranged, depending on the circumstances, in intraaxonal colonies of variable architecture. The hypothesis of the neurobiones, which explained many of the structural changes in neurons, was received with interest by the authors."*

These four points represent distinct observations. The first three points are discussed in the paragraph below and indicate that microtubules, composed of the tubulin polymers, may be the molecular mechanism responsible for the observations of Cajal. **Point 1** pinpoints the distal end of axons as the site of the first sprouts. The growth takes place at the site most distal to the cell body and most intimately exposed to environmental factors present near the damage. **Point 2** raises the important observation that sprouts can form in the isolated distal portion of a severed axon. This axonal fragment is separate from the cell body, yet it is able to assemble and extend sprouts. Although these sprouts are transient, they are organized and dynamic without instructions or factors coming from the cell body. In other words, the signals and material necessary for sprouting are contained in the terminal itself and does not depend on continuity with the cell body. Thus, Cajal's observations do not lend support to theories requiring nuclear DNA signaling for initiation of sprouting. **Point 3** provides a subcellular observation on the nature of the neurofibrillar structure. Cajal saw cytoskeletal components, which formed rings, hooks and handles at their ends when damaged. Interestingly, when tubulin polymers (microtubules) are depolymerizing in a cell-free system (Madelkow et al., 1984) they generate structures that resemble rings, hooks and handles (Fig. 7).

The final point, **Point 4**, the most intriguing as Cajal envisioned an autonomous *"life force"* inside the axon. His concept of *neurobiones* arose because of the special properties of this cytoskeletal component. The neurofibrils, because of their dynamic properties, appeared to have a *"life"* independent of the neuron. In studies of axons after sudden traumatic injury, Cajal could see the isolated distal portion of the axon form a ball and

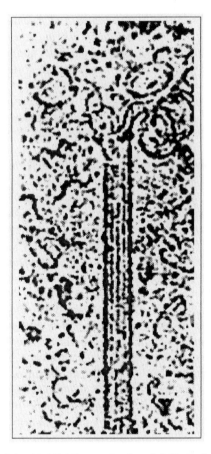

Fig. 7. [Fig. 23-11] Micrograph of a shrinking microtubule. (Modified Fig. 23-11, b; Lodish et al., 1995). Note that at the frayed ends, the tubulin polymers appear as hooks, handles and rings. Microtubules have been quickly frozen in liquid ethane and examined in the frozen state in a cryoelectron microscope. The contrast in the image is generated by the difference in density between protein (darken) and water (light). In disassembly conditions the protofilaments splay apart at microtubular ends, giving the ends a frayed appearance (Copied with permission from W.H. Freemand Company).

attempt to sprout. He wrote *"The large balls detached by autonomy from robust axons, maintain a central neurofibrillary core which in certain exceptional cases offer evidence of signs of survival and intraprotoplasmic sprouting. The cores are the Neurobiones."* (pp. 60–61, Cajal, 1917). Later he returned to this idea and attributed to these neurofibrils the source of life within the protoplasm of the neuron. *"The various acts of multiplication, degeneration, raveling, dispersion and segregation or autonomy of the neurofibrils, described so far in this thesis... lead us to believe that in the neurofibrils of the nerve cells there are ultra-microscopic units, i.e., invisible granules, which have the fundamental attributes of living protoplasm... named Neurobiones... [with a] capacity... to form lineal chains and colonies... [and] migrate... [having] extreme sensitivities to physical agents ... and, finally a certain polarity... Even though the neurobione is nourished in loco and multiplies independently of the cells.... During shrinkage [they form] handles, rings etc... [but ultimately] the well being of the colonies requires the co-operation of dynamic stimuli originating in the soma.*" (p. 368, Cajal, 1913–14) To Cajal, the neurobiones, neurofibrillary structures that are living and changing, were a major discovery that provided the basis and rationale for neuronal plasticity. He states "*How erroneous is the doctrine of those neurologists for whom the neurofibrils are a fixed and stable element...*" (p. 624, Cajal, 1913–14).

Obviously, Cajal was wrong in believing the cytoskeleton is alive, but the cytoskeleton, especially the microtubules have similar autonomous properties. Microtubules, forming the major part of the cytoskeleton, support the complex and intricate structure of neurons. Tubulin, a 450 amino acid protein, forms microtubules by spontaneously polymerizing. Cajal said the neurofibrils were "*lineal chains*", had "*polarity*", and were "*dynamic*". The strands of tubulin, when they exist *in vitro*, are long chains, highly polarized and are dynamic, growing at one end by polymerization or shrinking at the other end by depolymerization (Kirschner and Mitchison, 1986). To repeat, when the microtubules are depolymerizing they form structures similar to rings, handles, and hooks (Fig. 7).

The cytoskeleton and the spindle apparatus utilize the same pool of tubulin. Normally, proliferating cells lose their mature phenotype prior to undergoing mitosis, and, in fact, use the tubulin from their microtubules in processes to form the cell body spindle apparatus necessary for nuclear separation. The decrease in shape, length and complexity induced by tubulin depolymerization does not imply cell injury, but a form of dedifferentiation. Thus, depolymerization is a normal process for most cells, and loss of the mature morphology is a prelude to cell division and not an indication of injury. As Cajal said "*... material in the protoplasm is an extremely unstable product that changes very rapidly from the semi-solid to the liquid state when the dynamics of the neuron suffers the least perturbation... [and is] almost always reparable, which is perfectly compatible with cellular life*" (p. 197, Cajal, 1899).

Microtubule-associated proteins (MAPs) stabilize tubulin polymers in the polymerized state. *In vitro*, the microtubular stabilization leads to longer polymers of tubulin and *in vivo* to longer processes. These MAPs attach to the tubulin polymers only when they are unphosphorylated. The Ca^{++} activated protein kinase (PKC) and c-AMP activated protein kinase (PKA) phosphorylation of MAP proteins disrupts their binding to microtubules (Jameson and Caplow, 1981). MAPs are localized to different parts of the cell, and this is especially developed in neurons. MAP-2 is found primarily in dendrites and tau is found primarily in axons. In dendrites, phosphorylation of MAP-2 encourages the formation of dendritic spines (Aoki and Siekevitz, 1988) and dendritic arborization (Diez-Guerra and Avila, 1993). When phosphorylation of MAP-2 by PKC is extensive, studies show neuronal dendritic retraction (Matesic and Lin, 1994). The loss of microtubules leads to a corresponding loss of cognitive function in the animal's behavior (Johnson and Jope, 1992).

Neurotropic hypothesis

In the second part of this chapter, we try to expand the concepts of Cajal on plasticity to incorporate modern concepts of the cytoskeleton and the actions of S-1000β, the major neurite extension factor (NEF) from PNS Schwann cells and CNS astrocytes. We know of no previous attempt to connect Cajal's theory of *neurobiones* with his ideas of *chemoaffinity*. The observations made by Cajal during his career led to several modifications of his theory of *chemoaffinity*. The neurotropic hypothesis was first proposed in 1892 by Cajal. Initially he argued that neurotropic factors were chemicals that functioned as attractants, and as late as 1917 he wrote: "*The new axons are irreversibly attracted by the neurotropic substances elaborated by the cells of Schwann*" (p. 51, Cajal, 1917).

However, he appeared to greatly modify his original hypothesis by the time he published *Degeneration and Regeneration of the Nervous System* in 1913 at the age of 62. In the Introduction to the Spanish edition he said "*When I set to work [on the book], however, I saw that if the undertaking was to do justice to the magnitude and dignity of the subject, it could not merely consist of a compilation of published facts. ... I set myself the task, at the expense of laboratory work, of revisiting all the investigations previously published, and also making a*

retarded after PCPA treatment of developing rats (Blue et al., 1991). Injections of rats with PCPA at postnatal days 10–20 produces changes in brain dendritic maturation which appear to last throughout life (Mazer et al., 1997). Thus, low levels of serotonin during early development retards many of the events associated with brain differentiation and maturation: neurogenesis, synaptogenesis and cortical organizations.

In the adult brain, withdrawal of 5-HT or S-100β not only blocks growth, it promotes neurite retraction. The removal of 5-HT from the brains of mature rats produces profound changes in morphology and function, suggestive of loss of maturation. In adult rats, PCPA treatment for one week results in a 30–50% loss of cortical synaptic density (Fig. 9) (Cheng et al., 1994). PCPA treatment in adult rats decreases hippocampal and cortical immunolabeling with antibodies against synaptophysin and MAP-2 (Whitaker-Azmitia et al., 1995). Furthermore, a 5-HT1A receptor agonist can induce the re-appearance of the synaptic protein markers lost after para-chloroamphetamine (PCA) in adult (Azmitia et al., 1995) and neonate hippocampus (Haring and Yan, 1999). The neuroactive action of the 5-HT1A receptor appears to be mediated, at least in part, through release of S-100β from glial cells. Anti-S-100β infusion into the lateral ventricle of adult rats for seven days results in a significant ($p < 0.01$) decrease in synapses (Wilson et al., 1998). NAN-190 administration, a specific 5-HT1A receptor antagonist, also reduces the number of synapses. The actions of NAN-190 and anti-S-100β antibodies are not additive, providing further support for a common mechanism of these two treatments. These authors conclude that S-100β levels, controlled by 5-HT stimulation of astrocytic 5-HT1A receptors, regulate the maintenance of synaptic connections in the dentate molecular layer. Mice with extra copies of S-100β show clear evidence of accelerated maturation throughout the brain, but premature degeneration (Whitaker-Azmitia, 1997). This pattern is reminiscent of Down's children, who have excess S-100β, show accelerated maturation and early onset of Alzheimer's disease (Griffin et al., 1998).

Behavioral studies indicate that the regression of neuronal morphology has functional consequences. Faber and Haring (1999) found neonatal serotonin depletion (PCA or 5,7-DHT) or 5-HT1A receptor blockade (NAN-190) results in a reduction in the number of dentate granule cell dendritic spines and synaptic profiles in

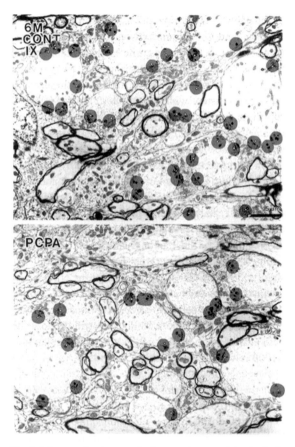

Fig. 9. Micrograph of rat cerabral cortex in normal (top) of after PCPA injections (see Cheng et al., 1994). The synapses are outlined in shade. Picture provided by Dr Nubuo Okado.

the molecular layer on P14 and P21. The granule cell responses in P60 rats showed reduced paired pulse facilitation in these groups, reflecting a diminished synaptic drive (Haring and Yan, 1999). Animals depleted of 5-HT from postnatal day 10–29 have pronounced learning deficits (Mazer et al., 1997). Finally, removal of brain 5-HT by PCA in the adult rat produced a loss of hippocampal synapses (Matsukawa et al., 1997). Similarly, removal of acetylcholine also resulted in a loss of synapses. Both these treatments alone produce small changes in memory function. However, when the treatments are combined, there is an additive loss of synapses, and a dramatic disruption of memory in the rats. Therefore, the loss of morphology produced by loss of 5-HT results in functional deficits in the animals.

We hypothesize that the Schwann cell factor described by Cajal and S-100β are the same molecule. However, despite the fact that S-100β is not a survival factor, it is antiapoptotic.

Colchicine, which disrupts microtubules, induces apoptosis in a number of cells, including neurons (Brewton et al., 2001). In addition, H_2O_2, a strong anti-oxidant, induces apoptosis. Finally, staurosporine, can also induce apoptosis (Ahlemeyer et al., 2000). In all three conditions, addition of S-100β can prevent programmed cell death. In our studies (Brewton et al., 2001), we expose the neuroblastoma cell line, N-18, to colchicine for 30 min and followed these cells for several hours (Fig. 10). The cells are visualized with a Nissl stain or reacted with TUNEL stain, which shows which cells are apoptotic. Colchicine exposure results in altered cell appearance and a significant increase in TUNEL staining. Treatment with S-100β of the N-18 cells after they are exposed to colchicine results in a dramatic reversal in the morphology and in the number of cells which stain with TUNEL. Thus, S-100β, a molecule found in high levels in astrocytes and Schwann cells, is a neurite extension, differentiating and anti-apoptotic factor. Clearly, the distribution, regulation, and properties identified for S-100β and 5-HT1A receptors encompasses and extend those envisioned by Cajal in his neurotropic hypothesis (see Fig. 11).

Conclusion

The phenomenon of brain plasticity was well described and understood at both the cellular and functional level by Ramón y Cajal. He described the growth and retraction of dendrites in reptiles, birds and mammals during cold, injury and starvation. He emphasized the dramatic retraction of dendrites during hibernation, a phenomenon recently confirmed. He was among the first to accept that various forms of mental illness could be accompanied by dendritic retraction. He held the optimistic view that these dynamic changes were "*almost always reparable*". Cajal's theory of memory formation supposed an increase in fiber growth and connections. In his Croonian lecture of 1894 he said: "*Brain activity is unlikely to improve the organization of the brain through an increase in cell number, because, we know that the neurons have lost, since the embryonic stage, the ability to proliferate; however, one can admit as very likely that*

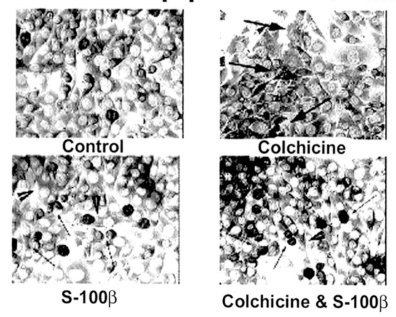

S-100 Blocks Apoptosis in N-18 Cells

Control **Colchicine**

S-100β **Colchicine & S-100β**

Fig. 10. Colchicine exposure for 30 min at a concentration of 10^{-7} M can induce cell death in N-18 cells within 2 h and S100β at a dose of 20 ng/ml applied after the colchicine can blocks this process. (See Brewton et al., 2001).

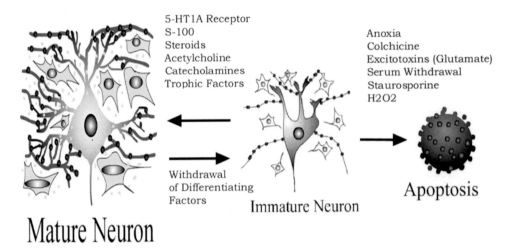

5-HT1A Receptor
S-100
Steroids
Acetylcholine
Catecholamines
Trophic Factors

Anoxia
Colchicine
Excitotoxins (Glutamate)
Serum Withdrawal
Staurosporine
H2O2

Withdrawal
of Differentiating
Factors

Immature Neuron

Apoptosis

Mature Neuron

Fig. 11. A summary cartoon showing the actions of serotonin and S-100β on neuronal morphology and apoptosis.

mental activity provokes a greater development of the protoplasmic apparatus and of the nerve collaterals in the part of the brain most utilized. In this way, preexisting connections between groups of cells could be notably reinforced by multiplication of the terminal branches of protoplasmic appendices and nerve collaterals; and, in addition, novel intercellular connections could be established thanks to the new formation of collaterals and protoplasmic expansions.

One objection immediately presents itself: how can the volume of brain remain constant if there is a multiplication and even new formation of terminal branches of protoplasmic appendices and nerve collaterals?

In response to this objection, we cannot dismiss the possibility of either a corresponding diminution (retraction) of cell bodies or a proportional compression of the regions of the brain whose functions do not correspond directly to intelligent activity" (pp. 466–467, Cajai 1894.

All of these ideas of expansion and retraction were expressed in the late nineteenth century, but were largely ignored by the mainstream of neuroscience research in the 20th century. In fact, Cajal himself in later years became pessimistic about neuroplasticity in the CNS. He wrote *"Adult cells of Schwann, ectodermal elements like those of the glia, the neurons themselves when they are necrosed or degenerating, the remnants of axons and of the medullary sheath, the exudates with their leucocytes, etc., are impotent to elaborate these stimuli [for growth]. Perhaps during the ontogenetic process the neuroblasts or neurons had a phase of specific neurotropic secretion; perhaps the*

ependymal elements also collaborated chemically in the tutorial and orienting process. But the functional specialization of the brain imposed on the neurons two great lacunae: proliferation inability and irreversibility of intraprotoplasmic differentiation. It is for this reason that, once the development was ended, the founts of growth and regeneration of the axons and dendrites dried up irrevocably. In adult centers, the nerve paths are something fixed, ended, immutable. Everything may die, nothing may be regenerated." (p. 750, Cajal 1913–14)

Today, Cajal's earlier views are experiencing a rediscovery as new techniques demonstrate increases and decreases in brain volume. Yet despite these observations of neuroplasticity in the normal and diseased brain, a comprehensive explanation of the neuronal basis of neuroplasticity is still lacking. Cajal's views of the cytoskeleton evolved from considering this fibrillary network as a passive conductor of electrical impulses. In his latter idea the neurites were described as *"neurobiones"* which represented an autonomous living forces within the neuron. Although both these ideas are wrong, the current knowledge about microtubules and the neuronal cytoskeleton reaffirms most of the observations Cajal made. As Cajal himself said, *"While we grant to the facts which are revealed by highly selective methods an unquestionable objective value, we do not extend this confidence to any hypothesis, our own or those of other investigators no matter how seductive they may appear. ... in biology theories are fragile and ephermeral constructions that are renewed every eight to ten years."*

(Cajal 75 years ago at the age of 75, 1913–14, p. vi, In English translation to Cajal by May in 1927).

In this review, we propose that the cytoskeleton of neurons, especially that microtubular component in dendritic processes, is a highly dynamic structural system which provides a molecular framework for understanding structural plasticity. We propose that S-100β, a neurite extension, differentiating and anti-apoptotic factor which is concentrated in PNS Schwann cells and CNS astrocyres, possesses many of the properties raised by Cajal in his "*Neurotropic Hypothesis*". The regulation of S-100β release from astrocytes by the 5HT1A receptor provides a neuronal-glial mechanism for neuronal instability which may help explain how neuroplasticity and mental illness are closely intertwined in the mammalian brain. Cajal in 1933, at the age of 81, a year before his death said "*Regeneration does not take place in the nervous centers [but could be induced by transplanted Schwann cells]... This demonstrates that the impotence of the central axons to restore the peripheral segment is neither fatal nor irremediable, but that is due, perhaps, to the absence of Schwann's cells in the process of rejuvenation.*" (p. 94, Cajal, 1933). If S-100β is the neurotropic factor, then astrocytes, not Schwann cells, could be awakened, possibly by manipulation of the 5-HT1A receptor, to aid in the process of rejuvenation.

References

Ahlemeyer, B., Beier, H., Semkova, I., Schaper, C. and Krieglstein, J. (2000) S-100beta protects cultured neurons against glutamate- and staurosporine-induced damage and is involved in the antiapoptotic action of the 5 HT(1A)-receptor agonist, Bay x 3702. *Brain Res.*, 858: 121–128.

Adayev, T., El-Sherif, Y., Barua, M., Penington, N.J. and Banerjee, P. (1999) Agonist stimulation of the serotonin1A receptor causes suppression of anoxia-induced apoptosis via mitogen-activated protein kinase in neuronal HN2-5 cells. *J. Neurochem.*, 72: 1489–1496.

Aoki, C. and Siekevitz, P. (1988) Plasticity in brain development. *Scientific American*, 259: 56–64.

Azmitia, E.C. (1999) Serotonin neurons, neuroplasticity and homeostasis of neural tissue. *Neuropsychopharmacology*, 21(2 Suppl): 33S–45S.

Azmitia, E.C., Dolan, K. and Whitaker-Azmitia, P.M. (1990) S-100$_b$ but not NGF, EGF, insulin or calmodulin functions as a CNS serotonergic growth factor. *Brain Research*, 516: 354–356.

Azmitia, E.C., Rubinstein, V.J., Strafaci, J.A., Rios, J.C. and Whitaker-Azmitia, P.M. (1995) 5-HT$_{1A}$ agonist and dexamethasone reversal of para-chloroamphetamine induced loss of MAP-2 and synaptophysin immunoreactivity in adult rat brain. *Mol. Brain Res.*, 677: 181–192.

Azmitia, E.C. and Whitaker-Azmitia, P.M. (1997) Development and neuroplasticity of central serotonergic neurons. In: H.G. Baumgarten and M. Gothert (Eds.), *Handbook Of Experimental Pharmacology. Serotonergic Neurons and 5-HT Receptors in the CNS*, Chpt. 1: Springer-Verlag, Berlin, pp. 1–39.

Baudier, J. and Cole, R.D. (1988) Interactions between the microtubule-associated tau proteins and S100b regulate tau phosphorylation by the Ca^{2+}/calmodulin-dependent protein kinase II. *J. Biol. Chem.*, 263: 5876–5883.

Blue, M.E., Erzurumlu, R.S. and Jhaveri, S. (1991) A comparison of pattern formation by thalamocortical and serotonergic afferents in the rat barrel field cortex. *Cereb. Cortex*, 1: 380–389.

Brewton, L.S., Haddad, L. and Azmitia, E.C. (2001) Colchicine-induced cytoskeletal collapse and apoptosis in N-18 neuroblastoma cultures is rapidly reversed by applied S-100beta. *Brain Res.*, 912(1): 9–16.

Cajal, S.R. (1894) The Croonian Lecture: La fine Structure des Centres Nerveux. *Proc. Royal soc. (London)*, 55: 444–468.

Cajal, S.R. (1892) El Nuevo concepto de la histologia de los centros nervioso. *Rev. Cienc. Med. (Barcelona)*, 18: 457–476.

Cajal, S.R. (1899) *Texture of the Nervous System of Man and the Vertebrates*. Translation by P. Pasik and T. Pasik, (1999), Springer-Verlag, Wren, New York.

Cajal, S.R. (1913–14) *Degeneration and Regeneration of the Nervous System*. Translation by R.M. May, (1928), Oxford University Press, London.

Cajal, S.R. (1917) *Recuerdos de mi Vida*, translation by J. DeFelipe and E.G. Jones 1991, Oxford University Press, New York, Oxford.

Cajal, S.R. (1933) Neuron theory or reticular theory? Objective evidence of the anatomical unity of the nerve cells. Translated by M. Ubeda-Purkiss and C.A. Fox. Madrid, CSIC. Reproduced In: J. DeFelipe and E.G. Jones (Eds.), *Cajal's Degeneration and Regeneration of the Nervous System*, pp. 91–100, 1991 Oxford University Press, New York, Oxford.

Cheng, L., Hamaguchi, K., Ogawa, M., Hamada, S. and Okado, N. (1994) PCPA reduces both monoaminergic afferents and non-monoaminergic synapses in the cerebral cortex, *Neurosci. Res.*, 19: 111–115.

Deinum, J., Baudier, J., Briving, C. et al. (1983) The effect of S-100a and S-100b proteins and Zn^{2+} on the assembly of brain microtubule proteins *in vitro*. *FEES Lett.*, 163: 287–291.

Descartes, R. (1662) *Treatise on Man*. In: T. Hall (Ed. and Trans.), Treatise On Man. Harvard University Press, Cambridge. (Reproduced 1972).

Diez-Guerra, F.J. and Avila, J. (1995) An increase in phosphorylation of microtubule associated protein 2 accompanies dendrite extension during the differentiation of cultured hippocampal neurones. *Eur. J. Biochem.*, 227: 68–77.

Duvall, M. (1895) Hypotheses sur la physilogie des centres nerveux; theorie histologique du sommeil. *Compt Rend Hebd Sean. Mem. Soc. Biol*, 47: 74–77.

Dustin, A. (1910) Le role des tropisms et de l'odogenesis dans le regeneration du systeme nerveux. *Arch. de Biol.*, 25: 292–295.

Ebendal, T. (1981) Control of neurite extension by embryonic heart explants. *J. Embryol. Exp. Morphol*, 61: 289–301.

Faber, K.M. and Haring, J.H. (1999) Synaptogenesis in the postnatal rat fascia dentata is influenced by 5-HT1a receptor activation. *Dev. Brain Res.*, 114: 245–52.

Griffin, W.S., Sheng, J.G., McKenzie, J.E. et al. (1998) Life-long overexpression of S100beta in Down's syndrome: implications for Alzheimer pathogenesis. *Neurobiol. Aging*, 19: 401–405.

Haglid, K.G., Hamberger, A., Hansson, H.A. et al. (1976) Cellular and subcellular distribution of the S-100 protein in rabbit and rat central nervous system. *J. Neurosci. Res.*, 2: 175–191.

Haring, J.H. and Yan, W. (1999) Dentate granule cell function after neonatal treatment with parachloroamphetamine or 5,7-dihydroxytryptamine. *Dev. Brain Res.*, 114: 269–272.

Hesketh, J. and Baudier, J. (1986) Evidence that S100 proteins regulate microtubule assembly and stability in rat brain extracts. *Int. J. Biochem.*, 18: 691–695.

Jameson, L. and Caplow, M. (1981) Modification of microtubule steady-state dynamics by phosphorylation of the microtubule-associated proteins. *Proc. Natl. Acad. Sci. USA*, 78: 3413–3417.

Johnson, G.V. and Jope, R.S. (1992) The role of microtubule-associated protein 2 (MAP-2) in neuronal growth, plasticity and degeneration. *J. Neurosci. Res.*, 33: 505–512.

Kirschner, M.W. and Mitchison, T. (1986) Microtubule dynamics. *Nature*, 324: 621–623.

Kligman, D. and Hsieh, L.S. (1987) Neurite extension factor induces rapid morphological differentiation of mouse neuroblastoma cells in defined medium. *Brain Res.*, 430(2): 296–300.

Kligman, D. and Marshak, D.R. (1985) Purification and characterization of a neurite extension factor from bovine brain. *Proc. Natl. Acad. Sci. U S A*, 82(20): 7136–7139.

Kligman, D. (1982) Isolation of a protein from bovine brain which promotes neurite extension from chick embryo cerebral cortex neurons in defined medium. *Brain Res.* 250(1): 93–100.

Landry, C.F., Ivy, G.O., Dunn, R.J. et al. (1989) Expression of the gene encoding the betasubunit of S-100 protein in the developing rat brain analyzed by *in situ* hybridization. *Brain Res. Mol. Brain Res.*, 6: 251–262.

Lauder, J.M. and Krebs, H. (1976) Effects of p-chlorophenylalanine on time of neuronal origin during embryogenesis in the rat. *Brain Res.*, 107: 638–644.

Lodish, H., Baltimore, D., Berk, A. et al. (1995). *Molecular Cell Biology*. Publ. Scientific American Inc. New York, Oxford.

Lucaites, V.L. Nelson, D.L. Wainscott, D.B. and Baez, M. (1996) Receptor subtype and density determine the coupling repertoire of the 5-HT2 receptor subfamily. *Life Sci.*, 59: 1081–1095.

Mandelkow, E., Schltheiss, R. and Mandelkow, E.-M. (1984) Reconstruction of Tubulin protofilaments: different appearance of the same structure. *Ultrastructure*, 13: 125–136.

Matesic, D.F., Lin, R.C. (1994) Microtubule-associated protein 2 as an early indicator of ischemia-induced neurodegeneration in the gerbil forebrain. *J. Neurochem.*, 63: 1012–1020.

Matsukawa, M., Ogawa, M., Nakadate, K. et al. (1997) Serotonin and acetylcholine are crucial to maintain hippocampal synapses and memory acquisition in rats. *Neurosci. Lett*, 230: 13–16.

Mazer, C., Muneyyirci, J., Taheny, K. et al. (1997) Serotonin depletion during synaptogenesis leads to decreased synaptic density and learning deficits in the adult rat: a possible model of neurodevelopmental disorders with cognitive deficits. *Brain Res.*, 760: 68–73.

Muller, H.W. and Seifert, W. (1982) A neurotrophic factor (NTF) released from primary glial cultures supports survival and fiber outgrowth of cultured hippocampal neurons. *J. Neurosci. Res.*, 8: 195–204.

Nishi, M., Kawata, M. and Azmitia, E.C. (2000) Trophic interactions between brain-derived neurotrophic factor and s100beta on cultured serotonergic neurons. *Brain Research*, 868: 113–118.

Nishi, M., Poblete, J.C., Whitaker-Azmitia, P.M. and Azmitia, E.C. (1996) Brain derived neurotrophic factor and S100β; trophic interactions on cultured serotonergic neurons. *Neurosci. Net*, 10003 (www.neuroscience.com).

Nishi, M., Kawata, M. and Azmitia, E.C. (1997) S100β promotes the extension of microtubule associated protein 2 (MAP2)-immunoreactive neurites retracted after colchicine treatment in rat spinal cord culture. *Neurosci. Lett.*, 229: 212–214.

Sano, M. and Kitajima, S. (1998) Activation of mitogen-activated protein kinases is not required for the extension of neurites from PC12D cells triggered by nerve growth factor. *Brain Res.*, 785(2): 299–308.

Shenker, A., Maayani, S., Weinstein, H. and Green, J.P. (1985) Two 5-HT receptors linked to adenylate cyclase in guinea pig hippocampus are discriminated by 5-carboxamidotryptamine and spiperone. *Eur. J. Pharmacol.*, 109(3): 427–429.

Sheu, F.-S., Azmitia, E.C., Marshak, D.R. et al. (1994) Glial-derived S100b protein selectively inhibits recombinant protein kinase C (PKC) phosphorylation of neuron-specific protein F1IGAP43. *Mol. Brain. Res.*, 21: 62–66.

Stefansson, K., Wollmann, R.L. and Moore B.W. (1982) Distribution of S-100 protein outside the central nervous system. *Brain Res.*, 234(2): 309–317.

Watts, S.W., Cox, D.A. and Johnson, B.G. et al. (1994) Contractile serotonin-2A receptor signal transduction in guinea pig trachea: importance of protein kinase C and extracellular and intracellular calcium but not phosphoinositide hydrolysis. *J. Pharmacol. Exp. Ther.*, 271: 832–844.

Whitaker-Azmitia, P.M. and Azmitia, E.C. (1986) ^{3}H-serotonin binding to brain astroglial cells: differences between intact and homogenized preparations and mature and immature cultures. *J. Neurochem.*, 46: 1186–1189.

Whitaker-Azmitia, P.M., Borella, A. and Raio, N. (1995) Serotonin depletion in the adult rat causes loss of the dendritic marker MAP-2: a new animal model of schizophrenia? *Neuropsychopharmacology*, 12: 269–272.

Whitaker-Azmitia, P.M., Murphy, R.B. and Azmitia, E.C. (1990) S-100 protein release from astrocytic glial cells by stimulation of 5-HT$_{1A}$ receptors and regulates the development of serotonergic neurons. *Brain Res.*, 528: 155–158.

Whitaker-Azmitia, P.M., Wingate, M., Borella, A. et al. (1997) Transgenic mice overexpressing the neurtrophic factor S-100β show neuronal cytoskeletal and behavioral signs of altered aging processes: implications for Alzheimer's disease and Down's Syndrome. *Brain Res.*, 776(1–2): 51–60.

Wilson, C.C., Faber, K.M. and Haring, J.H. (1998) Serotonin regulates synaptic connections in the dentate molecular layer of adult rats via 5-HT1 a receptors: evidence for a glial mechanism. *Brain Res.*, 782: 235–239.

Yin, Q.W., Johnson, J., Prevette, D. and Oppenheim, R.W. (1994) Cell death of spinal motoneurons in the chick embryo following deafferentation: rescue effects of tissue extracts, soluble proteins, and neurotrophic agents. *J. Neurosci.*, 14: 7629–7640.

E.C. Azmitia, J. DeFelipe, E.G. Jones, P. Rakic and C.E. Ribak (Eds.)
Progress in Brain Research, Vol. 136

CHAPTER 9

Changing views of Cajal's neuron: the case of the dendritic spine

Menahem Segal*

Deparment of Neurobiology, The Weizmann Institute, Rehovot 76100, Israel

Abstract: Ever since dendritic spines were first described in detail by Santiago Ramón y Cajal, they were assumed to underlie the physical substrate of long term memory in the brain. Recent time-lapse imaging of dendritic spines in live tissue, using confocal microscopy, have revealed an amazingly plastic structure, which undergoes continuous changes in shape and size, not intuitively related to its assumed role in long term memory. Functionally, the spine is shown to be an independent cellular compartment, able to regulate calcium concentration independently of its parent dendrite. The shape of the spine is instrumental in regulating the link between the synapse and the parent dendrite such that longer spines have less impact on the dendrite than shorter ones. The spine can be formed, change its shape and disappear in response to afferent stimulation, in a dynamic fashion, indicating that spine morphology is an important vehicle for structuring synaptic interactions. While this role is crucial in the developing nervous system, large variations in spine densities in the adult brain indicate that tuning of synaptic impact may be a role of spines throughout the life of a neuron.

Dendritic spines were first described by Santiago Ramón y Cajal already in the 19th century. He found them first in Purkinje cells of the cerebellum and later in cerebral cortical neurons. Like with other major discoveries related to the creation of the neuronal dogma, it involved heated debates on whether the spine is a genuine structure, or an artifact of the fixation procedure. Being a fine structure, at the limit of optical resolution, it was quite impossible in those early days, to resolve this issue. The importance of these arguments stems from the fact that the spine is the postsynaptic end of the synapse, the focus of the debate between reticularists and neuronalists that lasted from the late 19th century, all the way to the 50's of the 20th century. This debate was finally settled when electron microscopic (EM) studies showed that the presynaptic terminals and the postsynaptic region are clearly separable entities. Cajal used his familiar sharp

tongue in this debate; "*It is difficult not to see in this completely arbitrary hypothesis a great deal of ego involvement in an attempt to defend an earlier mistake*" he referred to Semi Meyer's proposal that the spines are silver salt precipitates in a lymphatic space surrounding dendrites (Cajal, 1995 English translation).

Beyond the initial description of the spine, Cajal was already puzzled by this unique organelle, and assumed that "the receptive surface of dendrites is increased tremendously by the presence of spines and that, because of them, contacts between terminal arborizations of axons and dendrites could be more intimate" (Cajal, 1995). This simple view is surprisingly one of a handful of recent hypotheses of why dendritic spines exist (Harris and Kater, 1994; Segal, 1995a). Interestingly, Cajal already noticed that spines vary in shape and density in different types of neurons, and that their shape is strikingly influenced by age and by formation of synapses with afferent fibers, such that immature spines have a 'filopodium' like morphology, different from that of the

*Corresponding author: Tel.: 972 89342553; Fax: 972 89344140; E-mail: menahem.segal@weizmann.ac.il

102

mature spine, which receive afferent input (Fig. 1). However, he drew the spines as having the same shape and length along the dendritic segment, failing to make a point that there is actually a great heterogeneity among spines even in the same neuron (Fig. 2). The spine was realized as a genuinely complex structure many years later, when it was finally seen at the EM level (Gray, 1959) and could be reconstructed in 3D (Harris and Stevens, 1989; Segev et al., 1995). It was then recognized that the spine contains certain subcellular organelles, including, for example, actin filaments. These were assumed, but not demonstrated until recently, to underlie mechanical 'twitches', much like muscles (see below). A protein synthetic machinery is found in the vicinity of the spine stem, which is probably responsible for supplying the spine with proteins associated with urgent changes in spine shape and functions (Steward and Schuman, 2001). More interestingly, the spine does not contain some critical subcellular organelles (e.g., mitochondria). This lack of mitochondria may hint to possible functions of the spine (see below). The extensive use of immunocytochemical methods have caused a rapid rate of identification of over 70 families of molecules, in a recent count (Zhang and Benson, 2000). Among these are receptors,

ion channels, transduction mechanisms, adhesion molecules and scaffolding proteins.

For many years, analysis of changes in spine structure was restricted to the postmortem, fixed tissue, where changes in spine shape/size and density were measured in populations of neurons, typically in relation to learning and memory or developmental and aging processes (Globus et al., 1973; Feldman and Dowd, 1975; Purpura, 1974; Scheibel et al., 1975). These early observations were conducted with Golgi material at the light microscopic or the EM level. While being extremely tedious and time consuming, these studies did not reach a clear consensus as to what are the changes that the spine undergoes in processes related to plasticity. Assuming that morphological changes in spines will reflect functional changes occurring, for example, following learning, there was little agreement as to what exactly are these changes (Lowndes and Stewart, 1994; Jones et al., 1997; O'Malley et al., 1998) except for the intuitive generalization that more spines probably mean better functions of the neuron. More formal attempts to correlate structural changes with functional ones involved application of a tetanic stimulation and the production of LTP, followed by a search for changes in the spines.

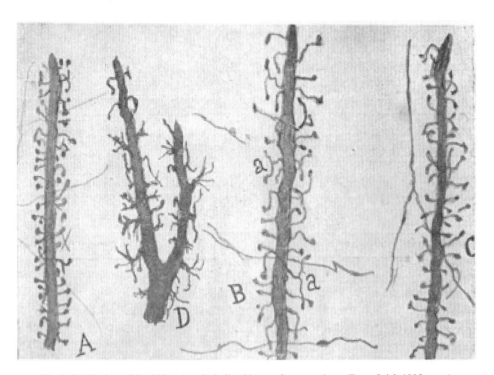

Fig. 1. Cajal's view of dendritic spines including his own figure captions. (From Cajal, 1995 trans.)

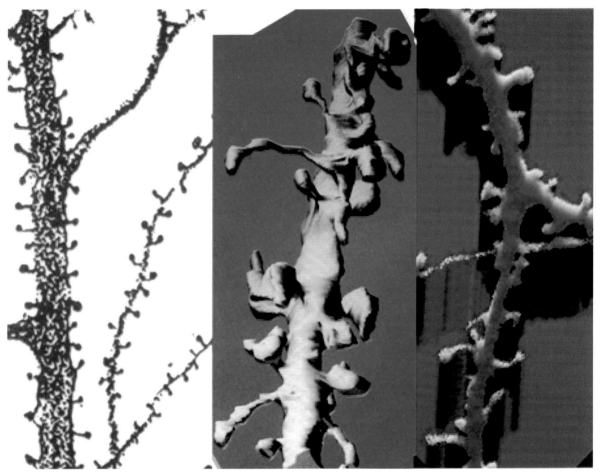

Fig. 2. Comparison of dendritic spines of pyramidal neurons, across generations of studies. Left, original drawing of Cajal, showing dendritic spines of same size, evenly distributed along a dendritic shaft. Middle, EM reconstruction of spines and dendrites (modified from Harris and Stevens, 1989) and Left, spines of cultured hippocampal neurons, reconstructed from serial optical sections taken with a confocal laser scanning microscope (courtesy of E. Korkotian).

Experiments like this, conducted both *in-vivo* and in slice preparations also did not yield a coherent view on what is actually changing structurally in correlation with the functional change (Lee et al., 1980; Desmond and Levy, 1983; Trommald et al., 1996; Rusakov et al., 1997).

It was only recently, when spines could be visualized in living neurons in both *in-vitro* and *in-vivo* (Segal, 1995a; Yuste and Denk, 1995), that the research of spine structure and function began to gain momentum. Recent studies contributed to a radical change of the traditional view of the spine as a rigid locus of synaptic interaction, subjected perhaps to long-term modification in relation to plasticity, to a dynamic structure, which undergoes rapid,

continuous changes in shape and possibly in function (Segal, 1995c; Fischer et al., 1998; Halpain et al., 1998). The initial observations made with live neurons, involved imaging of variations of intracellular calcium concentrations ($[Ca^{2+}]i$) in spines and their parent dendrites (Segal, 1995a; Yuste and Denk, 1995). Besides the confirmation that spines are genuine structures, that can be observed in live neurons, and thus are not a product of fixation, these observations also demonstrated that the spine is a unique calcium compartment, capable of independent regulation of $[Ca^{2+}]i$. This indicates that while the spine may not be a unique electrical compartment, responsible for variations in the charge transferred from the synapse to the dendrite, as was predicted by theoreticians (Segev et al., 1995; Shepherd, 1996), it may very well regulate calcium-dependent processes, that are linked to synaptic receptors and the complex machinery associated with them.

Two issues related to dendritic spine functions were analyzed extensively by us and others in the past decade; the first one focuses on the factors which govern changes in $[Ca^{2+}]i$ in the spine ($[Ca^{2+}]s$); Initially, it was found that changes produced in dendritic $[Ca^{2+}]$ are not always reflected in $[Ca^{2+}]s$ (Guthrie et al., 1991), indicating that the spine may contain independent calcium-regulating mechanisms. It was also found that minimal synaptic stimulation can evoke $[Ca^{2+}]i$ changes that are restricted to individual spines (Muller and Connor, 1991). The spine contains NMDA and AMPA receptors, as well as voltage-gated calcium channels (Segal, 1995b). In addition, it contains local calcium stores, that may contribute significantly to the calcium rise seen in response to synaptic stimulation (Emptage et al., 1999; Korkotian and Segal, 1998). These studies helped to delineate the possible mechanisms responsible for synaptic plasticity, known to involve changes in $[Ca^{2+}]i$ at or near the synapse. In essence, they propose that the spine is a unique compartment, where $[Ca^{2+}]i$ can rise to high levels, to allow local changes in synaptic functions, without involving dendritic mechanisms (Volfovsky et al., 1999).

A second series of studies was aimed at the rules that govern the formation of novel dendritic spines, and the variations in their shape and functions. The main motivation for these studies is the intuitive feeling that morphological changes in spines underlie long-term changes in synaptic activity, associated with learning and memory. The two basic questions related to this issue are, what is the nature of the stimuli that govern changes in spine morphology, and what are the functional consequences of such changes. Early studies have shown that exposure of dendrites to high concentration of glutamate, resulting in a large and continuous rise in $[Ca^{2+}]s$, causes shrinkage of the exposed spines, to their complete elimination (Segal, 1995; Halpain et al., 1998). Exposure to stimuli which cause lower rises in [Ca]s resulted in elongation of existing spines, and occasionally also formation of novel ones (Korkotian and Segal, 1999). In fact, the same spine could be seen to shrink after high glutamate concentration, and to expand following low glutamate exposure. The functional relevance of these morphological variations was indicated in studies that

examined the spine/dendrite interaction, showing that longer spines are more detached functionally from the parent dendrite than short ones (Volfovsky et al., 1999).

The ability to time lapse-photograph morphological changes in the same dendrite/spines over time re-ignited the search for a spine-associated morphological basis of memory. In a pioneering study, Engert and Bonhoeffer (1999) described the formation of novel spines in a neuron undergoing long term potentiation of reactivity to afferent stimulation. Novel spines were formed in response to plasticity-producing stimuli in a manner that is selective for the stimulated dendritic segment, and was not found throughout unstimulated segments of the dendritic tree of the stimulated cell. This indicates that postsynaptic activity or a global rise in [Ca]i are not sufficient to produce a novel spine, but an association between pre- and postsynaptic activity, as is the case with the 'Hebbian' synapse is the stimulus that leads to formation of novel spines. Still, it was not clear that the novel spines are at all functional, or that they contribute to the enhanced synaptic currents observed in the affected cells. While these observations are still awaiting confirmation by other research groups, we (Goldin et al., 2001) have found that a transient elevation of network activity can trigger a massive formation of novel dendritic spines without a need to selectively activate a specific pathway. This increase in network activity does not involve electrical stimulation, which is alien to the network, or an activation of extrasynaptic receptors, but it involves a continuous change in synaptic activity in many neurons in the network. Subsequent to this change in activity, there is formation of dendritic spines (Fig. 3), and pruning of others. The novel spines are indeed functional, in that they are innervated by active presynaptic terminals (Goldin et al., 2001). The mechanisms underlying the formation of these novel spines are currently being investigated but they may involve activation of MAP-kinases and the nuclear cyclic AMP response element binding protein (CREB) as suggested by others (Wu et al., 2001).

Concomitant with the formation of novel spines, there is a marked pruning of existing ones. The pruning of spines, originally thought to be present only in developing neurons, has been found recently to be an active process, involving activation of the NMDA receptor (Bock and Braun, 1999). In our current studies, pruning has also been associated with activation of the NMDA receptor, and to correlate with an enhanced

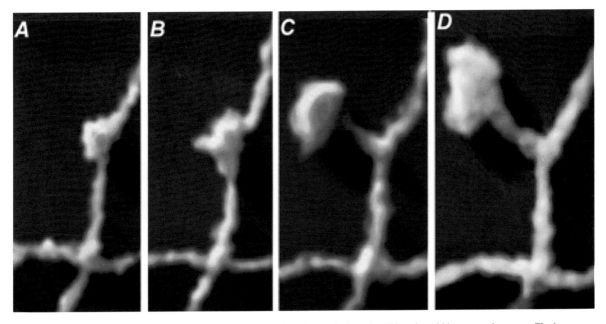

Fig. 3. The formation of a dendritic spine following exposure to plasticity producing stimuli in cultured hippocampal neurons. The images are taken every 30 minutes, before (A) and after (B–D) exposure to recording medium which enhances activation of the NMDA receptor. 1 h after exposure to the conditioning medium, there is formation of novel dendritic spines (modified from Goldin et al., 2001).

network activity. Unlike novel spines, pruned ones seem not to be associated with an active presynaptic terminal (Goldin et al., 2001), indicating that the presence of an active terminal tends to enhance existing synapses, and its absence tends to cause elimination of present but not functional dendritic spines.

An interesting and potentially important behavior of developing dendritic spines is their local motility. Young dendritic spines are highly motile (Ziv and Smith, 1996; Dunaevsky et al., 1999) and this motility is probably instrumental in making synaptic contacts with incoming afferents. More recently, Matus and his colleagues have demonstrated that dendritic spines of neurons that have been transfected with actin-linked green fluorescent protein (GFP) express considerable local motility even after synaptic contacts are made, as indicated by the presence of presynaptic marker synaptophysin, next to the motile spine (Fischer et al., 1998). This motility can be minimized by exposing the spine to glutamate. We (Korkotian and Segal, 2001a) have confirmed and extended these observations and found that motility is independent of postsynaptic spontaneous calcium transients, but that motility of dendritic spines are highly correlated with the

presence of *active* presynaptic terminals, labeled with the fluorescent dye FM4-64 in living cultures. When presynaptic terminals adjacent to the spine are active to the extent that they take up the dye, spines do not move. It is important to distinguish between structural presynaptic terminals, which are marked by immunolabeling with synaptophysin, a presynaptic marker, and functional synapses which are marked with FM4-64 dye. We have indications that the latter group is only a subgroup of the former one. There are a number of studies showing that even when a presynaptic terminal is present, it may not be functional, in that it may produce no electrical impact on the postsynaptic neuron (Vicario-Abejón et al., 1998). Once spike activity is blocked with tetrodotoxin, spines begin to express local motility (Korkotian and Segal, 2001a). Our observations do not necessarily contradict those of Matus', because the possible differences in the growth conditions may allow more spontaneous activity among the neurons in our cultures than in theirs, and allow the detection of more spontaneous motility in their cells than in ours. In either case, spine motility is negatively correlated with network activity in culture. The role of these fine movements of the spine head is still obscure, but they seem to be dependent on the age of the cell, and may have some role in trafficking synaptic proteins into and out of the spine head (Shi et al., 1999).

In addition to the slow movement in space (Ziv and Smith, 1996) and the faster local movement (Fischer et al., 1998; Korkotian and Segal, 2001a) we have recently characterized fast twitches of dendritic spines, associated with back propagating action potentials evoked in these cells by depolarizing the soma (Korkotian and Segal, 2001b). During a large transient rise of $[Ca^{2+}]$s which accompanies the action potentials, the spine shrinks momentarily. This twitch is small, at the limit of optical resolution, and brief, lasting at times less than 1 second. It is dependent on actin polymerization in the spine head, and is absent when actin polymerization is blocked by the selective drug, latrunculin. Since this drug also has an effect on reactivity of the spine head to glutamate (unpublished observations), it may hint to a possible role of the spine twitch in long-term regulation of reactivity of the spine head to synaptic stimulation (Kim and Lisman, 1999). Further experiments are needed to analyze this possibility.

Current studies on the molecular composition of the spine (Sala et al., 2001) bring us closer to understanding the mechanisms that underlie the morphological hetero-geneity of spines, and high resolution imaging of living spines bring us closer to understanding the functions of this unique organelle, seen first over a hundred years ago, and yet still constitutes an enigma. While Cajal's hypothesis, that the spine simply increases cell surface is still as viable as any other hypothesis, it becomes apparent that this static view of the spine is not accurate, and a more dynamic view is more appropriate. In any case, the spine is not just a cytoplasmic extension of the dendrite, or an artifact of silver salt precipitate, but an extremely complex machinery that awaits the best tools in the market for it to be finally understood.

Acknowledgments

Supported by a grant from the Binational Science foundation.

References

Bock, J. and Braun K. (1999) Blockade of *N*-methyl-D-aspartate receptor activation suppresses learning-induced synaptic elimination. *Proc. Natl. Acad. Sci. USA*, 96: 2485–2490.

Cajal, S.R. (1995 English Translation) *Histology of the Nervous System of Man and Vertebrates*. Oxford University Press, New York.

Desmond, N.L. and Levy, W.B. (1983) Synaptic correlates of associative potentiation/depression: an ultrastructural study in the hippocampus. *Brain Res.*, 265: 21–30.

Dunaevsky, A., Tashiro, A., Majewska, A., Mason, C. and Yuste, R. (1999) Developmental regulation of spine motility in the mammalian central nervous system. *Proc. Nat. Acad. Sci. USA*, 96: 13438–13443.

Emptage, N., Bliss, T.V. and Fine, A. (1999) Single synaptic events evoke NMDA receptor mediated release of calcium from internal stores in hippocampal dendritic spines. *Neuron*, 22: 115–124.

Engert, F. and Bonhoeffer, T. (1999) Dendritic spine changes associated with hippocampal long-term synaptic plasticity. *Nature*, 399: 66–70.

Feldman, M.L. and Dowd, C. (1975) Loss of dendritic spines in aging cerebral cortex. *Anat. Embryol.*, 148: 279–301.

Fischer, M., Kaech, S., Knutti, D. and Matus, A. (1998) Rapid actin based plasticity in dendritic spines. *Neuron*, 20: 847–854.

Globus, A., Rosenzweig, M.R., Bennett, E.L. and Diamond, M.C. (1973) Effects of differential experience on dendritic spine counts in rat cerebral cortex. *J. Comp. Physiol. Psychol.*, 82: 175–181.

Gray, E.G. (1959) Axosomatic and axodendritic synapses of the cerebral cortx: an electron-microscopic study. *J. Anat.*, 93: 420–433.

Goldin, M., Segal, M. and Avignone, E. (2001) Functional plasticity triggers formation and pruning of dendritic spines in cultured hippocampal networks. *J. Neurosci.*, 21: 186–193.

Guthrie, P.B., Segal, M. and Kater, S.B. (1991) Independent regulation of calcium revealed by imaging dendritic spines. *Nature*, 354: 76–80.

Halpain, S., Hipolito, A. and Saffer, L. (1998) Regulation of F-actin stability in dendritic spines by glutamate receptors and calcineurin. *J. Neurosci.*, 18: 9835–9844.

Harris, K.M. and Kater, S.B. (1994) Dendritic spines: cellular specializations imparting both stability and flexibility to synaptic function. *Ann. Rev. Neurosci.*, 17: 341–371.

Harris, K.M. and Stevens, J.K. (1989) Dendritic spines of CA1 pyramidal cells in the rat hippocampus: serial electron microscopy with reference to their biophysical characteristics *J. Neurosci.*, 9: 2982–2997.

Jones, T.A., Klintsova, A.Y., Kilman, V.L., Sirevaag, A.M. and Greenough, W.T. (1997) Induction of multiple synapses by experience in the visual cortex of adult rats. *Neurobiol. Learning Memory*, 68: 13–20.

Kim, C.H. and Lisman, J.E. (1999) A role of actin filament in synaptic transmission and long-term potentiation. *J. Neurosci.*, 19: 4314–4324.

Korkotian, E. and Segal, M. (1998) Fast confocal imaging of calcium released from stores in dendritic spines. *Eur. J. Neurosci.*, 10: 2076–2084.

Korkotian, E. and Segal, M. (1999a) Release of calcium from stores alters the morphology of Dendritic spines in cultured hippocampal neurons. *Proc. Nat. Acad. Sci. USA*, 96: 12068–12072.

Korkotian, E. and Segal, M. (1999b) Bidirectional regulation of dendritic spine dimensions by glutamate receptors. *Neuroreport*, 10: 2875–2877.

Korkotian, E. and Segal, M. (2001a) Regulation of dendritic spine motility in cultured hippocampal neurons. *J. Neurosci.*, 21: 6115–6124.

Korkotian, E. and Segal, M. (2001b) Spike-associated fast twitches of dendritic spines in cultured hippocampal neurons. *Neuron*, 30: 751–758.

Lee, K.S., Schottler, F., Oliver, M. and Lynch, G. (1980) Brief bursts of high-frequency stimulation produce two types of structural change in rat hippocampus. *J. Neurophysiol.*, 44: 413–422.

Lowndes, M. and Stewart, M.G. (1994) Dendritic spine density in the lobus parolfactorius of the domestic chick is increased 24 h after one-trial passive avoidance training. *Brain Res.*, 654: 129–136.

Moser, M.B., Trommald, M., Egeland, T. and Andersen, P. (1997) Spatial training in a complex environment and isolation alter the spine distribution differently in rat CA1 pyramidal cells. *J. Comp. Neurol.*, 380, 373–381.

Muller, W. and Connor, J.A. (1991) Dendritic spines as individual neuronal compartments for synaptic Ca^{2+} responses. *Nature*, 354(6348): 73–76.

Murphy, D.D. and Segal, M. (1996) Regulation of dendritic spine density in cultured rat hippocampal neurons by steroid hormones. *J. Neurosci.*, 16: 4059–4068.

Murphy, D.D. and Segal, M. (1997) Morphological plasticity of dendritic spines in central neurons is mediated by activation of cAMP response element binding protein. *Proc. Natl. Acad. Sci. USA*, 94: 1482–1487.

O'Malley, A., O'Connell, C. and Regan, C.M. (1998) Ultrastructural analysis reveals avoidance conditioning to induce a transient increase in hippocampal dentate spine density in the 6 hour post-training period of consolidation. *Neurosci.*, 87: 607–613.

Papa, M., Bundman, M.C., Greenberger, V. and Segal, M. (1995) Morphological analysis of the development of dendritic spines in primary cultures of hippocampal neurons. *J. Neurosci.*, 15: 1–11.

Popov, V.I., Bocharova, L.S. and Bragin, A.G. (1992) Repeated changes of dendritic morphology in the hippocampus of ground squirrels in the course of hibernation. *Neurosci.*, 48: 45–51.

Purpura, D.P. (1974) Dendritic spine dysgenesis and mental retardation. *Science*, 186: 1126–1128.

Rampon, C., Tang, Y.P., Goodhouse, J., Shimizu, E., Kyin, M. and Tsien, J.Z. (2000) Enrichment induces structural changes and recovery from nonspatial memory deficits in CA1 NMDAR1-knockout mice. *Nature Neuroscience*, 3: 238–244.

Rusakov, D.A., Richter-Levin, G., Stewart, M.G. and Bliss, T.V. (1997) Reduction in spine density associated with long-term potentiation in the dentate gyrus suggests a spine fusion-and-branching model of potentiation. *Hippocampus*, 7: 489–500.

Sala, C., Piech, V., Wilson, N.R., Passafaro, M., Liu, G. and Sheng, M. (2001) Regulation of dendritic spine morphology and synaptic function by Shank and Homer. *Neuron*, 31: 115–130.

Scheibel, M.E., Lindsay, R.D., Tomiyasu, U. and Scheibel, A. (1975) Progressive dendritic changes in aging human cortex. *Exptl. Neurol.*, 47: 392–403.

Segal, M. (1995a) Imaging of calcium variations in dendritic spines of cultured hippocampal neurons. *J. Physiol.*, 486: 285–296.

Segal, M. (1995b) Fast imaging of [Ca]i reveals presence of voltage gated calcium channels in dendritic spines of cultured hippocampal neurons. *J. Neurophysiol.*, 74: 484–488.

Segal, M. (1995c) Morphological alternations in dendritic spines of rat hippocampal neurons exposed to NMDA. *Neurosci. Lett.*, 193: 73–75.

Segal M. (1995d) Dendritic spines for neuroprotection. *Trends in Neurosci.*, 11: 468–471.

Segal, M.E. Korkotian and Murphy, D.D. (2000) Dendritic spine induction and pruning-common cellular mechanisms? *Trends in Neuroscience*, 23: 53–57.

Segev, I., Friedman, A., White, E.L. and Gutnick, M.J. (1995). Electrical consequences of spine dimensions in a model of a cortical spiny stellate cell completely reconstructed from serial thin sections. *J. Comput. Neurosci.*, 2: 117–130.

Shepherd, G.M. (1996) The dendritic spine: A multifunctional integrative unit. *J. Neurophysiol.*, 75: 2197–2210

Shi, S.H., Hayashi, Y., Petralia, R.S., Zaman, S.H., Wenthold, R.J., Svoboda, K. and Malinow, R. (1999) Rapid spine delivery and redistribution of AMPA receptors after synaptic NMDA receptor activation. *Science*, 284: 1811–1816.

Steward, O. and Schuman, E.M. (2001) Protein synthesis at synaptic sites on dendrites. *Annu. Rev. Neurosci.*, 24: 299–325.

Trommald, M. Hulleberg, G. and Andersen, P. (1996) Long term potentiation is associated with new excitatory spine synapses on rat dentate granule cells. *Learning and Memory*, 3: 218–228.

Van Harreveld, A. and Fifkova, E. (1975) Swelling of dendritic spines in the fascia dentata after stimulation of the perforant fibers as a mechanism of post-tetanic potentiation. *Exptl. Neurol.*, 49: 736–749.

Vicario-Abejón, C., Collin, C., McKay, R.D.G. and Segal, M. (1998) Neurotrophins induce formation of functional excitatory and inhibitory synapses between cultured hippocampal neurons. *J. Neurosci.*, 18: 7256–7271.

Volfovsky, N., Parnas, H., Segal, M. and Korkotian, E. (1999) Geometry of dendritic spines affects calcium dynamics in hippocampal neurons: theory and experiments. *J. Neurophysiol.*, 82: 450–462.

Wu, G.Y., Deisseroth, K. and Tsien, R.W. (2001) Spaced stimuli stabilize MAPK pathway activation and its effects on dendritic morphology. *Nat. Neurosci.*, 4(2): 151–158.

Yuste, R. and Denk, W. (1995) Dendritic spines as basic functional units of neuronal integration. *Nature*, 375: 682–684.

Zhang, W. and Benson, D.L. (2000) Development and molecular organization of dendritic spines and their synapses. *Hippocampus*, 10: 512–526.

Ziv, N.E. and Smith, S.J. (1996) Evidence for a role of dendritic filopodia in synaptogenesis and spine formation. *Neuron*, 17: 91–102.

E.C. Azmitia, J. DeFelipe, E.G. Jones, P. Rakic and C.E. Ribak (Eds.)
Progress in Brain Research, Vol. 136

CHAPTER 10

Spine distribution in cortical pyramidal cells: a common organizational principle across species

Guy N. Elston[1,2,*] and Javier DeFelipe[2]

[1]*Vision, Touch and Hearing Research Centre, Department of Physiology and Pharmacology, The University of Queensland, St. Lucia, QLD 4072, Australia*
[2]*Instituto Cajal (CSIC), Avenida del Doctor Arce 37, 28002 Madrid, Spain*

Introduction

Dendritic spines were initially described by Cajal (1888) from his observations of Golgi preparations (Fig. 1). From early on in his scientific career he was keenly aware of the distinction between CNS neurons which bore dendritic spines and those that did not. His own observations, and those of his contemporaries (Retzius, 1891; Schaffer, 1892; Edinger, 1893; Berkley, 1895), led him to propose that they play an integral role in the functioning of spiny cells. However, various of Cajal's contemporaries were more skeptical and suggested that spines were merely artifacts, resulting from crystalization during processing (Golgi, 1886; Meyer, 1895). Hearsay has it that such was Camilo Golgi's conviction that spines were artifacts that he forbode his students from drawing them (Fig. 2). Ultimately, Cajal's conclusions have come to be widely accepted, and the study of dendritic spines has developed into an active field of research. As new methodologies are developed, it is becoming more apparent that these minute dendritic protrusions are highly complex in function. Due to their ubiquity in the nervous system, their significance in excitatory transmission and their putative involvement in memory and plasticity, more is surely to come. There are many excellent reviews on spine types, their use in

neuronal classification, their development, and factors which influence spine number. Readers are directed to reviews by Peters and Jones (1984), Horner (1993), Shepherd (1996) and Harris (1999) for discussion of these topics. In this review we focus on the distribution of spines in the dendritic arbors of neocortical pyramidal cells.

Spine types

Despite the technology of his time, Cajal was able to distinguish different types of dendritic spines. As can be seen from Fig. 3, several different types are illustrated on the apical dendrite of a cortical pyramidal cell. Subsequent classification included pedunculated and sessile spine types (Jones and Powell, 1969). The pedunculated spine is defined as 'the classical dendritic spine of the cerebral cortex; a narrow pedicle of varying length is attached at one end to its parent dendrite, and at the other expands into a cup-like or prism-shaped bulb with a flattened side receiving an axon terminal at a typical synaptic complex'. A sessile spine is 'broad and there is little or no constriction at its junction with the parent dendrite' (Jones and Powell, 1969). Sessile spines include two of the three types described by Peters and Kaiserman-Abramof (1970). Shepherd and Greer (1988) described three types of dendritic spines: nubbins, mushrooms, and whispy wands. Various other dendritic processes have also been described (see Fialia and Harris, 1999, for a review).

*Corresponding author: Tel.: +617 3365 4108; Fax: +617 3365 4522;
E-mail: g.elston@vthrc.uq.edu.au

110

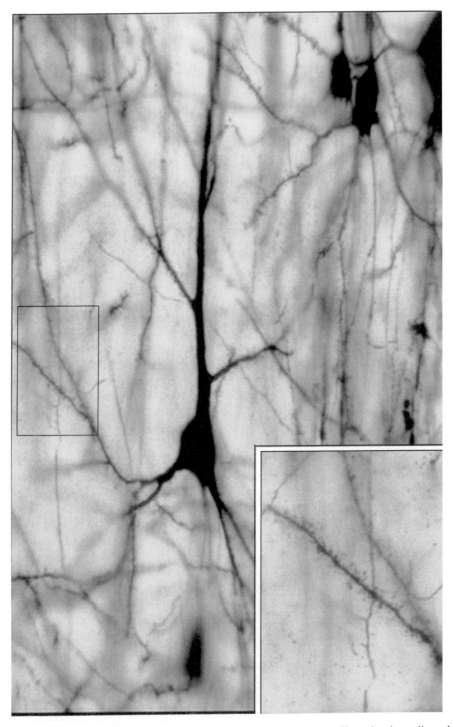

Fig. 1. Photomicrograph of one of Cajal's original Golgi-Cox preparations of cat cerebral cortex, illustrating the quality and completeness of staining of pyramidal cell dendritic arbors. Dendritic spines are easily distinguished at high magnification (inset, higher magnification of the boxed area). Scale bar = 27 μm; inset 10 μm.

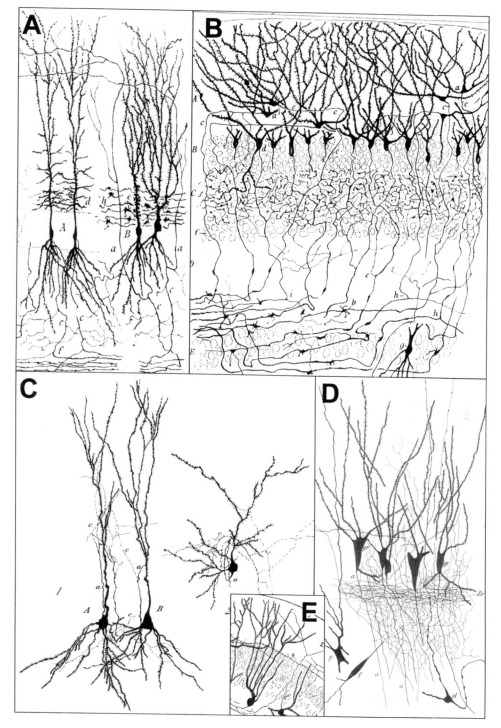

Fig. 2. Examples of original illustrations published by Cajal (A, B), Athias (C), Schaffer (D), Edinger (E), Golgi (F, G), Schiefferdecker and Kossel (H) and Meyer (I) at the turn of the 20th century. Differences in opinion led some to believe that dendritic spines were a fundamental component of neurons (A–E), whereas others were of the opinion that spines were artifacts of processing (F–I).

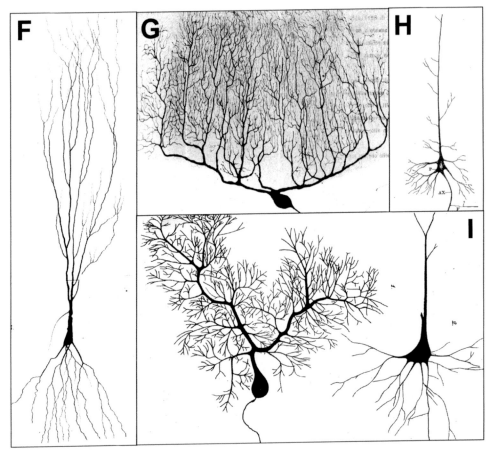

Fig. 2. (*Continued*)

Function of spines

Various functions have been ascribed to dendritic spines: biophysical and biochemical (see Shepherd, 1996 and Koch, 1999, for reviews). Here, we place emphasis on the finding that spines are a major site of synapses to cells such as pyramidal neurons and spiny stellate cells. Synapses can be classified into two basic types: type I and type II (Gray, 1959), (asymmetrical and symmetrical types, respectively, in the nomenclature of Colonnier (1968)) (Fig. 4). The presynaptic terminal of type I asymmetrical synapses in the cerebral cortex typically contain the excitatory transmitter glutamate (DeFelipe et al., 1988; Kharazia and Weinberg, 1993, 1994), whereas that of type II symmetrical synapses contain the GABA synthesizing enzyme GAD (Ribak et al., 1977; Ribak, 1978) (Fig. 5). Different receptor subunits have also been shown to be localized in the synaptic terminals of type I and type II synapses (Fig. 5B, D), consistent with their proposed role in excitation and inhibition (Petralia and Wenthold, 1992; Petralia et al., 1994a–c; Kharazia et al., 1996; Somogyi et al., 1996; Kharazia and Weinberg, 1999). In addition, type I and type II synapses appear to target different sites, at least for cortical spiny cells. Type I synapses are predominantly found on the heads of dendritic spines, whereas type II synapses target spine necks, dendrites, somata and axon initial segments of neurons (see White, 1989; DeFelipe and Fariñas 1992; Somogyi, et al., 1998, for reviews).

The majority of cortical spines reportedly receive a single asymmetrical synapse; however, occasionally (5–20% of axo-dendritic synapses) double or multiple synapses do occur (e.g., see Jones and Powell, 1969;

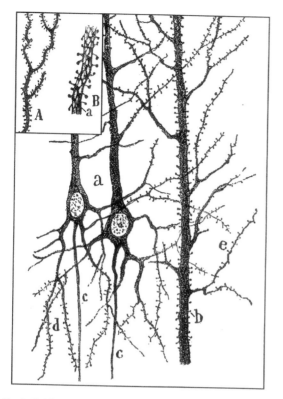

Fig. 3. Cajal not only understood the importance of dendritic spines, he recognized different spine types. Examples of pedunculated and stubby spines are clearly seen in this figure originally published by Cajal (1899).

Peters and Kaiserman-Abramof, 1970; Sloper and Powell, 1979; Koch and Poggio, 1983; Beaulieu and Colonnier, 1985; Somogyi and Soltesz, 1986; Quian and Sejnowski, 1989, 1990; Andersen et al., 1998). In the case of multiple synaptic innervation of individual spines, asymmetrical/excitatory synapses are found most often on the spine head, whereas the symmetrical/inhibitory synapses are usually found on the pedicle or in the immediate association of the dendritic shaft (Jones and Powell, 1969). However, variations on this pattern have been demonstrated in different regions of the CNS. For example, olfactory bulb granule cells possess 'reciprocal' synapses: the asymmetrical synapse projects to the spine whereas the symmetrical synapse originates in the spine (Shepherd and Greer, 1988; Woolf et al., 1991; Fifkova et al., 1992; see Shepherd and Greer, 1998, for a review).

Spine number—functional implications

Recent studies have shown marked differences in the density of spines found on pyramidal cells in different cortical areas (Elston and Rosa, 1997, 1998a, 2000; Jacobs et al., 1997, 2001; Elston et al., 1999a,b, 2001a; Elston, 2000) (Figs. 6 and 7). The different spine densities and branching patterns of layer III pyramidal cells result in a 2.6 fold difference in the number of

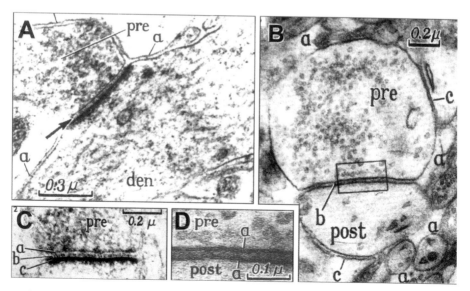

Fig. 4. High-power photomicrographs of cortical synapses illustrating examples of asymmetrical (A, C) and symmetrical (B, D) synapses (taken from Gray, 1959).

114

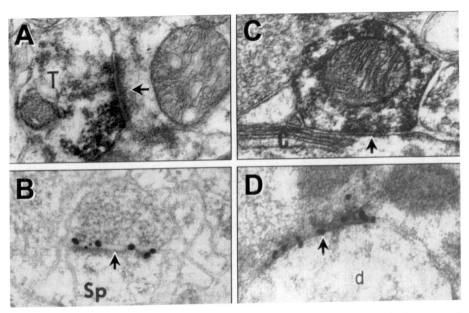

Fig. 5. High-power photomicrographs showing the presence of the excitatory neurotransmitter glutamate in the presynaptic terminal of an asymmetrical synapse (A) and the GABAergic synthesizing enzyme GAD in the presynaptic terminal of asymmetrical synapse (C). Glutamatergic receptors have been localized at asymmetrical synapses (B) and GABAergic receptors at symmetrical synapses (D) by immuno-gold immunohistochemistry (taken from, repectively, DeFelipe et al., 1988; Ribak, 1978; Kharazia et al., 1996; Somogyi et al., 1996).

spines on cells in the middle temporal area (MT) and the primary visual area V1 of the macaque monkey. Cells in cytoarchitectonic area TE have 11 fold more spines, and those in prefrontal cortex have up to 16 times more spines, than those in V1 (Elston et al., 1999a; Elston, 2000). In addition, cross species comparisons reveal that cells in human prefrontal cortex have, on average, 23 times more dendritic spines than those in V1 of the macaque (Elston et al., 2001a) (Fig. 8). As the majority of spines receive at least one asymmetrical synapse (Colonnier, 1968; Jones, 1968; White, 1989; Peters et al., 1991), differences in the number of spines within the dendritic arbors of different cortical areas/species likely reflect differences in the number of excitatory inputs they integrate. These findings confirm and extend previous reports of cytological heterogeneity in cortex (Fig. 9).

In addition, varying spine densities reported on the basal dendrites of pyramidal cells in different cortical areas may also affect electrical and biochemical compartmentalization, cooperativity between inputs and shunting inhibition (Koch et al., 1982; Shepherd et al., 1985; Rall and Segev, 1987; Shepherd and Brayton, 1987; Koch and Zador, 1993; Mainen, 1999). Differences in total length, number of branches, and

diameters of the dendrites determine: the cable properties (Rall, 1959); the degree of nonlinear compartmentalization (Rall, 1964; Koch et al., 1982); and the propagation of potentials (Stuart and Sackman, 1994; Spruston et al., 1995; Markram et al., 1997; Vetter et al., 2001) within the arbor (for reviews, see Rall, et al., 1992; Stuart et al., 1997; Koch, 1999; Mel, 1999; Spruston et al., 1999; Häusser et al., 2000). Modeling studies have also shown that a greater potential for electrical compartmentalization in highly branched dendritic arbors may result in a significant increase in a neuron's capacity for learning and memory by increasing the representational power of the cell (Poirazi and Mel, 2000).

Therefore, it appears likely that regional differences in pyramidal cell morphology contribute to area-specific aspects of cellular and systems function such as discharge properties and contrasting synaptic plasticity (Fuster and Alexander, 1971; Kubota and Niki, 1971; Fuster and Jervey, 1981; Ashford and Fuster, 1985; Funahashi et al., 1989; Miyashita et al., 1993a; Murayama et al., 1997). As a logical extension, species differences in pyramidal cell morphology in corresponding brain regions are likely to contribute to species-specific differences in

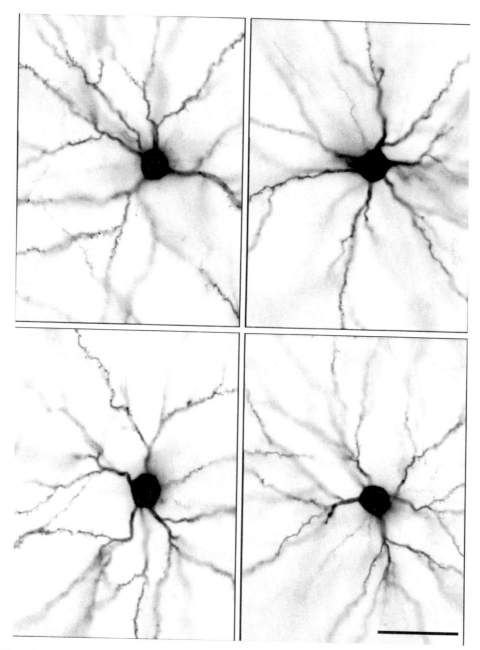

Fig. 6. (*Left*) Photomicrographs of four different layer III pyramidal cells intracellularly injected with Lucifer Yellow in tangential slices taken from macaque area 4, and processed for a DAB reaction product. (*Right*) High-power photomicrographs of horizontally projecting dendrites of layer III pyramidal neurons in the primary visual area (V1), the dorsomedial area (DM), the middle temporal area (MT) and inferotemporal (IT) cortex of the marmoset monkey. Differences in the type and density of dendritic spines on the basal dendrites are so marked that they are easily observed in photomicrographs, despite the limited focal depth of the images. In all examples, the cell body is located to the left and the middle two thirds of the dendrite is illustrated (taken from Elston et al., 1999b). Scale bar = 50 μm.

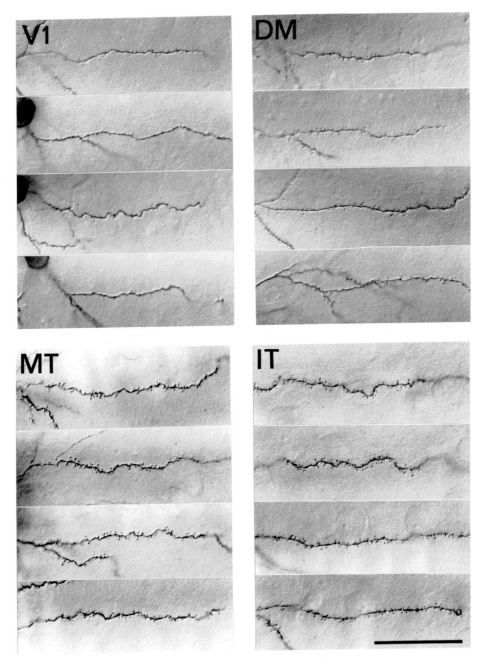

Fig. 6. (*Continued*)

cortical function (Elston et al., 2001a). More specifically, cells in human prefrontal cortex (PFC) potentially compartmentalize a greater number of inputs within their dendritic arbors than those in the PFC of the macaque, and those in the PFC of macaque more than those in the PFC of the marmoset. Moreover, cells in human PFC may integrate a greater diversity of inputs than those in other species. Similar observations, although not quantified, led Cajal to speculate that the structural complexity of the human cortical pyramidal cell

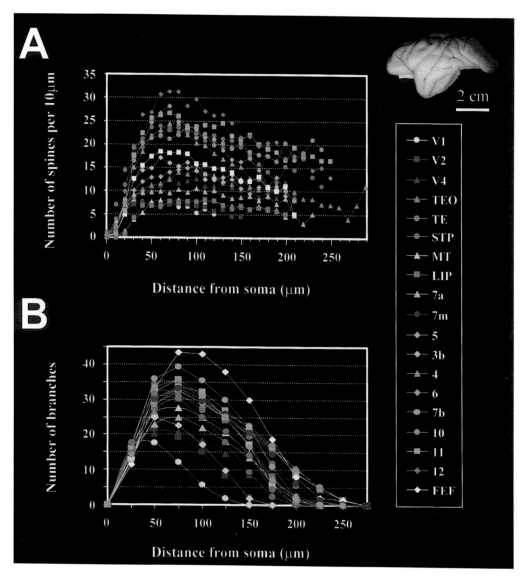

Fig. 7. Plots of the number spines (A) and branches (B) in the basal dendritic arbor of layer III pyramidal cells in 19 different cortical areas of the macaque monkey. Differences in arbor structure are not merely the result of scaling, but represent fundamental differences in their structure (data taken from Elston and Rosa, 1997, 1998a,b; Elston et al., 1999a,c; Elston, 2000; Elston and Rockland, 2002).

underlies man's cognitive abilities, and led him to consider the modified phenotype to be the "*psychic*" cell (Cajal, 1894a,b).

Distribution of spines

Despite these impressive differences in spine density, number of dendritic branches, and the absolute number of spines found in the basal dendritic arbors of pyramidal cells in different cortical regions, normalized cumulative spine distribution (as a function of relative distance from the soma to the distal tips of the dendrites) is remarkably constant for all cells. The normalized distribution in pyramidal cells in 19 different cortical areas of the macaque monkey cortex are tightly grouped and have similar gradients (Fig. 10). Furthermore, comparison

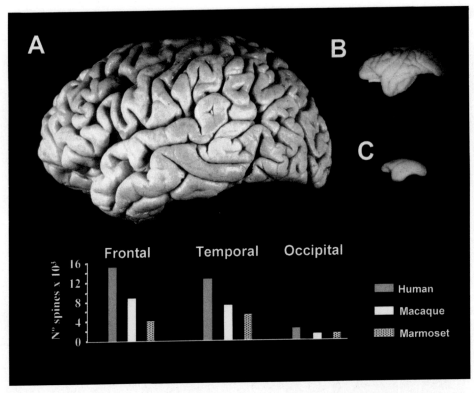

Fig. 8. Diagram showing the number of spines in the basal dendritic arbor of the 'average' layer III pyramidal cell in selected cortical areas of the human (A) and macaque (B) and marmoset (C) monkey cortex. Cells in layer III of human prefrontal area 10 have, on average, 23 times more spines than those in the primary visual area (V1) of macaque and marmoset monkeys (15138, 643 and 699, respectively) (data taken from Elston et al., 2001a).

of data obtained from cells in human, the New World marmoset monkey and those sampled from phyolgenetically remote species, such as the mouse and the platypus, with those of macaque monkey reveal that normalized spine distribution is remarkably constant across species of different orders (Fig. 11).

Mechanisms that determine the distribution of inputs to CNS neurons are controversial. Two general theories prevail: (1) that synapse distribution is determined by the target neurons themselves; or (2) that synapse distribution is determined locally by the inputs. Both of these theories have been attributed variously to activity-dependent and activity-independent mechanisms (see Berry et al., 1978; Sotelo, 1978, 1990; Easter et al., 1985; Rossi and Strata, 1995; Steward, 1995, 1997, for reviews). Studies on cerebellar Purkinje cells suggest that the distribution of different sets of excitatory inputs may be determined by different mechanisms. For example, climbing fiber inputs are reportedly mediated by activity-dependent mechanisms, whereas the parallel fiber inputs are thought to be determined by genetically programmed activity-independent mechanisms (Sotelo et al., 1975; Annis et al., 1993, 1994; Baptista et al., 1994; Takács and Hámori, 1994; Kossel et al., 1997; Bravin et al., 1999; Drakew et al., 1999; Frotscher et al., 2000; Schmidt et al., 2000). Studies on the retina, thalamus and neocortex suggest that spine formation is dependent on input activity (see Jones, 1985; Kalil, 1990; Shatz, 1990; Goodman and Shatz, 1993; Segal et al., 2000, for reviews). Moreover, the structural differences in neocortical pyramidal cell dendritic arbors (Table 1) make it unlikely that the uniformity in normalized input distribution results from a cell mediated, activity-independent genetically encoded program. Cells in each cortical region would necessarily express a different program resulting in a constant excitatory input distribution profile despite different branching structure and spine density.

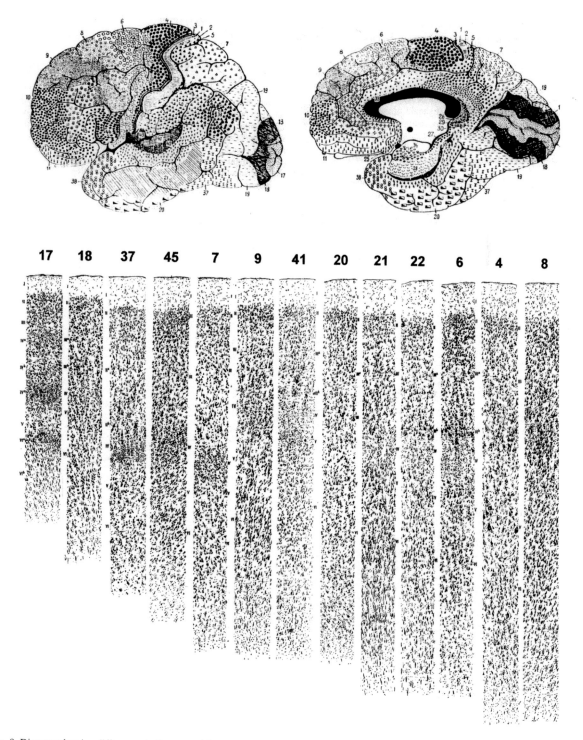

Fig. 9. Diagram showing differences in the cytoarchitecture of different cortical areas in the human brain. Regional variations in cytoarchitecture reflect structural differences in cortical organization fundamental in determining the functional characteristics of cells within. Taken from Brodmann (1905). Translated by Garey (1994). See also Brodmann (1907, 1908), Vogt and Vogt (1919) and Walker (1940).

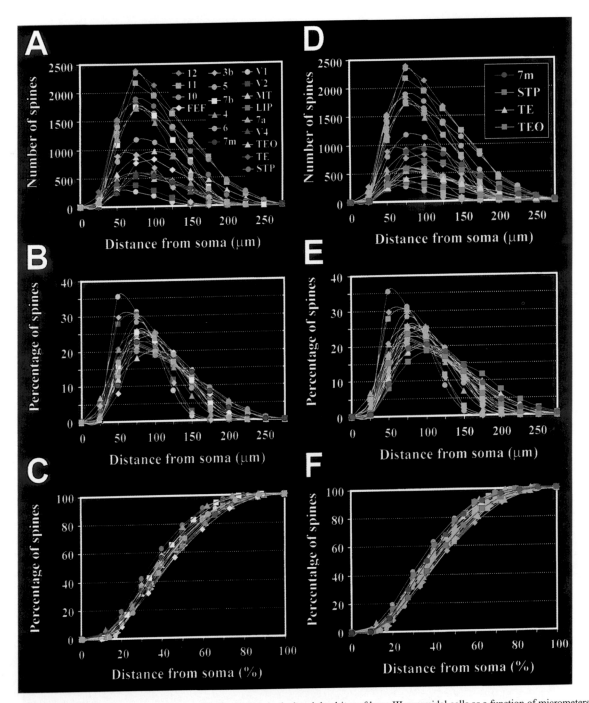

Fig. 10. Plots of the number (A) and proportion (B, C) of spines in the basal dendrites of layer III pyramidal cells as a function of micrometers (A, B) and relative distance (C) from the soma to the distal tips of the dendrites. The same trends are plotted for layer V pyramidal cells (D–F). Data were reconstructed from a sample of over 1000 neurons in 19 different cortical areas of the macaque monkey. Note that the normalized cumulative spine profiles (C, F) are remarkably uniform (taken from Elston and Rosa, 1997, 1998a,b, 2000; Elston et al., 1999a,c; Elston, 2000; Elston and Rockland, 2002).

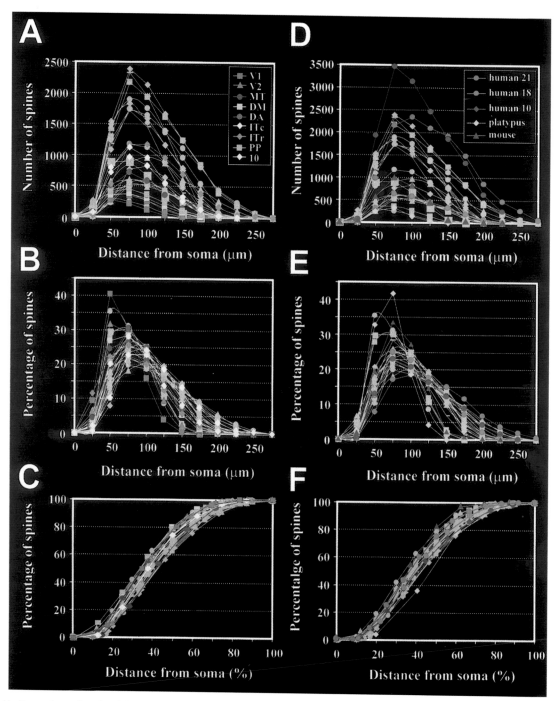

Fig. 11. Comparison of number (A) and percentage (B, C) of spines in the basal dendrites as a function of micrometers (A, B), and relative distance (C) from the cell body to distal tips of dendrites, of layer III pyramidal cells in the marmoset (color) and macaque (gray) monkeys. Similar plots for data obtained from humans, mice and the platypus (color) are illustrated (D–F). Note that the normalized cumulative spine profiles (C, F) are remarkably uniform for data taken from all brain regions and species. The normalized cumulative spine profiles of cells in the somatoelectrosensory cortex of the platypus, however, differ somewhat from those taken from other species (data taken from Elston et al., 1999a–d, 2001a; Benavides-Piccione et al., 2002).

Table 1. Statistical comparisons of fractal dimensions of cells in different cortical areas. Cortical areas are grouped according to the study of Felleman and van Essen (1991). Neurons in V1 and V2 are included in both pathways: data from layer IIIc of V1 and the cytochrome oxidase-rich thick bands of V2 are included in the dorsal stream, while those of middle and upper layer III in V1 and the cytochrome oxidase-rich thin bands in V2 are included in the ventral stream.

	V1	V2	V4	TEO	TE	V1	V2	MT	LIP	7a
V2	+									
V4	+	−								
TEO	+	+	+							
TE	+	+	+	−						
V1	+	−	−	+	+					
V2	+	+	−	+	+	−				
MT	+	+	+	−	−	+	+			
LIP	+	+	+	−	−	+	+	−		
7a	+	+	+	+	+	−	−	+	+	
STP	+	+	+	+	−	+	+	−	−	+

$+ \; p < 0.05$; $- \; p > 0.05$
Taken from Jelinek and Elston (2001), see also Elston and Jelinek (2001).

The constancy in the normalized spine distribution in the arbors of cortical pyramidal cells in different layers and different cortical regions in different species, suggests a common principle determines the location of excitatory inputs. A likely candidate for determining the distribution of inputs is the backpropagating potential. Backpropagation (Stuart and Häusser, 1994; Stuart and Sackman, 1994; Spruston et al., 1995; Buzsáki et al., 1996; Svoboda et al., 1997; Helmchen et al., 1999) reportedly serves to potentiate synchronously active inputs which result in the firing of action potential at the cell body (Magee and Johnston, 1997; Markram et al., 1997), thus stabilizing synaptic inputs by Hebbian type (Hebb, 1949) synaptic reinforcement (see Stuart et al., 1997; Spruston et al., 1999; Häusser et al., 2000, for reviews). If the backpropagating potential is responsible for stabilizing excitatory inputs, its spread throughout the dendritic arbor may determine the distribution of these inputs (Fig. 12).

The spread of the action potential throughout the arbor may occur according to two different principles, which act in concert. In the first instance, the arbor can be considered as a passive structure (such as a cable), with decay of the potential occurring in a linear manner (Rall, 1959; see also Goldstein and Rall, 1974). In the second instance, the arbor itself actively determines propagation of potentials, resulting in nonlinear decay (Markram et al., 1998; Segev and Schneidman, 1999). Mechanisms that determine such active propagation in dendrites have been the subject of intense research in recent years. Vetter and colleagues (2001) reported that the decay of the backpropagating potential throughout the arbor is crucially dependent on the number of bifurcations within the arbor. However, as seen in Figs. 10 and 11, the normalized distribution of spines is remarkably consistent for cortical pyramidal cells, despite marked differences in the number of branches in the arbors. Thus, if the backpropagating potential does determine the distribution of spines within the arbor of cells of markedly different size and branching patterns, its decay must occur according to nonlinear properties, or have varying amplitude. Indeed, Vetter and colleagues noted the influence of nonlinear properties on the decremental decay of the backpropagating potentials, suggesting that the decay is influenced by spine density, particularly in more branched cells. While it has not been demonstrated empirically that the larger pyramidal cells in areas such as TEO and TE contain more voltage-gated ion channels than smaller cells, such as those in V1, converging data suggest that this is likely to be the case. For example, there is a decrease in neuron density (Kondo et al., 1999), and an increase in the density of glutamate receptors (Xu et al., 1997), through cortical areas of the ventral visual pathway of the macaque monkey. Further electrophysiological

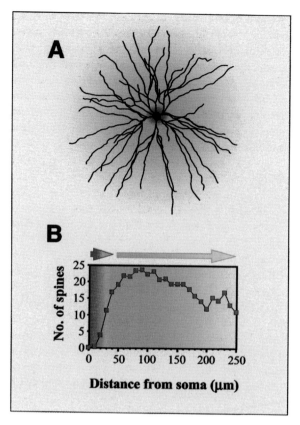

Fig. 12. Diagram illustrating possible mechanisms which determine the distribution of excitatory inputs to mature pyramidal cell dendrites. The same mechanisms are illustrated in the tangential (A) and transverse (B) planes. Excitatory inputs are excluded from the soma and proximal dendrites (red). The excluding factor/s become less pronounced with radial progression, resulting in a transition zone (red/green) where excitatory inputs localize. As the exclusion factor/s progressively decay with radial progression, the density of excitatory inputs increases (blue profile in B) to a maximum where the characteristics of the backpropagating potentials are most conducive to excitatory input localization (solid green). This region typically occurs at approximately one-third the distance from the soma to the distal tips of the basal dendrites. The decay of the backpropagating potential with progression to the distal tips (dark green/light green transition) results in decreasing spine density (blue profile in B). At least two possible mechanisms may determine the zone of exclusion: (1) the mature membrane is nonpermissive to localization of excitatory inputs; or (2) characteristics the backpropagating potential preclude excitatory synapse localization on the soma and proximal dendrites.

studies of cells in the different cortical areas are required to determine to what extent linear and nonlinear properties may determine the distribution of spines within their dendritic arbors.

Plasticity of dendritic processes

It has long been known that cortical circuitry is highly plastic in developing cortex. Cajal himself was fascinated in the ability of neurons to reshape and grow new processes following nerve injury and/or changes in environmental conditions (see DeFelipe and Jones, 1991, for a translation of Cajal's works). His nerve transsection and grafting experiments clearly demonstrated the ability of the developing nervous system to regenerate following injury. His observations on cortical pyramidal cells led him to conclude:

> ... l'ecorce cérébrale est pareille a un jardin peuplé d'arbres innombrables, les cellulae pyramidales, qui, grace a une culture intelligente, peuvent multiplier leurs branches, enfocer plus lion leurs racines, et produir des fleurs et des friuts chaque fois plus variés et exquis (Cajal, 1894a).

> ...la corteza cerebral semeja un jardin poblado de innumerables árboles, las células pirimidales, que gracias un cultivo inteligente pueden multiplicar sus ramas, hundir más lejos sus raíces y producir flores y frutos cada día más exquisitos (Cajal, 1894b).

> ... the cerebral cortex is similar to a garden filled with trees, the pyramidal cells, which, thanks to intelligent culture, can multiply their branches, sending their roots deeper and producing more and more varied and exquisite flowers and fruits (p. 87, DeFelipe and Jones, 1988).

The data represented in Figs. 7, 8, 10 and 11 represent a 'snapshot' in time. Studies in the developing and mature CNS reveal that spines change their shape, new spines grow and existing spines disappear (see Crick, 1982 and Matus, 2000, for reviews). Thus, it could be argued that structural changes related to rearing conditions, differing maturation rates across cortical regions, or inter-individual variation (Valverde, 1967, 1968; Volkmar and Greenough, 1972; Greenough et al., 1973; Bourgeois et al., 1994; Huttenlocher and Dabholkar, 1997) may underlie the phenotypic variation in pyramidal cell morphology. However, this is clearly not the case for human data (Elston et al., 2001; Jacobs et al., 1997, 2001; see also Conel, 1947, 1955, 1959, 1963, 1967), as these data were sampled from the same hemisphere of individuals that died sudden and unexpected death. Moreover, these data have been replicated in different animals, revealing that consistency in the trends for phenotypic variation and that inter-areal differences in cell morphology are greater than inter-individual differences in age/sex matched animals (Elston et al., 1999b; Jacobs et al., 2001).

In addition, systematic regional differences in pyramidal cell structure have been reported by a number of independent laboratories, by different methods, in different species (Lund et al., 1993; Elston, 2000; Jacobs et al., 2001; Elston et al., 2001a). Thus, while the data represent single time points, the continuous turnover of spines/ synapses which occurs during normal cortical functioning appears to reach a different equilibrium in pyramidal cells in different cortical areas/species (see Craig, 1998; Turrigiano 1999; Turrigiano and Nelson, 2000; Craig and Boudin, 2001, for reviews on mechanisms which determine synapse formation and stabilization). How, then, might such plasticity of individual spines effect their overall distribution within the arbor?

(i) Environmentally induced changes

Various studies have demonstrated that animals raised under different environmental conditions have different numbers of dendritic spines (Fig. 13). Animals raised in an enriched environment have more spinous cells than those raised in control, or impoverished, environments (see Bailey and Kandel, 1993; Horner, 1993; Harris and Karter, 1994; Kintsova and Greenough, 1999, for

reviews). Comparison of spine distributions in the basal dendritic arbors of layer III pyramidal cells in frontal cortex of rats reared in an enriched environment, with those raised under control conditions, revealed that the "average" neuron in the former group had twice the number of spines as that of the latter group (Benavides-Piccione et al., 2002). Nonetheless, the normalized cumulative distributions of spines within their basal dendritic arbors were similar (Fig. 14).

(ii) Age-related changes

It has also been well-documented that there is a decrease in spine density and dendritic atrophy (Scheibel et al., 1975; Lund et al., 1977; Boothe et al., 1979; Nakamura et al., 1985; Anderson and Rutledge, 1996) as well as a decrease in the number of excitatory synapses in the cortex (Huttenlocher, 1979; Huttenlocher et al., 1982; Huttenlocher and de Courten, 1987; Bourgeois and Goldman-Rakic, 1993; Missler et al., 1993; Bourgeois et al., 1994) during senescence. Comparison of layer III pyramidal cells in extrastriate visual association areas 7m and STP (superior polysensory area) obtained from a 11-year-old animal, with those of an

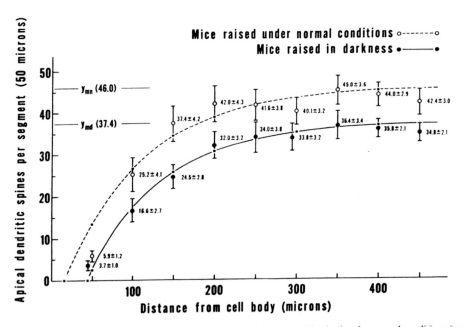

Fig. 13. Plots of spine density of the apical dendrites of layer V pyramidal cells in mouse V1 raised under normal conditions (open circles), and raised in the dark (closed circles). Dark reared mice clearly had fewer spines on their apical shafts, as compared with controls (taken from Valverde, 1968).

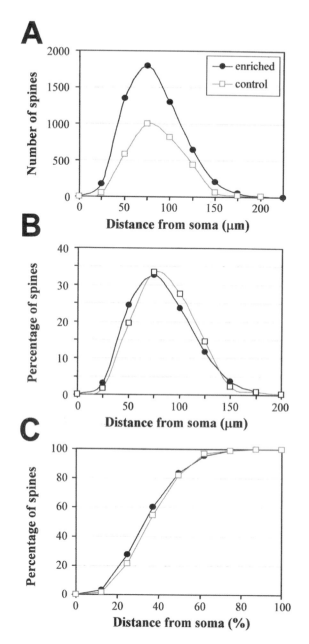

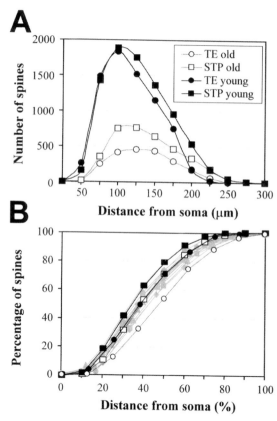

18-month-old animal, revealed a 50% decrease in spine number in the basal dendritic arbor of the 'average' cell in each cortical area. Despite the 50% decrease, the normalized distribution of spines within the arbors of cortical pyramidal cells remains relatively unchanged (Fig. 15).

(iii) Experimentally induced changes

Mature adult circuitry is capable of large-scale structural reorganization (see Kaas, 1991; Buonomano and

Fig. 14. (A) Plots of spine density, and dendritic branching patterns of layer III pyramidal cells in the frontal cortex of mice raised in normal (squares) and enriched (circles) environments. (B) Mice raised in enriched environment clearly had a greater number of spines in their dendritic arbors, as compared with controls. Nonetheless, despite the marked increase in the absolute number of spines, their normalized distributions (C) were remarkably similar (data taken from Benavides-Piccione et al., 2002).

Fig. 15. (A) Plots of the number of spines (per 25 μm) showing the effects of aging. In both cytoarchitectonic areas TE and STP (the superior temporal polysensory area) of the macaque monkey there was more than a 50% decrease in spine density when comparing animals of 18 months of age with those of 11 years of age. (B) Normalized plots of the cumulative percentage of spines as a function of distance from the cell body to the distal tips of the dendrites. Despite the 50% reduction in spine density, the normalized cumulative spine distribution (as a function of relative distance from the soma to the distal dendritic tips) is similar for both age groups, suggesting spatially regulated spine loss within the arbor.

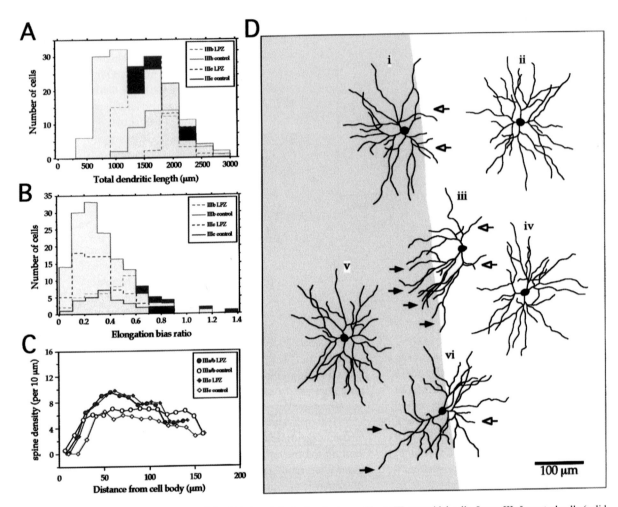

Fig. 16. (A) Frequency histograms of the total dendritic length in the basal arbors of layer III pyramidal cells. Layer IIIa/b control cells (solid red outline and light-red infill) had a smaller total dendritic length than those in the region of cortex affected by the retinal lesion (the lesion projection zone; LPZ) (dashed red outline). Solid red infill shows the putative increase in the total dendritic length. Similarly, layer IIIc control cells (solid blue outline and light-blue infill) had a smaller total dendritic length than those in the LPZ (dashed blue outline). The solid blue infill shows the putative increase in the total dendritic length. (B) Frequency histograms of the elongation ratios of the basal dendritic arbors of layer III pyramidal neurons. Layer IIIa/b control cells illustrated in solid red outline and light-red infill. Layer IIIa/b LPZ cells illustrated in dashed red outline. Layer IIIc control cells (solid blue outline and light blue infill) were less elongated than those in the LPZ (dashed blue outline). Solid blue infill shows the putative increase in the degree of elongation. (C) Plots of dendritic spine densities of control (open symbols) and LPZ (solid symbols) cells in sublaminae IIIa/b (blue) and sublamina IIIc (red) showing an increase in spine density at most distances from the cell body of LPZ cells. Error bars = standard deviations. (D) In addition to these structural changes, cells located near a border of an ocular dominance column (i, iii and vi) appeared to show a regression of dendrites which projected toward the center of the CO-poor column (open arrows) and an elongation of dendrites toward the CO-rich column (closed arrows). On the other hand, cells located in the centers of the OD columns (ii, iv and v) appeared to be relatively symmetrical (taken from Elston et al., 1998).

Merzernich, 1998; Calford et al., 1998; Gilbert, 1998, for reviews). The mature sensory cortex undergoes large-scale functional reorganization following disruption of peripheral receptors (Merzenich et al., 1983a,b; Calford and Tweedale, 1988; Kaas et al., 1990; Pons et al., 1991).

In addition to functional and molecular changes reported in adult circuitry, mature dendrites and axons have been shown to undergo active sprouting (Darian-Smith and Gilbert, 1994; Jones et al., 1996; Kossut, 1998; Elston et al., 2001b). Factors involved in such functional reorganization remain controversial, with both excitatory and inhibitory circuitry being implicated (Kano, 1991; Clarey et al., 1996; Garraghty and Muja, 1996; Arkens et al., 2000a; Meyers et al., 2000). Activity-dependent triggering of molecular cascades in mature cortex, involving up- and/or down-regulation of receptor subunits, neurotrophins, kinases and synapsins (Hendry and Jones, 1988; Hendry et al., 1990; Benson et al., 1991, 1994; Obata et al., 1999; Arkens et al. 2000a,b; Muñoz et al., 2000), are thought to be directly involved (see Jones, 1990, for a review). The extent to which mature neocortical pyramidal cells can reshape their arbors is impressive. Elston and colleagues (1998) recently demonstrated dendritic growth and spine acquisition in V1 cells following retinal lesioning (Fig. 16) resulting in up to a 65% increase in spines. In spite of this marked increase in number, the normalized cumulative distribution of spines in their dendritic arbors is remarkably constant (Fig. 17).

In summary, the normalized cumulative spine distribution in the basal dendritic arbors of cortical pyramidal cells is remarkably similar in different brain regions in different species, despite marked differences in arbor size, branching structure and spine density. In addition, the normalized cumulative spine distribution is not grossly altered during aging, by environment enrichment or by experimentally induced changes in input activity. In conjunction, these data suggest a common activity-dependent mechanism determines the distribution of excitatory inputs to pyramidal cells. The most likely candidate appears to be the backpropagating potential.

Caveats

All of our data were derived from two-dimensional reconstructions of the basal dendritic arbors of pyramidal cells. Inaccuracies are inevitably introduced when reducing three-dimensional cell morphology to two dimensions (see Uylings et al., 1986, for a review). For example, calculations of the total number of spines found in the basal dendritic arbor of the 'average' pyramidal cell in different cortical areas were made by determining the spine density of horizontally projecting dendrites, and multiplying the average spine density by the average number of dendritic branches in the corresponding region (Elston, 2001). These calculations are likely to be underestimates of the true values, due to trigonometric

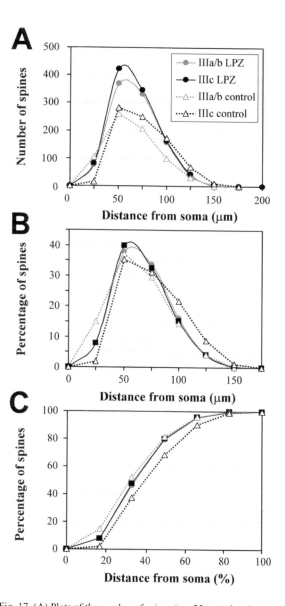

Fig. 17. (A) Plots of the number of spines (per 25 μm) showing the effects of adult-induced plastic changes of cortical pyramidal cells. Cells in both sublaminae IIIa/b and IIIc of V1 showed an increased spine density following retinal lesioning. (B) Normalized plots of the cumulative percentage of spines as a function of distance from the cell body to the distal tips of the dendrites. Despite the 50% increase in the total number of spines in the arbors of lesioned animals as compared with controls, the normalized cumulative spine distribution (as a function of relative distance from the soma to the distal dendritic tips) is similar for both groups (data taken from Elston et al., 1998).

128

truncation of downward projecting dendrites. Moreover, the extent of the underestimation is likely to be greater for cells with more branches (i.e., those in higher cortical areas, such as areas TE and STP). Thus, the 23-fold difference in the number of spines between cells in macaque V1 and human PFC, for example, is likely to be an underestimate of the average interareal differences in the integrative abilities of the basal dendritic arbors of pyramidal cells. Nonetheless, the methodology employed in these studies has revealed new data not necessarily detectable by other methodologies, and provides some advantages when used as a relative measure of various morphological features of individual cortical cells.

Various studies have used correction factors to overcome problems in determining spine density of cortical dendrites, as the dendritic shaft obscures many spines from view (Feldman and Peters, 1979; Larkman, 1991b). This is particularly a problem when analyzing apical dendrites of pyramidal cells revealed by the Golgi method. No such correction was used in the present study because: (1) the dendritic spines on the basal dendrites of pyramidal neurons of this study were characterized by relatively large spine necks, so spines which issued from the under side of the parent dendrite could be seen (e.g., Figs. 1 and 3 of Elston et al., 1999b); and (2) the DAB reaction product is more opaque than the Golgi reaction product, allowing identification of smaller 'stubby' type spines which were partially obscured by the dendrite.

Conclusions

(a) There are marked differences in the density and number of spines in the dendritic arbors of cortical pyramidal cells in different cortical areas. Despite these differences, their normalized cumulative distribution is remarkably constant.

(b) The constancy in normalized spine distribution holds true for cortical pyramidal cells in primates, rodents and monotremes.

(c) Environment enrichment, manipulation of inputs, and aging do not grossly affect the normalized distribution of spines in the dendritic arbors of cortical pyramidal cells.

(d) Spine distribution in cortical pyramidal cells is likely to be determined by epigenetic activity-dependent mechanisms.

(e) The most probable activity-dependent mechanism appears to be the backpropagating potential.

(f) Relatively small variations in normalized distribution of spines in the arbors of pyramidal cells may be related to linear and/or non-linear properties of the cells.

Acknowledgments

Supported by a CJ Martin Fellowship (GNE) from the National Health and Medical Research Council of Australia, and a DGCYT grant (PM99-0105) from Spain.

References

Anderson, J.C., Binzegger, T., Martin, K.A.C. and Rockland, K.S. (1998) The connection from cortical area V1 to V5: A light and electron microscopic study. *J. Neurosci.*, 18: 10525–10540.

Anderson, B. and Rutledge, V. (1996) Age and hemisphere effects on dendrite structure. *Brain*, 119: 1983–1990.

Annis, C.M., O'Dowd, D.K. and Robertson, R.T. (1994) Activity-dependent regulation of dendritic spine density on cortical pyramidal neurons in organotypic slice cultures. *J. Neurobiol.*, 25: 1483–1493.

Annis, C.M., Robertson, R.T. and O'Dowd, D.K. (1993) Aspects of early postnatal development of cortical neurones that proceed independently of normally present extrinsic influences. *J. Neurobiol.*, 24: 1460–1480.

Arkens, L., Schweigart, G., Qu, Y., Wouters, G., Pow, D.V., Vandesande, F., Eysel, T.H. and Orban, G. (2000) Cooperative changes in GABA, glutamate and activity levels: the missing link in cortical plasticity. *Eur. J. Neurosci.*, 12: 4222–4232.

Ashford, J.W. and Fuster, J.M. (1985) Occipital and inferotemporal responses to visual signals in the monkey. *Exp. Neurol.*, 90: 444–446.

Athias, M. (1905) *Anatomia da Cellula Nervosa*. Lisboa.

Bailey, C.H. and Kandel, E.R. (1993) Structural changes accompanying memory storage. *Ann. Rev. Physiol.*, 55: 397–426.

Baptista, C.A., Hatten, M.E., Blazeski, R. and Mason, C.A. (1994) Cell–cell interactions influence survival and differentiation of purified Purkinje cells *in vivo*. *Neuron*, 12: 243–260.

Beaulieu, C., and Colonnier, M. (1985) A laminar analysis of the number of round-asymmetrical and flat-symmetrical synapses on spines, dendritic trunks, and cell bodies in area 17 of the cat. *J. Comp. Neurol.*, 231: 180–189.

Benavides-Piccione, R., Elston, G.N., DeFelipe, J., Dierssen, M. and Flórez, J. (2002) The effects of environment enrichment on circuit maturation in the Ts65Dn trisomic mouse model of Down syndrome. *Abstracts Int. J. Dev. Neurosci.*, 19: 726.

Benson, D.L., Huntsman, M.M. and Jones, E.G. (1994) Activity-dependent changes in GAD and preprotachykinin mRNAs in visual cortex of adult monkeys. *Cereb. Cortex*, 4: 40–51.

Benson, D.L., Isackson, P.J., Gall, C.M. and Jones, E.G. (1991) Differential effects of monocular deprivation on glutamic acid decarboxylase and type II calcium-calmodulin-dependent protein kinase gene expression in the adult monkey visual cortex. *J. Neurosci.*, 11: 31–47.

Berkley, J. (1895) Studies on the lesions produced by the action of certain poisons on the nerve cell. *Medical News*, 1: 1–24.

Berry M., Bradley P. and Borges S. (1978) Environmental and genetic determinants of connectivity in the central nervous system—an approach through dendritic field analysis. *Prog. Brain Res.*, 48: 133–146.

Boothe, R.G., Greenough, W.T., Lund, J.S. and Wrege, K. (1979) A quantitative investigation of spine and dendrite development of neurons in visual cortex (area 17) of *Macaca nemistrina* monkeys. *J. Comp. Neurol.*, 186: 473–489.

Bourgeois, J.-P. and Goldman-Rakic, P.S. (1993) Changes of synaptic density in the primary visual cortex of the macaque monkey from fetal to adult stage. *J. Neurosci.*, 13: 2801–2820.

Bourgeois, J.-P., Goldman-Rakic, P.S. and Rakic, P. (1994) Synaptogenesis in the prefrontal cortex of rhesus monkeys. *Cerebr. Cortex*, 4: 78–96.

Bravin, M., Morando, L., Vercelli, A., Rossi, F. and Strata, P. (1999) Control of spine formation by electrical activity in the adult rat cerebellum. *Proc. Natl. Acad. Sci. USA*, 96: 1704–1709.

Brodmann, K. (1905) Beiträge zur histologischen Lokalisation der Großhirnrinde. *J. Psychol. Neurol.*, 4: 177–226.

Brodmann, K. (1907) Beiträge zur histologischen Lokalisation der Großhirnrinde. *J. Psychol. Neurol.*, 10: 1–16.

Brodmann, K. (1908) Über Rinbdenmessungen. *Zent. Nerv. Psych.*, 19: 781–798.

Buonomano, D.V. and Merzenich, M.M. (1998) Cortical plasticity: from maps to synapses. *Ann. Rev. Neurosci.*, 21: 149–186.

Buzsáki, G., Penttonen, M., Nádasdy, Z. and Bragin, A. (1996) Pattern and inhibition-dependent invasion of pyramidal cell dendrites by fast spikes in the hippocampus *in vivo*. *Proc. Natl. Acad. Sci. USA*, 93: 9921–9925.

Cajal, S.R. (1888) Estructura de los centros nerviosos de las aves. *Rev. Trim. Histol. Norm. Patol.*, 1: 305–315.

Cajal, S.R. (1894a) The Croonian lecture: la fine structure des centres nerveux. *Proc. R. Soc. Lond.*, 55: 445–467.

Cajal, S. R. (1894b) Estructura intima de los centros nerviosos. *Rev. Ciencias Méd.*, 20: 145–160.

Cajal, S.R. (1899) Textura del Sistema Nervioso del Hombre y de los Vertebrados. Madrid, Moya.

Calford, M.B., Clarey, J.C. and Tweedale, R. (1998) Short-term plasticity in adult somatosensory cortex. In: J. Morley (Ed.), *Advances in Psychology: Neural Aspects of Tactile Sensation*, Vol. 11, Elsevier, Amsterdam, pp. 299–350.

Calford, M.B. and Tweedale, R. (1988) Immediate and chronic changes in responses of somatosensory cortex in adult flying-fox after digit amputation. *Nature*, 332: 446–448.

Clarey, J.C., Tweedale, R. and Calford, M.B. (1996) Interhemispheric modulation of somatosensory receptive fields: evidence for plasticity in primary somatosensory cortex. *Cerebr. Cortex*, 6: 196–206.

Colonnier, M. (1968) Synaptic patterns on different cell types in the different laminae of the cat visual cortex. *Brain Res.*, 9: 268–287.

Conel, J.L. (1947) The cortex of a three month old infant. In: *The Post Natal Development of the Human Cerebral Cortex*, Vol. III, Harvard University Press, Cambridge.

Conel, J.L. (1955) The cortex of a fifteen month old infant. In: *The Post Natal Development of the Human Cerebral Cortex*, Vol. V, Harvard University Press, Cambridge.

Conel, J.L. (1959) The cortex of a twenty-four month old infant. In: *The Post Natal Development of the Human Cerebral Cortex*, Vol. VI, Harvard University Press, Cambridge.

Conel, J.L. (1963) The cortex of a four year old child. In: *The Post Natal Development of the Human Cerebral Cortex*, Vol. VII, Harvard University Press, Cambridge.

Conel, J.L. (1967) The cortex of a six year old child. In: *The Post Natal Development of the Human Cerebral Cortex*, Vol. VIII, Harvard University Press, Cambridge.

Craig, A.M. (1998) Activity and synaptic receptor targeting: the long view. *Neuron*, 21: 459–462.

Craig, A.M. and Boudin, H. (2001) Molecular heterogeneity of central synapses: afferent and target regulation. *Nature Neurosci.*, 4: 569–578.

Crick, F. (1982) Do dendritic spines twitch? *Trends Neurosci*, 5: 44–46.

Darian-Smith, C. and Gilbert, C.D. (1994) Axonal sprouting accompanies functional reorganization in adult striate cortex. *Nature*, 368: 737–740.

DeFelipe, J. and Fariñas, I. (1992) The pyramidal neuron of the cerebral cortex: morphological and chemical characteristics of the synaptic inputs. *Prog. Neurobiol.*, 39: 563–607.

DeFelipe, J. and Jones, E.G. (1988) *Cajal on the Cerebral Cortex*. Oxford University Press, New York.

DeFelipe, J. and Jones, E.G. (1991) *Cajal's Degeneration and Regeneration of the Nervous System*, Oxford University Press, New York.

DeFelipe, J., Conti, F., Van Eyck, S.L. and Manzoni, T. (1988) Demonstration of glutamate-positive axon terminals forming asymmetric synapses in cat neocortex. *Brain Res.*, 455: 162–165.

Drakew A., Frotscher M. and Heimrich B. (1999) Blocade of neuronal activity alters spine maturation of dentate granule cells but not their dendritic arborization. *Neuroscience*, 94: 767–774.

Easter, S.S., Purves, D., Rakic, P. and Spitzer, N.C. (1985) The changing view of neural specificity. *Science*, 230: 507–511.

Eayrs, J.T. and Goodhead, B. (1959) Postnatal development of the cerebral cortex in the rat. *J. Anat.*, 93: 385–402.

Edinger, L. (1893) Vergleichend-entwickelungsgeschichtliche und anatomische Studien im Breiche der Hirnanatomie. *Anat. Anzeiger*, 8: 305–321.

Elston, G.N. (2000) Pyramidal cells of the frontal lobe: all the more spinous to think with. *J. Neurosci.*, 20RC95: 1–4.

Elston, G.N. (2001) Interlaminar differences in the pyramidal cell phenotype in cortical areas 7 m and STP (the superior temporal polysensory area) of the Macaque monkey. *Exp. Brain Res.*, 138: 141–151.

Elston, G.N. and Jelinek, H.F. (2001) Dendritic branching patterns of pyramidal cells in the visual cortex of the New World marmoset monkey, with comparative notes on the Old World macaque monkey. *Fractals*, 9: 297–303.

Elston, G.N. and Rockland, K. (2002) The pyramidal cell in sensorimotor cortex of the macaque monkey: systematic variation of cell structure. *Proc. Aust. Neurosci. Soc.*, 13: 209.

130

Elston, G.N. and Rosa, M.G.P. (1997) The occipitoparietal pathway of the macaque monkey: comparison of pyramidal cell morphology in layer III of functionally related cortical visual areas. *Cereb. Cortex*, 7: 432–452.

Elston, G.N. and Rosa, M.G.P. (1998a) Morphological variation of layer III pyramidal neurones in the occipitotemporal pathway of the macaque monkey visual cortex. *Cereb. Cortex*, 8: 278–294.

Elston, G.N. and Rosa, M.G.P. (1998b) Complex dendritic fields of pyramidal cells in the frontal eye field of the macaque monkey: comparison with parietal areas 7a and LIP. *Neuroreport*, 9: 127–131.

Elston, G.N. and Rosa, M.G.P. (2000) Pyramidal cells, patches, and cortical columns: a comparative study of infragranular neurons in TEO, TE, and the superior temporal polysensory area of the macaque monkey. *J. Neurosci.*, 20: RC117 (1–5).

Elston, G.N., Benavides-Piccione, R. and DeFelipe, J. (2001a) The pyramidal cell in cognition: a comparative study in human and monkey. *J. Neurosci.*, 21: RC163 (1–5).

Elston, G.N., Manger, P.R. and Pettigrew, J.D. (1999d) Morphology of pyramidal neurones in cytochrome oxidase modules of the S-I bill representation of the platypus. *Brain Behav. Evol.*, 53: 87–101.

Elston, G.N., Rosa, M.G.P. and Calford, M.B. (1998) Reorganization of neuronal dendritic fields in adult monkey V1 following retinal lesions. *Proc. Fed. Eur. Neurosci.*, 10: 227P.

Elston, G.N., Tweedale, R. and Rosa, M.G.P. (1999a) Cortical integration in the visual system of the macaque monkey: large scale morphological differences of pyramidal neurones in the occipital, parietal and temporal lobes. *Proc. R. Soc. Lond. Ser. B*, 266: 1367–1374.

Elston, G.N., Tweedale, R. and Rosa, M.G.P. (1999b) Cellular heterogeneity in cerebral cortex. A study of the morphology of pyramidal neurones in visual areas of the marmoset monkey. *J. Comp. Neurol.*, 415: 33–51.

Elston, G.N., Tweedale, R. and Rosa, M.G.P. (1999c) Supragranular pyramidal neurones in the medial posterior parietal cortex of the macaque monkey: morphological heterogeneity in subdivisions of area 7. *Neuroreport*, 10: 1925–1929.

Feldman, M.L. and Peters, A. (1979) A technique for estimating total spine numbers on Golgi-impregnated dendrites. *J. Comp. Neurol.*, 188: 527–542.

Felleman, D.J. and Van Essen, D.C. (1991) Distributed hierarchical processing in primate cerebral cortex. *Cerebr. Cortex*, 1: 1–47.

Fialia, J.C. and Harris, K.M. (1999) Dendritic structure. In: G. Stuart, N. Spruston and M. Häusser (Eds.), *Dendrites*, Oxford University Press, New York, pp. 1–34.

Fifkova, E., Eason, H. and Schane, P. (1992) Inhibitory contacts on dendritic spines of the dentate fascia. *Brain Res.*, 577: 331–336.

Frotscher, M., Drakew, A. and Heimrich, B. (2000) Role of afferent innervation and neuronal activity in dendritic development and spine maturation of fascia dentata granulae cells. *Cerebr. Cortex*, 10: 946–951.

Funahashi, S., Bruce, C.J. and Goldman-Rakic, P.S. (1989) Mnemonic coding of visual space in the monkey's dorsolateral prefrontal cortex. *J. Neurophysiol.*, 61: 331–349.

Fuster, J.M. and Alexander, G.E. (1971) Neuron activity related to short-term memory. *Science*, 173: 652–654.

Fuster, J.M. and Jervey, J.P. (1981) Inferotemporal neurons distinguish and retain behaviorally relevant features of visual stimuli. *Science*, 212: 952–955.

Garey, L.J. (1994) *Brodmann's 'Localisation in the Cerebral Cortex'*. Smith-Gordon, London.

Garraghty, P.E. and Muja, N. (1996) NMDA receptors and plasticity in adult primate somatosensory cortex. *J. Comp. Neurol.*, 367: 319–26.

Gilbert, C.D. (1998) Adult cortical dynamics. *Physiol. Rev.*, 78: 467–485.

Goldstein, S.S. and Rall, W. (1974) Changes in action potential shape and velocity for changing core conductor velocity. *Biophys. J.*, 14: 731–757.

Golgi, C. (1886) *Sulla Fina Anatomia delgi Organi Centrali del Sistema Nervoso*. Milan, Ulrico Hoepli.

Goodman, C.S. and Shatz, C.J. (1993) Developmental mechanisms that generate precise patterns of neuronal activity. *Cell*, 72: 77–98.

Gray, E.G. (1959) Axo-somatic and axo-dendritic synapses of the cerebral cortex: an electron microscope study. *J. Anat.*, 93: 420–433.

Greenough, W., Volkmar, F.R. and Juraska, J.M. (1973) Effects of rearing complexity on dendritic branching in frontolateral and temporal cortex in the rat. *Exp. Neurol.*, 41: 371–378.

Harris, K.M. (1999) Structure, development, and plasticity of dendritic spines. *Curr. Opin. Neurobiol.*, 9: 343–348.

Harris, K.M. and Karter, S.B. (1994) Dendritic spines: cellular specializations imparting both stability and flexibility to synaptic function. *Ann. Rev. Neurosci.*, 17: 341–371.

Häusser, M., Spruston, N. and Stuart, G.J. (2000) Diversity and dynamics of dendritic signalling. *Science*, 290: 739–744.

Hebb, D.O. (1949) *The Organization of Behaviour*. John Wiley and Sons, New York.

Helmchen, F., Svoboda K., Denk, W. and Tank, D.W. (1999) *In vivo* dendritic calcium dynamics in deep-layer cortical pyramidal neurons. *Nature Neurosci.*, 2: 989–996.

Hendry, S.H.C. and Jones, E.G. (1988) Activity-dependent regulation of GABA expression in the visual cortex of adult monkeys. *Neuron*, 1: 701–712.

Hendry, S.H.C., Fuchs, J., deBlas, A.L. and Jones, E.G. (1990) Distribution and plasticity of immunocytochemically localized $GABA_A$ receptors in adult monkey visual cortex. *J. Neurosci.*, 10: 2438–2450.

Horner, C.H. (1993) Plasticity of the dendritic spine. *Prog. Neurobiol.*, 41: 281–321.

Huttenlocher, P.R. (1979) Synaptic density in human frontal cortex-developmental changes and effects of aging. *Brain Res.*, 163: 195–205.

Huttenlocher, P.R. and Dabholkar, A.S. (1997) Regional differences in synaptogenesis in human cerebral cortex. *J. Comp. Neurol.*, 387: 167–178.

Huttenlocher, P.R. and de Courten, C. (1987) The development of synapses in striate cortex of man. *Hum. Neurobiol.*, 6: 1–9.

Huttenlocher, P.R., de Courten, C., Garey, L.G. and Van der Loos, H. (1982) Synaptogenesis in human visual cortex: Evidence for synapse elimination during normal development. *Neurosci. Lett.*, 33: 247–252.

Jacobs, B., Larsen-Driscoll, L. and Schall, M. (1997) Lifespan dendritic and spine changes in areas 10 and 18 of human cortex: a quantitative Golgi study. *J. Comp. Neurol.*, 386: 661–680.

Jacobs, B., Schall, M., Prather, M., Kapler, L., Driscoll, L., Baca, S., Jacobs, J., Ford, K., Wianwright, M. and Treml, M. (2001) Regional dendritic and spine variation in human cerebral cortex: a quantitative study. *Cereb. Cortex*, 11: 558–571.

Jelinek, H.F. and Elston, G.N. (2001) Pyramidal neurones in macaque visual cortex: interareal phenotypic variation of dendritic branching patterns. *Fractals*, 7: 287–295.

Jones, E.G. (1968) An electron microscopic study of the terminations of afferent fiber systems onto the somatic sensory cortex of the cat. *J. Anat.*, 103: 595–597.

Jones, E.G. (1985) *The Thalamus*, Plenum Press, New York.

Jones, E.G. and Powell, T.P.S. (1969) Morphological variations in the dendritic spines of the neocortex. *J. Cell Sci.*, 5: 509–529.

Jones, E.G., Benson, D.L., Hendry, S.H.C. and Isackson, P.J. (1990) Activity-dependent regulation of gene expression in adult monkey visual cortex. *Cold Spring Harb. Symp. Quant. Biol.*, 55: 481–490.

Jones, T.A., Kleim, J.A. and Greenough, W.T. (1996) Synaptogenesis and dendritic growth in cortex opposite unilateral sensorimotor cortex damage in adult rats: a quantitative electron microscopic examination. *Brain Res.*, 733: 142–148.

Kaas, J.H. (1991) Plasticity of sensory and motor maps in adult mammals. *Ann. Rev. Neurosci.*, 14: 137–167.

Kaas, J.H., Krubitzer, L.A., Chino, Y.M., Langston, A.L., Polley, E.H. and Blair, N. (1990) Reorganization of retinotopic cortical maps in adult mammals after lesions of the retina. *Science*, 248: 229–231.

Kalil, R.E. (1990) The influence of action potentials on the development of the central visual pathway in mammals. *J. Exp. Biol.*, 153: 261–276.

Kano, M., Lino, K., and Kano, M. (1991) Functional reorganization of adult cat somatosensory cortex is dependent on NMDA receptors. *Neuroreport*, 2: 77–80.

Kharazia, V.N. and Weinberg, R.J. (1993) Glutamate in terminals of the thalamocortical fibers in rat somatic sensory cortex. *Neurosci. Lett.*, 157: 162–166.

Kharazia, V.N. and Weinberg, R.J. (1994) Glutamate in thalamic fibers terminating in layer IV of primary sensory cortex. *J. Neurosci.*, 14: 6021–6032.

Kharazia, V.N. and Weinberg, R.J. (1999) Immunogold localization of AMPA and NMDA receptors in somatic sensory cortex of albino rat. *J. Comp. Neurol.*, 412: 292–302.

Kharazia, V.N., Phend, K.D., Rustioni, A. and Weinberg, R.J. (1996) EM colocalization of AMPA and NMDA receptor subunits at synapses in rat cerebral cortex. *Neurosci. Lett.*, 210: 37–40.

Kintsova, A.Y. and Greenough, W. (1999) Synaptic plasticity in cortical systems. *Curr. Opin. Neurobiol.*, 9: 203–208.

Koch, C. (1999) *Biophysics of Computation. Information Processing in Single Neurons*, Oxford University Press, New York.

Koch, C. and Poggio, T. (1983) A theoretical analysis of electrical properties of spines. *Proc. Roy. Soc. Lond. B*, 218: 455–477.

Koch, C. and Zador, A. (1993) The function of dendritic spines: devices subserving biochemical rather than electrical compartmentalization. *J. Neurosci.*, 13: 413–422.

Koch, C., Poggio, T. and Torre, V. (1982) Retinal ganglion cells: A functional interpretation of dendritic morphology. *Phil. Trans. R. Soc. Lond. B.*, 298: 227–264.

Kondo, H.T., Tanaka, K., Hashikawa, T. and Jones, E.G. (1999) Neurochemical gradients along monkey sensory cortical pathways: calbindin-immunoreactive pyramidal neurons in layers II and III. *Eur. J. Neurosci.*, 11: 4197–4203.

Kossel, A.H., Williams, C.V., Schweizer, M. and Kater, S.B. (1997) Afferent innervation influences the development of dendritic branches and spines via both activity-dependent and non-activity-dependent mechanisms. *J. Neurosci.*, 17: 6314–6324.

Kossut, M. (1998) Experience-dependent changes in function and anatomy of adult barrel cortex. *Exp. Brain Res.*, 123: 110–116.

Kubota, K. and Niki, H. (1971) Prefrontal cortical unit activity and delayed alternation performance in monkeys. *J. Neurophysiol.*, 34: 337–347.

Larkman, A.U. (1991a) Dendritic morphology of pyramidal neurones in the visual cortex of the rat: I. Branching patterns. *J. Comp. Neurol.*, 306: 307–319.

Larkman, A.U. (1991b) Dendritic morphology of pyramidal neurones in the visual cortex of the rat: III. Spine distributions. *J. Comp. Neurol.*, 306: 332–343.

Lund, J.S., Boothe, R.G. and Lund, R.D. (1977) Development of neurons in the visual cortex (area 17) of the monkey (*Macaca nemistrina*): a Golgi study from fetal day 127 to postnatal maturity. *J. Comp. Neurol.*, 176: 149–188.

Lund, J.S., Yoshioka, T. and Levitt, J.B. (1993) Comparison of intrinsic connectivity in different areas of macaque monkey cerebral cortex. *Cerebr. Cortex*, 3: 148–162.

Magee, J.C. and Johnston, D. (1997) A synaptically controlled, associative signal for Hebbian plasticity in hippocampal neurons. *Science*, 275: 209–213.

Mainen, Z.F. (1999) Development of dendrites. In: G. Stuart, N. Spruston and M. Häusser, (Eds.), *Dendrites*. Oxford University Press, New York, pp. 310–338.

Matus A. (2000) Actin-based plasticity in dendritic spines. *Science*, 290: 754–758.

Markram, H., Lübke, J., Frotscher, M. and Sackman, B. (1997) Regulation of synaptic efficacy by coincidence of postsynaptic APs and EPSPs. *Science*, 275: 213–215.

Markram, H., Wang, Y. and Tsodyks, M. (1998) Differential signaling via the same axon of neocortical pyramidal neurons. *Proc. Natl. Acad. Sci. USA*, 95: 5323–5328.

Mel, B. (1999) Why have dendrites? A computation perspective. In: G. Stuart, N. Spruston and M. Häusser (Eds.), *Dendrites*. Oxford University Press, New York, pp. 271–289.

Merzenich, M.M., Kaas, J. H., Wall, J., Nelson, R.J., Sur, M. and Felleman, D. (1983a) Topographic Reorganization of somatosensory cortical areas 3b and 1 in adult monkeys following restricted deafferentation. *Neuroscience*, 8: 33–55.

Merzenich, M.M., Kaas, J.H., Wall, J.T., Sur, M., Nelson, R.J., and Felleman, D.J. (1983b) Progression of change following median nerve section in the cortical representation of the hand in areas 3b and 1 in adult owl and squirrel monkeys. *Neuroscience*, 10: 639– 665.

Meyer, S. (1895) Die Subcutane Methylenblauinjection, ein Mittel zur Darstellung der Elemente des Centralnervensystems. *Arch. Mikros. Anat.*, 46: 282–290.

Meyers, W.A., Churchill, J.D., Muja, N. and Garraghty, P.E. (2000) Role of NMDA receptors in adult primate cortical somatosensory plasticity. *J. Comp. Neurol.*, 418: 373–382.

Missler, M., Eins, S., Merker, H.-J., Rothe, H. and Wolff, J.R. (1993) Pre- and postnatal development of the primary visual cortex of the common marmoset. I. A changing space for synaptogenesis. *J. Comp. Neurol.*, 333: 41–52.

Miyashita, Y., Okuno, H. and Hasegawa, I. (1993a) Tuning and association—neural memory mechanisms of complex visual forms in monkey temporal cortex. *Biomed. Res.*, 14: 89–94.

Muñoz, A., DeFelipe, J. and Jones, E.G. (2000) Patterns of GABA$_B$r1a-b receptor gene expression in monkey and human visual cortex. *Cereb. Cortex*, 11: 104–113.

Murayama, Y., Fujita, I. and Kato M. (1997) Contrasting forms of synaptic plasticity in monkey inferotemporal and primary visual cortices. *Neuroreport*, 8: 1503–1508.

Nakamura, S., Akiguchi, I., Kameyama, M. and Mizuno, N. (1985) Age-related changes of pyramidal cell basal dendrites in layers III and V of human motor cortex: a quantitative Golgi study. *Acta Neuropathol.*, 65: 281–284.

Obata, S., Obata, J., Das, A. and Gilbert, C. (1999) Molecular correlates of topographic reorganization in primary visual cortex following retinal lesions. *Cereb. Cortex*, 9: 238–248.

Peters, A. and Jones, E.G. (1984) Classification of cortical neurons. In: A. Peters and E.G. Jones (Eds.), *Cerebral Cortex: Cellular Components of the Cerebral Cortex,* Vol. 1, Plenum, New York, pp. 107–122.

Peters, A. and Kaiserman-Abramof, I.R. (1970) The small pyramidal neuron of the rat cerebral cortex. The perikaryon, dendrites and spines. *Am. J. Anat.*, 127: 321–356.

Peters, A., Palay, S.L. and Webster, H. (1991) *The Fine Structure of the Nervous System. Neurons and their Supporting Cells*, Oxford University Press, New York.

Petralia, R.S. and Wenthold, R.J. (1992) Light and electron immunocytochemical localization of AMPA-selective glutamate receptors in the rat brain. *J. Comp. Neurol.*, 318: 329–354.

Petralia, R.S., Yokotani, N. and Wenthold, R.J. (1994a) Light and electron microscope distribution of the NMDA receptor subunit NMDAR1 in the rat nervous system using a selective antipeptide antibody. *J. Neurosci.*, 14: 667–696.

Petralia, R.S., Wang, Y.X. and Wenthold, R.J. (1994b) The NMDA receptor subunits NR2A and NR2B show histological and ultrastructural localization patterns similar to those of NR1. *J. Neurosci.*, 14: 6102–6120.

Petralia, R.S., Wang, Y.-X. and Wenthold, R.J. (1994c) Histological and ultrastructural localization of kainate receptor subunits, KA2 and GluR6/7, in the rat nervous system using selective antipeptide antibodies. *J. Comp. Neurol.*, 349: 85–110.

Poirazi, P. and Mel, B. (2000) Impact of active dendrites and structural plasticity on the storage capacity of neural tissue. *Neuron*, 29: 779–796.

Pons, T.P., Garraghty, P.E., Ommaya, A.K., Kaas, J.H., Taub, E. and Mishkin, M. (1991) Massive cortical reorganization after sensory deafferentation in adult macaques. *Science*, 252: 1857–1860.

Quian, N. and Sejnowski, T.J. (1989) An electro-diffusion model for computing membrane potentials and ionic concentrations in branching dendrites, spines and axons. *Biol. Cybern.*, 62: 1–15.

Quian, N. and Sejnowski, T.J. (1990) When is an inhibitory synapse effective? *Proc. Natl. Acad. Sci. USA*, 87: 8145–8149.

Rall, W. (1959) Branching dendritic trees and motorneuron membrane resistivity. *Expt. Neurol.*, 1: 491–527.

Rall, W. (1964) Theoretical significance of dendritic tree for input–output relation. In: R.F. Reiss, (Ed.), *Neural Theory and Modeling*. Stanford University Press, Stanford, pp. 73–97.

Rall, W. and Segev, I. (1987) Functional possibilities for synapses on dendrites and on dendritic spines. In: G.M. Edelman, W.E. Gall and W.M. Cowan (Eds.), *Synaptic Function*. Wiley, New York, pp. 605–636.

Rall, W., Burke, R.E., Holmes, W.R., Jack, J.J.B., Redman, S.R. and Segev, I. (1992) Matching dendritic neuron models to experimental data. *Physiol. Rev.*, 72: 159–186.

Retzius (1891) Ueber den Bau der Oberflachenschichte der Grosshirnrinde beim menschen und bei den Saugethiere. *Biologiska Foreningens Förhandlinger*, 3: 90–102.

Ribak, C.E. (1978) Aspinous and sparsely-spinous stellate neurons in the visual cortex of rats contain glutamic acid decarboxylase. *J. Neurocytol.*, 7: 461–478.

Ribak, C.E., Vaughn, J.E., Saito, K., Barber, R. and Roberts, E. (1977) Glutamate decarboxylase localization in neurons of the olfactory bulb. *Brain Res.*, 126: 1–18.

Rossi, F. and Strata, P. (1995) Reciprocal trophic interactions in the adult climbing fiber-Purkinje cell system. *Prog. Neurobiol.*, 47: 341–369.

Schaffer (1892) Beitrag zur Histologie des Ammonshornformation. *Arch. f. Mickros. Anat.*, 39: 611–

Scheibel, M.E., Lindsay, R.D., Tomiyasu, U. and Scheibel, A.B. (1975) Progressive dendritic changes in the ageing human cortex. *Exp. Neurol.*, 47: 392–403.

Schiefferdecker, P. and Kossel, A. (1891) *Gewebelehre mit Besonderer Berücksichtigung des Menschlichen Körpers*. Harald Bruhn, Braunschweig.

Segal, M., Korkatian, E. and Murphy, D.D. (2000) Dendritic spine formation and pruning: common cellular mechanisms? *Trends Neurosci.*, 23: 53–57.

Segev, I. and Schneidman, E. (1999) Axons as computing devices: basic insights gained from models. *J. Physiol.*, 93: 263–270.

Shatz, C.J. (1990) Impulse activity and the pattering of connections during CNS development. *Neuron*, 5: 745–756.

Shepherd, G.M. (1996) The dendritic spine: a multifunctional integrative unit. *J. Neurophysiol.*, 75: 2197–2210.

Shepherd, G.M. and Brayton, R.K. (1987) Logic operations are properties of computer-simulated interactions between excitable dendritic spines. *Neuroscience*, 21: 151–165.

Shepherd, G.M. and Greer, C.A. (1988) The dendritic spine: adaptations of structure and function for different types of synaptic intergration. In: R.J. Lasek and M.M. Black (Eds.), *Intrinsic Determinants of Neuronal Form and Function*. Liss, New York, pp. 245–262.

Shepherd, G.M. and Greer, C.A. (1998) Olfactory Bulb. In: G.M. Shepherd (Ed.), *The Synaptic Organization of the Brain*. Oxford University Press, New York, pp. 159–204.

Shepherd, G.M., Brayton, R.K., Miller, J.P., Segev, I., Rinzel, J. and Rall, W. (1985) Signal enhancement in distal cortical dendrites by means of interactions between active dendritic spines. *Proc Natl Acad Sci USA*, 82: 2192–2195.

Sloper, J.J. and Powell, T.P.S. (1979) An electron microscopic study of afferent connections to the primate motor and somatic sensory corticies. *Phil. Trans. Roy. Soc. B*, 19: 1051–1065.

Somogyi, P. and Soltesz, I. (1986) Immunogold demonstration of GABA in synaptic terminals of intracellularly recorded horse raddish peroxidase-filled basket cells and clutch cells in the cats visual cortex. *Neuroscience*, 19: 1051–1065.

Somogyi, P., Fritschy, J.-M., Benke, D., Roberts, J.D.B. and Sieghart, W. (1996) The γ2 subunit of the GABA$_A$ receptor is concentrated in synaptic junctions containing the γ1 and β2/3 subunits in hippocampus, cerebellum and globus pallidus. *Neuropharmacol.*, 35: 1425–1444.

Somogyi, P., Tamas, G., Lujan, R. and Buhl, E.H. (1998) Salient features of synaptic organisation in the cerebral cortex. *Brain Res. Rev.*, 26: 113–135.

Sotelo, C. (1978) Purkinje cell ontogeny: formation and maintenance of spines. *Prog. Brain Res.*, 48: 149–168.

Sotelo, C. (1990) Cerebellar synaptogenesis: what can we learn from mutant mice. *J. Exp. Biol.*, 153: 225–249.

Sotelo, C., Hillman, D.E., Zamora, A.J. and Llinás, R. (1975) Climbing fiber deafferentation: its action on Purkinje cell dendritic spines. *Brain Res.*, 98: 574–581.

Spruston, N., Schiller, Y., Stuart, G. and Sackman, B. (1995) Activity-dependent action potential invasion and calcium influx into hippocampal CA1 dendrites. *Science*, 268: 297–300.

Spruston, N., Stuart, G. and Häusser, M. (1999) Dendritic integration. In: G. Stuart, N. Spruston and M. Häusser (Eds.), *Dendrites*. Oxford University Press, New York, pp. 231–270.

Steward, O. (1995) Targeting of mRNAs to subsynaptic microdomains in dendrites. *Current Biol.*, 5: 55–61.

Steward, O. (1997) mRNA localization in neurons: a multipurpose mechanism? *Neuron*, 18: 9–18.

Stuart, G.J. and Häusser, M. (1994) Initiation and spread of sodium action potentials in cerebellar Purkinje cells. *Neuron*, 13: 703–712.

Stuart, G.J. and Sackman, B. (1994) Active propagation of somatic action potentials into neocortical pyramidal cell dendrites. *Nature*, 367: 69–72.

Stuart, G.J., Spruston N., Sackman, B. and Häusser, M. (1997) Action potential initiation and backpropagation in neurons of the mammalian CNS. *Trends Neurosci.*, 20: 125–131.

Svoboda, K., Denk W., Kleinfeld D. and Tank, D.W. (1997) *In vivo* calcium dynamics in neocortical pyramidal neurons. *Nature*, 385: 161–165.

Takács, J. and Hámori, J. (1994) Developmental dynamics of Purkinje cells and dendritic spines in rat cerebellar cortex. *J. Neurosci. Res.*, 38: 515–530.

Turrigiano, G.G. (1999) Homeostatic plasticity in neuronal networks: the more things change the more they stay the same. *Trends Neurosci.*, 22: 221–227.

Turrigiano, G.G. and Nelson, S.B. (2000) Hebb and homeostasis in neuronal plasticity. *Curr. Opin. Neurobiol.*, 10: 358–364.

Uylings, H.B., Ruiz-Marcos, A. and van Pelt, J. (1986) The metric analysis of three-dimensional dendritic tree patterns: a methodological review. *J. Neurosci. Meths.*, 18: 127–151.

Valverde, F. (1967) Apical dendritic spines of the visual cortex and light deprivation in the mouse. *Exp. Brain Res.*, 3: 337–352.

Valverde, F. (1968) Apical dendritic spines of the visual cortex and light deprivation in the mouse. *Exp. Brain Res.*, 5: 274–.

Valverde, F. (1978) The organization of area 18 in the monkey: A Golgi study. *Anat. Embryol.*, 154: 305–334.

Vetter, P., Roth, A. and Häusser, M. (2001) Propagation of action potentials in dendrites depends on dendritic morphology. *J. Neurophysiol.*, 85: 926–937.

Vogt, C. and Vogt, O. (1919) Allgemeine ergebnisse unserer hirnforschung. *J. Psychol. Neurol.*, 25: 279–462.

Volkmar, F.R. and Greenough, W. (1972) Rearing complexity affects branching compexity in the visual cortex of the rat. *Science*, 176: 1445–1447.

Walker, A.E. (1940) A cytoarchitectural study of the prefrontal areas of the macaque monkey. *J. Comp. Neurol.*, 73: 59–86.

White, E.L. (1989) *Cortical Circuits: Synaptic Organization of the Cerebral Cortex. Structure, Function and Theory*. Birkhaüser, Boston.

Woolf, T.B., Shepherd, G.M. and Greer, C.A. (1991) Local information processing in dendritic trees: subsets of spines in granule cells of the mammalian olfactory bulb. *J. Neurosci.*, 11: 1837–1854.

Xu, L.-H., Tanigawa, H. and Fujita, I. (1997) Distribution of AMPA-type glutamate receptors along the ventral visual cortical pathway in the macaque: a gradient reflecting the cortical hierarchy. *Soc. Neurosc. Abstr.*, 23: 2062p.

E.C. Azmitia, J. DeFelipe, E.G. Jones, P. Rakic and C.E. Ribak (Eds.)
Progress in Brain Research, Vol. 136

CHAPTER 11

Modification of dendritic development

Alfredo Feria-Velasco[1,*], Alma Rosa del Angel[2] and Ignacio Gonzalez-Burgos[3]

[1]*Division of Pathology, CIATEJ (SEP-CONACyT), Guadalajara, Jal., Mexico,*
[2]*Division of Neurosciences, CIBO, I.M.S.S., Guadalajara, Jal., Mexico, and*
[3]*Laboratory of Psychobiology, CIBIMI, I.M.S.S., Morelia, Mich., Mexico*

Abstract: Since 1890 Ramón y Cajal strongly defended the theory that dendrites and their processes and spines had a function of not just nutrient transport to the cell body, but they had an important conductive role in neural impulse transmission. He extensively discussed and supported this theory in the Volume 1 of his extraordinary book *Textura del Sistema Nervioso del Hombre y de los Vertebrados*. Also, Don Santiago significantly contributed to a detailed description of the various neural components of the hippocampus and cerebral cortex during development. Extensive investigation has been done in the last Century related to the functional role of these complex brain regions, and their association with learning, memory and some limbic functions. Likewise, the organization and expression of neuropsychological qualities such as memory, exploratory behavior and spatial orientation, among others, depend on the integrity and adequate functional activity of the cerebral cortex and hippocampus. It is known that brain serotonin synthesis and release depend directly and proportionally on the availability of its precursor, tryptophan (TRY). By using a chronic TRY restriction model in rats, we studied their place learning ability in correlation with the dendritic spine density of pyramidal neurons in field CA1 of the hippocampus during postnatal development. We have also reported alterations in the maturation pattern of the ability for spontaneous alternation and task performance evaluating short-term memory, as well as adverse effects on the density of dendritic spines of hippocampal CA1 field pyramidal neurons and on the dendritic arborization and the number of dendritic spines of pyramidal neurons from the third layer of the prefrontal cortex using the same model of TRY restriction. The findings obtained in these studies employing a modified Golgi method, can be interpreted as a trans-synaptic plastic response due to understimulation of serotoninergic receptors located in the hippocampal Ammon's horn and, particularly, on the CA1 field pyramidal neurons, as well as on afferences to the hippocampus which needs to be further investigated.

Don Santiago Ramón y Cajal, an illustrious Spanish scientist, masterly described back at the end of the century before last, the cytoarchitectural configuration of practically every area of the central nervous system (CNS) of mammals, including humans, employing metallic impregnation techniques for light microscopy designed by Camilo Golgi; likewise through variants to such procedures and other methods to study the nervous system structure designed by Don Santiago himself. It is well known that Cajal contributed not only to the knowledge of the structural bases of the interactions among the various CNS regions, but also to the structural configuration of the components of different types of individual neurons, particularly their dendritic arborizations (Cajal and Tello y Muñoz, 1940). Don Santiago wisely decided to study the different nervous system components during development because the dendritic and axonal ramifications and complexity of their course in the mature stages makes their study highly difficult. It should also be noted that metallic impregnations do not stain simultaneously all the neurons of a certain region (Cajal, 1899). Subsequent to

---

*Corresponding author: CIATEJ, Division of Pathology, Av. Normalistas 800, 44270 Guadalajara, Jal., Mexico; Tel. and Fax: (52-33) 3345-5200; E-mail: aferia@ciatej.net.mx

Don Santiago's studies, the normal development of dendritic configuration were studied employing metallic impregnations, injection of intracellular dyes, confocal microscopy and transmission electron microscopy techniques.

The present work deals with modifications of the dendritic tree of neurons during development, in two regions of the CNS: hippocampus and cerebral cortex using a model of selective nutrient restriction in the diet. Special emphasis is made to correlate these modifications with the basic functions in which those two regions are importantly involved.

As a constituent part of the nervous cell, the dendritic tree represents that region where most of the synaptic contacts with axon terminals of fibers originating from various neural pathways are established. Notwithstanding the multiplicity of contacts, these are not randomly distributed; there is a compartmentalization of such afferent fibers over specific dendritic zones, related to the neural region of origin, and to the nature of the neurotransmitter released in the synaptic cleft. Furthermore, in general terms, axosomatic synapses and those established on the dendritic area proximal to the soma are usually inhibitory in nature, including those making contact with the axon hillock and axon initial segment; while those synapses over distal zones of the dendritic arborization are predominantly excitatory (Edwards, 1995). In the case of neurons presenting spines on their dendritic surface, this is particularly true in that dendritic spines represent the preferential neuronal postsynaptic site of excitatory stimuli (Harris, 1999a; Hendry, 1996; Koch and Zador, 1993), while those of the inhibitory type establish contact predominantly on the dendritic trunk (Hendry, 1996).

Since the nerve impulses flow from its dendritic origin to the soma, the excitatory synaptic activation could be considered as the entrance of 'crude' excitatory information, analyzed and integrated afterwards by inhibitory and/or modulatory stimuli. This implicates that neurons with large amounts of spines integrate a big deal of information; moreover, these neurons constitute the exit source of such information to other CNS regions.

Just as much as in number and length of dendritic ramifications, as in the absence or presence, density, distribution and shape of their spines, the cytoarchitectural pattern of the dendritic tree under normal conditions, is characteristic of each neuron lineage. Atypical modifications in such parameters, either under

pathologic conditions or experimentally induced for their study, constitute changes that could be interpreted as a part of a degenerative process or otherwise as a plastic phenomenon with a tendency to reestablish this microsystem performance (Brailowsky et al., 1998). Both, neurodegenerative processes and neuronal plastic changes, theoretically with a tendency to rehabilitation, might show functional sequels to be expressed eventually by means of aberrant behaviors. Thus, the experimental study of the modifications in the structural neuronal elements and their results in behavior has given rise to a better knowledge of brain function, as well as its correlation with specific psychoneural profiles.

In recent years, we have used a model of tryptophan (TRY) restriction for rodent diet (Fernstrom, 1981), to study the functional role of serotonin (5-HT) on the regulation of hippocampus and prefrontal cerebral cortex activity. Cajal (1904) masterly described the cytoarchitecture of these zones in a diversity of vertebrate species, both in the adult stage and during their development, mainly at postnatal ages.

It is known that the hippocampus plays an important role in the organization of cognitive processes such as place learning through the establishment of cognitive maps related to the visuospatial signals in the surroundings (Jarrad, 1993). The hippocampus also participates in the accomplishment of instrumental processes such as exploratory behavior by means of individual adaptation skills and to dominate a new field (Campbell and Raskin, 1978; Gentsch et al., 1991; Myhrer, 1988). Correspondingly, prefrontal cerebral cortex is closely related to the organization of short-term memory by structuring diagrams of temporary sequences of motion actions tending to the performance of tasks requiring to evoke memories in the short term (Fuster, 1997, 2000). For this effect, the prefrontal cortex might require the spatial information that in fact emanates from hippocampal efferents innervating the medial prefrontal cortical zone (Cajal, 1904; Verwer et al., 1997).

For data presented in this communication, Sprague-Dawley rats just after weaning (21-day-old) were fed a diet restricted in TRY (0.15 g TRY/23 g protein/100 g of diet) on a free access bases. The development of their place learning capability was studied with a Morris labyrinth. A progressive impairment of this capacity was noticed, characterized by a lack of a defined spatial strategy, a disability to reduce the distance they went through during the attempts the test consisted of (Fig. 1),

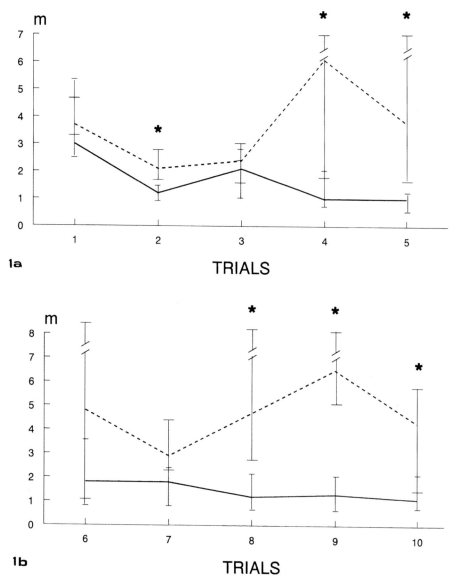

Fig. 1. Comparison of distances swum by control (continuous line) and TRY-restricted (discontinuous line) animals at 60 days of age (40 days after the study began) during the first (1–5) (1a) and second (6–10) (1b) attempt blocks for testing place learning using the Morris labyrinth. During the second series of attempts, both, the point of entry and the platform position were inverted to evaluate the task relearning process. m: meters. Medians ± quartils. Significantly different from control at $p < 0.05$ (asterisks) (Modified from: Olvera-Cortés et al., 1998).

and also, a remarkable irregularity of the learning curves (Olvera-Cortés et al., 1998). Afterwards, by using a modified Golgi method (González-Burgos et al., 1992) the density of spines on the apical and basal dendrites of pyramidal neurons of the CA1 hippocampal field (Pérez-Vega et al., 1998) of the same rats used for the behavioral tests was evaluated (Fig. 2). The pyramidal hippocampal neurons constitute the exit pathway for the processed information in the hippocampal trisynaptic circuit, which is known to be involved in the spatial information process (Shen et al., 1994).

138

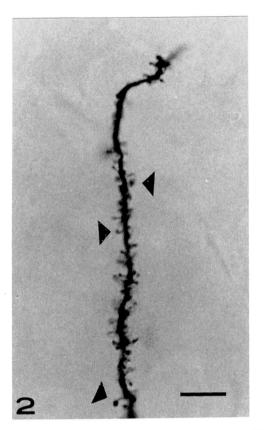

Fig. 2. Segment of an oblique dendrite of a hippocampal CA1 field pyramidal neuron of an adult rat, where large amount of dendritic spines are depicted (arrow heads). Modified Golgi technique. Bar = 20 μm.

In the morphological study, the apical dendrite was divided into three equal segments, and the dendritic spines seen along 25 μm of the mid portion of each segment were counted. Likewise, spines seen along 25 μm of the middle region in a primary basal dendrite of each impregnated pyramidal neuron were also counted. A lesser amount of spines on the distal two-thirds was observed in the TRY restricted animals in comparison with data obtained from the control group, while on the proximal third there were no significant differences when data from both groups of animals were compared. Basal dendrites of pyramidal cells in the TRY restricted group also showed less spines than corresponding dendrites in the control group (Table 1). Thus, taking into account that spines represent the entrance site of excitatory information, that loss of spines observed in animals under TRY restriction could explain in part the deficiency of their behavioral performance observed during the task. Based on this, the information entrance to pyramidal neurons of the hippocampal CA1 field derived from ambient sensory stimuli related to space demand, could have been insufficient, and therefore its integration to generate responses according to those demands had the possibility of being equally deficient. Such morphological findings could underlie the alterations in the pattern of behavioral response to give an efficient solution to the assigned spatial task because of a decrement in brain 5-HT concentration, and consequently on the serotoninergic activity in

Table 1 Dendritic spine density of the pyramidal neurons from the hippocampal CA1 field of control (C) and tryptophan-restricted (R) rats

Dendritic segment age	Apical			basal middle
	proximal	middle	terminal	
21 days				
C	14.3 ± 0.8	24.7 ± 0.4	24.9 ± 0.7	18.3 ± 1.0
R	12.1 ± 1.2	25.0 ± 0.5	26.1 ± 0.8	20.5 ± 1.3
40 days				
C	18.2 ± 1.5	33.4 ± 0.7	32.7 ± 0.4	25.0 ± 0.9
R	15.7 ± 1.8	32.4 ± 1.1	28.0 ± 0.9 *	23.8 ± 1.2
60 days				
C	17.1 ± 1.5	28.9 ± 0.7	24.8 ± 1.6	25.2 ± 0.8
R	14.0 ± 1.1	24.7 ± 1.2 *	25.2 ± 1.7	20.4 ± 0.9 *

Data represent the means ± SEM.
* $p < 0.05$

hippocampus. Neurochemical and electrophysiologic mechanisms corresponding to those morphologic alterations subjacent to an impairment of spatial learning are presently under study in our laboratory employing a model of a selective pharmacological lesion to interfere with the serotoninergic input to the hippocampus.

The organization of exploratory behavior is another functional attribute of the hippocampus. Its objective is the adjustment to novel ambiances an individual is exposed to, and it is formed by different instrumental skills; among them is the ability to avoid useless motor actions. The capacity of spontaneous alternation in a 'T' labyrinth was studied by means of TRY restriction design resembling the one mentioned above. It was noticed that the animals on a TRY restricted diet elected the alternative option in the second instance of the test in a greater percentage compared to what was seen in animals fed a well- balanced diet (Fig. 3) (González-Burgos et al., 1995). That is to say, they were able—to an abnormal degree— to suppress a useless action (to persevere over an alternative which did not represent any meaningful stimulus) and, at the same time 'to go forward' on the adaptation process through the exploration of a second alternative which was novel for the animals. It has been proposed that hippocampal cholinergic activity is strictly related to the conduct inhibition (Moorcroft, 1971). Moreover, we are aware about the existence of serotoninergic terminals which establish synaptic contact with cholinergic fibers, both at the hippocampus and at the prefrontal cerebral cortex, and it has been proposed that the result of such neurochemical interaction becomes the presynaptic inhibition of acetylcholine (ACh) release (Richter-Levin and Segal, 1991; Yukihiro et al., 1991). Thus, the behavioral findings related to the greater capability for spontaneous alternation seen in TRY-restricted animals could be associated with a submodulation of ACh release in such a way that cholinergic activity is significantly increased. In consequence, such ability to avoid useless conducts would be affected with a tendency to increase. To this effect, our results are congruent with the aforementioned proposal.

Continuing with this same scheme of TRY restriction, we have also studied the effects of low cerebral concentration of 5-HT on the short-term memory, employing the labyrinth of Biel of stable surface (Vorhes, 1986). We found out that the TRY restriction provoked a more efficient conduct performance, in terms of a significant reduction in the number of errors made during the labyrinth resolution from the second or third trial throughout five consecutive attempts; while

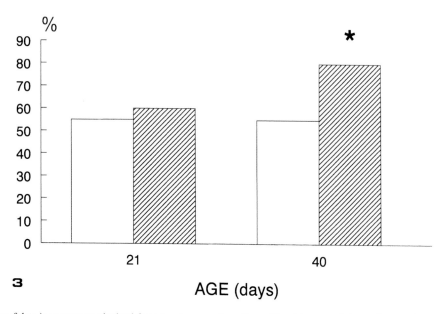

Fig. 3. Comparison of data in percentage obtained from spontaneous alternation achieved by control (empty bars) and TRY-restricted (striped bars) animals, at 21 and 40 days of age. Significantly increased proportion of the task resolution was seen in the TRY-restricted animals (asterisk) at 40 days of age. (Modified from: González-Burgos et al., 1995).

140

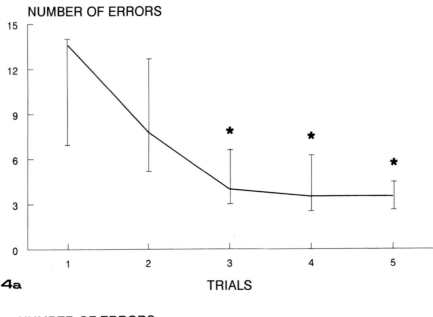

4a

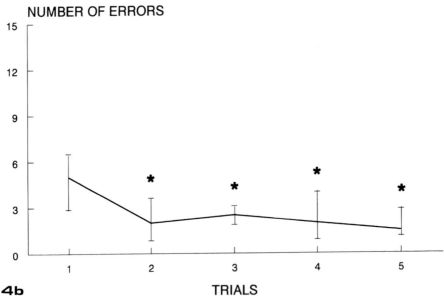

4b

Fig. 4. Number of errors made by animals from the control (4a) and TRY-restricted (4b) groups, during the Biel labyrinth resolution, 40 days after the study began. Significantly different from the number of errors made in the first attempt, at $p < 0.05$ (asterisks) (Modified from: González-Burgos et al., 1998).

the control animals made the same from the third or fourth attempt (Fig. 4 and B in Fig. 6) (González-Burgos et al., 1998). It has been demonstrated that pyramidal neurons of the third layer of prefrontal cortex 'associate' to conform the so-called 'memory fields' where the structure of patterns of action temporary

sequences lies, which are responsible for the coordinated performance of motor actions tending to a task resolution which call for memories on the short term (Fuster, 1998).

Figure 5 shows the structure of a pyramidal neuron from the prefrontal cerebral cortex, impregnated by a

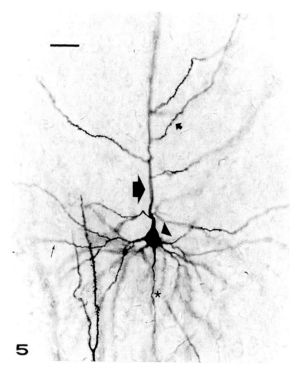

5

Fig. 5. Pyramidal neuron from the rat prefrontal cerebral cortex third layer, impregnated by a modified Golgi technique. The soma (arrow head), axon (asterisk), apical dendrite (large arrow), oblique (small arrow) and basal (thin arrow) dendrites are clearly identified. Spines can be depicted in some oblique and basal dendrites of this neuron, and in the apical dendrite of another pyramidal nerve cell. Bar = 50 μm.

modified Golgi technique. The pyramidal cell cytoarchitecture analysis revealed a reduced pattern of dendritic arborization, as well as an increase of the dendritic spine density, and an abnormal growth in length of both, apical and basal dendrites in the TRY-restricted animals (Fig. 6) (González-Burgos et al., 1996). Subsequent studies performed under a scheme of pharmacological lesion of the serotoninergic system afferent to the prefrontal cerebral cortex confirmed the behavioral results, and the previous data regarding the increment of the spine density. The shape of dendritic spines was also studied observing an increment in thin spines in both oblique and basal dendrites, whereas in the proximal third of the apical dendrite of these same neurons, an increased number of spines and more stubby spines were observed (Fig. 6) (Pérez-Vega et al., 2000). It has been proposed that thin spines have a greater capacity to transmit the synaptic impulse compared to stubby

spines (Harris and Kater, 1994; Koch et al., 1992; Korkotian and Segal, 1999). Likewise, the presence of a greater number of spines along with a greater proportion of thin spines, suggest the existence of an excitatory stimulation above normal values even though it does not induce its collapse (Harris, 1999b; Segal, 1995), helped by a lack of serotoninergic inhibition in the microenvironment. On these bases, the greatest behavioral efficiency would be partially sustained on the 'liberation' of the excitatory activity; on the existence of a greater number of spines; and on the thin spines predominance. On the other hand, the stubby spines that predominate on the dendritic parts near the soma suggests the occurrence of a compensatory facilitation to diminish the presumed neuronal hyperexcitability, due to the fact that stubby spines do not transmit the synaptic impulse efficiently. Due to the localization of those stubby spines in the areas of integration of predominantly inhibitory stimuli, this finding could represent a postsynaptic modulatory mechanism of neuronal excitability. Additionally and from a behavioral point of view, a lack of serotoninergic presynaptic inhibitions over the cholinergic activity could also contribute to the greater efficiency on the task resolution. This may be supported by the fact that the labyrinth of Biel is conformed by election alternatives resembling those stated as a conduct challenge in the spontaneous alternation labyrinth. In virtue of the cholinergic activity disinhibition, the animals would be able to make less errors during the labyrinth resolution, which in fact it happened. Likewise, the glutamatergic hippocampal output to the prefrontal cerebral cortex could have also contributed to the labyrinth resolution by means of the incorporation of spatial information to the proposed prefrontal memory fields, provided that the animals also had the possibility to appeal to fixed visuospatial signals available in the ambient. These, among other mechanisms involved in the dendritic and synaptic modeling pattern induced by the serotoninergic activity manipulation, are presently under study in our laboratory.

Acknowledgments

This work was supported in part by FUNSALUD. Cap. Jalisciense Grant # 101-001-003, and CONACYT Grant # 28646.

142

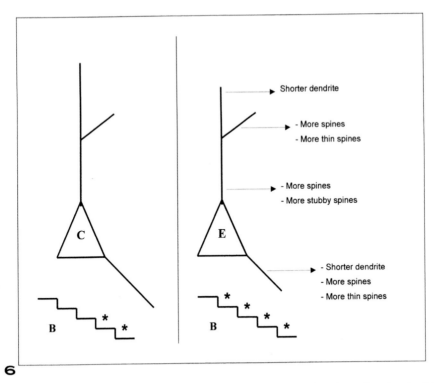

6

Fig. 6. Schematic representation of morphological modifications observed in pyramidal cells from the prefrontal cortex third layer of control (C) and pharmacologically lesioned (E) animals affecting the serotoninergic pathway originating at the dorsal raphe nucleus. Shorter apical and basal dendrites, more dendritic spines, more thin spines in oblique and basal dendrites, and more stubby spines in the initial segment of apical dendrite were seen in the experimental group when compared to data obtained from the control group. In the lower part (B) a reduction in the number of errors made during the Biel labyrinth resolution from the second attempt in the experimental group is shown; while the control animals made the same from the fourth attempt (asterisks) (Modified from: Pérez-Vega et al., 2000).

References

Brailowsky, S., Stein, D.G. and Will, B. (1998) El cerebro averiado. Plasticidad cerebral y recuperación funcional. México, CONACyT / Fondo de Cultura Económica, pp. 98–122.

Cajal, S.R. (1899) *Textura del Sistema Nervioso del Hombre y de los Vertebrados.* Vol. 1. Madrid, Imprenta y Librería de Nicolás Moya, pp. 41–76.

Cajal, S.R. (1904) *Textura del Sistema Nervioso del Hombre y de los Vertebrados.* Vol. 2, Part 2. Madrid, Imprenta y Librería de Nicolás Moya, pp. 792–864; 997–1042.

Cajal, S.R. and Tello y Muñoz, J.F. (1940) *Elementos de Histología Normal y de Técnica Micrográfica.* Madrid, Tipográfica Artística pp. 434–450.

Campbell, R.A. and Raskin, L.A. (1978) Ontogeny of behavioral arousal: the role of environmental stimuli. *J. Comp. Physiol. Psychol.*, 92: 176–184.

Edwards, F.A. (1995) Anatomy and electrophysiology of fast synapses lead to a structural model for long-term potentiation. *Physiol. Rev.*, 75: 759–787.

Fernstrom, J.D. (1981) Effects of the diet and other metabolic phenomena on brain tryptophan uptake and serotonin synthesis. *Ann. Rev. Med.*, 23: 413–425.

Fuster, J.M. (1997) The prefrontal cortex. *Anatomy, physiology, and Neuropsychology of the Frontal Lobe*, Lippincot–Raven, New York, pp. 66–149.

Fuster, J.M. (1998) Cellular dynamics of network memory. *Z. Naturforsch.*, 53c, 670–676.

Fuster, J.M. (2000) The prefrontal cortex of the primate: a synopsis. *Psychobiol.*, 28: 125–131.

Gentsch, C., Lichtsteiner, M. and Feer, H. (1991) Genetic and environmental influences on the active and spontaneous locomotor activities in rats. *Experientia*, 47: 998–1008.

González-Burgos, I. Olvera-Cortés, E., Del Angel-Meza, A.R. and Feria-Velasco A. (1995) Serotonin involvement in the spontaneous alternation ability: a behavioral study in tryptophan-restricted rats. *Neurosci. Lett.*, 190: 143–145.

González-Burgos, I., del Angel-Meza, A.R., Barajas-López, G. and Feria-Velasco, A. (1996) Tryptophan restriction causes long-term plastic changes in corticofrontal pyramidal neurons. *Int. J. Develop. Neurosci.*, 14: 673–679.

González-Burgos, I., Pérez-Vega, M.I., Del Angel-Meza, A.R. and Feria-Velasco, A. (1998) Effect of tryptophan restriction on short-term memory. *Physiol. Behav.*, 63: 165–169.

González-Burgos, I., Tapia-Arizmendi, G. and Feria-Velasco, A. (1992) Golgi method without osmium tetroxide for the study of the central nervous system. *Biotech. Histochem.*, 67: 288–296.

Harris, K.M. (1999a) Structure, development, and plasticity of dendritic spines. *Curr. Op. Neurobiol.*, 9: 343–348.

Harris, K.M. (1999b) Calcium from internal stores modifies dendritic spine shape. *Proc. Natl. Acad. Sci. USA.*, 96: 12213–12215.

Harris, K.M. and Kater, S.B. (1994) Dendritic spines: cellular specializations imparting both stability and flexibility to synaptic function. *Ann. Rev. Neurosci.*, 17: 341–371.

Hendry, S.H.C. (1996) The anatomy of the cerebral cortex: aspects of neuronal morphology and organization. In: F. Conti and T.P. Hicks, (Eds.), *Excitatory amino acids and the cerebral cortex.* The MIT Press, Boston, pp. 3–20.

Jarrad, L.E. (1993) On the role of the hippocampus in learning and memory in the rat. *Behav. Neural Biol.*, 60: 9–26.

Koch, Ch. and Zador, A. (1993) The function of dendritic spines. Devices subserving biochemical rather than electrical compartmentalization. *J. Neurosci.*, 13: 413–422.

Koch, Ch., Zador, A. and Brown, T.H. (1992) Dendritic spines: convergence of theory and experiment. *Science*, 256: 973–974.

Korkotian, E. and Segal, M. (1999) Release of calcium from stors alters the morphology of dendritic spines in cultured hippocampal neurons. *Proc. Natl. Acad. Sci. USA*, 96: 12068–12072.

Moorcroft, W.H. (1971) Ontogeny of forebrain inhibition or behavioral arousal in the rat. *Brain Res.*, 35: 513–522.

Myhrer, T. (1988) Exploratory behavior and reaction to novelty in rats with hippocampal perforant path systems disrupted. *Behav. Neurosci.*, 102: 356–362.

Olvera-Cortés, E., Pérez-Vega, M.I., Barajas-López, G., Del Angel-Meza, A.R., González-Burgos, I. and Feria-Velasco, A. (1998) Place learning impairment in chronically tryptophan-restricted rats. *Nutr. Neurosci.*, 1: 223–235.

Pérez-Vega, M.I., Barajas-López, G., Del Angel-Meza, A.R., González-Burgos, I. and Feria-Velasco, A. (1998) Dendritic spine density of pyramidal neurons in field CA1 of the hippocampus decreases due to chronic tryptophan restriction. *Nutr. Neurosci.*, 1: 237–242.

Pérez-Vega, M.I., Feria-Velasco, A. and González-Burgos, I. (2000) Prefrontocortical serotonin depletion results in plastic changes of prefrontocortical pyramidal neurons, underlying a greater efficiency of short-term memory. *Brain Res. Bull.*, 53: 291–300.

Richter-Levin, G. and Segal, M. (1991) The effects of serotonin depletion and raphe grafts on hippocampal electrophysiology and behavior. *J. Neurosci.*, 11: 1585–1596.

Segal, M. (1995) Morphological alterations in dendritic spines of rat hippocampal neurons exposed to N-methyl-D-aspartate. *Neurosci. Lett.*, 193: 273–276.

Shen, Y., Specht, S.M., Ghislain, I.D.S. and Li, R. (1994) The hippocampus: a biological model for studying learning and memory. *Prog. Neurobiol.*, 44: 485–496.

Verwer, R.W.H., Meijer, R.J., Van Vum, H.F.M. and Witter, M.P. (1997) Collateral projections from the rat hippocampal formation to the lateral and medial prefrontal cortex. *Hippocampus*, 7: 397–402.

Vorhes, Ch.V. (1986) Methods for assessing the adverse effects of foods and other chemicals on animal behavior. *Nutr. Rep. Suppl.*, 44: 185–192.

Yukihiro, N., Yoshiaki, O., Etsuko, S. and Makoto, O. (1991) Involvement of central cholinergic mechanisms in RU-24969-induced behavioral deficits. *Pharmacol. Biochem. Behav.*, 38: 441–446.

E.C. Azmitia, J. DeFelipe, E.G. Jones, P. Rakic and C.E. Ribak (Eds.)
Progress in Brain Research, Vol. 136

CHAPTER 12

Electron microscopic immunolabeling of transporters and receptors identifies transmitter-specific functional sites envisioned in Cajal's neuron

Virginia M. Pickel[1],*, Miguel Garzón[2] and Elisa Mengual[3]

[1]*Division of Neurobiology, Department of Neurology and Neuroscience, Weill Medical College of Cornell University, 411 East 69th St., New York, NY 10021, USA*
[2]*Departamento de Morfología, Facultad de Medicina, Universidad Autónoma de Madrid (UAM), Madrid, Spain*
[3]*Departmento de Anatomía, Facultad de Medicina, Universidad de Navarra, Irunlarrea 1, Pamplona 31008, Navarra, Spain*

Abstract: Neuronal arborizations that were so elegantly demonstrated in the early drawings of Santiago Ramón y Cajal can now be viewed by high resolution electron microscopic immunocytochemical localization of vesicular and plasmalemmal neurotransmitter transporters and receptors. The subcellular distribution of these proteins confers both chemical selectivity and functional specificity to the dendritic and axonal arborizations described by Cajal. This is illustrated by central dopaminergic and cholinergic neurons. Dopamine terminals in the striatum and ventral pallidum, as well as dendrites of midbrain dopaminergic neurons in the ventral tegmental area and substantia nigra express the plasmalemmal dopamine transporter (DAT) and the vesicular monoamine transporter (VMAT2). In forebrain regions, the dopamine D2 receptor (D2R) autoreceptor is localized to dopamine terminals, but also is targeted to pre- and postsynaptic neuronal profiles at a distance from the dopamine terminals. In somata and dendrites of the midbrain dopaminergic neurons, D2R labeling is expressed in most dendrites that contain VMAT2 storage vesicles, as well as in both excitatory and inhibitory afferents. Together, these observations indicate that dopamine is stored in and released from vesicles in both dendrites and axons, and may activate either local or more distant receptors through volume transmission. By analogy, the vesicular acetylcholine transporter (VachT) is similarly localized to the membranes of axon terminals and tubulovesicles in dendrites in the mesopontine tegmental cholinergic nuclei, suggesting that there also may be release of acetylcholine from both dendrites and axons. These results identify chemically selective functional sites for neuronal signaling envisioned by Cajal and redefined by modern technology.

Introduction

Neurons are polarized cells vividly portrayed with elaborate dendritic and axonal arborizations in Cajal's drawings of silver impregnated brain tissue. Observations from these drawings, led to the formulation of the law of interneuronal connections by which a functional synapse or useful effective contact between two neurons was postulated to mainly, or exclusively occur between collaterals or terminal axons of one neuron and the dendrites or cell body of another neuron (Swanson and Swanson, 1995). Neuronal polarity is largely attributed to the targeting of proteins to the axonal or somatodendritic domains through selective sorting and recycling of endocytosed plasma membrane proteins in highly mobile tubulovesicular organelles (Prekeris et al., 1999). Transporters responsible for the vesicular storage and plasmalemmal uptake of neurotransmitters, as well as the diversified subtypes of receptors are among those

*Corresponding author: Tel.: (212) 570-2900; Fax: (212) 988-3672; E-mail: vpickel@mail.med.cornell.edu

proteins that would be expected to have highly segregated distributions consistent with their role in axodendritic synaptic communication.

The identification of the functional sites for actions mediated by transporters and receptors, together with the corresponding transmitters was made possible by the development of an immunogold-silver and immunoperoxidase dual labeling method (Chan et al., 1990). This allowed the electron microscopic localization of high titer antisera against peptide sequences uniquely expressed in the relevant proteins, thus conferring chemical specificity and function to neuronal profiles seen in light microscopic silver stains. We have used electron microscopic immunocytochemistry for the localization of a large variety of neurotransmitter transporters and receptors, as well as peptide receptors in the central nervous system (CNS) (Garzón and Pickel, 2000; Pickel et al., 2000, 2001a,b; Rodriguez et al., 2000; Doherty and Pickel, 2001; Glass et al., 2001; Svingos et al., 2001; Wang and Pickel, 2002; Mengual and Pickel, 2002). For simplicity, we focus the present review on (1) striatal and pallidal dopaminergic terminals, (2) midbrain dopaminergic neurons in substantia nigra and VTA, and (3) mesopontine cholinergic neurons. Highlights of the results in each area are briefly summarized and then integrated into the emerging view of Cajal's neuron.

Striatal and pallidal dopaminergic terminals

DAT

Dopaminergic transmission is initiated through stimulation evoked vesicular release of dopamine and terminated largely by concentration-dependent plasmalemmal reuptake into dopaminergic neurons through the actions of the dopamine transporter (DAT; Horn, 1990; Pickel and Sesack, 1995). Thus, in regions where dopamine is the major catecholamine, the catecholamine synthesizing enzyme, tyrosine hydroxylase (TH) is extensively colocalized with DAT. This has been shown in both the motor (nucleus accumbens core and dorsal striatum or caudate-putamen nucleus) and limbic (nucleus accumbens shell) striatum (Nirenberg et al., 1996, 1997a). In these studies, the DAT plasmalemmal distribution was established by using immunoperoxidase or immunogold labeling for a sequence-specific antiserum against a cloned gene encoding a sodium- and chloride-dependent DAT (Giros et al., 1991).

In striatum, DAT is localized to the plasma membranes of axonal varicosities and terminals containing aggregates of synaptic vesicles, but is not seen within the presynaptic membrane specialization, and is often found at some distance from synaptic junctions (Nirenberg et al., 1996; Hersch et al., 1997). This localization of DAT to non-synaptic portions of plasma membranes may, in part reflect the fact that many monoaminergic terminals, including those that contain dopamine, lack well-defined synaptic junctions (Beaudet and Descarries, 1978; Pickel and Sesack, 1995). The location of DAT at a distance from synaptic junctions may play a significant role in the 'spatial buffering' of dopamine within the extracellular space (Nicholson and Rice, 1991).

VMAT2

In contrast with DAT, which is a highly selective plasmalemmal transporter of dopamine, the neuronal vesicular monoamine transporter (VMAT2) mediates the uptake of dopamine and other monoamines into acidic vesicles (Edwards, 1992). The differences in function between the plasmalemmal and vesicular transporters are directly reflected in their subcellular distribution in dopaminergic axons (Nirenberg et al., 1997b). In the striatum, immunogold labeling of an antipeptide raised against the C-terminus of rat VMAT2 (Peter et al., 1995) is discretely localized to membranes of mainly small synaptic vesicles in presumed dopaminergic axon terminals containing TH, and to large dense core vesicles in several other terminals without TH immunoreactivity (Nirenberg et al., 1997b) that are most likely serotonergic (Soghomonian et al., 1989). These results indicate that while small synaptic vesicles are the major storage organelles for dopamine, the large dense core vesicles are likely to be more actively involved in the storage of other monoamines such as serotonin.

D2R

The released dopamine elicits physiological actions through the activation of one of several subtypes (D1–D5) of dopamine receptor (Lachowicz and Sibley, 1997; Sibley, 1999; Sealfon and Olanow, 2000). Of these, the dopamine D2 receptor (D2R) has been most extensively examined for its role in the gating of information flow through limbic and motor systems implicated in normal reward and motor functions (Blum et al., 1996) as well as in the pathophysiology of schizophrenia (Moore et al., 1999; Grace, 2000). The cloning and sequencing of the D2R has permitted selective localization of the receptor in central neurons (Fisher et al., 1994; Lachowicz and Sibley, 1997). We have examined the electron microscopic immunolabeling of an antiserum against an amino acid sequence within the third cytoplasmic loop of the D2R that recognizes both short and long isoforms. This analysis was done in both the dorsal and ventral striatum (Sesack et al., 1994; Delle Donne et al., 1996) and in the ventral pallidum (Mengual and Pickel, 2002). In each region, D2R is localized to plasmalemma and vesicles in axon terminals, some of which are dopaminergic as indicated by their content of TH or DAT. In the striatum, D2R immunoreactivity is often localized to glutamatergic cortical afferents (Wang

and Pickel, 2002) and to dendritic spines and axon terminals of GABAergic neurons, which form exclusively symmetric, inhibitory-type synapses with dendrites (Delle Donne et al., 1997; Yung and Bolam, 2000). In the ventral pallidum, which receives major GABAergic input from the striatum, the D2R is also mainly localized to axon terminals that form inhibitory-type synapses on dendrites. The D2R-immunoreactive terminals sometimes appose dopaminergic afferents containing TH (Fig. 1A), but are more often seen at a distance from the TH-labeled terminals (Fig. 1B). These observations identify specific sites where activation of the D2R can not only autoregulate dopamine release (Cragg and Greenfield, 1997), but also modulate the release of both excitatory and inhibitory transmitters (Expósito et al., 1999). Interestingly, when expressed in striatal dendrites, the D2R is usually not seen in sites postsynaptic to dopaminergic terminals, but is

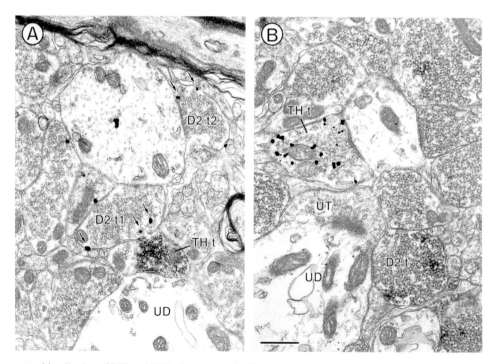

Fig. 1. Ultrastructural localization of D2R and TH in the rat ventral pallidum. **A**, Immunogold labeling for D2R (small arrows) is seen on the plasma membrane and associated with synaptic vesicles in two terminals (D2 t1 and D2 t2), both of which form symmetric synapses with a dendrite that also contains a single gold particle. D2 t1 is apposed to a small axon terminal containing immunoperoxidase labeling for TH (TH t), and forming a symmetric synapse with an unlabeled dendrite (LID). **B**, Immunoperoxidase labeling for D2R is localized to clusters of synaptic vesicles in an axon terminal (D2t) that forms a symmetric synapse with an unlabeled dendrite (UD). The terminal is apposed to an unlabeled terminal (UT) that forms what appears to be an asymmetric synapse with the same dendrite. Within the distant neuropil, immunogold labeling for TH is localized to another axon terminal (Th t) forming a symmetric synapse on a dendrite. Neither the TH-labeled terminal or dendrite show detectable labeling for D2R. Scale bars = 0.5 μm.

instead highly enriched within and near the asymmetric synapses formed by unlabeled excitatory terminals, many of which are of cortical origin (Wang and Pickel, 2002). The targeting of D2R to synaptic and nonsynaptic sites on the plasmalemma most likely reflects linkage of the receptor to downstream signaling molecules and the actin cytoskeleton (Smith et al., 1999).

Midbrain dopaminergic cell body regions

DAT

Dopaminergic neurons of the A8 and A9 groups located in the substantia nigra play an essential role in motor functions ascribed principally to the release of dopamine from axon terminals in the dorsal striatum or caudate-putamen nucleus (CPN) and core of the nucleus accumbens (Bjorklund and Lindvall, 1984; Lewis and Sesack, 1997). In contrast, the A10 dopaminergic neurons in the ventral tegmental area give rise mainly to cortical and limbic projections terminating in the nucleus accumbens shell and ventral pallidum and affecting reward and motivated behaviors [see above and Le Moal, (1995)]. Thus, the presence of DAT mRNA in somata and dendrites of midbrain dopaminergic neurons in the VTA (Ciliax et al., 1995; Freed et al., 1995) could exclusively represent the synthesis of proteins destined for functional sites in axon terminals. This hypothesis is refuted by our immunocytochemical studies of DAT distribution and by the presence of DAT binding sites in the substantia nigra and VTA, together with the known dendritic release of dopamine in these regions (Geffen et al., 1976; Nirenberg et al., 1997c; Cragg et al., 2001).

Immunolabeling for DAT in dopaminergic perikarya and proximal dendrites is mainly localized to intracellular tubulovesicles near the Golgi and distant from the plasma membrane. These sites are among those involved in the synthesis, and trafficking of surface proteins including transporters (Parton et al., 1992; Bradbury and Bridges, 1994). In contrast with somata, medium-small diameter dopaminergic dendrites in the substantia nigra and VTA (Nirenberg et al., 1996, 1997c) often express plasmalemmal labeling for DAT. The transport sites are often seen on membranes of apposed dopaminergic dendrites, and these appositions occur more commonly in the VTA than in the substantia nigra. Such appositional contacts are potential sites for dopamine release from storage vesicles or possibly by DAT reversal (Sulzer et al., 1993; Attwell et al., 1993).

The content of both TH and DAT varies significantly between pairs of dopaminergic dendrites in the VTA (Bayer and Pickel, 1990; Nirenberg et al., 1997c). Moreover, the more lightly TH immunoreactive dendrites receive proportionally less GABAergic input (Bayer and Pickel, 1991), and those dendrites containing the least DAT immunogold labeling are more frequently contacted by excitatory cholinergic terminals (Garzón, et al., 1999). Together, these observations suggest important differences in dendritic dopamine concentration and membrane potential, both of which affect DAT function (Sonders et al., 1997; Hoffman et al., 1999). Thus, the unique arrangement of dendrites differing in their dopamine and DAT concentrations could facilitate the uptake of dopamine into dendrites other than those of release in response to afferent stimulation. Such a novel functional coupling in the VTA (Nirenberg, et al., 1997c) would be expected to differ markedly from the electrotonic coupling that occurs between pairs of dopaminergic neurons in the substantia nigra (Grace and Bunney, 1983).

VMAT2

The expression of plasmalemmal DAT, together with studies showing calcium-dependent release of dopamine in both the substantia nigra and VTA (Kalivas et al., 1989; Jaffe et al., 1998) suggest that there also must be vesicular packaging of dopamine in these dendrites. This has been confirmed by the electron microscopic immunogold labeling of VMAT2 to membranes of dendritic tubulovesicles, which are the presumed storage vesicles (Figs. 2 and 3). Moreover, dual labeling showed extensive colocalization of VMAT2 and TH in somatodendritic profiles in both the substantia nigra and VTA dopaminergic neurons (Nirenberg et al., 1996). In dopaminergic somata, immunogold labeling for VMAT2 is associated mainly with membranes of the Golgi apparatus and tubulovesicles that resembled smooth endoplasmic reticulum (SER). In dopaminergic dendrites, VMAT2 also is mainly localized to tubulovesicles that are isolated, or seen in clusters near the plasma membrane (Fig. 2).

Functional involvement of VMAT2 in somatodendritic dopamine storage and release is supported by our demonstration that the levels of expression of VMAT2 in individual dendrites in the substantia nigra and VTA (Nirenberg et al., 1996) directly parallel the known region-specific differences in dopamine release (Rice et al., 1997).

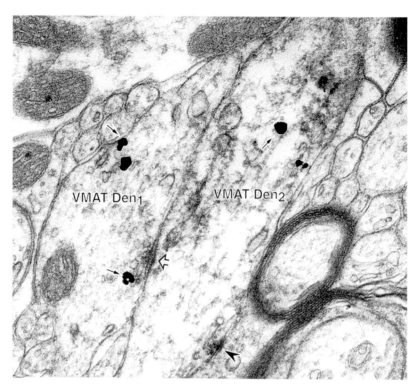

Fig. 2. Electron micrograph showing immunoperoxidase localization of D2-R (arrowhead) and VMAT2 immunogold (arrows) in dendrites in the paranigral VTA of rat brain. A dendrodendritic synapse (open arrow) is formed between the two dendrites, each of which contains immunogold labeling (small arrows) for VMAT2 (VMAT Den 1 and VMAT Dent). An aggregate of immunogold particles is seen within the cluster of vesicles in Den1; whereas Den2 shows a diffuse cytoplasmic and discrete plasmalemmal labeling for the D2R. Scale bars = 0.5 μm.

Compared with the dopaminergic dendrites in the substantia nigra, those in the VTA express higher levels of VMAT2, and have greater potential for evoked release of dopamine (Nirenberg et al., 1996). Within the VTA, there is also an enrichment of VMAT2 in dendrites within the parabrachial region that contributes mainly to mesocortical dopaminergic projections, as compared to those of the paranigral that project more extensively to the shell of the nucleus accumbens (Pickel et al., 2001). These VTA subdivisions also differ in their afferent inputs from the prefrontal cortex and other brain regions (Swanson, 1982). Together, these observations suggest that dendritic storage and release of dopamine is region specific and at least in part dependent on neuronal connectivity.

D2R

The D2R mRNA and binding sites are also prevalent in midbrain dopaminergic neurons (Chen et al., 1991) where the receptor is involved in autoregulation of the dopaminergic output to forebrain regions (Mercuri et al., 1997). In contrast with VMAT2, however, D2R mRNA is less abundant in cells of the VTA compared with the substantia nigra (Haber et al., 1995). Our initial electron microscopic study of D2R in midbrain dopaminergic neurons was not quantitative, and the diffuse peroxidase reaction product precluded the distinction between plasma membrane and cytoplasmic labeling (Sesack et al., 1994). Thus, we observed no significant cellular or regional differences in D2R immunoreactivity in midbrain neurons. More recently, we have used a higher dilution of the primary antiserum and improved labeling methods to show a more restricted, mainly extrasynaptic plasmalemmal distribution of the D2R in the VTA (Pickel et al., 2002). The D2R immunoreactivity was, however also frequently seen within and near asymmetric excitatory-type synapses formed by nonmonoaminergic terminals as indicated by their absence of detected labeling for VMAT2 (Pickel et al., 2002). This distribution suggests a role for the receptor in dopaminergic modulation of glutamatergic

150

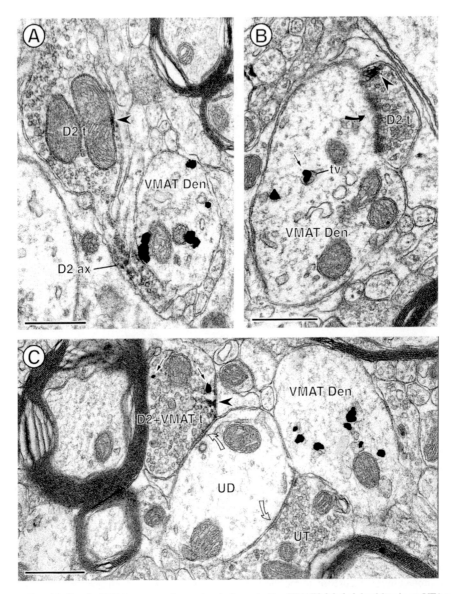

Fig. 3. Immunoperoxidase labeling for D2R in axons and axon terminals contacting VMAT2-labeled dendrites in rat VTA subdivisions. **A**, In paranigral region, D2R is intensely localized within a small axon that apposes a VMAT2 immunogold labeled dendrite (VMAT Den). More diffuse D2R peroxidase labeling is seen in the terminal D2t. **B**, In the parabrachial region, D2R peroxidase immunoreactivity (arrowhead) is localized to vesicles near the plasma membrane of an axon terminal (D2 t) that forms an asymmetric synapse (black curved arrow) with a dendrite (VMAT Den) that shows immunogold labeling of tubulovesicles (tv). **C**, In the parabrachial region, D2R peroxidase (arrowhead) and immunogold for VMAT2 (arrows) are localized to an axon terminal that forms a symmetric synapse (curved clear arrow) with an unlabeled dendrite (UD). The dendrite also receives a symmetric synapse (curved clear arrow) from an unlabeled terminal and is apposed to a dendrite that contains immunogold labeling for VMAT2 (VMAT Den). Scale bars = 0.5 μm.

transmission, which could produce plasticity of excitatory postsynaptic responses in this region (Thomas et al., 2000).

D2R labeling in the VTA is also present in many small unmyelinated axons and axon terminals without VMAT2 immunoreactivity (Fig. 3). These terminals form asymmetric or symmetric synapses with dendrites many of which contain VMAT2 labeled tubulovesicles (Pickel et al., 2002). These observations suggest a role for D2 receptors in the VTA, which is similar to that in the striatum, namely presynaptic modulation of the release of excitatory and inhibitory amino acids that are preferentially contained in terminals that form symmetric or asymmetric synapses (Charara et al., 1996; Steffensen et al., 1998; Chatha et al., 2000; Rodriguez et al., 2000). Unlike the striatum, however, the changes in transmitter release evoked by activation of D2Rs in the VTA often affect dopaminergic, not GABAergic neurons; and the dopamine is of dendritic, not axonal origin. This may occur through actions similar to those previously demonstrated in other brain regions, where D2R activation can affect transmitter release through activation of presynaptic $G_{i/o}$-like proteins (Aronin and DiFiglia, 1992; Missale et al., 1998), ATP sensitive potassium channels (Neusch et al., 2000) or L-type calcium channels (Okita et al., 2000; Sanz et al., 2000). The presynaptic effects of D2R activation by dendritically released dopamine could account for the depression of dopaminergic neurons in the VTA by repetitive stimulation (Bond and Malenka, 1999). These actions are not likely to be restricted to glutamatergic terminals in the VTA, since D2R labeling is also seen in terminals in this region that form symmetric, inhibitory-type synapses that are typical of GABAergic neurons (Steffensen et al., 1998).

Somata and dendrites of mesopontine cholinergic neurons

Cholinergic neurons of the mesopontine tegmentum located within the pedunculopontine (PPT) and laterodorsal tegmental (LDT) nuclei are hyperpolarized by acetylcholine (Leonard and Llinas, 1994). The cholinergic autoregulation of cholinergic neurons in the PPT/LDT through activation of muscarinic receptors (Mathur et al., 1997) plays a major role in central regulation of locomotor activity and motivated behaviors (Bechara and van der Kooy, 1989, 1992; Winn et al., 1997; Inglis et al., 2000), and in the mechanisms of some psychotic states such as schizophrenia or antimuscarinic psychosis (Tandon et al. 1991; Yeomans, 1995). These cholinergic neurons are immunolabeled for the synthesizing enzyme choline acetyltransferase (ChAT), as well as the vesicular acetylcholine transporter (VAchT; Kimura et al., 1980; Maley et al., 1988; Gilmor et al., 1996). In cholinergic neurons, VAchT plays a role similar to that of VMAT2 in monoaminergic neurons, and specifically identifies the sites for vesicular

storage and release of acetylcholine (Gilmor et al., 1996). VAchT is present in somata and dendrites, but is most highly enriched on membranes of small synaptic vesicles in axon terminals as seen in the PPT/LDT (Fig. 4A) and other brain regions (Weihe et al., 1996; Schäfer et al., 1998; Garzón et al., 1999; Garzón and Pickel, 2000).

In the PPT/LDT, the axons and terminals containing VAchT immunoreactive vesicles are relatively sparse, as compared with somatodendritic profiles. Within somata and large dendrites, VAchT is associated with cytoplasmic membranes of the Golgi apparatus, smooth endoplasmic reticulum, and intracytoplasmic tubulovesicles. By far the most prevalent structures expressing VAchT are medium-small diameter dendrites, where the labeling is also principally membrane associated (Fig. 4B). Dendrodendritic contacts are also seen in which one or both dendrites show tubulovesicular labeling for VAchT, similar to that seen for DAT in the midbrain dopaminergic neurons. In other examples, VAchT-immunoreactive dendrites are postsynaptic to axon terminals containing VAchT. Together, these observations suggest that cholinergic neurons in the PPT and LDT may release acetylcholine from both dendrites and axon terminals to act at specialized synapses. Thus, our findings sustain the concept that tubulovesicles in medium-small cholinergic dendrites of PPT/LDT are storage sites for dendritic release of acetylcholine, in parallel to reported dendritic release of dopamine from midbrain dopaminergic dendrites. There is to our knowledge no direct *in vivo* evidence for release of acetylcholine from dendrites in the PPT/LDT or other central cholinergic cell groups. Acetylcholine, is however released from somata and/or dendrites of ciliary ganglion cells in response to depolarization (Johnson and Pilar, 1980). Moreover, primary embryonic septal cultures of cholinergic neurons show sustained potassium-evoked release of acetylcholine, which is dependent on extracellular choline and prevented by vesamicol, a well known blocker of VachT (Auld et al., 2000). Presumably at least some of the vesicular acetylcholine release from these cultures could occur at the level of somata and dendrites of the cholinergic neurons. These observations, together with the sparsity of axodendritic or dendrodendritic synapses between cholinergic neurons in the PPT/LDT suggest that the activation of autoreceptors on cholinergic neurons may occur largely by nonsynaptic vesicular release of acetylcholine.

152

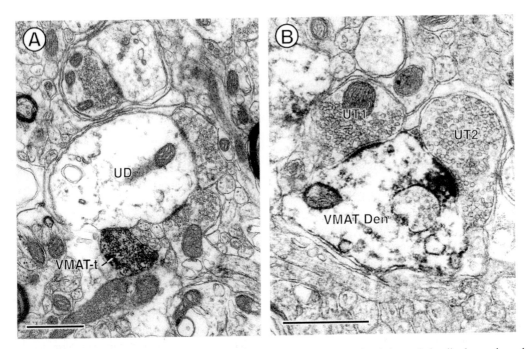

Fig. 4. Immunoperoxidase labeling for VAchT in the rat LDT. **A**, The peroxidase reaction product is intensely localized around membranes of small synaptic vesicles in an axon terminal (VachT) that forms a symmetric synapse with an unlabeled dendrite (UD). **B**, Immunolabeling is diffusely distributed throughout a dendrite (VAchT) that is postsynaptic to two unlabeled terminals (UT$_1$ and UT$_2$). The reaction product is prominently seen in associated with membranous structures near the contact formed by UT$_1$. Scale bars = 0.5 μm.

Conclusion

Electron microscopic immunocytochemistry has allowed the identification of functional sites for neurotransmitter transport and receptor activation as illustrated for neurons containing dopamine. The plasmalemmal dopamine transporters and receptors are expressed in both axons and dendrites, and do not have a restricted distribution at synapses formed by dopaminergic terminals. Moreover, the transporters responsible for the packaging of neurotransmitters into synaptic vesicles such as VMAT2 and VAchT are associated not only with synaptic vesicles in axon terminals, but also with tubulovesicles in dendrites. The presence of VAchT in dendrites comparable to the distribution of VMAT2 in dopaminergic dendrites suggests that dendritic transmitter release is a fundamental property of both cholinergic and dopaminergic neurons, and possibly neurons containing a variety of other neurotransmitters. The localization of receptors at distant sites from their transmitter pools gives evidence that receptor activation occurs by volume transmission in addition to classic local synapses. Thus, the axodendritic synapses

that were viewed by Cajal as the primary, or even exclusive means for interneuronal communication, must be expanded to include novel retrograde signaling from dendrites to axons, as well as local and long distance targeting of extrasynaptic receptors.

Acknowledgments

Supported by grants from the National Institutes of Health; Grant numbers: DA04600, MH40342, and MH00078 to V.M.P; a NIDA Invest Award to E.M.; and a Postdoctoral F.P.I. Program of the Spanish Education and Culture Ministry to M.G.

References

Aronin, N. and DiFiglia, M. (1992) The subcellular localization of the G-protein Gi alpha in the basal ganglia reveals its potential role in both signal transduction and vesicle trafficking. *J. Neurosci.*, 92: 3435–3444.

Attwell, D., Barbour, B. and Szatkowski, M. (1993) Nonvesicular release of neurotransmitter. [Review]. *Neuron*, 11: 401–407.

Auld, D.S., Day, J.C., Mennicken, F. and Quirion, R. (2000) Pharmacological characterization of endogenous acetylcholine release from primary septal cultures. *J. Pharmacol. Exp. Ther.*, 292: 692–697.

Bayer, V.E. and Pickel, V.M. (1990) Ultrastructural localization of tyrosine hydroxylase in the rat ventral tegmental area: Relationship between immunolabeling density and neuronal associations. *J. Neurosci.*, 10: 2996–3013.

Bayer, V.E. and Pickel, V.M. (1991) GABA-labeled terminals form proportionally more synapses with dopaminergic neurons containing low densities of tyrosine hydroxylase-immunoreactivity in rat ventral tegmental area. *Brain Res.*, 559: 44–55.

Beaudet, A. and Descarries, L. (1978) The monoamine innervation of rat cerebral cortex: Synaptic nonsynaptic axon terminals. *Neurosci.*, 3: 851–860.

Bechara, A. and van der, K.D. (1989) The tegmental pedunculopontine nucleus: a brainstem output of the limbic system critical for the conditioned place preferences produced by morphine and amphetamine. *J. Neurosci.*, 9: 3400–3409.

Bechara, A. and van der Kooy, D. (1992) Lesions of the tegmental pedunculopontine nucleus: effects on the locomotor activity induced by morphine and amphetamine. *Pharmacol. Biochem. Behav.*, 42: 9–18.

Bjorklund, A. and Lindvall, O. (1984) Dopamine-containing systems in the CNS. In: A. Bjorklund, and T. Hokfelt, (Eds.), *Handbook of Chemical Neuroanatomy*. Vol. 2 *Classical Transmitters in the CNS*, Part 1, Elsevier Science Publishers, Amsterdam, pp. 55–121.

Blum, K., Sheridan, P.J., Wood, R.C., Braverman, E.R., Chen, T.J.H., Cull, J.G., and Comings, D.E. (1996) The D_2 dopamine receptor gene as a determinant of reward deficiency syndrome. *J. R. Soc. Med.*, 89: 396–400.

Bond, A. and Malenka, R.C. (1999) Properties and plasticity of excitatory synapses on dopaminergic and GABAergic cells in the ventral tegmental area. *J. Neurosci.*, 19: 3723–3730.

Bradbury, N.A. and Bridges, R.J. (1994) Role of membrane trafficking in plasma membrane solute transport. *Am. J. Physiol.*, 267: C1–24.

Chan, J., Aoki, C. and Pickel, V.M. (1990) Optimization of differential immunogold-silver and peroxidase labeling with maintenance of ultrastructure in brain sections before plastic embedding. *J. Neurosci. Methods*, 33: 113–127.

Charara, A., Smith, Y. and Parent, A. (1996) Glutamatergic inputs from the pedunculopontine nucleus to midbrain dopaminergic neurons in primates: Phaseolus vulgaris-leucoagglutinin anterograde labeling combined with postembedding glutamate and GABA immunohistochemistry. *J. Comp. Neurol.*, 364: 254–266.

Chatha, B.T., Bernard, V., Streit, P. and Bolam, J.P. (2000) Synaptic localization of ionotropic glutamate receptors in the rat substantia nigra. *Neuroscience*, 101: 1037–1051.

Chen, I.F., Qin, Z.H., Szele, F., Bai, G. and Weiss, B. (1991) Neuronal localization and modulation of the D_2 dopamine receptor mRNA in brain of normal mice and mice lesioned with 6-hydroxydopamine. *Neuropharmacology*, 30: 927–941.

Ciliax, B.J., Heilman, C., Demchyshyn, L.L., Pristupa, Z.B., Ince, E., Hersch, S.M., Niznik, H.B. and Levey, A.I. (1995) The dopamine transporter: Immunochemical characterization and localization in brain. *J. Neurosci.*, 15: 1714–1723.

Cragg, S.J. and Greenfield, S.A. (1997) Differential autoreceptor control of somatodendritic and axon terminal dopamine release in substantia nigra, ventral tegmental area, and striatum. *J. Neurosci.*, 17: 5738–5746.

Cragg, S.J., Nicholson, C., Kume-Kick, J., Tao, L. and Rice, M.E. (2001) Dopamine-mediated volume transmission in midbrain is regulated by distinct extracellular geometry and uptake. *J. Neurophys.*, 85: 1761–1771.

Delle Donne, K.T., Sesack, S.R. and Pickel, V.M. (1996) Ultrastructural immunocytochemical localization of neurotensin and the dopamine D_2 receptor in the rat nucleus accumbens. *J. Comp. Neurol.*, 371: 552–566.

Delle Donne, K.T., Sesack, S.R. and Pickel, V.M. (1997) Ultrastructural immunocytochemical localization of the dopamine D_2 receptor within GABAergic neurons of the rat striatum. *Brain Res.*, 746: 239–255.

Doherty, M.D. and Pickel, V.M. (2001) Targeting of serotonin 1A receptors to dopaminergic neurons within the parabrachial subdivision of the ventral tegmental area in rat brain. *J. Comp. Neurol.*, 433: 390–400.

Edwards, R.H. (1992) The transport of neurotransmitters into synaptic vesicles. *Curr. Opin. Neurobiol.*, 2: 586–594.

Expósito, I., Del Arco, A., Segovia, G. and Mora, F. (1999) Endogenous dopamine increases extracellular concentrations of glutamate and GABA in striatum of the freely moving rat: Involvement of D1 and D2 dopamine receptors. *Neurochem. Res.*, 24: 849–856.

Fisher, R.S., Levine, M.S., Sibley, D.R. and Ariano, M.A. (1994) D_2 dopamine receptor protein location: Golgi impregnation-gold toned and ultrastructural analysis of the rat neostriatum. *J. Neurosci. Res.*, 38: 551–564.

Freed, C., Revay, R., Vaughan, R.A., Kriek, E., Grant, S., Uhl, G.R. and Kuhar, M.J. (1995) Dopamine transporter immunoreactivity in rat brain. *J. Comp. Neurol.*, 359: 340–349.

Garzón, M. and Pickel, V.M. (2000) Dendritic and axonal targeting of the vesicular acetylcholine transporter to membranous cytoplasmic organelles in laterodorsal and pedunculopontine tegmental nuclei. *J. Comp. Neurol.*, 419: 32–48.

Garzón, M., Vaughan, R.A., Uhl, G.R., Kuhar, M.J. and Pickel, V.M. (1999) Cholinergic axon terminals in the ventral tegmental area target a subpopulation of neurons expressing low levels of the dopamine transporter. *J. Comp. Neurol.*, 410: 197–210.

Geffen, L.B., Jessel, T.M., Cuello, A.C. and Iversen, L.L. (1976) Release of dopamine from dendrites in rat substantia nigra. *Nature (London)*, 260: 258–260.

Gilmor, M.L., Nash, N.R., Roghani, A., Edwards, R.H., Yi, H., Hersch, S.M. and Levey, A.I. (1996) Expression of the putative vesicular acetylcholine transporter in rat brain and localization in cholinergic synaptic vesicles. *J. Neurosci.*, 16: 2179–2190.

Giros, B., el Mestikawy, S., Bertrand, L. and Caron, M.G. (1991) Cloning and functional characterization of a cocaine-sensitive dopamine transporter. *FEBS. Lett.*, 295: 149–154.

Glass, M.J., Huang, J., Aicher, S.A., Milner, T.A. and Pickel, V.M. (2001) Subcellular localization of α-2A-adrenergic receptors in the rat medial nucleus tractus solitarius: regional targeting and relationship with catecholamine neurons. *J. Comp. Neurol.*, 433: 193–207.

Grace, A.A. (2000) Gating of information flow within the limbic system and the pathophysiology of schizophrenia. *Brain Res. Rev.*, 31: 330–341.

Grace, A. and Bunney, B.S. (1983) Intracellular and extracellular electrophysiology of nigral dopaminergic neurons-3. Evidence for electrotonic coupling. *Neurosci.*, 10: 333–348.

Haber, S.N., Ryoo, H., Cox, C. and Lu, W. (1995) Subsets of midbrain dopaminergic neurons in monkeys are distinguished by different levels of m RNA for the dopamine transporter: Comparison with the mRNA for the D_2 receptor, tyrosine hydroxylase and ca Ibindin immunoreactivity. *J. Comp. Neurol.*, 362: 400–410.

Hersch, S.M., Yi, H., Heilman, C.J., Edwards, R.H. and Levey, A.I. (1997) Subcellular localization and molecular topology of the dopamine transporter in the striatum and substantia nigra. *J. Comp. Neurol.*, 388: 211–227.

Hoffman, A.F., Zahniser, N.R., Lupica, C.R., and Gerhardt, G.A. (1999) Voltage-dependency of the dopamine transporter in the rat substantia nigra. *Neurosci. Lett.*, 260: 105–108.

Horn, A.S. (1990) Dopamine uptake: A review of progress in the last decade. *Prog. Neurobiol.*, 34: 387–400.

Inglis, W.L., Olmstead, M.C. and Robbins, T.W. (2000) Pedunculopontine tegmental nucleus lesions impair stimulus-reward learning in autoshaping and conditioned reinforcement paradigms. *Behav. Neurosci.*, 114: 285–294.

Jaffe, E.H., Marty, A., Schulte, A. and Chow, R.H. (1998) Extrasynaptic vesicular transmitter release from the somata of substantia nigra neurons in rat midbrain slices. *J. Neurosci.*, 18: 3548–3553.

Johnson, D.A. and Pilar, G. (1980) The release of acetylcholine from post-ganglionic cell bodies in response to depolarization. *J. Physiol. (Lond)*, 299: 605–619.

Kalivas, P.W., Bourdelais, A., Abhold, R. and Abbott, L. (1989) Somatodendritic release of endogenous dopamine: *in vivo* dialysis in the A10 dopamine region. *Neurosci. Lett.*, 100: 215–220.

Kimura, H., McGeer, P.L., Peng, F. and McGeer, E.G. (1980) Choline acetyltransferase-containing neurons in rodent brain demonstrated by immunohistochemistry. *Science*, 208: 1057–1059.

Lachowicz, J.E. and Sibley, D.R. (1997) Molecular characteristics of mammalian dopamine receptors. *Pharmacol. Toxicol.*, 81: 105–113.

Le Moal, M. (1995) Mesocorticolimbic do paminergic neurons: functional and regulatory roles. In: F.E. Bloom, and D.J. Kupfler, (Eds.), *Psychopharmacology: the Fourth Generation of Progress.* Raven Press, New York, pp. 283–204.

Leonard, C.S. and Llinas, R. (1994) Serotonergic and cholinergic inhibition of mesopontine cholinergic neurons controlling REM sleep: an in vitro electrophysiological study. *Neuroscience*, 59: 309–330.

Lewis, D.A. and Sesack, S.R. (1997) Dopamine systems in the primate brain. In: F.E. Bloom, A. Bjorklund and T. Hokfelt (Eds.) *Handbook of Chemical Neuroanatomy.* Amsterdam, Elsevier Science Publishers, pp. 261–373.

Maley, B.E., Frick, M.L., Levey, A.I., Wainer, B.H. and Elde, R.P. (1988) Immunohistochemistry of choline acetyltransferase in the guinea pig brain. *Neurosci. Lett.*, 84: 137–142.

Mathur, A., Shandarin, A., LaViolette, S.R., Parker, J. and Yeomans, J.S. (1997) Locomotion and stereotypy induced by scopolamine: contributions of muscarinic receptors near the pedunculopontine tegmental nucleus. *Brain Res.*, 775: 144–155.

Mengual, E. and Pickel, V.M. (2002) Ultrastructural immunocytochemical localization of the dopamine D_2 receptor and tyrosine hydroxylase in the rat ventral pallidum. *Synapse*, 43: 151–162.

Mercuri, N.B., Saiardi, A., Bonci, A., Picetti, R., Calabresi, P., Bernardi, G. and Borrelli, E. (1997) Loss of autoreceptor function in dopaminergic neurons from dopamine D_2 receptor deficient mice. *Neurosci.*, 79: 323–327.

Missale, C., Nash, S.R., Robinson, S.W., Jaber, M. and Caron, M.G. (1998) Dopamine receptors: from structure to function. *Physiological Rev.*, 78: 189–225.

Moore, H., West, A.R. and Grace, A.A. (1999) The regulation of forebrain dopamine transmission: relevance to the pathophysiology and psychopathology of schizophrenia. *Biological Psychiatry*, 46: 40–55.

Neusch, C., Runde, D. and Moser, A. (2000) G proteins modulate D2 receptor-coupled K(ATP) channels in rat dopaminergic terminals. *Neurochem. Res.*, 25: 1521–1526.

Nicholson, C. and Rice, M.E. (1991) Diffusion of ions and transmitters in the brain cell microenvironment. In: K. Fuxe and L.F. Agnati (Eds), *Volume Transmission in the Brain: Novel Mechanisms for Neural Transmission*, Raven Press Ltd., New York, pp. 279–294.

Nirenberg, M.J., Chan, J., Liu, Y.J., Edwards, R.H. and Pickel, V.M. (1996a) Ultrastructural localization of the vesicular monoamine transporter-2 in midbrain dopaminergic neurons: Potential sites for somatodendritic storage and release of dopamine. *J. Neurosci.*, 16: 4135–4145.

Nirenberg, M.J., Chan, J., Liu, Y. J., Edwards, R.H. and Pickel, V.M. (1997b) Vesicular monoamine transporter-2: Immunogold localization in striatal axons and terminals. *Synapse* 26: 194–198.

Nirenberg, M.J., Chan, J., Pohorille, A., Vaughan, R.A., Uhl, G.R., Kuhar, M.J. and Pickel, V.M. (1997a) The dopamine transporter: Comparative ultrastructure of dopaminergic axons in limbic and motor compartments of the nucleus accumbens. *J. Neurosci.*, 17: 6899–6907.

Nirenberg, M.J., Chan, J., Vaughan, R.A., Uhl, G.R., Kuhar, M.J. and Pickel, V.M. (1997c) Immunogold localization of the dopamine transporter: an ultrastructural study of the rat ventral tegmental area. *J. Neurosci.*, 17: 4037–4044.

Nirenberg, M.J., Vaughan, R.A., Uhl, G.R., Kuhar, M.J. and Pickel, V.M. (1996b) The dopamine transporter is localized to dendritic and axonal plasma membranes of nigrostriatal dopaminergic neurons. *J. Neurosci.*, 16: 436–447.

Okita, M., Watanabe, Y., Taya, K., Utsumi, H. and Hayashi, T. (2000) Presynaptic L-type Ca(2)+ channels on excessive dopamine release from rat caudate putamen. *Physiol. Behav.*, 68: 641–649.

Parton, R.G., Simons, K. and Dotti, C.G. (1992) Axonal and dendritic endocytic pathways in cultured neurons. *J. Cell Biol.*, 119: 123–137.

Peter, D., Liu, Y.J., Sternini, C., De Giorgio, R., Brecha, N. and Edwards, R.H. (1995) Differential expression of two vesicular monoamine transporters. *J. Neurosci.*, 15: 6179–6188.

Pickel, V.M., Chan, J., Delle Donne, K.T., Boudin, H., Pelaprat, D. and Rostene, W. (2001) High-affinity neurotensin receptors in the rat nucleus accumbens: Subcellular targeting and relation to endogenous ligand. *J. Comp. Neurol.*, 435: 142–155.

Pickel, V.M., Chan, J. and Nirenberg, M.J. (2002) Region-specific targeting of dopamine D2-receptors and somatodendritic vesicular monoamine transporter 2 (VMAT2) within the ventral tegmental area. *J. Neurosci.* (Submitted).

Pickel, V.M., Douglas, J., Chan, J., Gamp, P.D. and Bunnett, N.W. (2000) Neurokinin 1 receptor distribution in cholinergic neurons and targets of substance P terminals in the rat nucleus accumbens. *J. Comp. Neurol.*, 423: 500–511.

Pickel, V.M. and Sesack, S.R. (1995) Electron microscopy of central dopamine systems. In: F.E. Bloom and D.J. Kupfer (Eds.) *Psychopharmacology*, Raven Press Ltd., New York, pp. 257–268.

Prekeris, R., Foletti, D.L. and Scheller, R.H. (1999) Dynamics of tubulovesicular recycling endosomes in hippocampal neurons. *J. Neurosci.*, 19: 10324–10337.

Rice, M.E., Cragg, S.J. and Greenfield, S.A. (1997) Characteristics of electrically evoked somatodendritic dopamine release in substantia nigra and ventral tegmental area *in vitro*. *J. Neurophys.*, 77: 853–862.

Rodriguez, J.J., Doherty, M.D. and Pickel, V.M. (2000) N-methyl-D-aspartate (NMDA) receptors in the ventral tegmental area: Subcellular distribution and colocalization with 5-hydroxytryptamine (2A) receptors. *J. Neurosci Res.*, 60: 202–211.

Sanz, A.G., Badia, A, and Clos, M.V. (2000) Role of calcium on the modulation of spontaneous acetylcholine efflux by the D_2 dopamine receptor subtype in rat striatal synaptosomes. *Brain Res.*, 854: 42–47.

Schäfer, M.K., Eiden, L.E., and Weihe, E. (1998) Cholinergic neurons and terminal fields revealed by immunohistochemistry for the vesicular acetylcholine transporter. I. Central nervous system. *Neurosci.*, 84: 331–359.

Sealfon, S.C. and Olanow, C.W. (2000) Dopamine receptors: from structure to behavior. *Trends in Neurosci*, 23: S34–S40.

Sesack, S.R., Aoki, C., and Pickel, V.M. (1994) Ultrastructural localization of D_2 receptor-like immunoreactivity in midbrain dopamine neurons and their striatal targets. *J. Neurosci.*, 14: 88–106.

Sibley, D.R. (1999) New insights into dopaminergic receptor function using antisense and genetically altered animals. *Annu.Rev. Pharmacol. Toxicol*, 39: 313–341.

Smith, F.D., Oxford, G. S. and Milgram, S.L. (1999) Association of the D2 dopamine receptor third cytoplasmic loop with spinophilin, a protein phosphatase-1-interacting protein. *J. Biol. Chem.*, 274: 19894–19900.

Soghomonian, J.J., Descarries, L. and Watkins, K.C. (1989) Serotonin innervation in adult rat neostriatum. II. Ultrastructural features: a radioautographic and immunocytochemical study. *Brain Res.*, 481: 67–86.

Sonders, M.S., Zhu, S.J., Zahniser, N.R., Kavanaugh, M.P., and Amara, S.G. (1997) Multiple ionic conductances of the human dopamine transporter: The actions of dopamine and psychostimulants. *J. Neurosci*, 17: 960–974.

Steffensen, S.C., Svingos, A.L., Pickel, V.M. and Henriksen, S.J. (1998) Electrophysiological characterization of GABAergic neurons in the ventral tegmental area. *J. Neurosci.*, 18: 8003–8015.

Sulzer, D., Maidment, N.T. and Rayport, S. (1993) Amphetamine and other weak bases act to promote reverse transport of dopamine in ventral midbrain neurons. *J. Neurochem.*, 60: 527–535.

Svingos, A.L., Colago, E.E.O. and Pickel, V.M. (2001) Vesicular acetylcholine transporter in the rat nucleus accumbens shell: Subcellular distribution and association with μ-opioid receptors. *Synapse*, 40: 184–192.

Swanson, L.W. (1982) The projections of the ventral tegmental area and adjacent regions: a combined fluorescent retrograde tracer and immunofluorescence study in the rat. *Brain Res. Bull.*, 9: 321–353.

Swanson, N. and Swanson, L. W. (1995) Histology of the nervous system of man and vertebrates by S. Ramón y Cajal. *History of Neuroscience, (6).* 1995. Oxford University Press, New York.

Tandon, R., Shipley, J.E., Greden, J.F., Mann, N.A., Eisner, W.H. and Goodson, J. (1991) Muscarinic cholinergic hyperactivity in schizophrenia. Relationship to positive and negative symptoms. *Schizophr. Res.*, 4: 23–30.

Thomas, M.J., Malenka, R.C. and Bonci, A. (2000) Modulation of long-term depression by dopamine in the mesolimbic system. *J. Neurosci.*, 20: 5581–5586.

Wang, H. and Pickel, V.M. (2002) Dopamine D2-receptors are present in prefrontal cortical afferents and their targets in patches of rat caudate-putamen nucleus. *J. Comp. Neurol.*, 442: 392–404.

Weihe, E., Tao-Cheng, J.H., Schäfer, M.K.H., Erickson, J.D. and Eiden, L.E. (1996) Visualization of the vesicular acetylcholine transporter in cholinergic nerve terminals and its targeting to a specific population of small synaptic vesicles. *Proc. Natl. Acad. Sci. USA*, 93: 3547–3552.

Winn, P., Brown, V.J. and Inglis, W.L. (1997) On the relationships between the striatum and the pedunculopontine tegmental nucleus. *Crit. Rev. Neurobiol.*, 11: 241–261.

Yung, K.K.L. and Bolam, J.P. (2000) Localization of dopamine D1 and D2 receptors in the rat neostriatum: Synaptic interaction with glutamate- and GABA-containing axonal terminals. *Synapse*, 38: 413–420.

E.C. Azmitia, J. DeFelipe, E.G. Jones, P. Rakic and C.E. Ribak (Eds.)
Progress in Brain Research, Vol. 136
© 2002 Elsevier Science B.V. All rights reserved

CHAPTER 13

Synaptic and extrasynaptic GABA$_A$ receptor and gephyrin clusters

Sean B. Christie, Rong-Wen Li, Celia P. Miralles, Raquel Riquelme, Bih Y. Yang,
Erik Charych, Wendou-Yu, Stephen B. Daniels, Marie E. Cantino and Angel L. De Blas*

Department of Physiology and Neurobiology, 3107 Horsebarn Hill Road, U-4156, Storrs, CT 06269, USA

Introduction

Santiago Ramón y Cajal beautifully described and classified different types of specialized 'connections' between individual nerve cells. Cajal's descriptions revealed the morphological substrate for the concept of 'synapse', a term coined later by Sherrington in 1897 to explain the 'reflex latency'. The arrival of electron microscopy (EM) techniques confirmed Cajal's interpretations, showing that synapses are specialized structures mediating the 'connections' between neurons. Synapses have specific morphological features including synaptic vesicles in the presynaptic ending and a dense structure, the postsynaptic density (PSD) that is attached to the cytoplasmic side of the postsynaptic membrane. Dense material is also found at the synaptic cleft between the presynaptic and postsynaptic membranes and at the cytoplasmic side of the presynaptic membrane. Moreover, it has been shown that there are morphological differences between excitatory glutamatergic synapses (Gray's type I or asymmetric synapses) and inhibitory GABAergic or glycinergic synapses (Gray's type II or symmetric synapses). Excitatory glutamatergic synapses have spherical synaptic vesicles and a prominent postsynaptic density. Inhibitory GABAergic and glycinergic synapses have flattened synaptic vesicles and a less prominent postsynaptic density.

Cajal and his followers also described the morphologies and the extensive variety of what today are called interneurons. He referred to these cells as neurons with a small axon. He also described the complexity of their connections. Nevertheless, the concepts of inhibition and inhibitory transmission were absent in Cajal's models and hypotheses. Today we know that interneurons are inhibitory and use GABA and/or glycine as neurotransmitter(s). In the brain, most interneurons are GABAergic. Glycinergic neurons are mainly localized in the spinal cord. In addition to the neurotransmitter-mediated signaling that occurs between interneurons and between interneurons and principal neurons, interneurons can be electrically coupled to each other via gap junctions (Galarreta and Hestrin, 2001).

Nowadays powerful tools are being used to reveal the molecular organization of excitatory and inhibitory synapses and the various signaling pathways involved in these synapses. Recent developments in genomics and proteomics, gene knockout animal models, protein–protein interaction assays (such as yeast two-hybrid), and the production and application of novel specific antibodies in combination with immunofluorescence microscopy (confocal and two-photon) and electron microscopy immunogold techniques are advancing at a very rapid pace our knowledge of the organization of the molecular machinery of chemical synapses. These studies are revealing that the postsynaptic complex is not just a transmitter receptor-enriched membrane patch that senses the neurotransmitter released to the synaptic cleft. Besides specific ionotropic and metabotropic glutamate

---

*Corresponding author: Tel.: (860) 486-3285;
Fax: (860) 486-5439; E-mail: deblas@oracle.pnb.uconn.edu

receptors, the excitatory postsynaptic complex also contains receptor clustering proteins, scaffolding and adaptor proteins that anchor the postsynaptic receptors and clustering proteins to the cytoskeleton, various protein kinases and phosphatases, small G-proteins and modulators, transcription factors, voltage-dependent channels, cell adhesion molecules and various membrane proteins that interact with the presynaptic membrane proteins and that might be involved in synaptic recognition, among others (Husi et al., 2000; Walikonis et al., 2000; Husi and Grant, 2001; Sheng, 2001). In addition, the postsynaptic complex plays an important role in synaptic plasticity (i.e. LTP and LTD), by regulating both the activity of the transmitter receptors (i.e. via phosphorylation) and the number of receptors at the synapse (i.e. by receptor translocation between the postsynaptic membrane and receptor pools present in subsynaptic vesicular compartments). For review see Scannevin and Huganir (2000).

Our knowledge of the molecular machinery of the GABAergic postsynaptic complex (Kneussel and Betz, 2000; Moss and Smart, 2001) is much more limited than that of the glutamatergic synaptic complex. However, the available information on the GABAergic postsynaptic complex indicates that the molecular components of this structure are quite different from that of the glutamatergic postsynaptic complex. This difference adds to the aforementioned morphological differences between symmetrical and asymmetrical synapses and to the different neurotransmitter and neurotransmitter receptors present in each type of synapse.

Synaptic recognition and specificity in the matching between presynaptic and postsynaptic membrane molecules must also occur. This specificity must also contribute to the different molecular composition of the two types of synapses. Candidate cell adhesion molecules involved in the recognition of the pre- and postsynaptic glutamate synapse machinery at contact points are ephrins and Eph receptors (Bruckner and Klein, 1998; Torres et al., 1998), cadherins and protocadherins (Shapiro et al., 1995; Benson and Tanaka, 1998; Wu and Maniatis, 1999; Tanaka et al., 2000) and neurexins-neuroligins (Scheiffele et al., 2000). The large number of genes and alternatively spliced variants described for some of these molecules also make them attractive candidates for being involved in pre–postsynaptic membrane recognition at GABAergic synapses. Thus N-Cadherins and their β-catenin partners accumulate at

GABAergic synapses early in development (Benson and Tanaka, 1998). However, little is known about the identity, recognition and organizing role (if any) of the aforementioned molecules in GABAergic synapses.

In the present communication we will be mainly addressing the synaptic localization and clustering of two molecules highly concentrated at the postsynaptic complex at GABAergic synapses: GABA$_A$ receptors (GABA$_A$Rs) and gephyrin.

GABA$_A$ receptors of different subunit composition and properties are expressed in various brain regions and cell types

Mammalian brain GABA$_A$Rs are pentameric proteins comprised of combinations of various subunit classes and isoforms (α1-6, β1–3, γ1–3, δ, ϵ and θ), and known splice variants (i.e. γ2 long and γ2 short forms). For reviews, see McKernan and Whiting (1996); Barnard et al., (1998); Mehta and Ticku (1999); Whiting et al. (1999). The most common subunit combination contains two alpha subunits, two beta and one gamma (Im et al., 1995; Chang et al., 1996; Li and De Blas, 1997; Jechlinger et al., 1998) although combinations of two alpha, one beta and two gamma subunits also occur in the brain (Backus et al., 1993; Khan et al., 1994a,b, 1996). Some receptors have the delta subunit substituting for the gamma (Quirk et al., 1995; Araujo et al., 1998). The expression of the various GABA$_A$R subunits differs among brain regions and neuronal cell types as shown by *in situ* hybridization (Laurie, et al., 1992; Persohn et al., 1992; Wisden et al., 1992) light microscopy immunocytochemistry (Richards et al., 1987; De Blas et al., 1988; Turner et al., 1993; Moreno et al., 1994; Fritschy and Möhler, 1995; De Blas, 1996; Gutierrez et al., 1996; Sperk et al., 1997; Miralles et al., 1999; Pirker et al., 2000) and immunoprecipitation studies (De Blas, 1996; McKernan and Whiting, 1996).

Figures 1 and 2 show the differential expression of various GABA$_A$R subunits and gephyrin in the rat hippocampus as revealed by light microscopy immunocytochemistry using anti-GABA$_A$R subunit-specific antibodies raised in our laboratory. The α2, α5, γ2, β1 and β3 GABA$_A$R subunits (Figs. 1B, D, E and 2A and C) and gephyrin (Fig. 1F) are highly expressed in the hippocampus. The α1 and β2 subunits are also highly expressed in this part of the brain although to a lesser

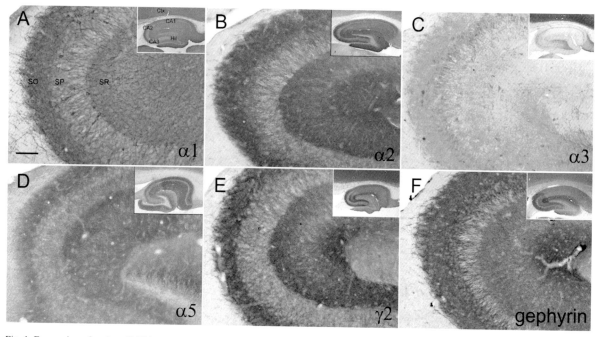

Fig. 1. Expression of various GABA$_A$ receptor isoforms and gephyrin in the rat hippocampus. Peroxidase immunocytochemistry (avidin-biotin) method. Each panel and inset show the distribution of a GABA$_A$R subunit in area CA3–CA2 of the hippocampus and in the whole hippocampus, respectively. Note the high expression levels of α2 (B), γ2 (E) and gephyrin (F) in the stratum oriens and the stratum radiatum. For these subunits, the expression in area CA3 is higher than in CA2 and CA1. However, the α5 subunit (D) shows higher expression in the stratum oriens and stratum radiatum of CA1 than that of CA2 or CA3. Note the high expression of α1 (A) in the interneurons localized in the stratum pyramidale and stratum radiatum and their processes. The α$_3$ subunit (C) is expressed at very low levels in the hippocampus, mainly in the hilus. Ctx, Cortex; SO, Stratum Oriens; SP, Stratum Pyramidale; SR, Stratum Radiatum; CA1, CA2 and CA3 are the corresponding areas of the Ammon's horn. Hil, Hilus. Scale bar is 0.1 mm.

level than α2, α5, γ2, β1 and β3 (Figs. 1A and 2B). Moreover, α1 and β2 are highly expressed by interneurons. The α3 subunit (Fig. 1C) is expressed at very low levels in the hippocampus, but it is highly expressed in the cortex (as shown in the insert). Note the various levels of subunit expression in the dentate gyrus and hippocampus and in the various areas of the latter (CA1, CA2 and CA3). Thus α2 and β3 are highly expressed in the dentate gyrus and area CA3 (Figs. 1B and 2C). The α5 and β1 subunits are highly expressed in CA1 and dentate gyrus (Figs. 1D and 2A). The γ2 subunit and gephyrin are highly expressed in CA3 (Fig. 1E and F). The α3 is mainly expressed in the hilus and less in CA3 and CA2 (Fig. 1C). The α1 and β2 show a more uniform distribution through the hippocampus and the dentate gyrus (Figs. 1A and 2B). The hippocampus shows very low levels of expression of α4, δ, γ1 and γ3 while the α6 subunit is not expressed at all (not shown).

The differential expression of receptor subunits and isoforms in various brain regions and cell types leads to the formation of GABA$_A$R subtypes with different pentameric subunit composition. Subunit composition affects the affinity of the receptor for the neurotransmitter GABA and for other ligands and modulators, such as benzodiazepines, barbiturates, steroids and ethanol. In addition, the properties of the Cl$^-$ channel (i.e. conductance and open time) depend on the subunit composition. The expression of specific receptor subtypes in restricted brain regions and neuronal circuits, together with the specific pharmacological properties of the various GABA$_A$R subtypes, account for the various effects of benzodiazepine drugs (i.e. diazepam or valium). Behavioral tests on mutant mice in which the diazepam-binding site of various alpha subunits have been targeted (by replacing an amino acid that is critical for the binding of diazepam to the receptor) have shown that GABA$_A$Rs containing the α2 subunit (this subunit is

164

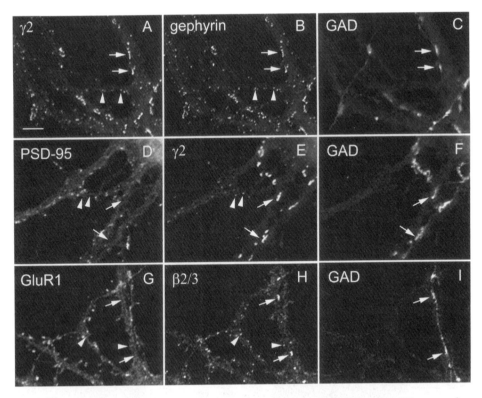

Fig. 6. Synaptic and extrasynaptic clustering of GABA$_A$Rs, gephyrin, AMPA receptors and PSD-95 in cultured hippocampal neurons as shown by triple-label immunofluorescence. Neurons were labeled with rabbit antibodies recognizing specific GABA$_A$R subunits γ2 (A and E) or β2/3 (H) and sheep anti-GAD (C, F, and I) in combination with mouse anti-gephyrin (B), PSD-95 (D) or GluR1 (G). Large GABA$_A$R clusters and/or aggregates of small clusters colocalize with GAD-containing presynaptic terminals from interneurons (arrows), while small GABA$_A$R clusters form in areas not receiving GABAergic contact (filled arrowheads). Note the lack of colocalization between GAD or GABA$_A$R clusters with the majority of the clusters of glutamatergic postsynaptic proteins PSD-95 or GluR1-containing AMPA receptors. Neurons are 3 weeks old, scale bar is 5 μm.

in the cerebellar granule cells, which have δ subunit (s) instead of the γ subunits, could not be detected in any GABAergic or any other type of synapse. The receptors having the δ subunit were extrasynaptically localized in dendrites and somatic membranes of granule cells (Nusser et al., 1998). In the granule cell layer of the cerebellum, α1, α6, β2/3 and γ2 were mainly localized at GABAergic type II Golgi synapses. The α1 and δ subunits were never detected in the granule cell membrane domains opposite to excitatory mossy fiber synapses. In contrast, the α6, γ2 and β2/3 GABA$_A$R subunits were sometimes present postsynaptic to excitatory type I mossy fiber synapses (Nusser et al., 1996b, 1998; Nusser and Somogyi 1997).

Gephyrin concentrates at the postsynaptic membrane of GABAergic synapses colocalizing with GABA$_A$Rs. Nevertheless, gephyrin also forms clusters outside GABAergic synapses

Gephyrin is a 93 KDa cytoplasmic protein that anchors glycine receptors to the postsynaptic membrane of the glycinergic synapses in the spinal cord and brainstem (Feng et al., 1998). In the brain, gephyrin frequently colocalizes with GABA$_A$Rs (Sassoe-Pognetto et al., 2000) and has been proposed to be involved in both the postsynaptic clustering of GABA$_A$Rs at GABAergic synapses and in the anchoring of these receptors to cytoskeletal elements such as microtubules and actin filaments (Essrich et al., 1998; Kneussel et al., 1999).

The clustering and colocalization of gephyrin and GABA$_A$Rs at GABAergic synapses were also observed in hippocampal neuronal cultures by using triple label immunofluorescence techniques. Figure 6 A–C and Fig. 7 A–I show that there is a very high degree of colocalization between gephyrin clusters and γ2, α1, α2 or α3 GABA$_A$R subunit clusters. Colocalization of gephyrin and GABA$_A$Rs occurs at the large synaptic clusters (arrows) formed at the contact points between the GAD-containing presynaptic endings of interneurons and the pyramidal neurons. In addition, GABA$_A$Rs and gephyrin also colocalize in the small clusters not associated with GABAergic synapses (arrowheads in Fig. 6 A and B and Fig. 7 G and H). Gephyrin and all GABA$_A$R subunits tested colocalized in 100% of the large clusters at GABAergic synapses. The small gephyrin and GABA$_A$R clusters that are present outside GABAergic synapses also showed a high degree of colocalization (Fig. 6A and B

and Fig. 7 G and H, filled arrowheads) but the colocalization was not complete since there was a significant number of small gephyrin clusters that did not colocalize with GABA$_A$R clusters and a significant number of small GABA$_A$R clusters that did not colocalize with gephyrin clusters (Fig. 7 G and H, empty arrowheads).

Colocalization of GABA$_A$Rs and gephyrin clusters has been previously demonstrated in hippocampal and spinal cord neuronal brain cultures (Craig et al., 1996; Essrich et al., 1998, Levi et al., 1999) as well as in slices of intact brain (Essrich et al., 1998; Giusteto et al., 1998; Sassoe-Pognetto et al., 2000) and retina (Sassoe-Pognetto et al., 1995). These studies were done by using immunofluorescence microscopy techniques. Although highly suggestive, the observed colocalization of gephyrin and GABA$_A$R clusters and puncta by light microscopy techniques is not sufficient to demonstrate that the two molecules colocalize at the postsynaptic membrane of

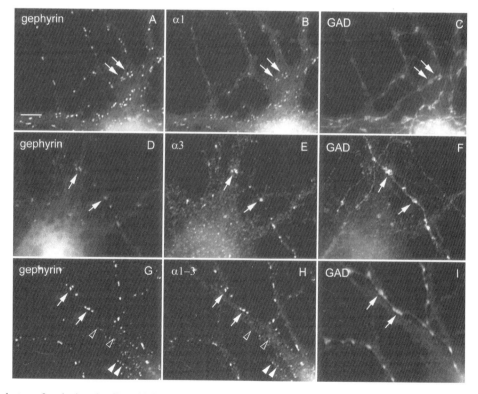

Fig. 7. Large clusters of gephyrin colocalize with large clusters of GABA$_A$Rs at GABAergic synapses, while many small clusters of gephyrin colocalize with small clusters of GABA$_A$Rs. Neurons were triple labeled with mouse anti-gephyrin (A, D and G), sheep anti-GAD (C, F and I) and either rabbit anti-α1 (B), rabbit anti-α3 (E) or a cocktail of rabbit anti-α1, α2 and α3 antibodies (H). The large clusters of gephyrin colocalize completely with all the large clusters of GABA$_A$Rs at GABAergic synapses (arrows, all panels). The small gephyrin clusters colocalize with most (filled arrowheads, G and H), but not all (empty arrowheads, G and H) the small GABA$_A$R clusters. Scale bar is 5 μm.

166

individual GABAergic synapses. Light microscopy does not have the necessary resolution.

By using double-labeling postembedding EM immuno-gold techniques we have shown (Fig. 8) that in the brain GABA$_A$Rs and gephyrin colocalize at the postsynaptic membrane of symmetric type II synapses. Figure 8 shows that gephyrin colocalizes with the α1, α2 or γ2 subunits of the GABA$_A$R at individual symmetric synapses. To the best of our knowledge, this is the first evidence at the EM level of (I) synaptic colocalization of α1, α2 and γ2 subunits with gephyrin at any CNS synapse; and (II) colo-calization of gephyrin and GABA$_A$Rs in brain synapses. A previous EM immunocytochemistry study has shown that, in the brain, gephyrin is localized postsynaptically to terminals containing the neurotransmitter GABA (Giusteto et al., 1998). Outside the brain, colocalization of gephyrin with the α3 subunit in retina (Giusteto et al., 1998) and the β3 in the spinal cord (Todd et al., 1996) had been previ-ously reported by using EM preembedding immunocyto-chemistry techniques that combined immunoperoxidase and immunogold labeling. We have also found some gephyrin extrasynaptically, which parallels the formation of the extrasynaptic gephyrin clusters observed in cultured neurons, as discussed above.

In a gephyrin knockout mouse mutant (Kneussel et al., 1999), the number and size of GABA$_A$R clusters were highly diminished and in a γ2 GABA$_A$R subunit knockout mouse (Essrich et al., 1998), the number and size of gephyrin clusters were also highly diminished as determined by light microscopy immunofluorescence techniques. These results suggest that the clustering of GABA$_A$Rs requires both the γ2 subunit and gephyrin. This hypothesis is consistent with the very high level of colocalization of γ2 (and other GABA$_A$R subunits) and gephyrin clusters both at GABAergic synapses (arrows) and outside GABAergic synapses (filled arrowheads) as Figs. 6 A–C, 7 A–I and 9 A–F show. See also Fig. 8 A. In addition, electrophysiological data (Brickley et al., 1999) support the notion that the presence of the γ2 subunit is necessary for the GABA$_A$Rs to be localized at the synapse. It has been proposed that gephyrin binds to β3 but not γ2 (Kirsch et al., 1993). Nevertheless, no direct binding of GABA$_A$Rs to gephyrin has been demonstrated. As shown above, we have found that some small GABA$_A$R clusters don't contain gephyrin. Therefore, gephyrin by itself can't be the only molecule responsible for the formation of all GABA$_A$R clusters. Even though most GABA$_A$R and gephyrin clusters

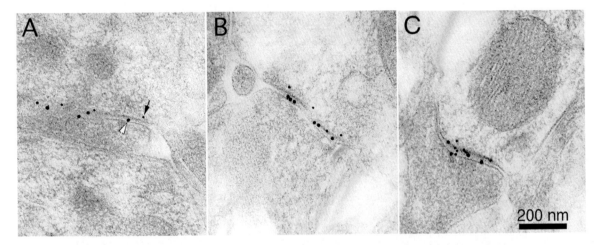

Fig. 8. Colocalization of GABA$_A$Rs and gephyrin at type II synapses. Double-label postembedding EM immunogold of mouse anti-gephyrin (A–C) with rabbit anti-γ2 (A); rabbit anti-α2 (B) and rabbit anti-α1 (C). Note the synaptic colocalization of gephyrin (small gold particles, black arrow) with γ2, α2 and α1 (larger particles, white arrow) in A–C, respectively. The secondary antibodies are goat anti-rabbit IgG and goat anti-mouse IgG labeled with 18 and 10 nm gold particles, respectively. The brain regions are cerebral cortex (A & C) and hippocampus (B). The α2 subunit in the hippocampus concentrates postsynaptically to terminals of parvalbumin-negative basket cells that innervate the soma and proximal dendrites of the pyramidal cells (Nyiri et al., 2001).The α2 subunit also concentrates on the axo-axonic synapses on the axon initial segment of the hippocampal CA1 pyramidal cells (Nusser et al., 1996a). Note that the larger immunogold particles are localized in the synap-tic cleft, as expected for extracellular GABA$_A$R epitopes. However, the gephyrin-labeling by smaller immunogold particles are mainly localized on the postsynaptic membrane or the subsynaptic cytoplasm. This localization is expected for a cytoplasmic protein involved in the direct or indirect attachment of GABA$_A$Rs to the synaptic cytoskeleton.

colocalize, proteins other than gephyrin might also be involved in GABA$_A$R clustering as discussed below (Knuesel et al., 1999, 2001; Wang et al., 1999; Fischer et al., 2000; Kneussel et al., 2000, 2001). One of these proteins, a protein named GABARAP (GABA$_A$R-associated protein, Wang et al., 1999) interacts with both the γ2 subunit of the GABA$_A$R and gephyrin (Kneussel et al., 2000) and was considered to be a candidate molecule for clustering both GABA$_A$Rs and gephyrin. Nevertheless, GABARAP doesn't seem to be involved in the clustering and anchoring of GABA$_A$R at the postsynaptic membrane. Instead, recent evidence suggests that it might be involved in the intracellular trafficking of the GABA$_A$R (Kneussel et al., 2000; Kittler et al., 2001). Gephyrin binds to other molecules such as collybistin, Raft1 and Profilin (Kneussel and Betz, 2000). However, there is no evidence that these proteins bind to GABA$_A$Rs. Gephyrin also binds to microtubules and actin filaments as indicated above.

Development of gephyrin and GABA$_A$ receptor clusters in hippocampal cultures in GABAergic synapses and outside GABAergic synapses

Figure 9 shows that very soon after plating (3.5 DIV, the earliest time tested), some hippocampal pyramidal cells express both small gephyrin and GABA$_A$R clusters that colocalize with each other (filled arrowheads). No GABAergic innervation by GAD-containing axons or GAD-containing neurons was detected in the very early cultures (i.e. 3.5–5.5 DIV). The results show that the formation of small GABA$_A$R and gephyrin clusters did not require GABA or GABAergic innervation (see below). We couldn't find any neuron having only gephyrin clusters or having only GABA$_A$R clusters, though at 3.5 DIV over 90% of the neurons had neither. These results also suggest that the clustering of both GABA$_A$Rs and gephyrin occurs simultaneously and that both molecules are necessary for the formation of the clusters. However, as indicated above, the presence of small GABA$_A$R clusters that don't have gephyrin suggests the existence of additional clustering molecules.

In the early cultures, we couldn't completely rule out the presence of immature interneurons that don't express GAD but which still innervate pyramidal cells and induce the clustering of gephyrin and GABA$_A$Rs at the contact points. Therefore, we studied the formation of GABA$_A$R and gephyrin clusters in microcultures of single pyramidal cells. These are glutamatergic neurons and therefore, no GABAergic synapses are formed in these microcultures. Nevertheless, these pyramidal cells make autaptic glutamatergic synapses with themselves. Figure 10 A and C show that small gephyrin and GABA$_A$R clusters are formed in isolated pyramidal cells that don't receive GABAergic innervation. These and the previous results support the notion that the formation of small GABA$_A$R and gephyrin clusters doesn't require GABA or GABAergic innervation.

Some gephyrin clusters that are not associated with GABAergic synapses are associated with glutamate receptor clusters

Figure 10 A, B, E and F shows that a subpopulation of the small gephyrin clusters (not associated with GABAergic synapses) are juxtaposed to AMPA receptor clusters. We have observed this association of gephyrin clusters and AMPA receptor clusters in both pyramidal cells in isolation (microcultures, Fig. 10 A and B, filled arrowheads) and pyramidal cells that receive limited GABAergic innervation from interneurons (Fig. 10 E and F, filled arrowheads). Nevertheless, many small gephyrin clusters are not associated with GluR1-containing AMPA receptor clusters (Fig. 10 A, B, E and F, empty arrowheads). We have recently found that some small GABA$_A$R clusters are juxtaposed to AMPA receptor clusters and NMDA receptor clusters in glutamatergic synapses (Christie et al., 2002). Given the high degree of colocalization of small gephyrin and GABA$_A$R clusters, one can safely conclude that some small gephyrin clusters are juxtaposed to glutamate receptors at glutamatergic synapses. This hypothesis is also consistent with the observed colocalization of the synaptic vesicle marker synaptophysin with GABA$_A$R clusters in microcultures of single pyramidal cells (Fig. 10 C and D). These cells have no GABAergic innervation. They only have autaptic glutamatergic innervation. Therefore, the observed colocalization of the presynaptic marker synaptophysin with GABA$_A$R clusters in the microcultures of single pyramidal cells plus the observed high degree of colocalization of gephyrin clusters and GABA$_A$R clusters suggest that some GABA$_A$R and gephyrin clusters might be associated with glutamatergic synapses. If that were the case, the presence of gephyrin and GABA$_A$R clusters in some glutamatergic synapses in

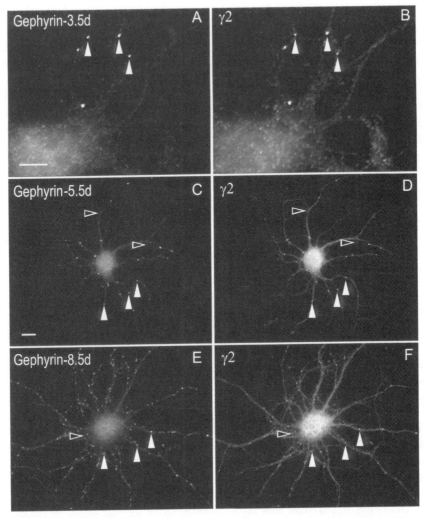

Fig. 9. Clusters of gephyrin and γ2 subunit-containing GABA$_A$Rs are expressed and colocalize during the early development of hippocampal neurons in culture. Hippocampal neurons double labeled with mouse anti-gephyrin (A, C and E) and rabbit anti-γ2 (B, D, F) at 3.5 DIV (A and B), 5.5 DIV (C and D), or 8.5 DIV (E and F) have small clusters of gephyrin and GABA$_A$Rs that colocalize with each other (filled arrowheads). Only a small fraction of the gephyrin or γ2 subunit containing GABA$_A$R clusters don't colocalize (empty arrowheads, C–F). Scale bar in A is 5 μm for panels A and B, scale bar in C is 10 μm for C–F.

hippocampal cultures would have a counterpart in the intact brain where, and as discussed above, EM immunogold experiments have shown that some GABA$_A$Rs are associated with type I synapses. Rao et al., (2000) have reported that some GABA$_A$R/gephyrin clusters might be mismatched (where no glutamate receptors are present) to presynaptic glutamate-releasing terminals in autaptic synapses. As indicated above, instead of mismatched GABA$_A$Rs, we find GABA$_A$R clusters associated with glutamatergic synapses that contain glutamate receptors.

A gephyrin antisense oligonucleotide significantly reduces the density of the small gephyrin and GABA$_A$R clusters outside GABAergic synapses but it has little effect on the large gephyrin and GABA$_A$R clusters at GABAergic synapses

Figure 11 shows that hippocampal cultures treated for a week with a gephyrin antisense oligonucleotide (5 μM) between 14–21 DIV showed significantly reduced density of both small gephyrin and GABA$_A$R clusters by

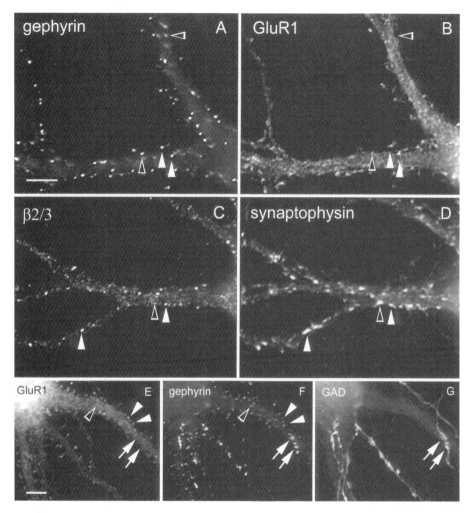

Fig. 10. Association of some small gephyrin clusters with glutamatergic synapses in both microisland cultures of hippocampal pyramidal neurons and regular hippocampal cultures. Neurons were double or triple labeled with mouse anti-gephyrin (A and F), rabbit anti-GluR1 (B and E), mouse anti-GABA$_A$R β2/3 subunit (C), rabbit anti-synaptophysin (D) and GAD (G) in either microisland cultures of pyramidal neurons (A–D) or low density hippocampal cultures (E–G). The association of some (filled arrowheads) but not all (empty arrowheads) small gephyrin clusters with clusters of GluR1-containing AMPA receptors occurs in pyramidal neurons whether the cells do (E–G) or do not (A and B) receive GABAergic innervation from interneurons (arrows). In microisland cultures of pyramidal neurons (therefore in the absence of GABAergic innervation), a significant number (filled arrowheads, C and D) but not all (empty arrowheads, C and D) small β2/3-containing GABA$_A$R clusters are associated with synaptophysin-containing synaptic vesicles in presynaptic terminals, presumably from glutamatergic autapses. Cultured pyramidal cells that have limited GABAergic innervation have large synaptic clusters of gephyrin that colocalize with GAD containing terminals of interneurons (arrows in F and G), and numerous small clusters that neither colocalize with GAD-containing terminals nor associate with clusters of GluR1-containing AMPA receptors (empty arrowhead, E and F). Scale bar in A is 5 μm for A–D, scale bar in E is 5 μm for E–G.

46–55%. However, the same antisense oligonucleotide had a much smaller effect on the density of the large gephyrin and GABA$_A$R clusters at GABAergic synapses (14–27%). In a similar experiment, Essrich et al., (1998) reported a reduction of the 'punctate' staining of the gephyrin (36%) and GABA$_A$R subunits α2 (43%) and γ2

(28%). Nevertheless, these authors did not distinguish between the large clusters present at GABA synapses and the small GABA$_A$R clusters that are located outside GABA synapses on the cell surface. Our results show that the main effect of the gephyrin antisense oligonucleotide is on the small gephyrin and GABA$_A$R clusters

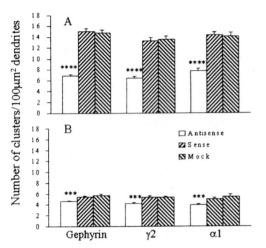

Fig. 11. Gephyrin antisense oligonucleotide treatment of hippocampal cultures highly decreases the density of small gephyrin and GABA$_A$R clusters (A). The density of large gephyrin and GABA$_A$R clusters at GABAergic synapses is also decreased but to a lesser extent (B). **A:** The number of small extrasynaptic clusters per 100 μm^2 of dendrite (mean + s.e.m.) for the cultures treated with antisense oligonucleotide was 6.9 ± 0.2 for gephyrin, 6.4 ± 0.3 for $\gamma 2$ and 7.7 ± 0.5 for $\alpha 1$. The density of the cultures treated with sense oligonucleotide was 15.1 ± 0.5 for gephyrin, 13.4 ± 0.5 for $\gamma 2$ and 14.4 ± 0.5 for $\alpha 1$. For the culture medium (mock) control the values were 14.8 ± 0.6 for gephyrin, 13.6 ± 0.5 for $\gamma 2$ and 14.2 ± 0.6 for $\alpha 1$. Thus antisense oligonucleotide treatment decreased the density of both gephyrin and GABA$_A$R clusters to 45–54% of the values obtained with the sense or mock controls (or 46–55% reduction). **B:** The number of large synaptic clusters per 100 μm^2 of dendrite (mean + s.e.m.) for the cultures treated with antisense oligonucleotide was 4.6 ± 0.2 for gephyrin, 4.0 ± 0.2 for $\gamma 2$ and 3.9 ± 0.2 for $\alpha 1$. For the cultures treated with the sense oligonucleotide cultures, the values were 5.4 ± 0.12 for gephyrin, 5.3 ± 0.3 for $\gamma 2$ and 5.0 ± 0.2 for $\alpha 1$. For the mock control the values were 5.7 ± 0.2 for gephyrin, 6.4 ± 0.3 for $\gamma 2$ and $5.5 + 0.4$ for $\alpha 1$. Thus, antisense oligonucleotide treatment decreased the density of both gephyrin and GABA$_A$R clusters to 73–86% of the values obtained with the sense or mock controls (or 14–27% reduction). Cultures were treated with gephyrin antisense or sense oligonucleotides as indicated in the methods section. The cultures were fixed and subjected to triple-label immunofluorescence as indicated in the methods, with anti-$\alpha 1$ (made in guinea pig), anti-gephyrin mouse monoclonal antibody (or anti-$\gamma 2$ made in rabbit) and anti-GAD made in sheep. Synaptic gephyrin and GABA$_A$R clusters were identified by colocalization with GAD-containing boutons. Three experiments were used for each treatment and four cultures per experiment. A total of 48-60 dendritic segments were observed (see methods) and an average of 521 synaptic and 1199 extrasynaptic clusters for each treatment were used in the analysis. ***, $P < 0.001$, ****, $P < 0.0001$ in Student's t test.

while also affecting large synaptic clusters to a lesser extent. In a gephyrin-deficient mouse mutant (Kneussel et al., 1999), GABA$_A$R clusters are highly diminished from the neuronal surface, while the intracellular pool of GABA$_A$Rs didn't change. The same authors have proposed that gephyrin prevents receptor endocytosis therefore stabilizing the GABA$_A$R clusters at synapses. Gephyrin antisense oligonucleotides also block the clustering of glycine receptors in spinal cord neurons (Kirsch et al., 1993).

The GABA$_A$R and gephyrin clustering and/or anchoring mechanisms operating at the GABAergic synapses are different from the ones that operate outside these synapses

The results shown above indicate that hippocampal pyramidal cells in culture make large GABA$_A$Rs and gephyrin clusters that are located at the postsynaptic membrane of the GABAergic synapses. This synaptic clustering/anchoring depends on GABAergic innervation by GAD-containing axons from interneurons. Large GABA$_A$R and gephyrin clusters are formed exactly at the synaptic sites and they are relatively resistant to gephyrin antisense oligonucleotide treatment.

Outside GABAergic synapses, gephyrin and GABA$_A$Rs also form clusters but they are small and independent of GABAergic innervation. These clusters are quite sensitive to gephyrin antisense oligonucleotide treatment (perhaps because these clusters turn over more rapidly than the synaptic clusters and/or because there are differences in the clustering mechanisms involved in the formation of large clusters at GABAergic synapses vs. the ones involved in the formation of small clusters outside these synapses). Some of these small GABA$_A$R/gephyrin clusters are associated with glutamatergic synapses. These differences indicate that the GABA$_A$R/gephyrin clustering and/or anchoring mechanisms operating at GABAergic synapses differ from those outside GABAergic synapses.

Unidentified proteins that interact with GABA$_A$ receptors might be involved in GABA$_A$ receptor trafficking, clustering or targeting to GABA synapses

There are several proteins that are tightly associated with the GABA$_A$Rs and that could be involved in trafficking, clustering and/or targeting of the GABA$_A$R to the GABA synapses. Thus, some cytoskeletal proteins such as tubulin and actin copurify with GABA$_A$Rs (Item and Sieghart, 1994; Kannenberg et al., 1997). Immunoprecipitation of the GABA$_A$Rs from bovine brain with an anti-α1 antibody (bd24) coprecipitated actin, tubulin and other still unidentified proteins (Kannenberg et al., 1997). Interestingly, gephyrin is absent from the affinity-purified GABA$_A$R preparations. Microtubule depolymerization also affects GABA$_A$R function (Whatley et al., 1994). Thus, the data suggest the existence of a connection between GABA$_A$Rs and the cytoskeleton, probably through adaptor proteins. It has been proposed that gephyrin is one of these adaptor proteins (Kneussel and Betz 2000). Nevertheless, microtubules and microfilaments don't seem to be directly involved in GABA$_A$R clustering because depolymerization of microtubules or actin did not affect GABA$_A$R or gephyrin clustering in hippocampal cultures (Allison et al., 2000).

As indicated above, the application of the yeast two-hybrid technology has led to the identification of GABARAP as a GABA$_A$R-interacting protein (Wang et al., 1999) that binds to both the large intracellular loop of the γ2 subunit of the GABA$_A$R and to gephyrin (Kneussel et al., 2000). GABARAP also interacts with the cytoskeleton (Wang and Olsen, 2000). GABARAP has homology to the light chain-3 of microtubule-associated proteins (MAPs) 1A and 1B and with the protein p16 or late-acting intra Golgi transport factor (Kneussel et al., 2000). GABARAP promotes GABA$_A$R clustering (Chen et al., 2000). Nevertheless, GABARAP doesn't seem to be involved in the synaptic or extrasynaptic clustering of gephyrin or GABA$_A$Rs. Instead, it seems to be involved in GABA$_A$R trafficking in intracellular organelles (Kneussel et al., 2000; Kittler et al., 2001). Yeast two-hybrid assays have also identified MAP-1B as a GABA$_C$ receptor-interacting protein. MAP-1B binds to the large intracellular loop of the ρ1 subunit but it does not bind to any of the GABA$_A$R subunits. Thus, MAP-1B is an adaptor protein linking GABA$_C$ receptors to the cytoskeleton (Hanley et al., 1999).

We are currently following two approaches for the identification of GABA$_A$R-interacting proteins: (1) We have raised monoclonal antibodies (mAbs), after immunizing mice with either affinity-purified GABA$_A$Rs or a synaptic plasma membrane-enriched fraction. Some of the prepared mAbs don't recognize GABA$_A$R subunits but they precipitate the affinity-purified GABA$_A$R complex, presumably by recognizing a GABA$_A$R-interacting protein that copurifies with GABA$_A$Rs; (2) We have done yeast two-hybrid library screenings using as baits the large intracellular loop of the β3, γ2 or α1 subunits.

Monoclonal antibody approach

The hypothesis is that antibodies that precipitate the affinity-purified GABA$_A$Rs (as determined by precipitation of [^{3}H]muscimol and [^{3}H]flunitrazepam binding activity), but that don't recognize GABA$_A$R subunits, are likely to recognize proteins that are tightly bound to the GABA$_A$R. These putative GABA$_A$R-interacting proteins co-purify and co-precipitate with the GABA$_A$Rs. In earlier publications, we have reported the generation of several mAbs with these characteristics such as the mAbs 62-5F6, 62-3F7 and 62-1H3, which were obtained by immunizing mice with GABA$_A$Rs that were affinity-purified by immobilized benzodiazepine (Vitorica et al., 1988). The hybridoma lines 62-5F6, 62-3F7 and 62-1H3 were generated in the same fusion experiment as the 62-3G1 hybridoma line, which produces a mAb that is specific for the β2/3 subunits of the GABA$_A$Rs (Vitorica et al., 1988; De Blas et al., 1988). Immunoblots with mAbs 62-5F6, 62-3F7 and 62-1H3 did not show immunoreactivity of any of these antibodies with any protein band, suggesting that these mAbs recognized conformation-dependent epitopes that were denatured by SDS-electrophoresis and blotting. These antibodies recognized native proteins since they precipitated the solubilized native GABA$_A$R complex. The mAbs could recognize epitopes located in one or more GABA$_A$R subunits, however light microscopy immunocytochemistry with brain tissue slices (not shown) and double-labeling immunofluorescence experiments using hippocampal cultures, show that this is not likely the case (see also below, Fig. 12).

The mAbs 4-7E10 and 7-3B8 were obtained by immunizing mice with purified synaptic plasma membranes (De Blas et al., 1984). Of the 72 hybridoma lines that produce mAbs recognizing antigens present in purified synaptic plasma membranes, hybridoma lines 4-7E10 and 7-3B8 produce mAbs that immunoprecipitate the affinity-purified GABA$_A$Rs (Vitorica and De Blas, unpublished results). In immunoblots of synaptic plasma membranes, mAb 4-7E10 recognizes a

172

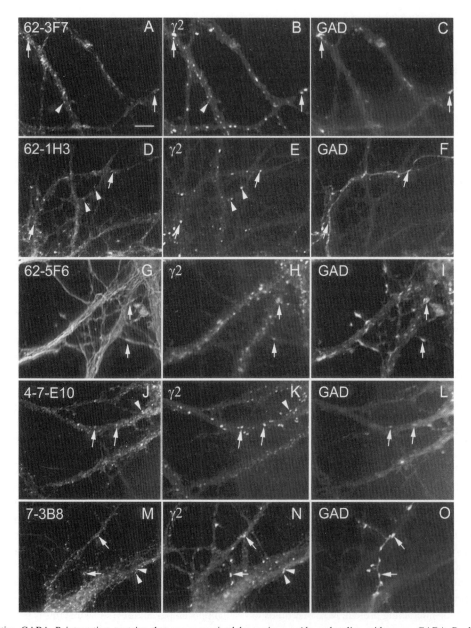

Fig. 12. Putative GABA$_A$R-interacting proteins that are recognized by various mAbs colocalize with some GABA$_A$R clusters at both GABAergic synapses and outside GABAergic synapses. Triple-label immunofluorescence of hippocampal cultures with mouse mAb (left column panels A, D, G, J, M), rabbit anti-γ2 GABA$_A$R subunit (middle column panels B, E, H, K, N) and sheep anti-GAD (right column panels C, F, I, L, O). Colocalization of the mAb with GABA$_A$R clusters at GABAergic synapses is shown by arrows and colocalization with GABA$_A$R clusters outside GABAergic synapses is shown by arrowheads. Scale bar is 5 µm.

protein of 105kDa (De Blas et al., 1984), while mAb 7-3B8 does not reveal any protein band. We don't know yet the molecular identities of the proteins recognized by any of the mAbs.

We have investigated whether the antigens recognized by the aforementioned mAbs that precipitate the GABA$_A$Rs were present in the synaptic and extrasynaptic GABA$_A$R clusters displayed by cultured hippocampal neurons. For this purpose, we have used double or triple-labeling immunofluorescence assays. The hypothesis is that GABA$_A$R-associated proteins recognized by these mAbs, if they are involved in GABA$_A$R clustering, should colocalize with the GABA$_A$R clusters. Figure 12 shows that mAbs 62-3F7, 62-1H3, 63-5F6, 4-7E10 and 7-3B8 recognized antigens that colocalize with GABA$_A$R clusters as shown with an anti-γ2 GABA$_A$R subunit antibody (Fig. 12 B, E, H, K, N). Colocalization was found with a significant number of both large GABA$_A$R clusters located at GABAergic synapses (as determined by colocalization with GAD-containing boutons, arrows) and the small GABA$_A$R clusters that are located outside these synapses (arrowheads). Nevertheless, none of the mAbs revealed a clustering pattern identical to that of any of the GABA$_A$R subunits or gephyrin. Thus, the proteins recognized by these mAbs are neither GABA$_A$Rs nor gephyrin. The mAbs 62-3F7, 62-1H3, 4-7E10 and 7-3B8 show both clusters that colocalize with GABA$_A$R clusters and clusters that don't. Thus,

the results indicate that these proteins are not exclusively involved in GABA$_A$R clustering and/or GABAergic synaptic function. Moreover, 62-3F7 not only showed colocalization with GABA$_A$R clusters but also colocalized with AMPA receptor clusters (Fig. 13 A and B). Another mAb (6-6A8) also recognized an antigen that showed significant colocalization with AMPA receptor clusters (Fig. 13 C and D). The mAb 62-5F6 (Fig. 12 G) showed a staining pattern with no clustering of the antigen. Instead, it suggested a cytoskeletal antigen. The 62-5F6 concentrated at and colocalized with large GABA$_A$R clusters at GABAergic synapses (Fig. 12 G, H, I, arrows). We don't know yet the molecular identities of any of the putative GABA$_A$R-associated proteins recognized by these mAbs.

The yeast two-hybrid approach

We have also done screenings of a rat brain cDNA library with the yeast two-hybrid assay using as bait the large intracellular cytoplasmic loop (IL) of the GABA$_A$R subunit β3, γ2 or α1. We are concentrating on the IL of the GABA$_A$R subunit(s) because that's the region predicted to be involved in the interaction with cytoplasmic proteins. It is through the IL where the interaction between the γ2 subunit of the GABA$_A$Rs and GABARAP occurs, as well as the interactions between the glycine receptor and gephyrin, between the nicotinic acetylcholine receptor and rapsyn and between the GABA$_C$ receptor and MAP1-B. In addition, the IL of various GABA$_A$R subunits can be phosphorylated by various protein kinases. This phosphorylation might regulate the strength of the interactions of the receptors with other proteins. We have isolated several cDNA clones encoding putative GABA$_A$R-interacting proteins that in the yeast two-hybrid assay interact with some of the IL baits. One of these clones, B91 (isolated with the β3IL bait), encoded a peptide that specifically interacts with the IL of the three β–subunit isoforms (β1, β2 and β3) but it doesn't interact with the IL of any of the alpha and gamma subunit isoforms. We have additional clones, GS6, GS8 and GS11, that encode proteins that interacted with the IL of γ2S but not with that of the IL of γ2L. We are currently identifying and characterizing the proteins encoded by these and other clones isolated with the yeast two-hybrid assay and their interaction with the GABA$_A$Rs.

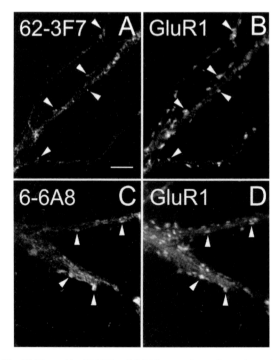

Fig. 13. The mAbs 62-3F7 and 6-6A8 recognize antigens that colocalize with AMPA receptor clusters. Double label immunofluorescence of hippocampal cultures with mouse mAb (panels A and C) and rabbit anti-GluR1 (panels B and D). Colocalization is shown by arrowheads. Scale bar is 5 μm.

Conclusions

GABA$_A$Rs and gephyrin colocalize in the brain at the postsynaptic membrane of GABAergic symmetric (type II) synapses. The clustering and accumulation of GABA$_A$Rs and gephyrin at GABAergic synapses is also observed in hippocampal cultures. In these cultures, large GABA$_A$R and gephyrin clusters are formed in pyramidal cell bodies and dendrites at the postsynaptic sites where GAD-containing presynaptic endings from interneurons contact and synapse on pyramidal cells. In addition, smaller clusters of GABA$_A$Rs and gephyrin are also formed by cultured neurons receiving GABAergic innervation, in the areas of the soma and dendrites devoid of GABAergic synapses. The formation of small GABA$_A$R and gephyrin clusters also occurs in micro-cultures of single glutamatergic pyramidal cells that don't receive any GABAergic innervation. These results indicate that the process of GABA$_A$R and gephyrin clustering *per se* is independent of GABA and GABAergic innervation. The high level of colocalization of gephyrin and GABA$_A$R clusters is consistent with the hypothesis that both molecules are necessary for the formation of the clusters, although other molecules that interact with GABA$_A$Rs and/or gephyrin seem also to be involved because some GABA$_A$R clusters have no gephyrin. A different clustering/anchoring mechanism is necessary to account for the formation and targeting of large GABA$_A$R and gephyrin clusters exactly at the points where GAD-containing axons from interneurons contact pyramidal cells forming GABAergic synapses. Some small gephyrin and GABA$_A$R clusters (not associated with GABA synapses) are associated with glutamate receptor clusters at glutamatergic synapses. This result suggests the possibility that some signal(s) that originate at glutamatergic synapses trigger the formation of both glutamate receptor clusters and small GABA$_A$R /gephyrin clusters. Hippocampal cultures treated with a gephyrin antisense oligonucleotide showed a highly decreased density of small gephyrin and GABA$_A$R clusters with significant, but smaller, effect on the large gephyrin and GABA$_A$R clusters that were present at GABA synapses. These results indicate that the large gephyrin and GABA$_A$R clusters present at GABAergic synapses are more stable than the small clusters present outside these synapses. Perhaps the latter turned over faster than the larger clusters. All the combined findings are compatible with the notion that the molecular mechanisms that are involved in the formation and anchoring of the large gephyrin and GABA$_A$R clusters at GABAergic synapses (that are dependent on GABAergic innervation) and the mechanisms involved in the formation of the small clusters outside GABA synapses (that don't require GABAergic innervation) are different. Current research is aimed at identifying the various molecular mechanisms involved in GABA$_A$R and gephyrin clustering at GABAergic synapses and outside GABAergic synapses.

Methods

Antibodies

The primary antibodies, guinea pig anti-α1 (1–15 A.A.), rabbit anti-α1 (1–15 A.A.), rabbit anti-α2 (417–423 A.A.), rabbit anti-α3 (1–13 A.A.), rabbit anti-α5 (1–13), rabbit anti-γ2 (1–15 A.A.) and guinea pig anti-γ2, were raised and affinity purified in our laboratory against synthetic peptides made to unique extracellular epitopes (N-terminus for α1, α3 and γ2 and C-terminus for α2) of rat GABA$_A$R subunits (Miralles et al., 1999). The monoclonal mouse anti-β2/3 (62-3G1) was raised in our laboratory to affinity purified GABA$_A$Rs (De Blas et al., 1988; Vitorica et al., 1988). This antibody recognizes an extracellular N-terminus epitope that is common to β2 and β3 subunits (β2/3). Antibodies to fusion proteins of the intracellular loops of β1, β2 and β3 were also raised in rabbits in our laboratory, and affinity purified with purified intracellular loop of the respective isoform (Moreno et al., 1994; Li and De Blas 1997). All antibodies to GABA$_A$R subunits used in this study have been thoroughly characterized and their specificities determined elsewhere (De Blas et al., 1988; Vitorica et al., 1988; Moreno et al., 1994; Miralles et al., 1999). The monoclonal mouse anti-gephyrin (mAb 7a) was purchased from Cedarlane (Accurate Chemical & Scientific Corp., Westbury, NY). Rabbit anti-GluR1 was from Chemicon (Temecula, CA), mouse monoclonal anti-PSD-95 from Upstate Biotechnology (Lake Placid, NY), and mouse monoclonal anti-SV2 was a gift of Dr. Kathleen M. Buckley from Harvard Medical School. Sheep anti-GAD (gift of Dr. I. Kopin) or the GAD 65-specific mouse monoclonal GAD6 (Developmental

Studies Hybridoma Bank, University of Iowa) were used for identifying interneurons and GABAergic presynaptic processes.

Light microscopy immunocytochemistry with brain slices

The procedure has been described elsewhere (De Blas 1984; De Blas et al., 1988, Moreno et al., 1994). Briefly, 60-day-old Sprague-Dawley rats were perfused through the ascending aorta under anesthesia (80 mg/kg ketamine hydrochloride, 8 mg/kg xylazine, 2 mg/kg acepromazine maleate), with either 0.01M periodate, 0.075M lysine, 4% paraformaldehyde in 0.1 M phosphate buffer (PLP) fixative or Zamboni's fixative (0.2% picric acid, 4% paraformaldehyde in 0.1 M phosphate buffer pH 7.4). The brains were frozen and sliced in parasaggital sections (25 µm) with a freezing microtome. The free-floating tissue sections were incubated for 24 h at 4°C with affinity-purified rabbit anti-β2IL, anti-β3IL, anti-α1, anti-α2, anti-α3 anti-α5 or anti-γ2 (all at 1 µg/ml) in 0.3% Triton X-100 in 0.1 M phosphate buffer pH 7.4 or the mouse mAb 62-3G1 culture medium diluted $100 \times$ in the same buffer. The incubation with the primary antibody was followed by incubation with a biotin-labeled secondary antibody and avidin-biotin-horseradish peroxidase complex (ABC procedure, Vector laboratories). Reaction product was visualized by incubation with 3-3′ diaminobenzidine tetrahydrochloride (DAB) in the presence of cobalt chloride and nickel ammonium sulfate. Sections were washed and mounted on gelatin-coated glass slides. Specificity of the antibody reaction was demonstrated by specific displacement with the corresponding peptide or antigen as described elsewhere (Miralles et al., 1999). Control sections in which the primary antibody was omitted showed no immunolabeling.

Fluorescence immunocytochemistry with hippocampal cultures

Hippocampal cultures were fixed by incubating the glass coverslips in a phosphate buffered saline (PBS) solution containing 4% paraformaldehyde and 4% sucrose for 15 min at room temperature followed by permeabilization with 0.25% Triton X-100 in PBS. Nonspecific antibody labeling was minimized by treatment with 5% donkey

serum in PBS for 30 min, at room temperature. A mixture of primary antibodies raised in different species was diluted in 0.25% Triton X-100 PBS, and added to the cultures followed by incubation for 2 h at room temperature. Incubation with primary antibodies was followed by washes and incubation with the mixture of secondary antibodies raised in donkey (anti-species specific IgG) conjugated to either Texas Red, FITC, or AMCA fluorophores (1:150 dilution in 0.25% triton X-100 PBS, Jackson Immunochemicals) for 1 h at room temperature. The washed coverslips were mounted with Prolong antifade mounting solution (Molecular Probes; Eugene, Oregon). Specificity of the labeling with the various $GABA_AR$ subunit isoform antibodies was ensured by specific displacement of the antibody binding to the cultured cells by 20 µg/ml of the corresponding peptide. Control cultures in which the primary antibodies were omitted showed no immunolabeling.

Images were collected using a 60X pan-fluor objective on a Nikon Eclipse T300 microscope with a Sensys KAF 1401E CCD camera, driven by IPLab 3.0 acquisition software. Image files were then processed and merged for color colocalization figures using PhotoShop 4.01 (Adobe). Control slides in which one or more primary antibodies were omitted showed no spill over in the other two fluorescence channels. Random drift of the sample's fluorescence signal between channels was controlled by alignment of all channels using triple labeled fluorescent microspheres (0.1 µm and 0.4 µm diameter; Molecular Probes, Eugene, OR).

Low density and microisland hippocampal cultures

Hippocampal cultures were prepared as described by Banker and Goslin (1998). Briefly, embryonic day 18 Wistar rat pup hippocampi were dissected in Hanks Balanced Salts Solution (HBSS), followed by treatment with 0.25% trypsin (Sigma) and trituration using a fire polished Pasteur pipette. Dissociated cells were centrifuged in HBSS for 2 min at 1,500 rpm, and the pellet was suspended in plating medium [10% Horse serum (Gibco) in Dulbecco's modified eagle medium (DMEM) with 0.6% Glucose and 26 mM $NaHCO_3$] and plated in poly-L-lysine treated 18 mm diameter circular coverslip at a density of 5,000-10,000 per coverslip and placed in 5% CO_2 atmosphere at 37°C for 3–4 h to allow settling and attachment of cells. The coverslips with attached

Fritschy, J.M. and Möhler, H. (1995) GABA$_A$-receptor heterogeneity in the adult rat brain: differential regional and cellular distribution of seven major subunits. *J. Comp. Neurol.*, 359: 154–194.

Galarreta, M. and Hestrin, S. (2001) Electrical synapses between GABA-releasing interneurons. *Nature Rev. Neurosci.*, 2: 425–433.

Giustetto, M., Kirsch, J., Fritschy, J.M., Cantino, D. and Sassoe-Pognetto, M. (1998) Localization of the clustering protein Gephyrin at GABAergic synapses in the main olfactory bulb of the rat. *J. Comp. Neurol.*, 395: 231–244.

Gutierrez, A., Khan, Z.U. and De Blas, A.L. (1996) Immunocytochemical localization of the alpha 6 subunit of the gamma-aminobutyric acid A receptor in the rat nervous system. *J. Comp. Neurol.*, 365: 504–510.

Hanley, J.G., Koulen, P., Bedford, F., Gordon-Weeks P.R. and Moss, S. (1999) The protein MAP-1B links GABA$_C$ receptors to the cytoskeleton at retinal synapses. *Nature*, 397: 66–69.

Husi, H., Ward, M.A., Choudhary, J.S., Blackstock W.P. and Grant, S.G. (2000) Proteomic analysis of NMDA receptor-adhesion protein signaling complexes. *Nature Neurosci.*, 3: 661–669

Husi, H. and Grant, S.G. (2001) Proteomics of the nervous system. *Trends Neurosci.*, 24: 259–266.

Im, W.B., Pregenzer, J.F., Binder, J.A., Dillon, G.H. and Alberts, G.L. (1995) Chloride channel expression with the tandem construct of alpha 6-beta 2 GABAA receptor subunit requires a monomeric subunit of alpha 6 or gamma 2. *J. Biol. Chem.*, 270: 26063–26066.

Item, C. and Sieghart, W. (1994) Binding of GABA$_A$ receptors to tubulin. *J. Neurochem.*, 63: 1119–1125.

Jechlinger, M., Pelz, R., Tretter, V., Klausberger, T. and Sieghart, W. (1998) Subunit composition and quantitative importance of het-ero-oligomeric receptors: GABAA receptors containing alpha6 subunits. *J. Neurosci.*, 18: 2449–2457.

Jensen, K., Lambert, J.D.C. and Jensen, M.S. (1999) Activity-dependent depression of GABAergic IPSCs in cultured hippocampal neurons. *J. Neurophysiol.* 82: 42–49.

Kannenberg, K., Baur, R. and Sigel, E. (1997) Proteins associated with α1-subunit-containing GABA$_A$ receptors from bovine brain. *J. Neurochem.*, 68: 1352–1360.

Kannenberg, K., Sieghart, W. and Reuter, H. (1999) Clusters of GABAA receptors on cultured hippocampal cells correlate only partially with functional synapses. *Eur. J. Neurosci.*, 11: 1256–1264.

Khan, Z.U., Gutiérrez A. and De Blas, A.L. (1994a) Short and Long Form γ$_2$ Subunits of the GABA$_A$/Benzodiazepine Receptors. *J. Neurochem.*, 63: 1466–1476.

Khan, Z.U., Gutiérrez, A. and De Blas, A.L. (1994b) The Subunit Composition of a GABA$_A$/Benzodiazepine Receptor from Rat Cerebellum. *J. Neurochem.* 63: 371–374.

Khan, Z.U., Gutierrez, A. and De Blas, A.L. (1996) The alpha 1 and alpha 6 subunits can coexist in the same cerebellar GABAA receptor maintaining their individual benzodiazepine-binding specificities. *J. Neurochem.*, 66: 685–691.

Kirsch, J., Wolters, I., Triller A. and Betz, H. (1993) Gephyrin anti-sense oligonucleotides prevent glycine receptor clustering in spinal neurons. *Nature*, 366: 745–748.

Kirsch, J. Kuhse and Betz, H. (1995) Targeting of glycine receptor subunits to gephyrin-rich domains in transfected human embryonic kidney cells. *Mol. Cell Neurosci.*, 6: 450–461.

Kittler, J.T., Rostaing, P., Schiavo, G., Fritschy, J.M., Olsen, R., Triller, A. and Moss, S.J. (2001) The subcellular distribution of gabarap and its ability to interact with nsf suggest a role for this protein in the intracellular transport of gaba(a) receptors. *Mol. Cell Neurosci.*, 18: 13–25.

Kneussel, M., Bransdtatter, J.H., Laube, B., Stahl, S., Muller, U. and Betz, H. (1999) Loss of postsynaptic GABA(A) receptor clustering in gephyrin-deficient mice. *J. Neurosci.*, 19: 9289–9297.

Kneussel, M., and Betz, H. (2000) Clustering of inhibitory neurotransmitter receptors at developing postsynaptic sites: the membrane activation model. *Trends Neurosci.*, 23: 429–435.

Kneussel, M., Haverkamp, S., Fuhrmann, J.C., Wang, H., Wassle, H., Olsen, R.W. and Betz, H. (2000) The gamma-aminobutyric acid type A receptor (GABAAR)-associated protein GABARAP interacts with gephyrin but is not involved in receptor anchoring at the synapse. *Proc. Natl. Acad. Sci. USA*, 97: 8594–8599.

Kneussel, M., Helmut Brandstatter, J., Gasnier, B., Feng, G., Sanes J.R. and Betz, H. (2001) Gephyrin-independent clustering of postsynaptic gaba(a) receptor subtypes. *Mol Cell Neurosci.*, 2001 17: 973–982

Knuesel, I., Mastrocola, M., Zuellig, R.A., Bornhauser, B., Schaub M.C. and Fritschy, J.M. (1999) Short communication: altered synaptic clustering of GABA$_A$ receptors in mice lacking dystrophin (mdx mice). *Eur. J. Neurosci.*, 11: 4457–4462.

Knuesel, I., Zuellig, R.A., Schaub, M.C. and Fritschy, J.M. (2001) Alterations in dystrophin and utrophin expression parallel the reorganization of GABAergic synapses in a mouse model of temporal lobe epilepsy. *Eur. J. Neurosci.*, 13: 1113–1124.

Laurie, D.J., Seeburg, P.H. and Wisden, W. (1992) The distribution of 13 GABA$_A$ receptor subunit mRNAs in the rat brain II. Olfactory bulb and cerebellum. *J. Neurosci.*, 12: 1063–1076.

Levi, S., Chesnoy-Marchais, D., Sieghart, W. and Triller, A. (1999) Synaptic control of glycine and GABA(A) receptors and gephyrin expression in cultured motoneurons. *J. Neurosci.*, 19: 7434–7449.

Li, M. and De Blas, A.L. (1997) Coexistence of two beta subunit isoforms in the same gamma-aminobutyric acid type A receptor. *J. Biol. Chem.*, 272: 16564–16569.

Low, K., Crestani, F., Keist, R., Benke, D., Brunig, I., Benson, J.A., Fritschy, J.M., Rulicke, T., Bluethmann, H., Mohler, H. and Rudolph, U. (2000) Molecular and neuronal substrate for the selective attenuation of anxiety. *Science*, 290: 131–134.

McKernan, R.M. and Whiting, P.J. (1996) Which GABAA-receptor subtypes really occur in the brain? *Trends Neurosci.* 19: 139–143.

Mehta, A.K. and Ticku, M.K. (1999) An update on GABAA receptors. *Brain Res. Rev.*, 29: 196–217.

Miralles, C.P., Li, M., Mehta A.K., Kahn Z.U. and De Blas, A.L. (1999) Immunocytochemical localization of the beta(3) subunit of the gamma-aminobutyric acid(A) receptor in the rat brain. *J. Comp. Neurol.*, 413: 535–548.

Moreno, J.I., Piva, M.A., Miralles C.P. and De Blas, A.L. (1994) Immunocytochemical localization of the beta 2 subunit of the gamma-aminobutyric acidA receptor in the rat brain. *J. Comp. Neurol.*, 350: 260–271.

Moss, S.J. and Smart, T.G. (2001) Constructing inhibitory synapses. *Nat. Rev. Neurosci.*, 2: 240–250.

178

Nusser, Z., Sieghart W., Benke, D., Fritschy, J.M. and Somogyi, P. (1996a) Differential synaptic localization of two major gamma-aminobutyric acid type A receptor alpha subunits on hippocampal pyramidal cells. *Proc. Natl. Acad. Sci., USA* 93: 11939–11944.

Nusser, Z., Sieghart W., Stephenson F.A. and Somogyi, P. (1996b) The alpha 6 subunit of the GABAA receptor is concentrated in both inhibitory and excitatory synapses on cerebellar granule cells. *J. Neurosci.*, 16: 103–114

Nusser, Z. and Somogyi, P. (1997) Compartmentalized distribution of GABA$_A$ and glutamate receptors in relation to transmitter release sites on the surface of cerebellar neurons. *Prog. Brain Res.*, 114: 109–127.

Nusser, Z., Sieghart, W. and Somogyi, P. (1998) Segregation of different GABAA receptors to synaptic and extrasynaptic membranes of cerebellar granule cells. *J. Neurosci.*, 18: 1693–1703

Nyiri, G., Freund, T.F. and Somogyi, P. (2001) Input-dependent synaptic targeting of α_2-subunit-containing GABA$_A$ receptors in synapses of hippocampal pyramidal cells of the rat. *Eur. J. Neuroscience*, 13: 428–442.

Persohn, E., Malherbe, P., and Richards, J.G. (1992) Comparative molecular neuroatomy of cloned GABA$_A$ receptor subunits in the rat CNS. *J. Comp. Neurol.*, 326: 193–216.

Pirker, S., Schwarzer, C., Wieselthaler, A., Sieghart, W. and Sperk, G. (2000) GABA(A) receptors: immunocytochemical distribution of 13 subunits in the adult rat. *Neuroscience*, 101: 815–850.

Quirk, K., Whiting, P.J., Ragan, C.I. and McKernan, R.M. (1995) Characterisation of delta-subunit containing GABAA receptors from rat brain. *Eur. J. Pharmacol.*, 290: 175–181.

Rao, A., Cha, E.M. and Craig, A.M. (2000) Mismatched appositions of presynaptic and postsynaptic components in isolated hippocampal neurons. *J. Neurosci.*, 20: 8344–8353.

Richards, J.G., Schoch, P., Haring, P., Takacs, B. and Möhler, H. (1987) Resolving GABAA/benzodiazepine receptors: cellular and subcellular localization in the CNS with monoclonal antibodies. *J. Neurosci.*, 7: 1866–1886.

Rubio, M.E. and Wenthold, R.J. (1997) Glutamate receptors are selectively targeted to postsynaptic sites in neurons. *Neuron*, 18: 939–950

Rudolph, U., Crestani, F., Benke, D., Brunig, I., Benson J.A., Fritschy J.M., Martin J.R., Bluethmann, H. and Mohler, H. (1999) Benzodiazepine actions mediated by specific gamma-aminobutyric acid(A) receptor subtypes. *Nature*, 401: 796–800.

Sassoe-Pognetto, M., Kirsch, J., Grunert, U., Greferath, U., Fritschy. J.M., Mohler, H., Betz, H. and Wassle, H. (1995) Colocalization of gephyrin and GABA$_A$ receptor subunits in the rat retina. *J. Comp. Neurol.*, 357: 1–14.

Sassoe-Pognetto, M., Panzanelli, P., Sieghart, W. and Fritschy, J.M. (2000) Colocalization of multiple GABA(A) receptor subtypes with gephyrin at postsynaptic sites. *J. Comp. Neurol.*, 420: 481–498.

Scannevin, R.H. and Huganir, R.L. (2000) Postsynaptic organization and regulation of excitatory synapses. *Nat. Rev. Neurosci.*, 1: 133–141

Scheiffele, P., Fan, J., Choih, J., Fetter, R. and Serafini, T. (2000) Neuroligin expressed in nonneuronal cells triggers presynaptic development in contacting axons. *Cell*, 101: 657–669.

Scotti, A.L. and Reuter, H. (2001) Synaptic and extrasynaptic gamma-aminobutyric acid type A receptor clusters in rat hippocampal cultures during development. *Proc. Natl. Acad. Sci. USA*, 98: 3489–3494.

Segal, M.M. (1991) Epileptiform activity in microcultures containing one excitatory hippocampal neuron. *J. Neurophysiol.*, 65: 761–770.

Segal, M. and Barker, J.L. (1984) Rat hippocampal neurons in culture: Voltage clamp analysis of inhibitory synaptic connections, *J. Neurophysiol.*, 52: 469–487.

Shapiro, L., Fannon, A.M., Kwong, P.D., Thompson, A., Lehmann, M.S., Grubel, G., Legrand, J.F., Als-Nielsen, J., Colman DR and Hendrickson, W.A. (1995) Structural basis of cell-cell adhesion by cadherins. *Nature*, 374: 327–337.

Sheng, M. (2001) Molecular organization of the postsynaptic specialization. *Proc. Natl. Acad. Sci., USA.* 98: 7058–7061

Somogyi, P., Fritschy, J.M., Benke, D., Roberts, J.D.B. and Sieghart, W. (1996) The γ2 subunit of the GABA$_A$ receptor is concentrated in synaptic junctions containing the α1 and β2/3 subunits in hippocampus, cerebellum and globus pallidus. *Neuropharmacol.*, 35: 1425–1444.

Sperk, G., Schwarzer, C., Tsunashima, K., Fuch, K. and Sieghart, W. (1997) GABA$_A$ receptor subunits in the rat hippocampus immunocytochemical distribution of 13 subunits. *Neuroscience*, 80: 987–1000.

Tanaka, H, Shan, W., Phillips, G.R., Arndt, K., Bozdagi, O, Shapiro, L., Huntley, G.W., Benson, D.L. and Colman, D.R. (2000) Molecular modification of N-cadherin in response to synaptic activity. *Neuron.*, 25: 93–107.

Todd, A.J., Watt, C., Spike, R.C. and Sieghart, W. (1996) Colocalization of GABA$_A$, glycine and their receptors at synpses in the rat spinal cord. *J. Neurosci.*, 16: 974–982.

Torres, R., Firestein, B.L., Dong, H., Staudinger, J., Olson, E.N., Huganir, R.L., Bredt, D.S., Gale, N.W. and Yancopoulos, G.D. (1998) PDZ proteins bind, cluster, and synaptically colocalize with Eph receptors and their ephrin ligands. *Neuron.*, 21: 1453–1463.

Turner, J.D., Bodewitz, G., Thompson, C.L. and Stephenson, F.A. (1993) Immunohistochemical mapping of gamma-aminobutyric acid type-A receptor alpha subunits in rat central nervous system. *Psychopharmacol. Ser.*, 11: 29–49.

Vitorica, J., Park, D., Chin, G. and De Blas, A.L. (1988) Monoclonal antibodies and conventional antisera to the GABAA receptor/benzodiazepine receptor/Cl- channel complex. *J. Neurosci.*, 8: 615–622.

Walikonis, R.S., Jensen, O.N., Mann, M., Provance, D.W. Jr, Mercer, J.A. and Kennedy, M.B. (2000) Identification of proteins in the postsynaptic density fraction by mass spectrometry. *J. Neurosci.*, 20: 4069–4080.

Wang, H., Bedford, F.K., Brandon, N.J., Moss, S.J. and Olsen, R.W. (1999) GABA(A)-receptor-associated protein links GABA(A) receptors and the cytoskeleton. *Nature*, 397: 69–72.

Wang, H. and Olsen, R.W. (2000) Binding of the GABA(A) receptor-associated protein (GABARAP) to microtubules and microfilaments suggests involvement of the cytoskeleton in GABARAP/GABA(A) receptor interaction *J. Neurochem.*, 75: 644–655.

Whatley, V.J., Mihic, S.J., Allan, A.M., McQuilkin, S.J. and Harris, R.A. (1994) GABA$_A$ receptor function is inhibited by microtubule depolymerization. *J. Biol. Chem.*, 269: 19546–19552.

Wisden, W., Laurie, D.J., Monyer, H. and Seeburg, P.H. (1992) The distribution of 13 GABAA receptor subunit mRNAs in the rat brain. I. Telencephalon, diencephalon, mesencephalon. *J. Neurosci.*, 12(3): 1040–1062.

Whiting, P.J., Bonnert, T.P., McKernan, R.M., Farrar, S., Le Bourdelles, B., Heavens, R.P., Smith, D.W., Hewson, L.,

Rigby, M.R., Sirinathsinghji, D.J., Thompson, S.A. and Wafford, K.A. (1999) Molecular and functional diversity of the expanding GABA-A receptor gene family. *Ann. N. Y. Acad. Sci.*, 868: 645–653.

Wu, Q. and Maniatis, T. (1999) A striking organization of a large family of human neural cadherin-like cell adhesion genes. *Cell*, 97: 779–790.

Character and function of specific neurons

E.C. Azmitia, J. DeFelipe, E.G. Jones, P. Rakic and C.E. Ribak (Eds.)
Progress in Brain Research, Vol. 136

CHAPTER 14

Character and function of specific neurons: a Cajalian perspective

Pedro Pasik and Tauba Pasik*

Department of Neurology, Mount Sinai School of Medicine, New York, NY 10029, USA

Cajal remains the greatest neurohistologist of all times. The essence of this assertion, many times expressed in various forms, is based not only on the theoretical tenets of his interpretation of nervous system organization, but on the power of his observations on almost every single structure of both, the central and peripheral nervous systems. Having produced an annotated and edited translation of his *opera magna*, Texture of the Nervous System of Man and the Vertebrates (to be referred hereinafter as TNS), and being forced to go over it more than ten times from A to Z, we cannot feel but awe at the extent of his accomplishment. Is there any mystic element in this statement, that would therefore require a demystification for the further advancement of Neuroscience? We do not believe this to be the case, and the learned presentations at this gathering, and in particular, at the session which we had the honor to preside, bear to this negation.

The five contributions on the Characterization and Function of Specific Neurons are not strictly dealing with the purported theme of the meeting, namely *Changing Views of Cajal's Neuron*. Three of them represent invaluable *additions* to the foundations laid by Cajal in the fields of hippocampal circuitry (Freund) and cortical organization (DeFelipe, Goldman-Rakic—see section VI); the other two (Bennett, Vaney) are straight forward *challenges* to Cajal's more theoretical constructs.

Additions to Cajal's views

Freund moved forward our knowledge of hippocampal circuitry by single cell labeling combined with physiologic recordings and immuno-electronmicroscopy. The amount and quality of his work is indeed admirable in following the Lenhossék-Szentágothai-Somogyi tradition on information gathering and interpretation of exquisite neuroanatomical and neurophysiologic findings. Particularly exciting results derived from stereologic analysis leading to numerical estimates of input–output connectivity of both, pyramidal and short axon neurons, indicating very high degrees of convergence and divergence in the basic circuitry. Equally important are the findings from recordings of cell pairs, which allow us to define the role of different types of short axon cells. The chemical identification of neurons containing various neuroactive substances and calcium-binding proteins together with modern tracing methods, confirm to a great extent Cajal's views on the target selectivity of particular cell types in various regions. Finally, Freund reviewed his fascinating findings of the possible global modulatory role of non-synaptic mediators, and particularly the differential modulation of GABAergic transmission by endocannabinoids and acetylcholine.

Some of Freund's opinions on Cajal's work require, in our view, certain corrections. Regarding the output of the hippocampal circuitry, there is no error in his classic diagram, originally published in 1901 (Cajal, 1901). The plane of section did not allow him to record a more accurate description. Careful reading of the texts

*Corresponding author: Tel.: (+1) 212 241 7071;
Fax: (+1) 212 722 3223; E-mail: pedro@pasik.net

(Cajal, 1893, 1901) indicate that the hippocampal efferents taking the fimbria route to reach the septum correspond to axons of pyramidal cells of the *regio inferior* (~CA3-4), whereas those of the *regio superior* (~CA1-2) have both, collateral and terminal branches ramifying in the plexi of the strata oriens, radiatum and lacunosum (Cajal, 1901). Moreover, some of these axons can be traced to the "*vicinity of the subiculum where they end in free ramifications that cover an extensive area of the cortex*" (Cajal, 1893). And again: "*By these means, the axons of small pyramidal cells of the* regio superior *of the horn are related to the pyramidal cells of the adjoining cerebral cortex, namely the subiculum and sometimes part of the occipital region*" (Cajal, 1893). Here the occipital region corresponds to what is presently known as the medial entorhinal cortex.

The assertion that inhibition was not considered at all by Cajal has been repeated many times. It is true that Cajal was puzzled by the possible role of short axon cells (see DeFelipe, this volume), and that at some point he expressed "the difficulty in understanding how an impulse suppresses another impulse" (TNS Vol. I, p. 481). However, in addition to referring several times to the inhibition of reflexes, he even considered at the cellular level, the existence of inhibitory neurons mediating vasodilation (TNS Vol. I, p. 432), the possible action of retinal centrifugal fibers "*inhibiting perhaps the impulse strength at the axodendritic junction*" (TNS Vol. I, p. 536), and that "*corticothalamic connections may influence to define territories of the sensory field either inhibiting or exciting cutaneous impulses*" (TNS Vol. III, in press).

Finally, Cajal was far from considering the brain as a hard-wired network. In fact, regarding theories of brain function he states: "*The determination of the series of molecular processes occurring in neurons during intellectual activity, ... requires precise ideas about those extremely complex changes of connections and commutations which must precede each dynamic, associative, emotional or motor variation*" (TNS Vol. III, in press). Furthermore, on his own theory on the growth of neuronal connections as a means to refinement of mental processes, he discusses the possibility of coupling and uncoupling of neuronal junctions (the term synapses had not yet been invented) through ameboid movements particularly of axon terminals, retraction of spines, changes due to exercise, learning, sleep, etc., all examples of neuronal plasticity (TNS Vol. III, in press).

DeFelipe gave a brilliant characterization of short axon cells in the cerebral cortex in the best Cajalian tradition, to which he added the differential input of the various morphologic types to specific regions of the pyramidal cell. Moreover, the nature of short axon cells was defined in terms of their neuroactive substances and calcium-binding properties, and their approximate location in some cortical microcircuits. His discovery that chandelier cells are immunoreactive to parvalbumin further characterized this singular short axon cell, in fact the only type that escaped Cajal's observational powers. The chandelier cell was first described and named by a most distinguished Cajalian of our times, the late János (John) Szentágothai, who actually followed in Cajal's steps by producing a sequence of fundamental studies on the spinal cord, brain stem, hypothalamus, cerebellum, thalamus, and cerebral cortex. In the progression of his studies, he skipped over the basal ganglia as Cajal almost did (only 13 pages in TNS). His studies of the cerebral cortex produced the concept of microcircuits within cortical modules, in addition to the discovery of the chandelier cell (for a partial account see Szentágothai, 1974).

DeFelipe correctly points out that there is some confusion in the naming of cortical short axon cells. Of particular concern are the references to those that Cajal called "*bipenachadas*" and described as showing tufts of bipolar dendrites as well as ascending and descending axonal branches, the correct English translation being "bitufted." The problem originated in Azoulay's French translation of TNS as "*cellule à double bouquet dendritique*," which became in English simply "double bouquet cell." Why Azoulay chose this awkward designation, we do not know. He had correctly translated Cajal's "*empenachadas*" of the olfactory bulb as "*à panache*" or "*à houpette*", which translated into English as "tufted," and that is how this type of olfactory bulb neuron is designated. The problem apparently continues. DeFelipe names all of those cells which show bipolar dendritic tufts, bitufted cells, but retains the designation of "double bouquet" for neurons with tight bundles of ascending and descending axonal branches, although the original French referred obviously to dendritic morphology. Therefore, DeFelipe refers to a short axon cell type that is at the same time double bouquet *and* bitufted, another that is chandelier *and* bitufted, and yet another that is a Martinotti cell *and* bitufted. We hope that with this paragraph we have not contributed to the confusion and welcome DeFelipe's typology once the preceding discussion is taken into account.

Goldman-Rakic (see Section VI) recast Cajal's psychic cell concept, originally stated as: "*Because of* [the] *constant orientation and shape of the cerebral pyramidal cell, as well as its high hierarchical activity, we have dared to designate it as the* psychic cell" (Cajal, 1892, 1895), using electrophysiologic recordings from cells in the prefrontal cortex of behaving monkeys. She reviewed the work in her laboratory showing through very elegant behavioral paradigms, that the dorsolateral cortex contains differential microcircuits responding to visuo-spatial, object and auditory memory cues in the superior, postero-inferior, and antero-inferior regions, respectively. Moreover, dual-cell recordings in ferret brain slices defined two types of pyramidal-nonpyramidal microcircuits, and it was proposed that they are responsible for differential isodirectional and cross-directional inhibitory processes. We, of course, have come a long way since deficits in delayed response tests were shown in nonhuman primates after prefrontal decortications, as reviewed by Goldman-Rakic. Reminiscing about the subject, it was initially argued that it was difficult to attribute a particular function to a cortical area on the basis of lesion studies when such function was not adequately defined. Advances in Cognitive Psychology suggest such a definition as "working memory," and her results support this view. Although we seem to be on the way to understanding human cognition or in Cajal's words the "*completion of the Neurology edifice*" much earlier than his prediction of several centuries (TNS Vol. I, p. 18), we consider it somewhat premature to attribute a specific gnostic function to any cortical region as suggested in Goldman-Rakic's legend of Fig. 4. The concept of agnosia, as originally formulated by Freud (1891), is a modality-specific deficit in recognition, in the absence of dementia and of sensory alterations. Careful examination of patients with so-called visual agnosia, for example visual object agnosia including prosopagnosia, have failed to reveal intact sensorium (Teuber et al., 1960). To our knowledge no verified cases of prosopagnosia have been reported since that thorough study, without concomitant alterations in the visual fields, not necessarily in terms of anopsias, but of fluctuating thresholds, changes in perception of size, depth and motion, reduced critical flicker fusion, and abnormalities in the performance of the hidden-figure test.

Challenges to Cajal's views

The existence of electrical synapses, as well as dendro-dendritic, dendrosomatic and axoaxonic chemical synapses, even in the mammalian nervous system is by now beyond doubt. And so is the possibility of dendritic conduction away from the axon. Are these realities actual challenges to Cajal's tenets? The two remaining chapters in this section are indeed addressing this question.

Bennett's functional and structural characterization of electrical synapses is already a classic (Bennett et al., 1963). The controversy between reticularism and neuronism almost parallels that of the means of interneuronal communication. Electrical transmission favors reticularism, whereas chemical transmission prefers neuronism. It is not surprising that the champion of electrical synapses adopts a reticularist perspective. His neoreticularist view, or better yet neo-neoreticularist, has of course nothing to do with the original reticularism of Gerlach and Golgi, who claimed the existence of anastomoses between neuronal processes, or the neoreticularism of the Apáthy-Bethe-Held type, who called for the contemporarily discovered neurofibrils to cross over from one to another neuron, and even to glial cells. As Bennett points out, it is by now clear that the continuity between certain neurons of his favorite experimental animal, the Mormyrid fish, is only apparent, because in fact there are membranes separating them, in addition to gap junctions. [As an aside, the existence of the neuronal membrane, a requirement of neuronism, was amply shown by Cajal, who offered at least five findings to support it (TNS Vol. I, pp. 123–126), and eventually it was confirmed by electron microscopy]. Furthermore, the molecular structure of at least one gap junction suggests an end-to-end docking of precisely aligned oligomeres belonging to the membrane of each cell, thus contributing to form a pore (Unger et al., 1999), which is permeable to ions and small molecules, including ATP and second messengers as inositol triphosphate. Such structural arrangements together with some synaptic characteristics of the gap junction including its gating behavior, and the fact that macromolecules such as those that determine the genetic differences between cells remain locked within the individual cell, place significant limitations to the neo-neoreticularist view, and do not strain much the neuron theory.

Regarding the synchrony of activity of neuronal groups apparently mediated by gap junctions, it is interesting that it was not conceptually unknown to Cajal, who referred frequently to "isodynamic groups," i.e. sets of neurons reacting together. Thus, he mentioned their occurrence in the ventral cochlear nucleus (TNS Vol. II, p. 165), cerebellar cortex (TNS Vol. II, p. 362,), superior colliculus and optic lobe (TNS Vol. II, p. 536), and thalamus (TNS Vol. III, in press). Finally, the unity of visual space perception would require that each sensory afferent axon contributes a specific spatial sign, and be in constant relationship with a single isodynamic group of cortical pyramidal cells. A similar reasoning applies to the unity of other sense modalities (TNS Vol III, in press). Of course, Cajal envisioned the neurons of isodynamic groups as joined by short connections in keeping with the neuron theory.

In view of Bennett's opinion that, although chemical synapses are the most numerous, gap junctions have come to represent a "respectable" minority, it is appropriate to quote one of Cajal's last statements: "[we] *insist now that regarding neuronal morphology and connections, we must adhere to the law of large numbers, i.e. to a rigorous statistical criterion*" (Cajal, 1933). The need for quantification is obvious but difficult because numbers may vary under different physiologic conditions.

Concerning the intrinsic functional polarization of the neuron, Cajal's ideas, as in most instances, evolved in trying to incorporate his ever increasing amount of observations. Thus, the so-called law of dynamic polarization (Cajal, 1891) gave way to the law of axipetal polarization which included the possibility of propagation of the nerve impulse from the soma to the dendrite, as it occurs in the case of the axon originating from a dendrite at a considerable distance from the soma. Similarly, as Bennett points out, the unidirectionality of propagation gave way to bidirectionality under certain conditions. The initial naming of the peripheral process of spinal ganglion cells as a dendrite was a purely semantic issue in trying to strictly follow the neuron theory, so much so that Cajal conceived the nerve impulse as propagating along such a peripheral process and continuing through the central process to the spinal cord, with no major invasion of the cell body (TNS Vol. I, p. 122). This view is supported by contemporary findings.

Cajal initially considered the possible existence of dendrodendritic articulations as interdendritic dynamic communications, but just limited to a colony of neurons which would exhibit a certain functional solidarity comparable to that of a battery of electric cells. However, he soon discarded the idea, becoming convinced that they are very rare and probably lack an important physiologic significance (TNS Vol. I, p. 71). This view has been superceded by their electron microscopic confirmation in various structures, where they give rise to complex synaptic arrangements of the triadic, serial and reciprocal types. In addition, there is clear evidence of impulse initiation in various regions of the neuron and consequent propagation in all directions within a cell. Furthermore, small parts of a neuron may function as almost independent units, so that a functional unit may be a restricted portion of a neuron, the whole neuron, a set of neurons, or the entire nervous system. We remain, therefore, with the idea that apparent deviations from Cajal's tenets may reflect the co-existence of different organizational planes, as summarized by Shepherd when stating that the neuron "*contains several levels of local subunits, and is itself a part of a larger multineuronal unit*" (Shepherd, 1991, p. 291).

Vaney's scholarly survey of retinal cytology and his own studies on the further characterization and distribution of multiple types of amacrine cells provide a comprehensive view of retinal organization. The most dramatic aspect of his work is the demonstration of neuronal couplings, both homologous (between amacrines or ganglion cells) as well as heterologous (between ganglion and amacrine cells). The coupling occurs presumably through gap junctions which allow the passage of small cationic tracers. He concludes that these results have much in common with Dogiel's model of the retina, which included the existence of neuronal colonies formed by dendritic anastomoses, particularly of ganglion cells. However, Vaney considers such a view not as a challenge to Cajal's conclusion that the retina is composed of discrete cells that communicate by contact, and this is indeed puzzling. Most of our comments regarding the challenges to Cajal's neuronism have been exhausted on discussing Bennett's presentation, and to a great extent they apply to Vaney's, so that the meagerness of this last paragraph should not be taken as assigning less importance to this formidable article.

In reviewing the preceding discussion, we feel that there is general agreement regarding Cajal's fundamental legacy. It is time now to end the attacks and defenses of his tenets, and proceed instead without such distractions to accumulate new facts with the marvelous techniques at hand and those to come in the near future, much earlier indeed than Cajal ever imagined.

References

Bennett, M.V.L., Aljure, G., Nakajima, Y. and Pappas, G.D. (1963) Electrotonic junctions between teleost spinal neurons: electrophysiology and ultrastructure. *Science*, 141: 262–264.

Cajal, S.R. (1892) Nuevo concepto de la histología de los centros nerviosos. *Rev Cien Méd Barcelona*, 18: 457–476.

Cajal, S.R. (1893) Estructura del asta de Ammon y fascia dentata. *An. Soc. Españ. Hist. Nat.*, 22: 53–114.

Cajal, S.R. (1895) *Les Nouvelles Idées sur la Structure du Sytème Nerveux chez l'Homme et les Vertébrés. Translation by L. Azoulay*, Reinwald, Paris, 200pp.

Cajal, S.R. (1899–1911) *Texture of the Nervous System of Man and the Vertebrates. Annotated and edited translation by P. Pasik and T. Pasik*, Springer, Wien, New York, Barcelona. Vol. I (1999) 631pp., Vol. II (2000) 666pp., Vol. III (2002) in press.

Cajal, S.R. (1901) Estudios sobre la corteza humana. IV. Estructura de la corteza cerebral olfativa del hombre y mamíferos. *Trab. Lab. Inv. Biol. Univ. Madrid*, 1: 1–140.

Cajal, S.R. (1933) ¿Neuronismo o Reticularismo? Las pruebas objetivas de la unidad anatómica de las células nerviosas. *Arch. Neurobiol.*, 13: 1–144.

Freud, S. (1891) *Zur Auffassung der Aphasien; eine kritische Studie.* Deuticke, Leipzig, 107pp.

Shepherd, G. (1991) *Foundations of the Neuron Doctrine.* Oxford University Press, Oxford, New York, 338pp.

Szentágothai, J. (1974) From the last skirmishes around the neuron theory to the functional anatomy of neuron networks. In: F.G. Worden, J.P. Swazey and G. Adelman (Eds.), *The Neurosciences: Paths of Discovery.* MIT Press, Cambridge, MA, pp. 103–120.

Teuber, H.-L., Battersby, W.S. and Bender, M.B. (1960) *Visual Field Defects after Penetrating Missile Wounds of the Brain*, Harvard University Press, Cambrige, MA, 142pp.

Unger, V.M., Kumar, N.M., Gilula, N.B. and Yeager, M. (1999) Three-dimensional structure of a recombinant gap junction membrane channel. *Science*, 283: 1176–1180.

E.C. Azmitia, J. DeFelipe, E.G. Jones, P. Rakic and C.E. Ribak (Eds.)
Progress in Brain Research, Vol. 136

CHAPTER 15

Neoreticularism and neuronal polarization

Michael V.L. Bennett*

Department of Neuroscience, Albert Einstein College of Medicine, 1300 Morris Park Avenue, Bronx, NY 10804, USA

Abstract: Santiago Ramón y Cajal made immense contributions to neuroscience, and the era in which his work is cited is likely to be longer than that for any other present or future neuroscientist. This commentary notes that there is qualification to the doctrine that neurons are distinct entities rather than reticular. Namely, gap junctions provide a private pathway between coupled cells that, at an ultramicroscopic scale, can be considered cytoplasmic continuity. Cytoplasmic continuity permits, but does not require, conduction in either direction across an electrical synapse. Furthermore, sites of impulse initiation can differ in the same or different cells; there is no *universal* direction of impulse propagation and it may differ in the same cell under different conditions; thus, there are exceptions to the law of "dynamic polarization". Cajal leaves ample evidence in his writings that he would have no difficulty in accepting these very minor modifications to the vast body of his contributions.

Introduction

Santiago Ramón y Cajal, or more commonly just Cajal, can arguably be considered the Watson and Crick of neuroscience. He was the real founder of the modern study of nervous systems. His descriptions were generally accurate, and he left an immense corpus of knowledge that is unchanging. His illustrations are esthetically pleasing, and they are still often used in introductions to symposia and seminars. I doubt that the work of any physiologist has had or will have as long a scientific "life" as the contributions of Cajal. In part, this longevity is due to the superb maps of the nervous system that he left us, and the geography that he discovered has changed but little. His physiological insights were phenomenal, and he clearly thought function when he looked at structure. However, several of his functional and structural concepts require updating. I will address two of them, the cellular basis of the nervous system as reviewed in his seminal work *¿Neuronismo o Reticularismo?* and the doctrine of dynamic polarization.

---
*Corresponding author: Tel.: 718 430 2536; Fax: 718 430 8944;
E-mail: mbennett@aecom.yu.edu

Neuronismo

The doctrine that neurons were distinct cells had as its opponent principle, reticularism, which held that neurons were syncytial. Cajal obtained a vast amount of data in support of "neuronism", and it is one of the nice ironies of science that one of his most important tools was the Golgi method invented by the foremost proponent of reticularism. Nevertheless, until the invention of the electron microscope, it would have been possible to argue that many of Cajal's synapses and other contacts between neurons might in fact involve cytoplasmic continuity. Some invertebrate neurons, such as the squid giant axons and some annelid septate axons are syncytial and are formed by fusion of distinct cells (as opposed to being multinucleate and formed by nuclear division within a single cell). Some vertebrate neurons seem to show cytoplasmic continuity, for example, neurons controlling the electric organ in Mormyrid fishes (Fig. 1A). These neurons have contacts between thick dendrites that can appear to provide continuity, but electron microscopy demonstrates membranes between them, and of course gap junctions (Fig. 1B).

Neuronism requires tranmission between cells, which Cajal asserted was by "*contact or contiguity, not*

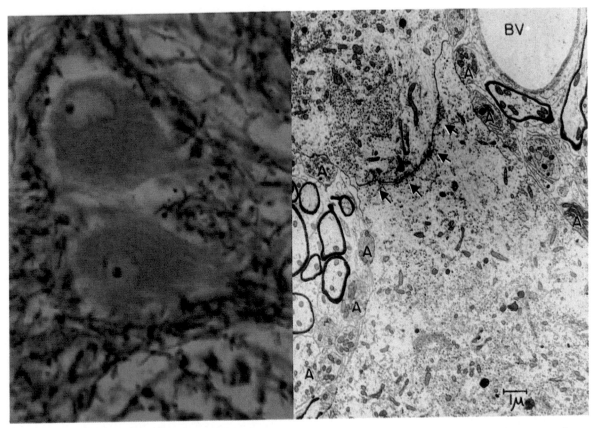

Fig. 1. Anastomoses between thick dendrites? Dendrodendritic connection between medullary electromotor relay neurons from a Mormyrid fish. The apparent cytoplasmic continuity seen in the (Cajal's) silver stained preparation (left panel) is shown by electron microscopy to be interrupted by a membrane containing gap junctions (right panel, arrows). A, axon terminals on the neurons. BV, blood vessel. From Bennett et al. (1967).

continuity". Electron microscopy establishes without doubt that chemically transmitting synapses involve a synaptic cleft and that there is no cytoplasmic continuity. Here of course we depend on our evidence that the cell membrane is a barrier that delimits the cytoplasm, a view not quite universally held. Moreover, there are proteins that extend into the synaptic gap and link the adjoining cells; thus, where one cell ends and the other begins can now be answered, no, requires an answer, at the molecular level.

The electrically transmitting synapses formed by gap junctions (Fig. 2A) provide a significant qualification to neuronism, since they provide cytoplasmic continuity for small molecules of the order of 1 kDa in molecular mass. (This is a rather soft number and depends on shape and charge as well as type of gap junction.) The continuity at the gap junction is not seen in thin sections with electron microscopy, but is inferred from electrical properties and intercellular movement of small molecules to which the non-junctional membranes are impermeable, as typified by dye coupling. The tracers that pass between cells do not enter when applied externally, and thus the passage between cells can be characterized as a private pathway, or, for small molecules, a region of cytoplasmic continuity (Fig. 2B). Some might bridle at calling a pathway with a diameter of 1.2 nm as cytoplasmic continuity. Still, frank cytoplasmic bridges may be impermeable to nuclei or mitochondria, and where does one draw the line? A common characterization of electrically coupled cells is that they form an electrical or functional syncytium, a reasonable characterization that preserves the basic tenet of neuronism that neurons are independent. The molecular subunits of gap junctions, the connexins, have been cloned and localized to gap junctions at light and electron microscopic levels (Fig. 2C, D).

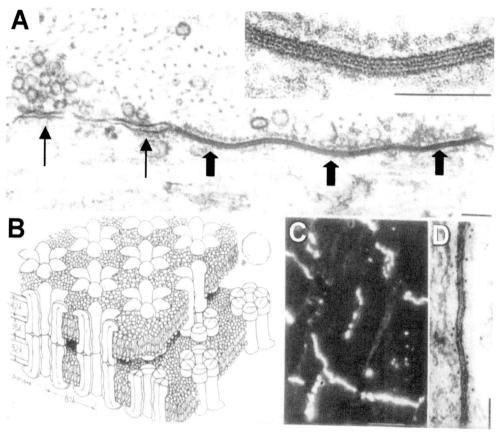

Fig. 2. Microscopy of electrical synapses. (**A**) An axodendritic synapse, axon to the top. A large gap junction, enlarged in the inset, is on the right of the image (wide arrows). Small active zones with presynaptic vesicles are on the left (narrow arrows). (**B**) A diagram of a gap junction showing the aqueous channel between cells (by D.L.D. Caspar and D.A. Goodenough). (**C**) An anti-connexin 43 antibody (with fluoresceinated secondary antibody) labels the intercalated disc of heart. (**D**) The same antibody with an immunogold secondary antibody shows localization to a gap junction at much higher resolution. (From Bennett et al., 1967).

Although the intercellular channels of gap junctions are not resolved by current techniques of preparation of tissue for thin sectioning, structures crossing the eponymous gap are seen by negative staining with extracellular markers. These stains often also label the central part of the gap junction molecule where the channel is presumed to be. This labeling occurs in cells that have not been deliberately permeabilized, suggesting that the membrane integrity is not as perfect as one might suppose from the lack of cytoplasmic staining. Freeze fracture electron microscopy of gap junctions often reveals a central pit in the intramembrane particles, which are generally in the P face in vertebrate junctions. A corresponding projection may be seen in the E face pits, although this structure is very sensitive to warming before shadowing, perhaps because it is ice. The most convincing images of gap junction channels are provided in reconstructed images from isolated gap junctions in which the channels can assume a two dimensional crystalline array (Unger et al., 1999).

Gap junctions are generally electrically linear for small transjunctional voltages, consistent with an aqueous pathway. This property facilitated the view of gap junctions as providing cytoplasmic continuity. Recent studies demonstrate that most gap junctions in fact are not electrically linear for larger voltages, and show gating behavior comparable to that of the classical voltage dependent channels of excitable membrane. (Here classical is relatively recent compared to Cajal's contributions. Hodgkin and Huxley propounded their equations in 1952, work still occasionally referenced, and single channel gating was demonstrated by Neher and Sakmann and colleagues in the late 1970's). Gap junctions may also show gating in response to various drugs and ions, properties in common with the channels of (electrically) excitable membrane. In addition to gating in response to various stimuli, gap junctions can exhibit selective permeability on the basis of charge as well as size (Verselis and Veenstra, 2000; Niessen et al., 2000).

Although electron microscopy has greatly refined our view of synapses, there remain important aspects that are not yet resolvable. In the early days of describing electrical transmission and identifying the morphological substrate as gap junctions, it became apparent that axosomatic and axodendritic synapses with gap junctions were for the most part "mixed", i.e., there were both gap junctions and apparent chemical synapses that had presynaptic active zones with associated vesicles, widening of the synaptic gap, and increased density of the postsynaptic membrane (Fig. 2A, narrow arrows; cf. Bennett, 1997; George Pappas, Yasuko Nakajiima, and later Konrad Akert and Clara Sandri were my anatomical collaborators in characterizing electrical synapses.) Yet these synapses transmitted entirely electrically; no chemical component could be identified in the postsynaptic potential, and they were more accurately described as "morphologically mixed". The missing chemical component in these synapses was not identified; it could have been in the synthesis of transmitter, in the release process or in the postsynaptic receptors. Since horseradish peroxidase was taken up by the presynaptic elements in several of these systems (Tokunaga et al., 1980; Bennett and Sandri, 1989), we suggested that the synapses were there to provide by membrane recycling uptake of molecules from the intercellular cleft for retrograde transport to the cell soma. Recently, it has been shown that at one site of morphologically mixed but purely electrical transmission, the postsynaptic cells lack glutamate receptors (Curti et al., 1999). Another and perhaps more damaging blow to prospects for morphological evaluation of synaptic efficacy is the presence of presynaptically silent synapses (Malgaroli et al., 1995; Malgaroli, 1999). These synapses look to be morphologically unexceptional chemical synapses, but apparently do not recycle membrane when their nerve fibers are activated. Constantino Sotelo also looked at many synapses with anatomical correlates of both chemical and electrical transmission. In one paper which we coauthored with Henri Korn

(Korn et al., 1977), the electrophysiological evidence was consistent with dual electrical and chemical transmission, but I persuaded him to leave the "morphologically" modifying the description of the synapses as mixed.

From a personal, neoreticularist perspective, I could at this point in the development of our knowledge feel somewhat superior to the devotee of chemical transmission, who could not rely on microscopy to identify a functional chemical synapse. This complacency was recently shattered by observations that gap junctions formed of connexins labeled with green fluorescent protein have no functional channels if they contain fewer than several hundred channels, and this measurement is made with single channel resolution (Bukauskas et al., 2000). As the number of associated particles in a junctional plaque increases, the fraction of functional channels increases, but never becomes greater than about 10–15%. An earlier report suggested that only about 1% of gap junction channels were functional at the club endings on the Mauthner cell (Tuttle et al., 1986). Although these synapses can transmit both chemically and electrically, the postsynaptic potentials often have no chemical component until potentiated (Lin and Faber, 1988). However, the chemical component can be increased by potentiation or by increasing the size of the afferent volley, apparently as a result of "antidromic" electrotonic spread of the electrical postsynaptic potential into the presynaptic fibers (Faber et al., 1991).

How would Cajal react to the existence of gap junctions? He wrote (Purkiss' and Fox's translation) "…[I]n accepting the most exaggerated syncytial hypotheses … everything that the physiologists, during 50 years of dogged and fruitful investigation, have taught us concerning localizations in the nervous centers is left without an explanation." But on the next page "I am neither exclusive nor dogmatic, I am proud of retaining a mental flexibility which is not afraid of corrections. Neuronal discontinuity … could sustain some exceptions."

Cajal was not aware of the synchrony that characterizes the activity of a number of groups of neurons. If so, he might have been more careful in asserting "localizations in the nervous centers". In a number of cases of synchronous firing, reticularism mediated by electrical continuity at gap junctions explains the synchronization (Bennett, 2000a,b). To be sure, mutual excitation can be mediated by chemical as well as by electrical transmission.

I have little doubt that Cajal, and also Sherrington, would have accepted axosomatic, axodendritic, and even dendrodendritic sites of electrical transmission as true synapses, whether they also transmitted chemically (and whether they transmitted in one or both directons, see next section). It is because of more recent history that many neuroscientists have had difficulty accepting that transmission might be of this form; indeed to this day, some do not consider gap junction based communication between neurons as synaptic. One source of this attitude is Occam's razor, which has nicked a number of prominent scientists when they assumed that the simplest answer must be the right one, ignoring that comparative physiology has demonstrated repeatedly that evolution finds multiple solutions to a given functional need (Bennett, 1985). Thus, when the controversy between electrical and chemical transmission was being resolved in most people's minds on the side of chemical transmission, it reduced their cognitive dissonance to define the newly discovered electrically transmitting contacts between neurons as non-synaptic. An outstanding exception was Paul Fatt, who pointed out in *Physiological Reviews* (1954) that there were synapses where electrical transmission was likely to be present. His prognosis, from a pioneer in demonstrating that inhibition was chemically mediated and who worked at the fountainhead of modern views of quantal transmission, was put forth when chemical transmission was clearly moving ahead of electrical transmission in the race for acceptance. Fatt hypothesized that a large presynaptic structure was required to excite a large postsynaptic structure, and he pointed to the giant motor synapse of the crayfish as satisfying that criterion. His suggestion bore fruit when Furshpan and Potter (1959) demonstrated that transmission at this site is electrical (and as an added bonus, rectifying).

Fatt's argument was not valid. Although he may have been inspired by the vertebrate neuromuscular synapse at which a small diameter presynaptic terminal excites a large postsynaptic cell, most chemical synapses do not simply relay an impulse from pre- to postsynaptic cell, and those that do have a large presynaptic terminal, e.g., the calyces of Held. The chick ciliary ganglion is another example where the presynaptic terminal is large, but in this case transmission is chemical in early development and becomes increasingly electrical in later life (Martin and Pilar, 1963). Whether the machinery of chemical transmission is lost is unclear; the terminal and cell become enveloped in myelin and inaccessible for microelectrode investigation; rapid transmission through the ganglion indicates that postsynaptic impulses are generated by

electrical transmission, but do not exclude the continued presence of a chemical component. To belabor the point: the actual interface at neuromuscular junctions is quite extensive, as the presynaptic fiber runs some distance along the fiber or branches profusely. Furthermore, the conductance of membranes is well correlated not with their areas but with the number of channels, and the conductance per unit area of activated postsynaptic membrane at chemical synapses is comparable to that of gap junctions and of nodal membrane of myelinated fibers, and the driving force of the presynaptic action potential is somewhat greater than that of the ligand gated channels; thus, a presynaptic terminal transmitting electrically can provide as much power as one transmitting electrically. To put a more modern face on it, the conductances of gap junction channels and of ligand gated channels can be comparable. Amplification from pre- to postsynaptic cell can be provided by ligand gated channels or by presynaptic action potentials.

Another reason for rejecting gap junctions as synapses arises from the view that synapses must exhibit unidirectional action, an attitude probably dating back to the time of Bell and Magendie and supported by Cajal's evidence for dynamic polarization of neurons, as discussed below. Stimulate fibers leading into or out of a nucleus, and impulses go in only one direction. Gap junctions are basically reciprocal, although a few are rectifying. Thus, if a connection between cells conducts impulses in both directions, it can't be a synapse. This argument to me is comparable to maintaining that if transmission is electrical, it can't be synaptic. Furthermore, most synapses generate small postsynaptic potentials; impulses in general do not propagate through nuclei, and signals are transformed by both divergence and convergence (as Cajal well knew). We now know of many specialized contacts between neurons that transmit reciprocally, by both chemical and electrical means, and there is even retrograde transmission at certain chemical synapses (e.g., Hawkins et al., 1998; Wilson and Nicoll, 2001). No one is arguing that these are not synapses, although the modes of retrograde transmission remain controversial.

Let me finally state here what I view to be the only defensible definition of a synapse. A synapse is a morphologically or molecularly specialized site of functional interaction between neurons or between neurons and other cells. (I specify molecularly specialized so as not to exclude possible cases where electron microscopy does not yet demonstrate differences in membrane properties.) Generally, a synapse must have a close physical approximation between the interacting cells. For chemical transmission we allow the existence of paracrine chemical transmission, where the secreting cell is somewhat separated from the sensing cell, and differentiate that from synaptic transmission. In extreme separation the transmission becomes endocrine, although between frank endocrine glands and paracrine varicosities, there are portal circulations. With respect to electrical transmission, gap junctions between neurons are unquestionably synaptic, and I am confident than Cajal and Sherrington would agree with me as would Eccles and Katz. There are also field effects without apparent morphological specialization, and one could consider these the equivalent of paracrine actions. An in between case is provided by close apposition of somata or dendrites without intervening glia. The absence of glia is a specialization compared to most other regions of the nervous system, and evidently there is some electrical interaction (Vigmond et al., 1997). Is the absence of glia enough to make these contacts synapses? Do we know whether there are specializations in the apposed membranes that make electrical interactions stronger?

In a discussion of electrical synapses, a small divergence from questions of reticularism might be permitted. [I follow the Master, Cajal; there are numerous digressions in *Recuerdos de mi Vida (1923)*.] There are electrically transmitting inhibitory synapses at the axon hillock of the Mauthner cell as described by Furukawa and Furshpan (1963), and subsequently Korn and Axelrad (1980) demonstrated a similar mechanism at basket cell synapses on the initial segment of Purkinje cells. The synapses have specializations of the associated glial cells resembling septate desmosomes and probably formed of homologous proteins. Transmission at the Mauthner cell inhibitory synapse is reciprocal (Korn and Faber, 1975), although the physiological meaning, if any, of the inhibition from Mauthner cell to inhibitory neuron has not been established. The highly specialized structures mediating the interaction unquestionably qualify them as synapses, by the above definition. The lack of close appositions between pre- and postsynaptic cells is required by their function and should not disqualify them as synapses; comparable widening of the intercellular cleft occurs at chemical synapses to reduce access resistance.

Although most gap junctions act as linear resistors under physiological conditions, electrical synapses need not conduct impulses in both directions because of low conductance, impedance mismatch or rectification (Bennett, 1966; Verselis and Veenstra, 2000). Thus, the older argument excluding electrical transmission on the basis of the doctrine of dynamic polarization is not valid. Pools of coupled neurons may also have sites of impulse initiation in different neurons and activity can then spread in all directions through the coupled network.

The recent discovery of neuron-specific connexins brings a currency to the topic of Cajal's views of "the neuron" (Condorelli et al., 1998; Teubner et al., 2001). He was a great general as well as comparative anatomist with uncommon physiological intuition. He would have been very interested in gap junctions and what they do.

In conclusion for this section, it has become clear that chemical transmission is the most common modality at synapses. However, the number of known electrical synapses is increasing, and they can be thought of as a respectable minority performing important roles in the operation of nervous systems, generally physiological but sometimes pathological. Although electrical synapses were thought to be primitive, molecular evolution suggests that they were later evolving than chemical synapses (cf. Bennett, 2000b). They are found not only in lower vertebrates, but in the neocortex of mammals (Fig. 3).

Dynamic polarization

In 1891 Cajal published:

> The transmission of the nervous impulse is always from the dendritic branches and the cell body to the axon or functional process. Every neuron, then, possesses a receptor apparatus, the body and the dendritic prolongations, an apparatus of emission, the axon, and an apparatus of distribution, the terminal arborization of the nerve fibers. I designated the foregoing principle: the theory of dynamic polarization. (*Recuerdos de mi Vida*, hereafter RdmV, p. 389)

Many of Cajal's drawings show little arrows indicating excitation flowing along dendrites toward the cell body. The primary evidence came from sensory inputs, where the activity indisputably came from the periphery (Fig. 4), but it was natural to extend the concept to neurons in other sites including the neocortex (Fig. 5). The general implication remains accurate, but in most neurons impulses arise in the cell body and propagate back out the dendrites. That impulses in mammalian neurons arise in the initial segment and from there invade the soma dendritic complex was first shown for spinal motoneurons of the cat (Coombs et al.; 1957; cf. Eccles, 1964).

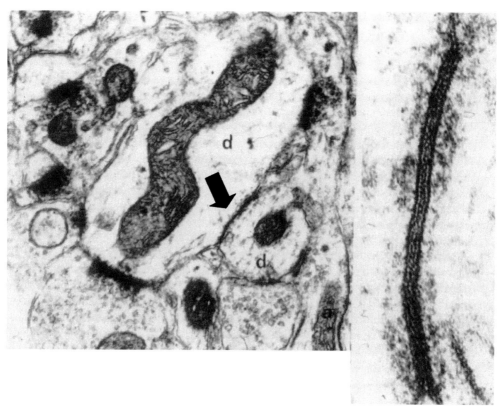

Fig. 3. A gap junction in the sensory cortex of a primate (Sloper, 1972). It is likely to mediate synchronous firing of inhibitory interneurons (cf. Bennett, 2000a,b).

The "back propagating" impulse was antidromic in that it went from axon towards the input part of the neuron, but orthodromic in that it was the normal direction for impulses to propagate. The finding was a little troublesome at the time because physiologists thought in terms of uniform membrane properties (Occam's kind of supposition), and synaptic inputs would be larger in the dendrites. The data were rapidly rationalized in terms of lower threshold in the initial segment, higher threshold or inexcitability of the dendrite, averaging of dendritic inputs, and integration of excitation and inhibition at a single site. Impulse initiation in or near the soma in response to dendritic inputs has now been shown by direct measurement in a number of other central neurons with simultaneous dendritic and somatic recordings (e.g., Fig. 6, Stuart and Sakmann, 1994). We showed for teleost oculomotor neurons that ipsilateral vestibular inputs initiate impulses in the dendrites and contralateral vestibular inputs initiate impulses in the soma, from where they presumably propagate somatofugally out the dendrites as well as out the axon (Korn and Bennett, 1975). More recently, multisite patch clamp recordings from dendrites and somata demonstrates that impulses can arise in the axon initial segment or dendrites, depending on the strength of the synaptic input; small depolarizations in the distal dendrite excite the cell near the soma, but large depolarizations reach the higher threshold of the local, dendritic membrane before the potential in the soma reaches threshold (Fig. 7, Chen et al., 1997; Larkum et al. 2001). The mitral cell, diagramed by Cajal in Fig. 4, is now directly shown to have bidirectional propagation along the apical dendrite.

In describing the evolution of his ideas on dynamic polarization, Cajal wrote:

Only later, in 1897, did I hit upon the realization that, contrary to the general opinion, the soma or cell body does not always take part in the conduction of the nerve impulses which are received. The afferent wave is sometimes propagated directly

196

Retina

Olfactory bulb

Spinal sensory

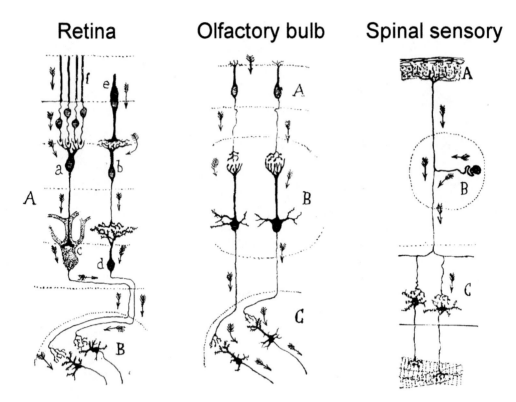

Fig. 4. Drawings of sensory pathways of retina, olfaction and cutaneous sensation with arrows indicating *dynamic polarization* of the conduction of impulses. For the actual flow of impulses in the mitral cell of the olfactory pathway, see Fig. 7. The spinal cutaneous sensory afferent has arrows leaving the soma, perhaps carrying impulses from a pericellular fiber not drawn here but present in Fig. 32 of TSN. Two of the central branches are shown as forming monosynaptic contacts on motoneurons. These diagrams are Fig. 47, 48 and 50 from Ramón y Cajal (1923).

from the dendrites to the axon. I had then to substitute for the preceding incorrect formula this other, which I designated *Theory of axipetal polarization: The soma and the dendrites conduct in an axipetal direction, that is, they transmit the waves of nervous excitation towards the axon. Inversely, the axon or axis cylinder conducts in a somatofugal or dendrifugal direction, carrying the impulses received by the soma or by the dendrites towards the terminal arborization of the nerve fibre.* (RdmV, p. 390)

Nevertheless, and always the comparative anatomist, he thought that:

in various nerve centres of vertebrates ... [there were] concentric zones in which only dendritic processes came together. In such cases it was necessary to admit contact between dendrites of diverse origins and hence conduction indifferently cellulipetal or cellulifugal. (RdmV, p. 385)

Cajal's brother subsequently found "*rich plexuses of axon terminations*" in these regions (RdmV, p. 388),

so that qualification could be excised. Nevertheless, dendrodendritic synapses, which we now know may be polarized or reciprocal, electrical and/or chemical, do not conform to those little arrows in a simple manner. Furthermore, Cajal, correctly, concluded that amacrine cells have multiple dendrites but no axon, thus suggesting conduction normally in either direction along the single processes.

We would now revise Cajal's view that, "*The three parts of the neuron: body, dendrites and axon, conduct equally the nerve impulse.*" (*Textura del Sistema nervioso...*, hereafter TSN, p. 88) We know that the excitability properties of the neuron vary over its surface. In some neurons dendrites appear to be inexcitable; in others there are varying degrees of excitability that modulate the input/output properties of the cell (e.g. Larkum et al., 2001).

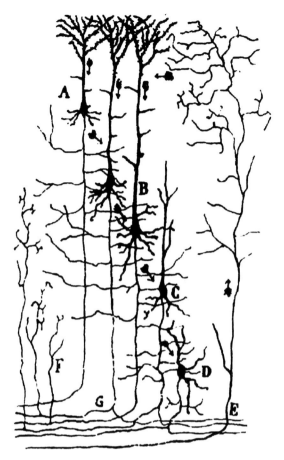

Fig. 5. Dynamic polarization in the neocortex? Cajal's legend: "The probable direction of current flow and the pattern of axodendritic connections between cells in the cerbral cortex. A: small pyramidal cell; B: large pyramidal cell; C and D: polymorph cells; E: terminal fiber arising in another center; F: white matter collaterals; G: an axon that bifurcates in the white matter." Fig. 16 from Ramon y Cajal (1933).

It is my impression, not based on an exhaustive reading of his works, that Cajal did not know that impulses can propagate in either direction along axons at the time he formulated the doctrine of dynamic polarization. Thus, the physiologists' concepts, and observations, of orthodromic and antidromic conduction would not have been in his mind. In writing the ultimate version of TSN (p. 114), however, he was fully cognizant that axons could conduct in both directions and his "opinion" was that dynamic polarization was a consequence of sensory receptors at the input part of the nervous system and muscles at the output. He recognized that conduction might go in the "wrong" direction in pathological states.

But when a change occurs in the neuronal connections, by experimental or pathologic lesions, so that the site of entry of the excitation in a nerve cell is now at the axonal apparatus, the direction of the propagation will change, and it will be possible for impulses to go from the axon to the cell body… (TSN, p. 115).

He was silent on whether impulses could cross contacts between cells in the wrong direction.

One of the difficulties for dynamic polarization was provided by the cells of the spinal sensory ganglia.

[T]he peripheral conducting branch, which is indisputably cellulipetal, is exceptional in that in the adult it takes on all the structural and morphological characters of the axis cylinder. (RdmV, p. 385)

As a student, I was never very happy with the term telo-dendron for the sensory axon distal to the spinal ganglion. It seemed perfectly reasonable to me to call it a sensory axon, but by that time the controversy about dynamic polarization and the role of dendrites had shifted to another facet: were dendrites electrically excitable and how much influence did distal synapses have on neuronal signaling? Cajal had no problem with calling the peripheral process a dendrite, although it was myelinated:

the possession of an insulating myelin sheath in the dendrites is related not so much to the direction of the nerve current as to the considerable length of the conductor. (RdmV, p. 388).

Coda

In preparing my contribution for this volume, *Changing Views of Cajal's Neuron*, it was my intention to examine two small areas in which it had appeared to me that Cajal had erred. In seeking documentation for my views, I have become much more aware of the breadth and subtlety of his views and more impressed with him as a scientist, thinker, and human being. He wrote about his development of the reduced silver stain:

I was inspired by the hope of procuring a powerful weapon with which to fence against many technical innovators who were irresistibly inclined to the anarchistic vice of denying in the name of a new truth the truths already discovered by others. (RdmV, p. 521)

And later:

Here was another hard battle won for the neuron doctrine. Will it be the last?

I doubt it very much. The morbid desire to assert and to make prominent one's own personality, to be original above all

198

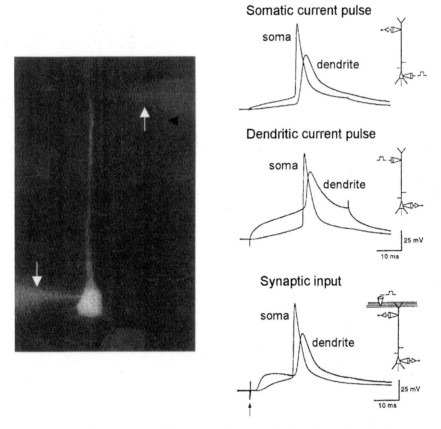

Fig. 6. In some neurons impulses arise in the soma or initial segment and propagate back out the dendrite. The fluorescence micrograph on the left shows the soma and apical dendrite of a neocortical pyramidal cell filled with Lucifer yellow through the patch pipette on the soma (arrow pointing up). The patch pipette on the dendrite is only faintly fluorescent (arrow pointing down). An impulse initiated by current applied in the soma propagates out the dendrite (upper record). An impulse initiated by current applied in the dendrite also appears first in the soma and then propagates out the dendrite, although the depolarization prior to the impulse is greater in the dendrite (middle record). An impulse evoked by synaptic activation due to electrical stimulation of afferent fibers also appears first in the soma and then the dendrite, although the excitatory postsynaptic potential is greater in the dendrites (lower record). From Stuart and Sakmann (1994).

things, wreaks ruin in our time. Following the course of least resistance, youth delights in reexamining values which it considers doubtful; and in the realm of science, instead of discovering new truths, it prefers to destroy its heritage of ideas from the past. (RdmV, p. 563)

There is no question that I was much younger at the time when gap junctions and electrical synapses were being described, and I admit to a somewhat iconoclastic predilection, now as then. Nonetheless, I maintain that I was taking pleasure in "discovering new truths" about synapses and neuronal connnectivity. Gap junctions do not contradict an old truth, although it is (for me) entertaining to pretend that they do so.

Much of what I have proposed here deals with teleology. Cajal often used teleological or functional arguments in interpreting his findings:

We have seen that the position of the soma as well as the direction and mode of origin of the axon, vary in different nerve cells. Are these variations merely whims of Nature, arrangements without importance, or have they some physiologic significance? All appears to indicate that such arrangements are of actual use to the dynamics of the organ that presents them. [A knowledge of the ontogeny of their development] would not give us a clue of the goal or utilitarian design pursued by Nature to adopt them only in certain foci of gray matter. These laws of economy must be considered as the teleological causes... (TSN, p. 102).

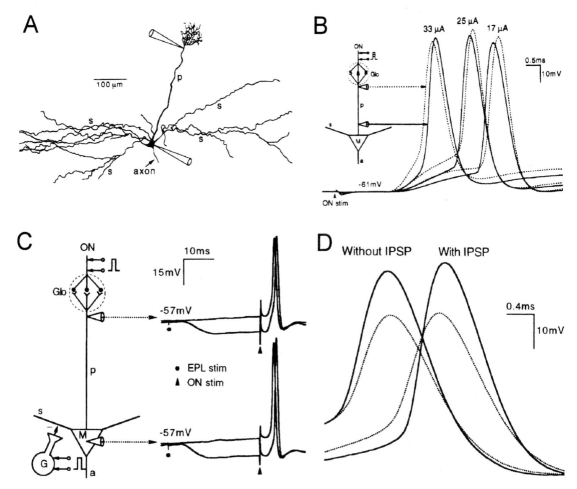

Fig. 7. In mitral cells of the olfactory bulb impulses can arise near the soma or out near the glomerular inputs, depending on strength of activation and inhibitory inputs. The apical dendrite can propagate impulses in either direction. (A) Drawing of a mitral cell filled with biocytin and recorded with patch electrodes on soma and distal apical (primary, p) dendrite. s: secondary dendrites. (B) Simultaneous recordings in proximal (continuous trace) and distal (dotted trace) apical dendrite. Olfactory nerve (ON) stimulation at the indicated strengths initiated impulses nearer the soma for weak stimulation (17 and 25 μA) and farther out the dendrite near the glomerulus (Glo) for stronger stimulation (33 μA). The synaptic depolarizations are larger near the glomerulus and for stimuli of 17 and 25 μA are superimposed on the synaptic depolarization near the soma evoked by the next stronger stimulus. (C, D) Inhibition alters the site of impulse initiation. Impulses evoked by ON stimulation alone arose first in soma and later in the dendrite; impulses evoked by ON stimulation during an IPSP evoked by stimulation of the external plexiform layer (EPL) arose first nearer the glomerulus (recordings from dendrite and from soma are superimposed with and without the IPSP in C); expanded sweeps of impulses in dendrite and soma are superimposed without the IPSP on the left of D and during the IPSP on the right of D. The larger impulse is that recorded from the soma. From Chen et al. (1997).

Lest the reader worries that Cajal was getting mystical, he states in a note:

Regarding final causes, we must declare that the terms *goal, designs, improvements*, etc. employed by us, are only expressions coined by usage. Indeed, according to us, there is no intentional direction, no preconceived plan in the evolution of Nature; only variations and adaptations which have prevailed because of their usefulness for survival. (TSN, p. 121).

Cajal is greatly deserving of homage. As autobiography, as well as scientific history, his *Recuerdos de mi Vida* is superb. I would like to include here a few quotes that I find wonderful.

[Neurons], those tiny cells, which keep hidden in the minuteness the mystery of life, are the whole man, in his two aspects, rational and physiological. Unified by the division of labour, they react to the stimuli of the environment, give us the illusion of free-will, and, in fine, perform our actions in their completeness. (RdmV, p. 446)

[I]ntellectual power, and its most noble expressions, talent and genius, do not depend on the size or number of the cerebral neurons, but on the richness of their connective processes. (RdmV, p. 459)

The perfection of function by exercise (physical education, speech, writing, piano-playing, mastery in fencing and other activities) [are] explained by either a progressive thickening of the nervous pathways…or the formation of new cell processes (non-congenital growth of new dendrites and extension and branching of axon collaterals) capable of improving the suitability and the extension of the contacts and even of making entirely new connections between neurons primitively independent. (RdmV, p. 459)

With respect to the Nobel Prize:

What a cruel irony of fate to pair, like Siamese twins united by the shoulders, scientific adversaries of such contrasting character! (RdmV, p. 553)

Finally, the prize for Peace was awarded to the American Theodore Roosevelt. This decision produced great surprise, especially in Spain.
Is it not the acme of irony and humor to covert into a champion of pacifism the man of the most impetuously pugnacious temperament and the most determined imperialist that the United States have ever produced? (RdmV, p. 550)

And as he described his aging:

The industrious young men to whom I refer [his students] are already legion, especially if we include those of the past with those of the present. Among the former ones (some dead in the flower of their youth and others unfortunately lost to national science in the *desert of the clinic*)… (RdmV, p. 592)

I repeat, let us cultivate our garden—as Voltaire used to say—fulfilling so far as we can the double and austere duty of men and patriots. For the biologist, the supreme ideal consists in solving the enigma of his own ego, contributing at the same time to clarifying the formidable mystery which surround us. It matters not that our work be premature or incomplete; incidentally, until the long sought ideal dawns, the world will gradually be made pleasanter for man. Nature is hostile to us because we do not know it; its cruelties represent revenge for our indifference. To listen to its inmost heartbeats with the fervour of passionate curiosity is the same as to decipher its secrets; it is to turn the ireful stepmother into the most tender mother.
In what nobler and more humanitarian enterprise could the intelligence be employed? (RdmV, p. 596)

If I were religious, I would say "Amen", but like Cajal, I am not.

References

Bennett, M.V.L. (1966) Physiology of electrotonic junctions. *Ann. N.Y. Acad. Sci.*, 37: 509–539.

Bennett, M.V.L., Pappas, G.D., Aljure and E., Nakajima, Y. (1967) Physiology and ultrastructure of electrotonic junctions. II. Spinal and medullary electromotor nuclei in mormyrid fish. *J. Neurophysiol.*, 30: 180–208.

Bennett, M.V.L. (1985) Nicked by Occam's razor: unitarianism in the investigation of synaptic transmission. *Biol. Bull.*, 168: 159–167.

Bennett, M.V.L. and Sandri, C. (1989) The electromotor system of the electric eel investigated with horseradish peroxidase as a retrograde tracer. *Brain Res.*, 488: 22–30.

Bennett, M.V.L. (1997) Gap junctions as electrical synapses. *J. Neurocytol.*, 26: 349–366.

Bennett, M.V.L. (2000a) Electrical synapses, a personal perspective (or history). *Brain Res. Brain Res. Rev.*, 32: 16–28.

Bennett, M.V.L. (2000b) Seeing is relieving: electrical synapses between visualized neurons. *Nat. Neurosci.*, 3: 7–9.

Bukauskas, F.F., Jordan, K., Bukauskiene, A., Bennett, M.V.L., Lampe, P.D., Laird, D.W. and Verselis, V.K. (2000) Clustering of connexin 43-enhanced green fluorescent protein gap junction channels and functional coupling in living cells. *Proc. Natl. Acad. Sci. USA*, 97: 2556–2561.

Cajal, S.R. (1899) *Textura del Sistema Nervioso del Hombre y de los Vertebrados. Texture of the Nervous System of Man and the Vertebrates.* Vol. 1. Translated and edited by P. Pasik and T. Pasik. Springer, New York, 1999.

Cajal, S.R. (1923) *Recuerdos de mi Vida. Recollections of My Life.* Translated by E. Horne Craigie with the assistance of Juan Cano. MIT Press, Cambridge, MA, 1966.

Cajal, S.R. (1933) *¿Neuronismo o Reticularismo?* Archivos de Neurobiología, XIII, Madrid. *Neuron Theory or Reticular Theory*, translated by U. Purkiss and C.A. Fox (1954). Consejo Superior de Investigaciones Científicas, Madrid.

Chen, W.R., Midtgaard, J. and Shepherd, G.M. (1997) Forward and backward propagation of dendritic impulses and their synaptic control in mitral cells. *Science*, 278: 463–467.

Condorelli, D.F., Parenti, R., Spinella, F., Trovato, Salinaro, A., Belluardo, N., Cardile, V. and Cicirata, F. (1998) Cloning of a new gap junction gene (Cx36) highly expressed in mammalian brain neurons. *Eur. J. Neurosci.*, 10: 1202–1208.

Coombs, J.S., Curtis, D.R. and Eccles, J.C. (1957) The interpretation of spike potentials of motoneurones. *J. Physiol. (London)*, 139: 198–231.

Curti, S., Falconi, A., Morales, F.R. and Borde, M. (1999) Mauthner cell-initiated electromotor behavior is mediated via NMDA and metabotropic glutamatergic receptors on medullary pacemaker neurons in a gymnotid fish. *J. Neurosci.*, 19: 9133–9140.

Eccles, J.C. (1964) *The Physiology of Synapses.* Springer Verlag, Berlin.

Faber, D.S., Lin, J.W., Korn, H. (1991) Silent synaptic connections and their modifiability. *Ann. N.Y. Acad. Sci.*, 627: 151–164.

Fatt, P. (1954) Biophysics of junctional transmission. *Physiol. Rev.*, 34: 674–710.

Furshpan, E.J., Potter, D.D. (1959) Transmission at the giant motor synapses of the crayfish. *J. Physiol. (London)*, 145: 289–325.

Furukawa, T., Furshpan, E.J. (1963) Two inhibitory mechanisms in the Mauthner neurons of goldfish. *J. Neurophysiol.*, 26: 140–176.

Hawkins, R.D., Son, H. and Arancio, O. (1998) Nitric oxide as a retrograde messenger during long-term potentiation in hippocampus. *Prog. Brain Res.*, 118: 155–72.

Korn, H. and Bennett, M.V.L. (1975) Vestibular nystagmus and teleost oculomotor neurons: functions of electrotonic coupling and dendritic impulse initiation. *J. Neurophysiol.*, 38: 430–451.

Korn, H. and Faber, D.S. (1975) An electrically mediated inhibition in goldfish medulla. *J. Neurophysiol.*, 38: 452–471.

Korn, H., Sotelo, C. and Bennett, M.V.L. (1977) The lateral vestibular nucleus of the toadfish, *Opsanus tau*: ultrastructural and electrophysiological observations with special reference to electrotonic transmission. *Neuroscience*, 2: 851–884.

Korn, H. and Axelrad, H. (1980) Electrical inhibition of Purkinje cells in the cerebellum of the rat. *Proc. Natl. Acad. Sci. USA*, 77: 6244–6247.

Larkum, M.E., Zhu, J.J. and Sakmann, B. (2001) Dendritic mechanisms underlying the coupling of the dendritic with the axonal action potential initiation zone of adult rat layer 5 pyramidal neurons. *J. Physiol.*, 533: 447–466.

Lin, J.W. and Faber, D.S. (1988) Synaptic transmission mediated by single club endings on the goldfish Mauthner cell. I. Characteristics of electronic and chemical postsynaptic potentials. *J. Neurosci.*, 8: 1302–1312.

Malgaroli, A., Ting, A.E., Wendland, B., Bergamaschi, A., Villa, A., Tsien, R.W. and Scheller, R.H. (1995) Presynaptic component of long-term potentiation visualized at individual hippocampal synapses. *Science,* 268: 1624–1628.

Malgaroli, A. (1999) Silent synapses: I can't hear you! Could you please speak aloud? *Nat. Neurosci.,* 2: 3–5.

Martin, A.R. and Pilar, G. (1963) Transmission through the ciliary ganglion of the chick. *J. Physiol. London*, 171: 454–475.

Niessen, H., Harz, H., Bedner, P., Kramer, K., and Willecke, K. (2000) Selective permeability of different connexin channels to the second messenger inositol 1,4,5-trisphosphate. *J. Cell Sci.*, 113: 1365–1372.

Sloper, J.J. (1972) Gap junctions between dendrites in the primate neocortex. *Brain Res.*, 44: 641–646.

Stuart, G.J. and Sakmann, B. (1994) Active propagation of somatic action potentials into neocortical pyramidal cell dendrites. *Nature*, 367: 69–72.

Teubner, B., Odermatt, B., Guldenagel, M., Sohl, G., Degen, J., Bukauskas, F., Kronengold, J., Verselis, V.K., Jung, Y.T., Kozak, C.A., Schilling, K. and Willecke, K. (2001) Functional expression of the new gap junction gene connexin47 transcribed in mouse brain and spinal cord neurons. *J. Neurosci.*, 21: 1117–1126.

Tokunaga, A., Akert, K., Sandri, C. and Bennett, M.V.L. (1980) Cell types and synaptic organization of the medullary electromotor nucleus in a constant frequency weakly electric fish, Sternarchus albifrons. *J. Comp. Neurol.*, 192: 407–426.

Tuttle, R., Masuko, S. and Nakajima, Y. (1986) Freeze-fracture study of the large myelinated club ending synapse on the goldfish Mauthner cell: special reference to the quantitative analysis of gap junctions. *J. Comp. Neurol.*, 246: 202–211.

Unger, V.M., Kumar, N.M., Gilula, N.B. and Yeager, M. (1999) Three-dimensional structure of a recombinant gap junction membrane channel. *Science*, 283: 1176–1180.

Verselis, V.L. and Veenstra, R. (2000) Gap junction channels, permeability and voltage gating. *Adv. Mol. Cell Biol.*, 30: 129–192.

Vigmond, E.J., Perez Velazquez, J.L., Valiante, T.A., Bardakjian, B.L. and Carlen, P.L. (1997) Mechanisms of electrical coupling between pyramidal cells. *J. Neurophysiol.*, 78: 3107–3116.

Wilson, R.I. and Nicoll, R.A. (2001) Endogenous cannabinoids mediate retrograde signalling at hippocampal synapses. *Nature*, 410: 588–592.

E.C. Azmitia, J. DeFelipe, E.G. Jones, P. Rakic and C.E. Ribak (Eds.)
Progress in Brain Research, Vol. 136

CHAPTER 16

Changes in the views of neuronal connectivity and communication after Cajal: examples from the hippocampus

Tamás F. Freund*

Institute of Experimental Medicine, Hungarian Academy of Sciences, Szigony u. 43, H-1083 Budapest, Hungary

Abstract: Intracellular recordings with concurrent visualization of the neuron as well as immunocytochemical studies in the last couple of decades confirmed the selectivity, and revealed additional complexity, in the synaptic connections in hippocampal circuits described by Santiago Ramón y Cajal. Even minor anatomical details began to gain functional meaning via the state-of-the-art combined approaches. The revolution of molecular biology brought about the rapid development of anatomy aimed at the localization of the numerous receptor subunits, ion channels, transporters and other proteins at the regional, cellular and subcellular levels that are being cloned every day (e.g. see Nusser, 2000). These fine-grain immunocytochemical data appear to have an immense predictive power for physiological and pharmacological studies and continue to serve as the ultimate test of hypotheses drawn from functional studies. Knowledge of the precise anatomical distribution of extrasynaptic receptors is required to understand the functional roles of various nonsynaptic mediators and diffuse pathways in the brain, as well as to the design of selective drugs for pharmacotherapy. Cajal would be delighted to see the revitalization of functional neuroanatomy, particularly of molecular anatomy, among the modern disciplines in the neurosciences today.

Introduction

One of the most famous arguments in neuroscience history was among Santiago Ramón y Cajal, Camillo Golgi and István Apáthy about whether the brain consists of enormous numbers of discrete cells, or is a continuous syncytium of nervous tissue (see Cajal, 1954). Cajal, using the silver impregnation technique of Golgi, correctly identified neurons as individual signaling elements of the brain. It has been over one hundred years ago when Cajal published his first diagrams on the neuron types, pathways and networks of the hippocampal formation. Most of those data are still valid, and extensively quoted in the literature. Even today, a lecture on hippocampal

circuits can hardly begin without a slide of the famous drawing of Cajal from his 1911 article grasping the most fundamental features of local connectivity, and the distribution of afferent input from the entorhinal cortex. There is one thing missing on this diagram, which delayed the discovery of the entorhinal-hippocampal-entorhinal reciprocal connections for decades. He thought, as it appears on his drawing, that the major output from CA1 is to the septal region, and from there to the hypothalamus. This view has been held for over 50 years, which explains why the hippocampus was not thought to be a memory-related structure, since its projection back to the cortex was unknown. The major reason for this mistake in his diagram is a technical problem inherent to Golgi impregnation, namely that myelinated axons cannot be visualized. Since most if not all outputs from cortical regions are carried by myelinated axons of pyramidal cells, these projections were

---
*Corresponding author: Tel.: 36-1-2109410; Fax: 36-1-2109412; E-mail: freund@koki.hu

often missed in adult animals, or juvenile animals had to be used with immature connectivity. Another disadvantage of the Golgi technique was its fortuitous nature, there was no way to influence which cell types would get impregnated. It was therefore very difficult to generalize conclusions without the visualization of several individual cells or connections of the same type. The question always arises which new finding should be considered a characteristic feature of a population or a rule in the connectivity, and which others are rather artifacts, a developmental abnormality or an exceptionally rare feature of the population. A third limitation of the Golgi technique is that it provides no information about the chemical nature or physiological properties of the stained neurons. These limitations have been overcome only 70–80 years after Cajal, just to demonstrate that in many cases Cajal was right in spite of the highly limited methodological repertoire used by him compared to what is available today. In the following sections some of the methodical advances will be illustrated by examples from the hippocampus, and the changes they caused in Cajal's views of hippocampal circuits will be pointed out.

Complete axon arbors revealed: advanced single cell labeling techniques with combined physiological characterisation

Single cell labeling techniques have gone through tremendous development in the last two decades. Golgi impregnation has been combined with high affinity uptake of radiolabelled transmitters or immunocytochemistry to provide neurochemical characterization of the morphologically identified neurons (for review, see Freund and Somogyi, 1989). A milestone in studies of cell types and connections was the intracellular filling of electrophysiologically recorded neurons by Schwartzkroin and Mathers (1978), which represents the beginning of the marriage of structure and function, i.e. of anatomical and physiological characterisation. The major benefit here was obviously the direct physiological data about firing patterns, electrical characteristics and pharmacology of inputs and postsynaptic actions of morphologically identified cell types. But at the same time, it also allowed the complete visualization of individual neurons for the first time, when an intracellular injection was made *in vivo* (Fig. 1). In the first years horseradish

peroxidase was used, but it was replaced later by smaller molecules (such as biocytin or neurobiotin) giving better electrical features for the intracellular electrodes. The extent of the axonal arbors of individual neurons (e.g. see Tamamaki et al., 1984; Sík et al., 1993) far exceeded the conservative estimates, and even the extrapolations of Cajal. According to recent calculations the number of axon terminals of a single pyramidal neuron in the CA3 region is between 15 and 40 thousand (Gulyas et al., 1993; Sik et al., 1993; Li et al., 1994). Since the connections between a pyramidal cell and a postsynaptic interneuron (Gulyas et al., 1993; Sik et al., 1993) and between two pyramidal cells (Sayer et al., 1990) are mostly mediated by a single contact, these numbers provide a close estimate of the number of target cells for a single pyramidal neuron. The entire synaptic coverage of single pyramidal neurons (Megias et al., 2001) and interneurons (Gulyas et al., 1999) has also been counted and calculated: a single pyramidal cell in the CA1 region, on average, receives a total of 30 thousand excitatory and 1700 inhibitory synapses, the inhibitory neurons containing parvalbumin receive a total of 15 thousand excitatory and 1000 inhibitory synapses, and other interneuron types receive a total of 1.5–3 thousand excitatory and 500–1200 inhibitory synapses. Thus, the degree of convergence and divergence in the quasi randomly connected ensemble of hippocampal principal cells is extremely high, such numbers rarely occur in the works of Cajal for obvious reasons: the incomplete visualization of axons, particularly the myelinated main trunks, and the lack of ultrastructural data (i.e. electron microscopy).

Visually guided whole cell patch clamp recordings using infrared DIC microscopy (Neher and Sakmann, 1992) allow the selection of the desired cell type for the investigation, thus, obtaining a large enough sample is not so difficult as with the blind approach. The selective sampling is further enhanced by the introduction of transgenic mice, where a fluorescent protein, eGFP, is coupled to the promoter of a selected marker gene, e.g. a calcium binding protein that is characteristically present in a specific interneuron type (Meyer and Monyer, 1999). Cells are then impaled under a fluorescent microscope. However, due to the limits of the thickness of the slices (usually between 250–400 micrometers) the neurons will be visualized only with a variable portion of their axonal and dendritic tree.

The inhibitory and excitatory synaptic interactions between identified neurons have been studied very

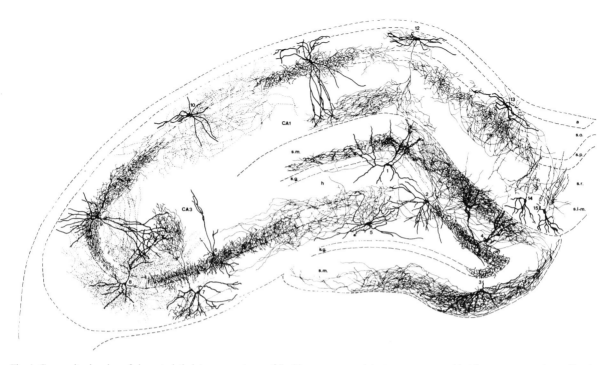

Fig. 1. Composite drawing of characteristic interneuron types of the hippocampus and dentate gyrus, assembled from reconstructions of *in vivo* (Nos. 5, 10–13) or *in vitro* (Nos. 1–3, 6–9) intracellularly labeled, or immunostained (Nos. 4, 14, 15) neurons in rat (Nos. 1–5, 10–15) and guinea pig (6–9). Thick lines represent the dendritic trees. 1) HICAP cell; 2) HIPP cell; 3) MOPP cell; 4) VIP-containing basket cell; 5) Trilaminar cell of CA3c; 6) axo-axonic (or chandelier) cell; 7) O-LM cell of CA3; 8) Bistratified cell of CA3; 9) Basket cell with axon in both CA3 and CA1; 10) Bistratified cell of CA1; 11) Basket cell of CA1; 12) O-LM cell of CA1; 13) Horizontal trilaminar cell of CA1; 14,15) IS-2 (Interneuron-Selective) VIP-containing cells. The figure also indicates that all subfields and layers in the hippocampal formation receive a massive GABAergic innervation from one or several interneuron types. The axons of some cells have been drawn by broken lines only in order to facilitate their distinction from axons of adjacent cells. Abbreviations: a, alveus; s.o., s.p., s.r., s.l-m., strata oriens, pyramidale, radiatum and lacunosum-moleculare of the hippocampus; s.m., s.g., h, strata moleculare, granulosum and hilus of the dentate gyrus; CA1, CA3, subfields of the hippocampus (Cornu Ammonis) according to Lorente de Nó. The original reconstruction derives from Freund and Buzsáki (1996), reproduced with permission from Wiley and Sons Ltd.

efficiently in the hippocampus (as well as in the neocortex) by recording from monosynaptically connected pairs of neurons under visual control (Gulyás et al., 1993; Buhl et al., 1994; Miles et al., 1996). These studies allowed direct conclusions to be drawn about their function, for example about the electrical features of single, anatomically verified glutamatergic synapses (Fig. 2), or the roles of different interneurons that have been morphologically described by Cajal a century ago (Buhl et al., 1994; for review, see Freund and Buzsáki, 1996). While inhibition was not considered at all by Cajal, today we can distinguish functionally distinct types of inhibition in the hippocampus mediated by Cajal's interneurons; i.e. dendritic inhibition controlling plasticity of excitatory synaptic inputs, versus perisomatic inhibition controlling

the output of large principal cell populations (Cobb et al., 1995; Miles et al., 1996).

Rules in connectivity unveiled by immunocytochemistry, electron microscopy and tract-tracing

Another limitation of classical Golgi studies is that neurons get impregnated randomly, and it is very difficult to collect a large enough sample of the same cell types or connections to describe typical consistent features of the network versus exceptions from the rule. Cajal partly managed to overcome this problem by working on very large samples over many years, and in most cases he had

206

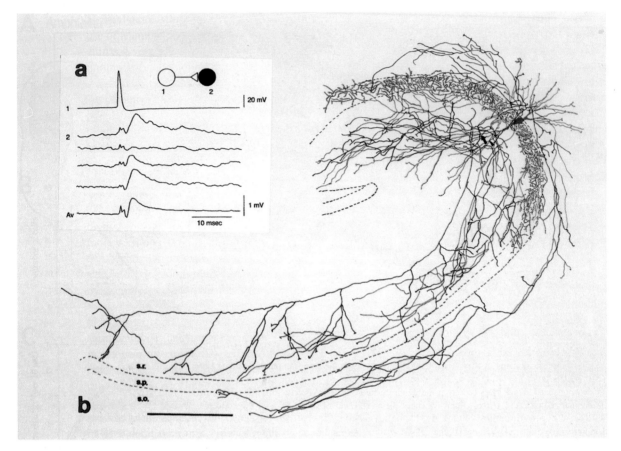

Fig. 2. Glutamatergic transmission (EPSPs) at single, anatomically verified synaptic contacts in the hippocampus between pyramidal cells and interneurons. a) Synaptic transmission between one of the filled pyramidal cells (1) and the postsynaptic basket cell (2). Single pyramidal cell action potentials evoked variable amplitude EPSPs in the inhibitory cell, and occasionally were associated with transmission failures (second trace). b) Camera lucida reconstruction of the axonal trees of two presynaptic pyramidal cells (black and blue) and a postsynaptic basket cell (red) simultaneously recorded and filled with biocytin in the CA3 region of the hippocampus *in vitro*. The axon of both pyramidal cells established a single contact on a mid-distal dendrite of the basket cell in stratum radiatum (arrow and arrowhead). From the original work of Gulyas et al. (1993). Reproduced from Freund and Buzsaki (1996) with permission from Wiley and Sons Ltd. Scale bar: 200 μm.

an extremely good eye to separate exceptions from the general rules. Today we are in a much easier situation, since immunocytochemistry allows us to visualize most if not all neurons belonging to a particular type. In several brain regions, in particular in the hippocampus and neocortex, various calcium binding proteins (parvalbumin, calbindin, calretinin) and neuropeptides (somatostatin, cholecystokinin, vasoactive intestinal polypeptide, neuropeptide Y, enkephalines, etc.) are present in functionally distinct cell types (for rev. see Freund and Buzsaki, 1996). Antisera against these proteins or peptides, and more recently, even antisera

against some transmitter receptors (that are selectively present in certain neurons) can be used to visualize the majority of neurons belonging to a functionally defined cell class (Fig. 3). This approach provides quantitative data on the frequency and distribution of a cell type, allows the identification of stereotyped features (e.g. input and output properties), and importantly, the changes associated with this cell type in certain neurological diseases or their animal models can also be established. Immunocytochemistry, however, provides a far more incomplete picture of the axonal and dendritic trees of individual neurons compared to Golgi impregnation or

207

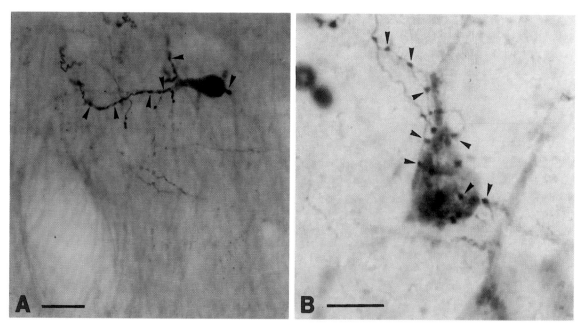

Fig. 3. Photomicrographs showing raphe-hippocampal (A) and basal forebrain-neocortical (B) afferents labeled with the anterograde tracer PHAL (black, Ni-DAB), and their postsynaptic targets. Postsynaptic targets were identified by immunostaining for calbindin (A) and somatostatin (B) using DAB as the chromogen (brown). A) Multiple contacts (arrowheads) are formed by median raphe afferents on a calbindin-positive interneuron in a climbing fiber-like manner in stratum radiatum of the CA1 region. B) A PHAL-labelled basal forebrain axon forms synaptic varicosities on a somatostatin-positive interneuron (arrowheads). Scales: A, B, 20 μm.

intracellular labeling techniques. Therefore, single cell labeling techniques should be combined with immuno-cytochemistry in order to obtain maximal information both at the single cell and at the population or network levels (see Somogyi and Freund, 1989; Freund and Somogyi, 1989; Kawaguchi and Kubota, 1996).

Drawing conclusions about connectivity and target selectivity from light microscopy alone is risky. Nevertheless, Cajal managed to provide a correct answer from his Golgi preparations for the targets of numerous cell types, particularly in the neocortex, hippocampus and cerebellum. There was only a single major cell type he missed in the cerebral cortex, the so called chandelier cells, which were discovered much later by Szentágothai (Szentágothai and Arbib, 1974), who was another major figure in neuroanatomy of the 20th century. In his first descriptions of the chandelier cell he claimed that this interneuron type with its radially oriented rows of bou-tons innervated apical dendrites of pyramidal cells. Electron microscopy of Golgi-impregnated neurons was required to identify the real targets of chandelier cells, the axon initial segments of pyramidal cells, which resulted

in a new name, "axo-axonic cell" (Somogyi, 1977). Conversion of the silver chromate crystals in the Golgi-impregnated neurons to metallic silver by a gold-toning procedure preserved the precipitate much better in the ultra-thin sections, and thereafter Golgi-electron microscopy became a widely used routine procedure (Fairén et al., 1977). Electron microscopy has been extensively used to demonstrate the existence of morphologically identifi-able synapses at most if not all sites of contacts where Cajal claimed an interaction between neurons. He described the hair-like appendages on axon terminals of dentate granule cells, similar to those he found on cerebel-lar mossy fibers, and took the liberty to call them by the same name. It was only recently that correlated light and electron microscopy of intracellularly filled dentate gran-ule cells in double-stained material demonstrated that these filopodia selectively innervate GABAergic interneurons as opposed to the large mossy boutons that terminate on pyramidal cell complex spines (Acsády et al., 1998). In addition to the target selection of output, informa-tion about total synaptic inputs could also be obtained by electron microscopy, replacing indirect reasoning

208

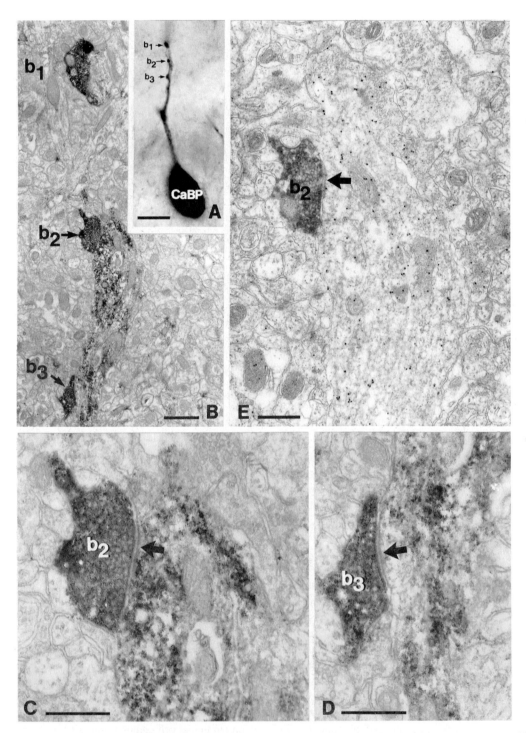

Fig. 4. Photomicrographs showing the postsynaptic targets of PHAL-labeled raphe-hippocampal afferents. Postsynaptic targets were identified using pre-embedding immunostaining for calbindin (CaBP) and postembedding immunogold staining for GABA. A) Light micrograph of a CaBP-positive interneuron that received multiple contacts (b1–3) from PHAL-labelled afferents arising from the median raphe. B) A correlated low power electron micrograph showing PHAL-labelled axon terminals (b1–3) making direct membrane contact with a calbindin-positive

based on light microscopy alone (Gulyás et al., 1999; Megias et al., 2001).

Golgi studies of Cajal revealed the termination pattern of certain afferent pathways in various brain regions, but in several of these studies the sources of those afferents could not be determined, and afferents from one particular source could not be labelled selectively. Today, in addition to anterograde degeneration, the transport of various lectins or other compounds (Phaseolus vulgaris leucoagglutinin, PHAL, biotinylated dextrane amine, neurobiotine) can be used to selectively label certain pathways (Gerfen and Sawchenko, 1984; Wouterlood and Jorritsma-Byham, 1993), and in combination with immunohistochemistry (Wouterlood et al., 1987), the synaptic targets can be directly identified (Figs. 3 and 4). The power of these approaches can be illustrated by an example taken from our own work in the hippocampus. Using a combination of anterograde tracing (PHAL) and immunostaining for markers of GABAergic interneurons and/or GABA itself we demonstrated that the GABAergic projection from the medial septum selectively innervates GABAergic interneurons in the hippocampus (Freund and Antal, 1988), similarly to the serotonergic raphe-hippocampal pathway, which was shown to distinguish even among different interneuron types (Figs. 3 and 4; Freund et al., 1990). These data paved the way to the physiological experiments identifying the mechanism of generation of hippocampal theta activity (Ylinen et al., 1995; Tóth et al., 1997). The data that emerged from these state-of-the-art tracing and immunocytochemical studies did not change Cajal's concept of neuronal networks, but rather confirmed his views about the remarkable target selectivity of connections among cell types in different regions.

Hard-wired networks modulated by diffusible messengers: specificity preserved by selective receptor distribution

As a neuroanatomist, and a father of the neuron theory, Cajal observed the brain as a hard-wired network of individual neurons that form specific connections with each other (Cajal, 1954). Even the direction of impulse propagation was marked by arrows along the axons in many of his diagrams, also indicating the potential target neurons, in most cases correctly. This traditional view of communication among neurons, i.e. exclusively via specific contacts or direct appositions (called synapses by Sherrington), was held by most neuroscientists even up to the last couple of decades. A fundamental change in this view took place when several pharmacological observations converged onto the conclusion that some diffusible neuronal messengers have to act at a distance from the site of release, i.e. at nonsynaptic receptors. A book by E. Sylvester Vizi (1984) entitled "Non-synaptic Interactions Between Neurons" represented a milestone in getting this new concept across to the neuroscience community, and today nonsynaptic interactions in the brain are widely accepted as an important way of communication among neurons in the nervous system (Agnati and Fuxe, 2000; Vizi, 2000). Superimposed on the hard-wired network, transmitters like monoamines, amino acids and neuropeptides, as well as less conventional mediators like nitric oxide, adenosine, endocannabinoids, may be released at synaptic or nonsynaptic sites, and diffuse to various distances from 1 to several hundred micrometers. They can exert their effects on extrasynaptic receptors present on the soma-dendritic membrane, or, more importantly, they influence transmitter release from terminals of various phenotypes that possess the appropriate receptors (for review, see Vizi, 2000). Even classical transmitters considered earlier to take part only in point-to-point synaptic signaling, like GABA and glutamate, have been shown to act extensively on extrasynaptic receptors, as in the case of the so called tonic GABAergic inhibition (Brickley et al., 1996; 2001). Endocannabinoids released by the postsynaptic neurons were found recently to be the mediators of retrograde synaptic signaling inhibiting transmitter release from GABAergic and glutamatergic axon terminals (Wilson and Nicoll, 2001; Kreitzer and Regehr, 2001). There are numerous examples also for cascades of synaptic and non-synaptic signaling, for example,

dendrite. Two of these juxtapositions (b2 and b3) are conventional synaptic contacts (arrows) at higher magnification in C and D. E) An adjacent ultrathin section stained for GABA with the immunogold procedure shows that the calbindin-positive dendrite is GABA-immunoreactive, whereas the PHAL-labelled raphe bouton (b2), which made a synaptic contact (arrow) with a dendrite, is GABA-negative. Reproduced from Freund and Buzsaki (1996) with permission from Wiley and Sons Ltd. Scales: A, 10 μm; B, 1 μm; C–E, 0.5 μm.

210

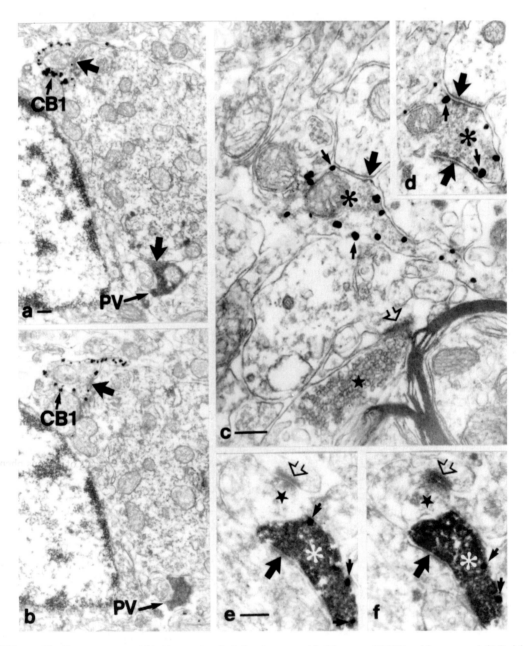

Fig. 5. CB1 cannabinoid receptors are restricted to axon terminals forming symmetrical (presumed GABAergic) synapses. (a,b) Serial sections cut from axon terminals of two different basket cell types forming symmetrical synapses (thick arrows) on a cell body in the CA3 subfield of the hippocampus. The upper bouton is immunoreactive for CB1 (see dense immunogold labeling around the membrane), whereas the lower terminal is positive for the calcium-binding protein parvalbumin (PV, see the dark, diffuse DAB precipitate of immunoperoxidase staining), but negative for CB1. Note that silver-gold particles representing CB1 protein nearly completely cover the axon terminal, as well as the pretermi-nal segment, but appear to avoid the synaptic active zone. Labeling is restricted to the inner surface of the bouton, where the intracellular C-terminus epitope of CB1 is located (see also c–f). (c,d) Thin, distal dendrites of pyramidal cells are also innervated by CB1-positive axon terminals (asterisks) as shown here in serial sections from the border of str. radiatum and str. lacunosum-moleculare in the CA1 subfield. In contrast, boutons (stars) forming asymmetrical (mostly glutamatergic) synapses (open arrows in e and f) on spine heads are always avoided by silver-gold particles (small arrows), and are therefore considered CB1-negative. (e,f) Combined immunogold (for CB1) and immunoperoxidase

glutamatergic synapses may trigger the diffuse release of NO, which, in turn, can modulate release from other transmitter-containing varicosities in relatively large tissue volumes (Kiss and Vizi, 2001).

An important implication of nonsynaptic transmission is that receptors and transporters mediating these effects often have affinities orders of magnitude higher than subsynaptic receptors or transporters, thus they likely mediate the majority of drug actions in pharmacotherapy. A drug will have influenced these receptors far earlier than it reaches sufficiently high concentrations in the synaptic cleft to activate low affinity receptors.

A major reason of skepticism about the importance of nonsynaptic transmission under physiological conditions is that diffusion of these messengers may mess up spatial and temporal specificity brought about by the hard-wired synaptic networks. Data demonstrate that even a few millisecond difference in firing synchrony may determine whether connections between neurons will be potentiated or depressed. The need for such temporal and spatial precision in synaptic interactions is obviously difficult to reconcile with diffuse transmitter release. A solution to this paradox may be that pathways operating via nonsynaptically released transmitters should be viewed as global modulators that function in a permissive manner, and do not convey information that requires a point-to-point specificity (e.g. the ascending monoaminergic systems involved in arousal and selective attention). Other mediators may provide an activity-dependent tuning or gain-control of specific synapses that are part of the point-to-point system. A key to the preservation of specificity even when hard-wired synaptic networks are under the global modulatory control of nonsynaptic mediators is the selective distribution of extrasynaptic receptors.

This specificity is well illustrated by the differential modulation of GABAergic transmission in the hippocampus by endocannabinoids and acetylcholine. Cajal's hippocampal basket cells turned out to be heterogenous regarding their neuropeptide/calcium binding protein-content, subcortical inputs and electrophysiological properties (for rev. see Freund and Buzsáki, 1996). Further complexity and selectivity is introduced into the operations of basket cells by the specific expression of presynaptic cannabinoid (CB1) and muscarinic (m2) receptors. We showed that the CB1 cannabinoid receptors are located selectively on GABAergic axon terminals that originate largely from CCK-containing basket cells (Fig. 5) both in rat and human hippocampus (Katona et al., 1999; 2000; Hájos et al., 2000). IPSCs evoked by stimulating these axons is blocked by CB1 receptor agonists, and this effect can be reversed by specific antagonists. Both receptor immunoreactivity and agonist effects were absent in CB1 knock-out mice (Hájos et al., 2000). In contrast, immunoreactivity for the m2 muscarinic receptor was confined to axon terminals of parvalbumin-containing basket and chandelier cells (Hájos et al., 1998), a population of interneurons that shows no overlap with those cells immunoreactive for CCK and CB1 (Freund and Buzsáki, 1996; Katona et al., 1999). The mutually exclusive distribution of CB1 and m2 receptors confirms that these two types of basket cells underlie distinct functions. Inhibition mediated by CCK basket cells may be attenuated by a Ca-dependent release of endocannabinoids from postsynaptic pyramidal cells (Wilson and Nicoll, 2001), e.g. during complex burst firing. In contrast, efficacy of inhibition exerted by the other basket cell type may be controlled largely by cholinergic input from the medial septum. Both types of basket cell appear to be involved in the generation of gamma frequency oscillations, since, while CB1 receptor agonists reduced the power, they did not abolish kainate-induced gamma in hippocampal slices (Hájos et al., 2000).

Glutamatergic transmission in the cerebellum is also under the control of retrograde signaling via endocannabinoids (Kreizer and Regehr, 2001), and recent evidence shows that a cannabinoid-sensitive receptor other than CB1 controls glutamatergic EPSCs in the hippocampus (Hájos et al., 2001)

(for the neuropeptide cholecystokinin, CCK) staining reveals that the axon terminals of CCK-containing interneurons bear presynaptic CB1 receptors. Serial sections in the stratum moleculare of the dentate gyrus show that gold particles (small arrows) representing CB1 are confined to a CCK-positive axon terminal (white asterisks) and avoid excitatory terminals (stars). Reproduced from Hájos et al. (2000) with permission from Blackwell Science Ltd. Scale bars: a (valid for a,b), c (valid for c,d), and e (valid for e,f), 0.2 μm.

Summary

All the above examples of changes in Cajal's views have been brought about by major technical advances in the second half of the last century, including intracellular filling of recorded neurons, immunohistochemistry, electron microscopy, tract-tracing and their combinations. It appears that we are once again in the middle of a profound change in our methodology, one that might lead to similarly major progress in our understanding of operational principles of the brain. These new approaches are largely brought about by the revolution in molecular biology and imaging, both of which cry out for neuroanatomy. A large number of molecules involved in neuronal signaling are cloned or discovered every day, and their cellular and subcellular localization is crucial for identifying their function. Imaging is basically functional neuroanatomy in itself, whether monitoring calcium concentration changes at the millisecond and single spine resolution, or voltage and metabolism at cellular, network or regional levels. Santiago Ramón y Cajal would be delighted with the fact that neuroanatomy, although considered a traditional discipline in neuroscience, is still indispensable in the 21st-century quest for understanding our brain.

References

Acsády, L., Kamondi, A., Sík, A., Freund, T.F. and Buzsáki, Gy. (1998) GABAergic cells are the major postsynaptic targets of mossy fibers in the rat hippocampus. *J. Neurosci.*, 18: 3386–3404.

Agnati, L.F. and Fuxe, K. (2000) Volume transmission as a key feature of information handling in the central nervous system possible new interpretative value of the Turing's B-type machine. *Prog. Brain Res.*, 125: 3–19.

Brickley, S.G., Revilla, V., Cull-Candy, S.G., Wisden, W. and Farrant, M. (2001) Adaptive regulation of neuronal excitability by a voltage-independent potassium conductance. *Nature*, 409: 88–92.

Brickley, S.G., Cull-Candy, S.G. and Farrant, M. (1996) Development of a tonic form of synaptic inhibition in rat cerebellar granule cells resulting from persistent activation of GABAA receptors. *J. Physiol.*, 497: 753–759.

Buhl, E.H., Halasy, K. and Somogyi, P. (1994) Diverse sources of hippocampal unitary inhibitory postsynaptic potentials and the number of synaptic release sites. *Nature*, 368: 823–828.

Cajal, S.R. (1893) Estructura del asta de Ammon y fascia dentata. *Ann. Soc. Esp. Hist. Nat.*, 22.

Cajal, S.R. (1911) *Histologie de systeme nerveux de I'Homme et des vertebres*. A. Maloine, Paris.

Cajal, S.R. (1954) Neuron theory or reticular theory? Objective evidence of the anatomical unity of nerve cells. (English translation by U. Purkiss and C.A. Fox). CSIC Instituto "Ramón y Cajal", Madrid.

Cobb, S.R., Buhl, E.H., Halasy, K., Paulsen, O. and Somogyi, P. (1995) Synchronization of neuronal activity in hippocampus by individual GABAergic interneurons. *Nature*, 378: 75–78.

Fairén, A., Peters, A. and Saldanha, J. (1977) A new procedure for examining Golgi impregnated neurons by light and electron microscopy. *J. Neurocytol.*, 6: 311–337.

Freund, T.F. and Antal, M. (1988) GABA-containing neurons in the septum control inhibitory interneurons in the hippocampus. *Nature*, 336: 170–173.

Freund, T.F. and Buzsáki, G. (1996) Interneurons of the hippocampus. *Hippocampus*, 6: 345–470.

Freund, T.F., Gulyás, A.I., Acsády, L., Görcs, T. and Tóth, K. (1990) Serotonergic control of the hippocampus via local inhibitory interneurons. *Proc. Natl. Acad. Sci. USA*, 87: 8501–8505.

Freund, T.F. and Somogyi, P. (1989) Synaptic relationships of Golgi impregnated neurons as identified by electrophysiological or immunocytochemical techniques. In: L. Heimer and L. Zaborszky (Eds.), *Neuroanatomical Tract-Tracing Methods II. Recent Progress.* New York: Plenum Publishing Corporation, pp. 201–238.

Gerfen, C.R. and Sawchenko, P.E. (1984) An anterograde neuroanatomical tracing method that shows the detailed morphology of neurons, their axons and terminals: immunohistochemical localization of an axonally transported plant lectin, Phaseolus vulgaris leucoagglutinin (PHA-L). *Brain Res.*, 290: 219–238.

Gulyás, A.I., Mégias, M., Emri, Zs. and Freund, T.F. (1999) Total number and ratio of excitatory and inhibitory synapses converging onto single interneurons of different types in the CA1 area of the rat hippocampus. *J. Neurosci.*, 19: 10082–10097.

Gulyás, A.I., Miles, R., Sík, A., Tóth, K., Tamamaki, N. and Freund T.F. (1993) Hippocampal pyramidal cells excite inhibitory neurons via single release sites. *Nature*, 366: 683–687.

Hájos, N., Cs. Papp, E., Acsády, L., Levey, A.I. and Freund, T.F. (1998) Distinct interneuron types express m2 muscarinic receptor immunoreactivity on their dendrites or axon terminals in the hippocampus. *Neuroscience*, 82: 355–376.

Hájos, N., Katona, I., Naiem, S.S., Mackie, K., Ledent, C., Mody, I. and Freund T.F. (2000) Cannabinoids inhibit hippocampal GABAergic transmission and network oscillations. *Eur. J. Neurosci.*, 12: 3239–3249.

Hájos, N., Ledent, C. and Freund, T.F. (2001) Novel cannabinoid-sensitive receptor mediates inhibition of glutamatergic synaptic transmission in the hippocampus. *Neuroscience*, 106: 1–4.

Katona, I., Sperlágh, B., Maglóczky, Zs., Sántha, E., Köfalvi, A., Czirjak, S., Mackie, K., Vizi, E.S. and Freund, T.F. (2000) GABAergic interneurons are the targets of cannabinoid actions in the human hippocampus. *Neuroscience*, 100: 797–804.

Katona, I., Sperlágh, B., Sík, A., Köfalvi, A., Vizi, E.S. and Freund, T.F. (1999) Presynaptically located CB1 cannabinoid receptors regulate GABA release from axon terminals of specific hippocampal interneurons. *J. Neurosci.*, 19: 4544–4558.

Kawaguchi, Y. and Kubota, Y. (1996) Physiological and morphological identification of somatostatin- or vasoactive intestinal polypeptide-containing cells among GABAergic cell subtypes in rat frontal cortex. *J. Neurosci.*, 16: 2701–2715.

Kiss, J.P. and Vizi, E.S. (2001) Nitric oxide: A novel link between synaptic and nonsynaptic transmission. *Trends Neurosci.*, 24: 211–215.

Kreitzer, A.C. and Regehr, W.G. (2001) Retrograde inhibition of presynaptic calcium influx by endogenous cannabinoids at excitatory synapses onto Purkinje cells. *Neuron*, 29: 717–727.

Li, X.-G., Somogyi, P., Ylinen, A. and Buzsáki, G. (1994) The hippocampal CA3 network: an in vivo intracellular labeling study. *J. Comp. Neurol.*, 339: 181–208.

Mégias, M., Emri, Zs., Freund, T.F. and Gulyás, A.I. (2001) Total number and distribution of excitatory and inhibitory synapses on hippocampal CA1 pyramidal cells. *Neuroscience*, 102: 527–540.

Meyer, A.H. and Monyer, H. (1999) Generation of transgenic mice expressing a green fluorescent protein in parvalbumin-positive neurons. *Soc. Neurosci. Abs.*, 25: 1973.

Miles, R., Tóth, K., Gulyás, A.I., Hájos, N. and Freund, T.F. (1996) Differences between somatic and dendritic inhibition in the hippocampus. *Neuron*, 16: 815–823.

Neher, E. and Sakmann, B. (1992) The patch clamp technique. *Sci. Am.*, 266: 44–51.

Nusser, Z. (2000) AMPA and NMDA receptors: similarities and differences in their synaptic distribution. *Curr. Opin. Neurobiol.*, 10: 337–341.

Sayer, R.J., Friedlander, M.J. and Redman, S.J. (1990) The time course and amplitude of EPSP's evoked at synapses between pairs of CA3/CA1 neurons in the hippocampal slice. *J. Neurosci.*, 10: 826–836.

Schwartzkroin, P.A. and Mathers, L.H. (1978) Physiological and morphological identification of a nonpyramidal hippocampal cell type. *Brain Res.*, 157: 1–10.

Sík, A., Tamamaki, N. and Freund, T.F. (1993) Complete axon arborization of a single CA3 pyramidal cell in the hippocampus, with special reference to the distribution of postsynaptic parvalbumin-containing interneurons. *Eur. J. Neurosci.*, 5: 1719–1728.

Somogyi, P. (1977) A specific 'axo-axonal' interneuron in the visual cortex of the rat. *Brain Res.*, 136: 345–350.

Somogyi, P. and Freund, T.F. (1989) Immunocytochemistry and synaptic relationships of physiologically characterized, HRP-filled neurons. In: L. Heimer and L. Zaborszky (Eds.), *Neuroanatomical Tract-Tracing Methods II. Recent Progress*, New York: Plenum Publishing Corporation. pp. 239–264.

Szentágothai, J. and Arbib, M.A. (1974) Conceptual models of neural organization. *Neurosci. Res. Program Bull.*, 12: 305–510.

Tamamaki, N., Watanabe, K. and Nojyo, Y. (1984) A whole image of the hippocampal pyramidal neuron revealed by intracellular pressure-injection of horseradish peroxidase. *Brain Res.*, 307: 336–340.

Tóth, K., Freund, T.F. and Miles, R. (1997) Disinhibition of rat hippocampal pyramidal cells by GABAergic afferents from the septum. *J. Physiol. (Lond.)*, 500: 463–474.

Vizi, E.S. (1984) Non-synaptic Interactions Between Neurons: Modulation of Neurochemical Transmission. Pharmacological and Clinical Aspects. John Wiley and Sons, Chichester, New York.

Vizi, E.S. (2000) Role of high-affinity receptors and membrane transporters in nonsynaptic communication and drug action in the central nervous system. *Pharmacol. Rev.*, 52: 63–89.

Wilson, R.I. and Nicoll, R.A. (2001) Endogenous cannabinoids mediate retrograde signalling at hippocampal synapses. *Nature*, 410: 588–592.

Wouterlood, F.G., Bol, J.G. and Steinbusch, H.W. (1987) Double-label immunocytochemistry: combination of anterograde neuroanatomical tracing with Phaseolus vulgaris leucoagglutinin and enzyme immunocytochemistry of target neurons. *J. Histochem. Cytochem.*, 35: 817–823.

Wouterlood, F.G. and Jorritsma-Byham, B. (1993) The anterograde neuroanatomical tracer biotinylated dextran-amine: comparison with the tracer Phaseolus vulgaris-leucoagglutinin in preparations for electron microscopy. *J. Neurosci. Methods*, 48: 75–87.

Ylinen, A., Soltész, I., Bragin, A., Penttonen, M., Sik, A. and Buzsáki, G. (1995) Intracellular correlates of hippocampal theta rhythm in identified pyramidal cells, granule cells, and basket cells. *Hippocampus*, 5: 78–90.

E.C. Azmitia, J. DeFelipe, E.G. Jones, P. Rakic and C.E. Ribak (Eds.)
Progress in Brain Research, Vol. 136

CHAPTER 17

Cortical interneurons: from Cajal to 2001

Javier DeFelipe*

Instituto Cajal (CSIC), Avenida del Doctor Arce 37, 28002 Madrid, Spain

Introduction

The detailed microanatomical study of the cerebral cortex began in the 1890s with Santiago Ramón y Cajal's master works on the structure of the cortex, using the *reazione nera* ("black reaction") method of Camillo Golgi (Golgi, 1873). Before the discovery of the Golgi method, the existence of two broad morphological types of cortical neurons was already recognized: *pyramidal* and *nonpyramidal* neurons (Jones, 1984). However, the methods of staining before the introduction of the Golgi method (mostly carmine staining) only allowed visualization of neuronal cell bodies and a small portion of their proximal processes, making further characterization of cortical neurons difficult. The complete staining of the neuron, that is, with all its parts (soma, dendrites and axon), and its finest morphological details were readily observed in Golgi-stained preparations. This led to the important breakthrough of full characterization and classification of neurons (Fig. 1).

Since the pioneer work of Cajal (see DeFelipe and Jones, 1988), nonpyramidal neurons are today subdivided into two large groups: *spiny nonpyramidal or stellate cells*, and *aspiny or sparsely spiny nonpyramidal cells*. Spiny stellate cells constitute the typical neurons of the middle cortical layers (especially layer IV). They form a morphologically heterogeneous group of neurons, and some of them project to other cortical areas, whereas others are short-axon cells or interneurons whose axons

are distributed within layer IV or in the layers above or below where their parent cell bodies are located (Lund, 1984). Aspiny or sparsely spiny nonpyramidal cells are interneurons (with some exceptions; e.g., Peters et al., 1990; Gonchar et al., 1995; Fabri and Manzoni, 1996; Kimura and Baughman, 1997) and show a great variety of morphological, biochemical and physiological types. They constitute the majority of short-axon cells and approximately 15–30% of the total neuron population (for reviews, see Fairén et al., 1984; Hendry, 1987; Peters, 1987; White, 1989; DeFelipe, 1993; Jones, 1993; Kawaguchi and Kubota, 1997; Thomson and Deuchars, 1997; Somogyi et al., 1998).

In this work, I will deal with aspiny nonpyramidal neurons with short-axon or aspiny interneurons in the neocortex, unless otherwise specified. The aim of this chapter is to provide some historical views whose roots lie in the observations of Cajal, and to discuss certain recent general aspects of neocortical aspiny interneurons, which, for simplicity, I shall refer to as *interneurons*.

Cajal and the classification of cortical neurons: short-axon cells

Golgi should be recognized not only as the discoverer of the method that bears his name, but also for his important early contributions to the study of the nervous system. For example, Golgi was the first to suggest that, in general, there were two morphologically and physiologically different types of neurons: *motor (type I) and sensory (type II)*. Motor neurons had long axons that gave rise to collaterals, but the main axon left the gray matter

---

*Corresponding author: Tel.: (+34) 91 585 4735; Fax: (+34) 91 585 4754; E-mail: defelipe@cajal.csic.es

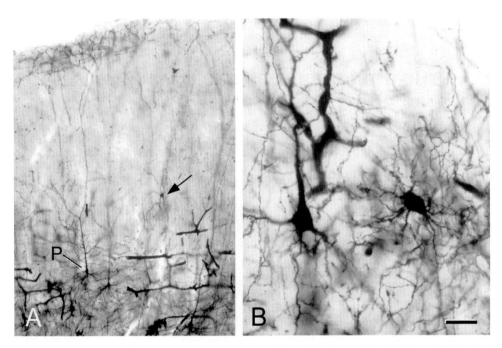

Fig. 1. Photomicrographs from Cajal's preparations of the postcentral gyrus of a newborn human (**A**) and of the occipital pole of a cat (**B**). **B**, photomicrograph showing a layer V pyramidal cell (P) whose apical dendrite forms a tuft in layer I. Arrow points to a small interneuron. (**B**) photomicrograph showing a pyramidal cell (*left*) and an interneuron (neurogliaform cell) (*right*). Scale bar: 130 μm for **A**; 20 μm for **B**. From DeFelipe and Jones (1988).

(projection neurons). Sensory neurons had short axons that arborized near the parent cell and did not leave the gray matter (intrinsic neurons). The former cells would have a motor function because their axons were considered to be in continuity with the motor roots, whereas the second type would be sensory because their axonal branches were linked with afferent fibers. According to Cajal (1892), it was not possible physiologically to maintain the distinction of the two Golgi types (for instance, the presence of a large number of cells with long axons in the retina). Furthermore, the motor type only differed morphologically from the sensory type in the length of the axon. Thus, Cajal designated Golgi's two types as *cells with a long axon* and *cells with a short axon*, avoiding any consideration of their possible physiological roles (Cajal, 1891, 1892). Since then, the term *short-axon cell* has commonly been used as synonymous with *interneuron*.

For Cajal, short-axon cells were "*condensers, or accumulators, of nervous energy*". He described (Cajal, 1901–1902) the possible mechanism of action as follows: "*The arrival of the current through a centripetal fiber would provoke the discharge of the cells with short axon, which would contribute to increasing the energy of the impulses that run through the chain of cells with long axon. The amount of this latent energy transformed into vital energy would depend on the intensity of the discharge received*". As explained below, the idea that interneurons are inhibitory and use GABA as a neurotransmitter arose in the 60s and 70s, after immunocytochemical studies and analyzing the morphology of the synapses they establish with other neurons.

Cajal described cortical neurons layer by layer in several cortical regions, mostly in the human, rat and cat (DeFelipe and Jones, 1988). He found a great variety of morphological types of interneurons, based on the morphology of their dendritic and/or axonal arborizations. However, with some exceptions (Fig. 2), he did not attempt to make a general classification of neurons, but rather he was describing the cells as he observed them in each layer. Cajal in his early studies of the cerebral cortex of small mammals (rabbit, guinea pig, rat and mouse) subdivided short-axon cells into two main categories (Fig. 2, *left*): *sensory cells of Golgi*, sometimes called

217

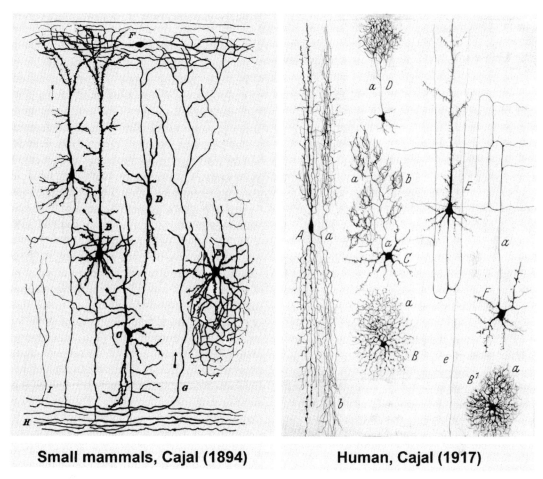

Small mammals, Cajal (1894)   **Human, Cajal (1917)**

Fig. 2. *Left*, The principal cellular types based on the works of Cajal (1890–1894) on the cerebral cortex of small mammals (rabbit, guinea pig, rat and mouse). **A**, pyramidal cell of medium size; **B**, giant pyramidal cell; **C**, polymorphic cell; **D**, cell whose axon is ascending; **E**, cell of Golgi; **F**, special cell of the molecular layer. From Cajal (1894). Right. The principal cellular types based on the works of Cajal (1899–1902) on the human cerebral cortex. **A**, bitufted cell; **B**, dwarf cell with short axon; **C**, basket cell; **D**, dwarf cell with axon resolving into a tuft; **E**, pyramidal cell with arciform collateral branches ("*small pyramidal cell characterized by exhibiting an axon that is almost completely exhausted in giving rise to very long arciform and recurrent collaterals*"); **F**, cell with ascending axon dividing into very long horizontal branches. From Cajal (1917); he says, referring to this figure, "*These cellular elements, particularly the first [A], second [B], fourth [E] and sixth [F], are extremely numerous and can be considered unique to the cerebrum of man.*"

Golgi-type, or Golgi's cells; and *cells with an ascending axon* or Martinotti cells. Golgi-type cells were distinguished because their axons give off collaterals at a short distance, forming a dense axonal arborization confined to or surpassing the dendritic arborization of the parent cell. Martinotti cells were characterized by their axons ascending towards layer I (where they frequently terminated), giving off the first collaterals at a relatively long distance, and by their main terminal axonal arborization being outside the dendritic arborization of the parent cell.

Furthermore, he distinguished a particular type of cell in layer I with long horizontal processes, which in his earlier studies he thought gave rise to two or more axons, calling them special cells of layer I (Cajal, 1890a,b, 1891). These special cells were the subject of numerous studies and they were considered by certain authors, like Retzius, to be a particular category of short-axon cells, some of which would give rise to one axon and others to two or multiple axons (Cajal, 1897). The special cells of layer I, which Cajal often referred to as *Cajal'sche Zellen*

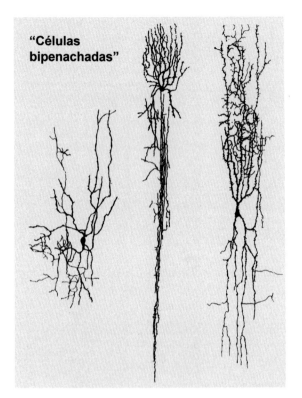

"Células bipenachadas"

Fig. 3. Composite of cells showing different dendritic and axonal morphologies, which Cajal called "*células bipenachadas*" in Spanish (bitufted cells in English) or "*double bouquet cells*" from the French. Taken from Figs. 10, 11 and 14 of Cajal (1899a,b and 1900, respectively).

of Retzius (now known as Cajal-Retzius cells), were later recognized by him as having a single axon (Cajal, 1911) (for recent reviews on this type of cell, see Marin-Padilla, 1998; Meyer et al., 1999).

Cajal was not consistent in his naming of the various morphological types of short-axon cells (Jones, 1975, 1984; Peters and Regidor, 1981; Fairén et al., 1984; DeFelipe and Jones, 1988). For example, Fig. 3 illustrates three "double bouquet cells" (células bipenachadas in Spanish; bitufted cells in English), which show different dendritic and axonal morphologies. Nevertheless, the studies of Cajal represent the first systematic and detailed description of the various types of neurons found in the cerebral cortex. His observations, together with accurate illustrations, had a great impact not only on the researchers of his time (Fig. 4), but, as we will see, also on modern studies on cortical organization (DeFelipe and Jones, 1988).

Modern classification of cortical interneurons

In spite of the notable recent discoveries in cortical circuitry, the problem of the classification of cortical interneurons remains without a satisfactory solution. The lack of consensus in classifying neurons is partially due to their great morphological, physiological and biochemical diversity, and to the fact that, with some exceptions, there are no rules for considering certain characteristics essential for individual neurons to belong to a given cell type. As examples, interneurons with the same somato-dendritic morphology may have different patterns of axonal arborization, or interneurons with the same axonal patterns may have different somato-dendritic morphologies (e.g., Jones, 1975; Fairén et al., 1984). Furthermore, interneurons with different morphological appearances may have the same general pattern of connectivity (e.g., Kisvárday, 1992), and different morphological types may have the same biochemical characteristics (DeFelipe, 1993, 1997a). In addition, because of the strong influence on cortical researchers regarding the concept of the existence of a basic circuit of cortical organization (Preuss, 2000), species differences in the morphology of interneurons are commonly considered to be superficial modifications rather than of kind. This has led to attempts to describe "basic" types of interneurons that are common to all species. However, as pointed out by Preuss (2000), most studies on cortical organization have been made on only a few species (mainly rats, cats and monkeys) and few cortical areas (mainly primary visual and somatosensory areas). Bearing these constraints in mind, certain interneurons can be readily recognized by their unique morphological characteristics, or they can be more generally divided into subgroups on the bases of their patterns of axonal arborization, synaptic connections both between themselves and with pyramidal cells, or biochemical characteristics (Fairén et al., 1984; DeFelipe, 1993, 1997a; Lund and Lewis, 1993; Condé et al., 1994; Jones et al., 1994; Nieuwenhuys, 1994; Gabbott and Bacon, 1996; Cauli et al., 1997; Gonchar and Burkhalter, 1997, 1999; Kawaguchi and Kubota, 1997; Reyes et al., 1998; Somogyi et al., 1998; DeFelipe et al., 1999; Gupta et al., 2000; González-Albo et al., 2001; Krimer and Goldman-Rakic, 2001). Below are described the main types of interneurons recognized in layers II–VI of the neocortex. Neurons in layer I and in the white matter have not yet been fully characterized and, therefore, I will not deal with them further.

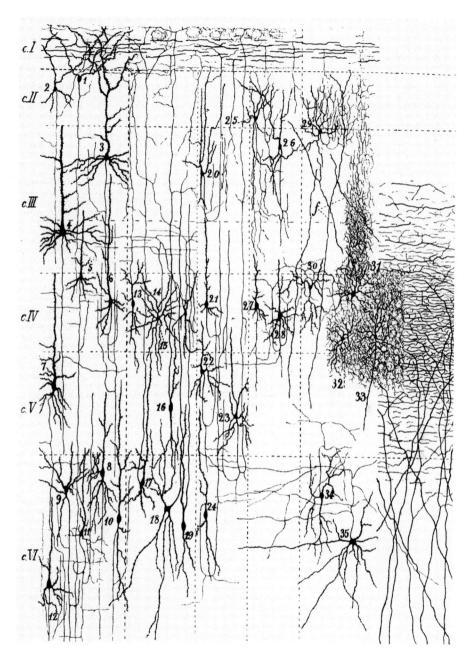

Fig. 4. Drawing showing the main types of cortical neurons and unmyelinated axons (*right*) described by Cajal. From Bonne (1906).

Classification based on morphologically distinct features

In general, interneurons are not distinguished by the specialization of their terminal axonal branches. The only interneuron that shows clearly recognizable terminal axonal specializations are chandelier cells, which originate candlestick, or chandelier, terminals. Basket formations, or the plexus of terminal axons that typically surround the cell bodies of pyramidal cells, originate from the convergence of several axons, but the individual, short curving, vertically or obliquely oriented branches that give rise to basket formations are not easily recognizable as basket terminals (Marin-Padilla, 1969; Jones, 1975; Fairén et al., 1984). Therefore, the neurons that originate such terminals (basket cells; see below) may pass unnoticed (Fairén et al., 1984).

All interneurons have more or less dense axonal arborizations distributed near their cell bodies, mainly within the areas occupied by their dendritic fields. However, some interneurons may display, in addition, prominent long horizontal or vertical axonal collaterals (Jones, 1975; Fairén et al., 1984; Lund, 1990; Jones et al., 1994). Accordingly, interneurons can be subdivided into three main groups on the basis of the general pattern of axonal arborization: *Group 1*, neurons with a mostly

restricted local axonal arborization within the dendritic field; *Group 2*, neurons with prominent long horizontal axonal collaterals; and *Group 3*, neurons whose axons give rise to conspicuous vertical axonal collaterals. Figure 5 illustrates the main morphological types of interneurons. Detailed descriptions of these types of cells by Cajal, and in modern studies, can be found in a number of articles (e.g., Colonnier, 1966; Marin-Padilla, 1969; Jones, 1975; Szentágothai, 1975; Valverde, 1978; Lund et al., 1979; Peters and Regidor, 1981; DeFelipe and Jones, 1988; Kisvárday, 1992; Somogyi et al., 1998; Budd, 2000). Thus, what follows is a brief description of these main types of interneurons.

Neurogliaform cells: Cells characterized by their multipolar morphology, small size and their very local dendritic and axonal arborization.

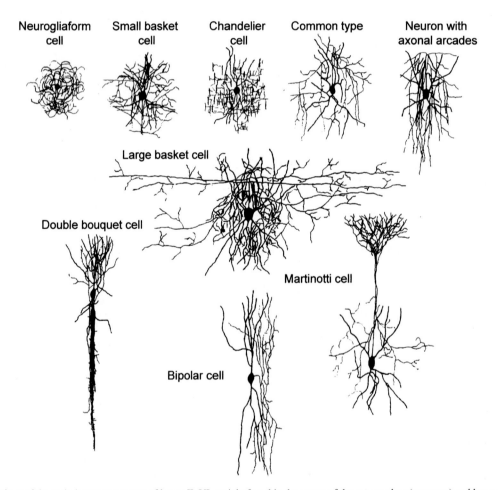

Fig. 5. Drawings of the main interneuron types of layers II–VI, mainly found in the cortex of the cat, monkey (macaque) and human.

Small basket cells: Multipolar cells of small or medium size, distinguished by the presence of numerous curving preterminal axonal branches.

Chandelier cells: Multipolar or bitufted cells which are distinguished by their preterminal axonal branches that form short vertical rows of boutons resembling candesticks.

Common type: Cells showing a multipolar or bitufted morphology. They are of small or medium size and their axons give rise to relatively short horizontal, oblique and vertical collateral branches without any apparent preference.

Neurons with axonal arcades: Multipolar cells whose axons give rise to axonal arcades, producing predominantly vertical axonal arborizations and relatively long descending collaterals.

Large basket cells: Multipolar cells characterized by their large somata, long dendrites and lengthy, horizontally oriented, myelinated axon collaterals that can reach several hundred microns.

Bipolar cells: Cells characterized by their long vertically oriented dendritic fields and by axons that originate a loose plexus of ascending and descending collaterals.

Double bouquet cells: Multipolar or bitufted cells, distinguished by axons that form tightly intertwined bundles of long descending vertical collaterals.

Martinotti cells: Multipolar, bitufted or bipolar cells with ascending axons that give rise to two plexuses, one near the cell body and the other at a variable distance above the cell body. This second plexus may be very dense (axonal tuft) or more widely distributed, and can be found within the same cortical layer of the cell of origin, or in the layers above (ascending axons can travel from layer VI to layer I).

Nevertheless, it should be pointed out that there are many other neurons which are difficult to classify, or that have not yet been recognized as belonging to a particular morphological type. Furthermore, the main types illustrated in Fig. 5 refer mostly to those found in the cat, monkey (macaque) and human cortex. In other commonly studied species, such as mice and rats (e.g., Lorente de Nó, 1922), basically the same types are found (Fairén et al., 1984), but with important exceptions and/or modifications. For example, there are no typical double bouquet cells in the mouse and rat (see section *Basic microcircuits*). Typical bipolar cells showing an ovoid or fusiform body giving rise to two principal, long vertically oriented dendrites (Peters, 1984), one

ascending from the upper pole and the other descending from the lower pole, are rather numerous in the mouse and rat, where the dendritic field may expand from layers II-III to layer VI (e.g., Morrison et al., 1984). However, in humans and monkeys they are less common and the cell bodies and dendrites are confined mainly to layers II-III. Other types, such as chandelier cells are found in a great variety of cortical areas and species, such as the hedgehog, mouse, rat, rabbit, cat, monkey and human (e.g., Somogyi et al., 1982; Valverde, 1983; Fairén et al., 1984; Marin-Padilla, 1987). Thus, some interneurons appear to be common to all species and, therefore, may be considered as basic elements of cortical circuits, whereas others may represent evolutionary specializations which are characteristic of particular mammalian subgroups and, thus, they cannot be taken as essential or general features of cortical organization.

Classification based on synaptic connections with pyramidal cells

All interneurons that have been studied in detail have been shown to form synapses with both pyramidal and nonpyramidal cells (for review, see Somogyi et al., 1998). In the rat hippocampus, there has been reported the existence of calretinin-immunoreactive and vasoactive intestinal polypeptide-immunoreactive interneurons specialized to contact other interneurons (Acsády et al., 1996; Gulyás et al., 1996). Similar results were reported in area 17 of the macaque monkey by Meskenaite (1997), who described calretinin-immunoreactive neurons that selectively formed synapses, mainly with other GABAergic neurons. However, in other studies also performed on the macaque and human cortex, it was found that calretinin-immunoreactive neurons innervated both pyramidal and nonpyramidal neurons (del Río and DeFelipe, 1997b; DeFelipe et al., 1999). Furthermore, with the exception of chandelier cells that form synapses exclusively with the axon initial segment of pyramidal cells, other types of interneurons have among their synaptic targets more than one type of postsynaptic element, including dendritic shafts, spines, somata and axon initial segments (e.g., Peters and Fairén, 1978; Peters and Proskauer, 1980; Somogyi et al., 1983; Kisvárday et al., 1985, 1986; DeFelipe and Fairén, 1988; Tamás et al., 1997, 1998). But, importantly, the degrees of preference

222

for these postsynaptic elements vary markedly between different types of interneurons. Based on the observation that different portions of a pyramidal cell are innervated by different types of interneurons (for reviews, see Peters, 1987; DeFelipe and Fariñas, 1992; Jones et al., 1994; DeFelipe, 1997b; Somogyi et al., 1998), the following main types of interneurons can be recognized (Fig. 6):

Axo-dendritic cells: Cells forming synapses only (or almost only) with dendrites; for example, cells with axonal arcades and double bouquet cells (e.g., Somogyi and Cowey, 1981; DeFelipe and Fairén, 1988; DeFelipe et al., 1989b).

Axo-somatic cells: Cells forming multiple synapses with both the dendrites and somata, but with different degrees of preference; for instance, large basket cells and small basket cells (e.g., DeFelipe and Fairén, 1982; Somogyi et al., 1983; Kisvárday et al., 1985, 1986).

Axo-axonic cells: Several types of neurons have been shown to include the axon initial segments among their

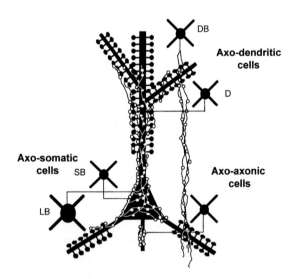

Fig. 6. Drawing illustrating the general synaptic relationships between interneurons with pyramidal cells. These interneurons represent a variety of types, which have been subdivided into three main groups: *axo-dendritic cells*, including double bouquet cells (DB) and other cells (D) that form synapses only, or almost only, with dendrites; *axo-somatic cells*, or cells which form numerous synapses with both dendrites and somata, but with different degrees of preference, and include small and large basket cells (SB and LB, respectively); *axo-axonic cells*, which form synapses with the axon initial segment, the chandelier cell being the only known neuron representative of this group to form synapses only with the axon initial segment. Modified from DeFelipe et al., (1999).

postsynaptic targets (e.g., Peters and Fairén, 1978; Somogyi et al., 1983; Kisvárday et al., 1985). However, most synapses on pyramidal cell axon initial segments arise from chandelier cells and, therefore, these cells are also called axo-axonic cells (e.g., Somogyi et al., 1982).

Classification based on the biochemical characteristics

Because in the cerebral cortex there are a large number of putative neurotransmitters or neuroactive substances, one of the problems in which many researchers are interested is to know if each of these morphological types can also be chemically characterized in order to get a more functional idea about possible roles that they play in processing intracortical information. After the early studies using immunocytochemistry for GAD (Ribak, 1978; Hendrickson et al., 1981), it was concluded that all or almost all interneurons are GABAergic and that the majority of these interneurons are multipolar (reviewed in Houser et al., 1984; see also Kisvárday et al., 1990; Prieto et al., 1994). Although the GABAergic nature appears to be true for most morphologically identified interneurons (Houser et al., 1984), there are some interneurons that do not contain GABA (e.g., Trottier et al., 1989; del Río and DeFelipe, 1997b), but it is not known what their proportion is.

In 1982, the first immunocytochemical colocalization study on the cerebral cortex appeared, showing the coexistence of the neuropeptides somatostatin and NPY in cortical neurons (Vincent et al., 1982). In 1984, several laboratories showed that different subpopulations of GABAergic neurons contained different neuropeptides (Hendry et al., 1984; Schmechel et al., 1984; Somogyi et al., 1984). The introduction of immunocytochemistry for the calcium-binding proteins calbindin, parvalbumin and calretinin (Celio, 1986, 1990; reviewed in Baimbridge et al., 1992; Andressen et al., 1993; DeFelipe, 1997a) represented another important step in the biochemical characterization of interneurons. Soon it was clear that most GABAergic neurons also expressed a number of different neurotransmitters (or their synthesizing enzymes), neuropeptides and calcium-binding proteins (Houser et al., 1984; Jones and Hendry, 1986; DeFelipe, 1993, 1997a; Jones et al., 1994). The main conclusion from these studies was that there are multiple biochemically definable subgroups of interneurons.

Interneurons and circuit diagrams of the cerebral cortex

Golgi method and early electron microscopy

The application of the Golgi method to the study of the cerebral cortex was not only useful for examining the morphology and distribution of interneurons, but also for revealing the connections between neurons, and between afferent fibers and neurons. These observations gave rise to another great advance, namely that of tracing the first circuit diagrams of the cerebral cortex (Fig. 7, *left*). These early diagrams, which increased in complexity as more data become available, reached a high point of complexity and refinement with Lorente de Nó (1938) (Fig. 7, *right*). However, after these early studies, there were very few articles about cortical circuits. Renewed interest in the method of Golgi arose in the 60s and 70s, mainly after the publication of several important contributions (e.g., Sholl, 1956; Colonnier, 1966; Marin-Padilla, 1969; Szentágothai, 1969; Scheibel and Scheibel, 1970; Valverde, 1970; Lund, 1973; Jones, 1975). Nevertheless, in the majority of cases, the exact intracortical connections could not be specified (see below).

The advent of electron microscopy, together with the development of techniques for the preparation of tissue for electron miscroscopy (for example, fixation in

osmium tetroxide and/or aldehydes, epoxy embedding, etc) (e.g., Robertson, 1953; Palade and Palay, 1954; De Robertis and Bennett, 1955; Palay, 1956; De Robertis, 1959; for review, see Robertson, 1987), constituted the next fundamental steps in the study of neuronal circuits. The first detailed ultrastructural studies and classification of synapses in the cerebral cortex were made by Gray (1959a,b) and, after that, a number of excellent studies on the ultrastructural characteristics of the neocortex appeared in the late 60s and early 70s (e.g., Colonnier, 1968; Peters and Kaiserman-Abramof, 1969, 1970; Jones and Powell, 1969, 1970; for review, see Peters et al., 1991). These early electron microscope studies culminated with the book of Peters, Palay and Webster (1970, 1976, 1991). The first attempts, after the works of Gray, to distinguish between excitatory and inhibitory synapses were soon followed by a number of authors (e.g., Andersen et al., 1963; Blackstad and Flood, 1963; Van der Loos, 1963, 1964). Synapses were classified into either types I and II (Gray, 1959b) or asymmetrical and symmetrical (Colonnier, 1968), a morphological distinction which is widely used at present to identify putatitive excitatory and inhibitory synapses, respectively (for reviews, see Colonnier, 1981; Peters, 1987; Peters et al., 1991; DeFelipe and Fariñas, 1992). Data from studies using the Golgi method and electron microscopy were combined by Szentágothai (1969, 1975, 1978), creating

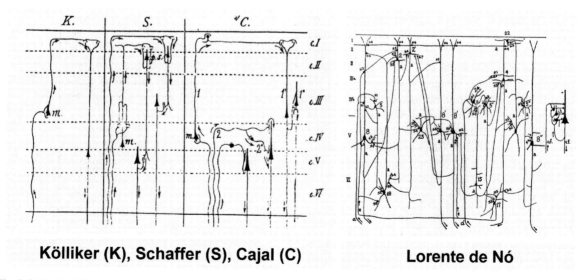

Kölliker (K), Schaffer (S), Cajal (C)   **Lorente de Nó**

Fig. 7. Early circuit diagrams of the cerebral cortex, based on studies using the Golgi method. *Left*, after Kölliker (K), Schaffer (S) and Cajal (C). *Right*, after Lorente de Nó. From Bonne (1906) (*left*) and Lorente de Nó (1938) (*right*).

cortical organization (Mountcastle, 1978). This minicol-umn is formed by a vertically oriented group of interconnected cells, which are contained in a vertical cylinder of tissue, with a diameter of about 30 μm, that crosses all cortical layers, about 600 million being the number of minicolumns present in the human neocortex (Mountcastle, 1978). The skeleton of the basic microcir-cuit is formed by a pyramidal cell and its input–output connections (Fig. 11). However, interneurons are differ-entiated into subtypes, some of which are lacking or display great modification in different species. One of the best examples is the double bouquet cell. Recent studies have emphasized the importance of studying this interneuron, because double bouquet cells form a widespread and regular microcolumnar structure, and because they appear to represent a key component of the

minicolumnar organization of the cortex as proposed by Mountcastle (DeFelipe et al., 1990; del Río and DeFelipe, 1997a; Peters and Sethares, 1997; reviewed in DeFelipe, 1997b; Jones, 2000).

As shown in Fig. 10, the regularity of spacing of dou-ble bouquet cell axons is one of their most impressive features. In various areas of the monkey and human cor-tex, it has been shown that double bouquet cell axons are so numerous (approximately 10 per 10,000 μm^2) and regularly distributed (mean center-to-center spacing of 30 μm) that they form a regular microcolumnar structure (DeFelipe et al., 1990, 1999; del Río and DeFelipe, 1995, 1997a). This distribution is rather similar to that shown by bundles of myelinated axons (radial fasciculi) (Fig. 12). These bundles of myelinated axons originate from pyramidal cells which form small vertical aggregates

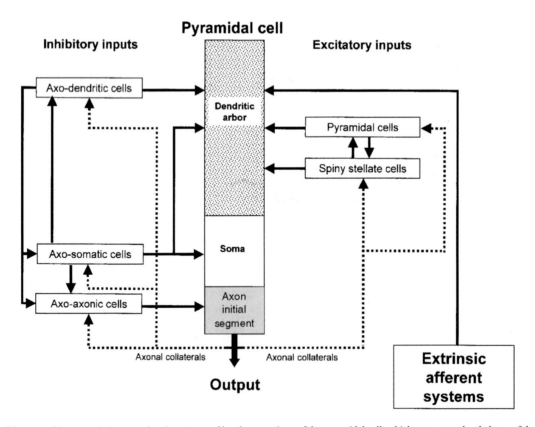

Fig. 11. Diagram of the synaptic inputs and main patterns of local connections of the pyramidal cell, which represents the skeleton of the basic microcircuit. Excitatory inputs arrive only to the dendritic arbor and originate from extrinsic afferent systems and spiny cells (which include other pyramidal cells and spiny stellate cells). Inhibitory inputs, which mostly originate from GABAergic interneurons, terminate on the den-drites, soma and axon initial segment. These interneurons are interconnected between themselves, with the exception of chandelier cells, which only form synapses with the axon initial segment of pyramidal cells. Modified from DeFelipe (1997b).

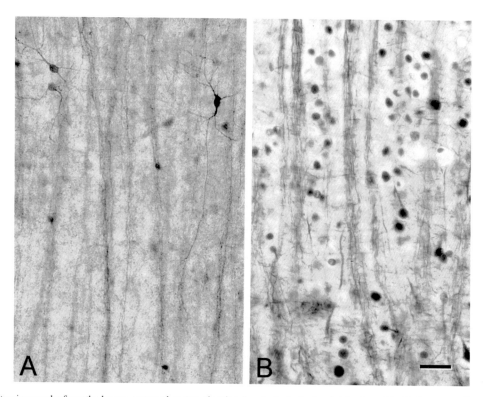

Fig. 12. Photomicrographs from the human temporal cortex, showing the similarity in the distribution of double bouquet cell axons and bundles of myelinated axons. These bundles originate from pyramidal cells which form small vertical aggregates. **A**, double bouquet cell axons immunostained for calbindin. **B**, bundles of myelinated axons (myelin staining). Scale bar: 50 μm for **A** and **B**.

(Peters and Sethares, 1996). Examination of the relationship between bundles of myelinated axons and double bouquet axons has revealed that there is one double bouquet cell axon per pyramidal cell module (del Río and DeFelipe, 1997a). Because double bouquet cells are very numerous and regularly distributed, and because of the long, vertical trajectory of their axons, and because they are GABAergic, double bouquet cells should constitute a widespread microcolumnar inhibitory system. Therefore, *double bouquet cells appear to represent a key component of the minicolumnar organization of the neocortex* (Fig. 13). However, these observations cannot be applied to all species. For instance, double bouquet cells in the human and monkey cortex show similar morphologies and distribution, whereas these "typical" double bouquet cells are less numerous in the cortex of other species (e.g., the cat), or they display great modification, or may even be absent (e.g., in the mouse and rat). Thus, differences in morphology, number and distribution of double bouquet cells may represent fundamental differences in cortical organization between primates and other species (Fig. 2). Other neurons have also been shown to differ between homologous cortical areas of different species. For example, pyramidal cells show a remarkable degree of variation in dendritic morphology (size, number of bifurcations and spine density) between different species (e.g., Elston et al., 2001; see Chapter 10), suggesting species variations in the cortical circuits that pyramidal cells form. Nimchinski and colleagues (1999) also reported that particular neuronal types are only found in the cortex of some primates, and not in other non-primate species.

Another problem for drawing a basic cortical microcircuit is that there are an indeterminate number of neurons which have not been characterized in detail. For instance, some large multipolar and horizontal bitufted NADPH-positive interneurons found in the human cortex (Fig. 14) cannot be included within any of the morphological types shown in the current general schemes of morphological types (Fig. 5). In addition, the number

Minicolumns

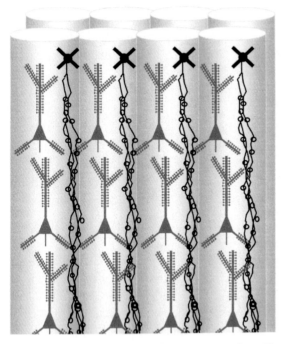

Fig. 13. Diagram showing the microcolumnar structure formed by double bouquet cells and their relationship with pyramidal cells.

and, in some cases, the proportion of morphological and biochemical types of neurons may differ between cortical layers and areas (e.g., see DeFelipe et al., 1999; Dombrowski et al., 2001 and references contained therein). Furthermore, combination immunocytochemistry for calcium-binding proteins with a variety of neurotransmitter-related substances, or other molecular markers, has revealed new anatomical and neurochemical aspects of cerebral cortex organization, increasing the complexity of cortical circuits (e.g., Freund and Gulyás, 1991; del Río and DeFelipe, 1994; 1997b; Gabbott and Bacon, 1996; Staiger et al., 1997; DeFelipe et al., 1999, 2001). For instance, we have found in the human cortex that calretinin-immunostained neurons innervate preferentially either the somata and proximal dendrites or the distal dendrites, depending on the neurochemical subpopulation of pyramidal cells (del Río and DeFelipe, 1997b). In Fig. 15A are shown pyramidal cells lightly labeled for calbindin that are highly innervated by calretinin-immunoreactive terminals at the level of the soma and proximal dendrites, whereas certain

pyramidal cells immunostained for non-phosphorylated neurofilament protein are innervated by calretinin-immunoreactive terminals mostly at the level of the distal dendrites (Fig. 15B). The lower pannels (C–F) of Fig. 15 illustrate a different experiment, showing a non-immunoreactive pyramidal cell soma innervated by both calretinin- and calbindin-immunoreactive terminals, but the cells and their axons that give rise to the pericellular terminals are not double-labeled. Therefore, different biochemically definable subgroups of interneurons may share not only the same general pattern of connectivity, but also the same synaptic targets.

Recent experiments using laser scanning photostimulation have further emphasized the complexity of cortical circuits (Dantzker and Callaway, 2000; Sawatari and Callaway, 2000). These studies have shown that there is a high diversity of input sources to individual interneurons and that distinct types of interneurons within a cortical layer receive different information. Finally, interneurons are not only connected by point-to-point chemical synapses (unidirectional connections), but they may also be coupled electrically (bidirectional) through gap junctions (Sloper, 1972; Sloper and Powell, 1978; for more recent publications, see Nadarajah et al., 1996; Galarreta and Hestrin, 1999; Gibson et al., 1999; Tamás et al., 2000; McBain and Fisahn, 2001; Szabadics et al., 2001). Moreover, the transmitter released at synaptic or non-synaptic sites may diffuse a certain distance and act on other synaptic contacts or on extrasynaptic receptors (for recent reviews, see Rusakov et al., 1999; Zoli et al., 1999; Agnati and Fuxe, 2000; Vizi, 2000). These different features represent further complexities in the system, making it even more difficult to establish information flow and wiring circuits.

As a whole, these observations suggest that intrinsic circuits are likely to be more complex than are currently thought, and that as more detailed studies on cortical microcircuits in different cortical areas and species are performed, more variations and complexities will be found. Thus, it is impossible to draw a "sufficiently" complete basic diagram of cortical microcircuitry that is valid for all cortical areas and species.

Summary and conclusions

After the collective work of many investigators, beginning with the early studies of Cajal, the following main

231

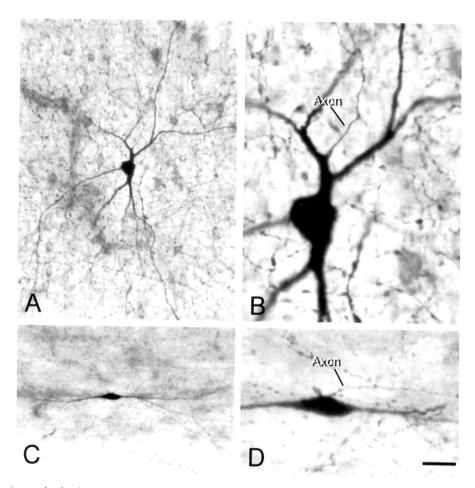

Fig. 14. Photomicrographs showing examples of NADPH diaphorase-positive neurons in the human temporal cortex that cannot be included within any of the morphological types shown in the diagram of Fig. 5. **A**, and **B**, low and high magnifications of a large multipolar NADPH-diaphorase neuron in layer III, which appears similar to a large basket cell; however, instead of giving rise to a myelinated axon, which is typical of large basket cells, this cell originates an unmyelinated axon with ascending and descending collaterals (**B**). **C**, and **D**, low and high magnifications of a horizontal bitufted NADPH-diaphorase neuron in layer VI, which gives rise to a horizontally oriented axon (**D**). Scale bar: 50 μm for **A** and **C**; 12 μm for **B**; 16 μm for **D**.

conclusions may be drawn regarding the morphology, biochemical characteristics and synaptic connections of interneurons:

1. Interneurons show a great variety of morphological, biochemical and physiological types. They constitute approximately 15–30% of the total population of neurons.
2. Because of the heterogeneity of interneurons and the lack of consensus as to which characteristics are essential for an individual neuron to be considered a member of a given cell type, there is no definitive classification of interneurons. Nevertheless, certain interneurons can be readily recognized by their unique morphological characteristics, or they can be more generally divided into subgroups on the basis of their biochemical characteristics, patterns of axonal arborization, or synaptic connections with pyramidal cells.
3. All interneurons have a more or less dense axonal arborization distributed near the cell body, mainly within the area occupied by their dendritic field. However, some interneurons may display, in addition, prominent long, horizontal or vertical axonal collaterals.

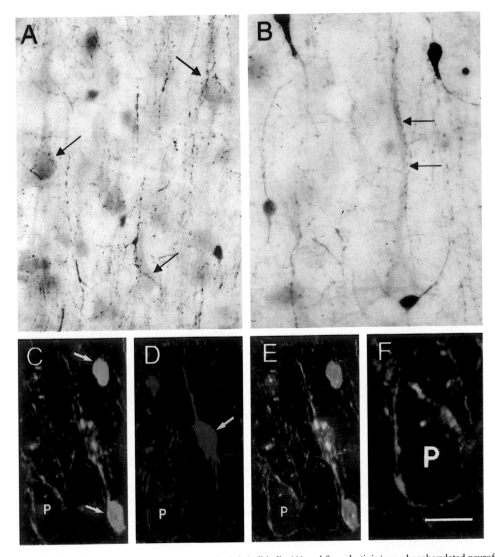

Fig. 15. **A**, and **B**, double immunocytochemical staining for calretinin/calbindin (**A**) and for calretinin/non-phosphorylated neurofilament protein. Calretinin-immunoreactive neurons innervate (arrows) the somata and proximal dendrites (**A**), or the distal dendrites (**B**), depending on the neurochemical subpopulation of pyramidal cells. **C**, and **D**, a pair of pseudocolored confocal images showing a pyramidal cell soma (p) innervated by axon terminals labeled for calretinin (green, **C**) and calbindin (red, **D**). Labeled neurons are indicated with arrows. **E**, pseudo-colored confocal image obtained after combining images **C** and **D**. **F**, high magnification of **E**. Note that none of the immunoreactive neurons are double-labeled and that the calretinin- and calbindin-immunoreactive perisomatic terminals are not double-labeled, which indicates that these axons have different origins. Scale bar: 52 μm for **A**; 23 μm for **B**; 20 μm for **C–D**; 10 μm for **F**. From del Río and DeFelipe (1997b).

4. Most interneurons form symmetrical synapses with both pyramidal cells and other interneurons, with the exception of chandelier cells, which only form synapses with the axon initial segment of pyramidal cells. Furthermore, interneurons are not only connected by chemical synapses (unidirectional connections), but they may also form electrical synapses through gap junctions (bidirectional) in a specific manner.

5. With the exception of chandelier cells, other types of interneurons include among their synaptic targets more than one type of postsynaptic element. But the degree of preference for these postsynaptic elements varies markedly between different types of interneurons.

6. The number of synapses made by a single axon originating from a given interneuron on another neuron is on the order of ten or less. Since, in general, cortical neurons receive many more interneuronal (symmetrical) synapses (on the order of a few hundred or thousand), a considerable convergence of various types of interneurons to pyramidal cells and interneurons appears to occur.

7. Most interneurons are GABAergic and also express a number of different neurotransmitters (or their synthesizing enzymes), neuropeptides and calcium-binding proteins. Thus, interneurons are, biochemically, widely heterogeneous.

8. Some of the morphologically identifiable neurons can be characterized by their particular biochemical characteristics, and some biochemically definable subgroups of interneurons display a particular morphology. However, different morphological types of GABAergic neurons may share one or several neurotransmitters, neuroactive substances and/or other molecular markers. Therefore, a great variety of subgroups of morphologically and biochemically identifiable neurons exist.

9. Some interneurons appear to be common to all species and, therefore, may be considered as basic elements of cortical circuits, whereas others may represent evolutionary specializations which are characteristic of particular mammalian subgroups and, thus, cannot be taken as essential, or general, features of cortical organization.

10. Given the complexity of cortical circuits and the areal and species differences, it is impossible to draw a "sufficiently" complete basic diagram of cortical microcircuitry that is valid for all cortical areas and species.

Acknowledgments

Supported by a DGCYT PM99-0105 grant and Comunidad Madrid grant 0.8.5/0036/2000.

References

Acsády, L., Görcs, T.J. and Freund, T.F. (1996) Different populations of vasoactive intestinal polypeptide-immunoreactive interneurons are specialized to control pyramidal cells or interneurons in the hippocampus. *Neuroscience*, 73: 317–334.

Agnati, L.F. and Fuxe, K. (2000) Volume transmission as a key feature of information handling in the central nervous system possible new interpretative value of the Turing's B-type machine. *Prog. Brain Res.*, 125: 3–19.

Andersen, P., Eccles, J.C. and Loyning, Y. (1963a) Recurrent inhibition in the hippocampus with identification of the inhibitory cell and its synapses. *Nature*, 198: 540–542.

Andressen, C., Blümcke, I. and Celio, M.R. (1993) Calcium-binding proteins: selective markers of nerve cells. *Cell Tiss. Res.*, 271: 181–208.

Baimbridge, K.G., Celio, M.R. and Rogers, J.H. (1992) Calcium-binding proteins in the nervous system. *Trends Neurosci.*, 15: 303–308.

Blackstad, T.W. (1965) Mapping of experimental axon degeneration by electron microscopy of Golgi preparations. *Z. Zellforsch.*, 67: 819–834.

Blackstad, T.W. and Flood, P.R. (1963) Ultrastructure of hippocampal axo-somatic synapses. *Nature*, 198: 542–543.

Bonne, Ch. (1906) L'écorce cérébrale. *Rev. Gén. Histol.*, 2: 291–581.

Budd, J.M.L. (2000) Inhibitory basket cell synaptic input to layer IV simple cells in cat striate visual cortex (area 17): a quantitative analysis of connectivity. *Visual Neurosci.*, 17: 331–343.

Buhl, E.H., Schwerdtfeger, W.K. and Germroth, P. (1990) Intracellular injection of neurons in fixed brain tissue combined with other neuroanatomical techniques at the light and electron microscopic level. In: A. Björcklund, T. Hökfelt, F.G. Wouterlood and A.N. van den Pool (Eds.), *Handbook of Chemical Neuroanatomy*, Vol. 8, *Analysis of Neuronal Microcircuits and Synaptic Interactions*, Elsevier, Amsterdam, pp. 273–304.

Cajal, S.R. (1890a) Textura de las circunvoluciones cerebrales de los mamíferos inferiores. Nota preventiva. *Gac. Méd. Catalana*, 1: 22–31.

Cajal, S.R. (1890b) Textura de las circunvoluciones cerebrales de los mamíferos inferiores. Nota preventiva. *Gac. Méd. Catalana*, 13: 737–739.

Cajal, S.R. (1891) Sur la structure de l'ecorce cérébrale de quelques mammifères. *La cellule*, 7: 125–176.

Cajal, S.R. (1892) El nuevo concepto de la histología de los centros nerviosos. *Rev. Ciencias Méd.*, 18: 457–476.

Cajal, S.R. (1894) The Croonian Lecture: La fine structure des centres nerveux. *Proc. Roy. Soc. London*, 55: 444–468.

Cajal, S.R. (1897) Las células de cilindro-eje corto de la capa molecular del cerebro. *Rev. Trim. Micrográf.*, 2: 105–127.

Cajal, S.R. (1899a) Estudios sobre la corteza cerebral humana I: Corteza visual. *Rev. Trim. Micrográf.*, 4: 1–63.

Cajal, S.R. (1899b) Estudios sobre la corteza cerebral humana II: Estructura de la corteza motriz del hombre y mamíferos superiores. *Rev. Trim. Micrográf.*, 4: 117–200.

Cajal, S.R. (1900) Estudios sobre la corteza cerebral humana III: Corteza acústica. *Rev. Trim. Micrográf.*, 5: 129–183.

Cajal, S.R. (1901–1902) Significación probable de las células nerviosas de cilindro-eje corto. *Trab. Lab. Invest. Biol. Univ. Madrid*, 1: 151–157.

Cajal, S.R. (1911) *Histologie du système nerveux de l'homme et des vertébrés*, Vol. 2, Maloine, Paris, pp. 519–598.

Cajal, S.R. (1917) *Recuerdos de mi vida*, Vol. 2. *Historia de mi labor científica*. Moya, Madrid.

Cauli, B., Audinat, E., Lambolez, B., Angulo, M.C., Ropert, N., Tsuzuki, K., Hestrin, S. and Rossier, J. (1997) Molecular and

234

physiological diversity of cortical nonpyramidal cells. *J. Neurosci.*, 17: 3894–3906.

Celio, M.R. (1986) Parvalbumin in most γ-aminobutyric acid-containing neurons of the rat cerebral cortex. *Science*, 231: 995–997.

Celio, M.R. (1990) Calbindin D-28k and parvalbumin in the rat nervous system. *Neuroscience*, 35: 375–475.

Chistensen, B.N. and Ebner, E.F. (1978) The synaptic architecture of neurons in opossum somatic sensory-motor cortex: a combined anatomical and physiological study. *J. Neurocytol.*, 7: 39–60.

Colonnier, M. (1966) The structural design of the neocortex. In: J.C. Eccles (Ed.), *Brain and Conscious Experience*, Springer-Verlag, Berlin, pp. 1–23.

Colonnier, M. (1968) Synaptic patterns on different cell types in the different laminae of the cat visual cortex. An electron microscope study. *Brain Res.*, 9: 268–287.

Colonnier, M. (1981) The electron-microscopic analysis of the neuronal organization of the cerebral cortex. In: F.O. Schmitt, F.G. Worden and S.G. Dennis (Eds.), *The Organization of the Cerebral Cortex*, MIT Press, Cambridge, pp. 125–152.

Condé, F., Lund, J., Jacobowitz, D.M., Baimbridge, K.G. and Lewis, D.A. (1994) Local circuit neurones immunoreactive for calretinin, calbindin D-28k or parvalbumin in monkey prefrontal cortex: distribution and morphology. *J. Comp. Neurol.*, 341: 95–116.

Cullheim, S. and Kellerth, J.O. (1976) Combined light and electron microscopic tracing of neurons, including axons and synaptic terminals, after intracellular staining with horseradish peroxidase. *Neurosci. Lett.*, 2: 307–313.

Dantzker, L.J. and Callaway, E.M. (2000) Laminar sources of synaptic input to cortical inhibitory interneurons and pyramidal neurons. *Nature Neurosci.*, 3: 701–707.

DeFelipe, J. (1993) Neocortical neuronal diversity: chemical heterogeneity revealed by co-localization studies of classic neurotransmitters, neuropeptides, calcium binding proteins and cell surface molecules. *Cereb. Cortex*, 3: 273–289.

DeFelipe, J. (1997a) Types of neurones, synaptic connections and chemical characteristics of cells immunoreactive for calbindin-D28K, parvalbumin and calretinin in the neocortex. *J. Chem. Neuroanat.*, 14: 1–19.

DeFelipe, J. (1997b) Microcircuits in the brain. In: J. Mira, R. Moreno-Díaz, J. Cabestany (Eds.), *Biological and artificial computation: from neuroscience to technology. Lecture Notes in Computer Science*, Vol. 1240, Springer, Berlin, pp. 1–14.

DeFelipe, J. (1999) Chandelier cells and epilepsy. *Brain*, 122: 1807–1822.

DeFelipe, J. and Fairén, A. (1982) A type of basket cell in superficial layers of the cat visual cortex: a Golgi-electron microscope study. *Brain Res.*, 244: 9–16.

DeFelipe, J. and Fairén, A. (1988) Synaptic connections of an interneuron with axonal arcades in the cat visual cortex. *J. Neurocytol.*, 17: 313–323.

DeFelipe, J. and Jones, E.G. (1988). *Cajal on the Cerebral Cortex*, Oxford University Press, New York.

DeFelipe, J. and Fariñas, I. (1992) The pyramidal neuron of the cerebral cortex: morphological and chemical characteristics of the synaptic inputs. *Prog. Neurobiol.*, 39: 563–607.

DeFelipe, J., Hendry, S.H.C., Jones, E.G. and Schmechel, D. (1985) Variability in the terminations of GABAergic chandelier cell axons on initial segments of pyramidal cell axons in the monkey sensory-motor cortex. *J. Comp. Neurol.*, 231: 364–384.

DeFelipe, J., Hendry, S.H.C. and Jones, E.G. (1989a) Visualization of chandelier cell axons by parvalbumin immunoreactivity in monkey cerebral cortex. *Proc. Natl. Acad. Sci. USA*, 86: 2093–2097.

DeFelipe, J., Hendry, S.H.C. and Jones, E.G. (1989b) Synapses of double bouquet cells in monkey cerebral cortex visualized by calbindin immunoreactivity. *Brain Res.*, 503: 49–54.

DeFelipe, J., Hendry, S.H.C., Hashikawa, T., Molinari, M. and Jones, E.G. (1990) A microcolumnar structure of monkey cerebral cortex revealed by immunocytochemical studies of double bouquet cell axons. *Neuroscience*, 37: 655–673.

DeFelipe, J., González-Albo, M.C., del Río, M.R. and Elston, G.N. (1999) Distribution and patterns of connectivity of interneurones containing calbindin, calretinin and parvalbumin in visual areas of the occipital and temporal lobes of the macaque monkey. *J. Comp. Neurol.*, 412: 515–526.

DeFelipe, J., Arellano, J., Gómez, A., Azmitia, E.C. and Muñoz, A. (2001) Pyramidal cell axon initial segments show a local specialization for GABA and 5-HT inputs in monkey and human cerebral cortex. *J. Comp. Neurol.*, 433: 148–155.

del Río, M.R. and DeFelipe, J. (1994) A study of SMI 32-stained pyramidal cells, parvalbumin-immunoreactive chandelier cells and presumptive thalamocortical axons in the human temporal neocortex. *J. Comp. Neurol.*, 342: 389–408.

del Río, M.R. and DeFelipe, J. (1995) A light and electron microscopic study of calbindin D-28k immunoreactive double bouquet cells in the human temporal cortex. *Brain Res.*, 690: 133–140.

del Río, M.R. and DeFelipe, J. (1997a) Double bouquet cell axons in the human temporal neocortex: relationship to bundles of myelinated axons and colocalization of calretinin and calbindin D-28k immunoreactivities. *J. Chem. Neuroanat.*, 13: 243–251.

del Río, M.R. and DeFelipe, J. (1997b) Synaptic connections of calretinin-immunoreactive neurons in the human neocortex. *J. Neurosci.*, 17: 5143–5154.

De Robertis, E. (1959) Submicroscopy morphology of the synapse. *Int. Rev. Cytol.*, 8: 61–96.

De Robertis, E. and Bennett, H.S. (1955) Some features of the submicroscopic morphology of synapses in frog and earthworm. *J. Biophys. Biochem. Cytol.*, 1: 47–58.

Dombrowski, S.M., Hilgetag, C.C. and Barbas, H. (2001) Quantitative architecture distinguishes prefrontal cortical systems in the rhesus monkey. *Cereb. Cortex*, 11: 975–988.

Eccles, J.C. (1984) The cerebral neocortex. A theory of its operation. In: E.G. Jones and A. Peters (Eds.), *Cerebral Cortex*. Vol. 2. *Functional Properties of Cortical Cells*, Plenum Press, New York, pp. 1–36.

Elston, G.N., Benavides-Piccione, R. and DeFelipe, J. (2001) The pyramidal cell in cognition: a comparative study in human and monkey. *J. Neurosci.*, 21RC163: 1–5.

Fabri, M. and Manzoni, T. (1996) Glutamate decarboxylase immunoreactivity in corticocortical projecting neurons of rat somatic sensory cortex. *Neuroscience*, 72: 435–448.

Fairén, A., Peters, A. and Saldanha, J. (1977) A new procedure for examining Golgi impregnated neurons by light and electron microscopy. *J. Neurocytol.*, 6: 311–337.

Fairén, A., DeFelipe, J. and Regidor, J. (1984) Nonpyramidal neurons. General account. In: A. Peters and E.G. Jones (Eds.), *Cerebral Cortex.* Vol. 1. *Cellular Components of the Cerebral Cortex*, Plenum Press, New York, pp. 201–253.

Freund, T.F. and Gulyás, A.I. (1991) GABAergic interneurons containing calbindin D28k or somatostatin are major targets of GABAergic basal forebrain afferents in the rat neocortex. *J. Comp. Neurol.*, 314: 187–199.

Freund, T.F., Martin, K.A.C., Smith, A.D. and Somogyi, P. (1983) Glutamate decarboxylase-immunoreactive terminals of Golgi-impregnated axoaxonic cells and of presumed basket cells in synaptic contact with pyramidal neurons of cat's visual cortex. *J. Comp. Neurol.*, 221: 263–278.

Gabbott, P.L.A. and Bacon, S.J. (1996) Local circuit neurones in the medial prefrontal cortex (areas 24a,b,c, 25 and 32) in the monkey: I. Cell morphology and morphometrics. *J. Comp. Neurol.*, 364: 567–608.

Galarreta, M. and Hestrin, S. (1999) A network of fast-spiking cells in the neocortex connected by electrical synapses. *Nature*, 402: 72–75.

Gibson, J.R., Beierlein, M., and Connors, B.W. (1999) Two networks of electrically coupled inhibitory neurons in neocortex. *Nature*, 402: 75–79.

Golgi, C. (1873) Sulla struttura della sostanza grigia del cervello (Comunicazione preventiva). Gazz Med Ital Lombardia 33: 244–246. Reimpress in: *Opera Omnia,* Vol. I. *Istologia Normale*, Ulrico Hoepli, Milano, pp. 91–98.

Gonchar, Y.A., Johnson, P.B. and Weinberg, R.J. (1995) GABA-immunopositive neurons in rat neocortex with contralateral projections to S-I. *Brain Res.*, 697: 27–34.

Gonchar, Y. and Burkhalter, A. (1997) Three distinct families of GABAergic neurons in rat visual cortex. *Cereb. Cortex*, 7: 347–358.

Gonchar, Y. and Burkhalter, A. (1999) Connectivity of GABAergic calretinin-immunoreactive neurons in rat primary visual cortex. *Cereb. Cortex*, 9: 683–696.

González-Albo, M.C., Elston, G.N. and DeFelipe, J. (2001) The human temporal cortex: characterization of neurons expressing nitric oxide synthase, neuropeptides, calcium-binding proteins, and their glutamate receptor subunit profiles. *Cereb. Cortex*, 11: 1170–1181.

Gray, E.G. (1959a) Electron microscopy of synaptic contacts on dendrite spines of the cerebral cortex. *Nature*, 183: 1592–1593.

Gray, E.G. (1959b) Axo-somatic and axo-dendritic synapses of the cerebral cortex: An electron microscopic study. *J. Anat.*, 93: 420–433.

Gulyás, A.I., Hájos, N. and Freund, T.F. (1996) Interneurons containing calretinin are specialized to control other interneurons in the rat hippocampus. *J. Neurosci.*, 16: 3397–3411.

Gupta, A., Wang, Y. and Markram, H. (2000) Organizing principles for a diversity of GABAergic interneurones and synapses in the neocortex. *Science*, 287: 273–278.

Hendrickson, A.E., Hunt, S.P. and Wu. J.-Y. (1981) Immunocytochemical localization of glutamic acid decarboxylase in monkey striate cortex. *Nature*, 292: 605–607.

Hendry, S.H.C. (1987) Recent advances in understanding the intrinsic circuitry of the cerebral cortex. In: S.P. Wise (Ed.), *Higher Brain Functions: Recent Explorations of the Brain's Emergent Properties*, Wiley, New York, pp. 241–283.

Hendry, S.H.C., Houser, C.R., Jones, E.G. and Vaughn, J.E. (1983) Synaptic organization of immunocytochemically identified GABA neurons in the monkey sensory-motor cortex. *J. Neurocytol.*, 12: 639–660.

Hendry, S.H.C., Jones, E.G., DeFelipe, J., Schmechel, D., Brandon, C. and Emson, P.C. (1984) Neuropeptide-containing neurons of the cerebral cortex are also GABAergic. *Proc. Natl. Acad. Sci. USA*, 81: 6526–6530.

Hendry, S.H.C., Jones, E.G., Emson, P.C., Lawson, D.E.M., Heizmann, C.W. and Streit, P. (1989) Two classes of cortical GABA neurons defined by differential calcium binding protein immunoreactivities. *Exp. Brain Res.*, 76: 467–472.

Hof, P.R., Glezer, L.I., Nimchinsky, E.A. and Erwin, J.M. (2000) Neurochemical and cellular specializations in the mammalian neocortex reflect phylogenetic relationships: evidence from primates, cetaceans, and artiodactyls. *Brain Behav. Evol.*, 55: 300–310.

Houser, C.R., Vaughn, J.E., Hendry, S.H.C., Jones, E.G. and Peters, A. (1984) GABA neurons in the cerebral cortex. In E.G. Jones and A. Peters (Eds.), *Cerebral Cortex,* Vol. 2. *Functional Properties of Cortical Cells*, Plenum Press, New York, pp. 63–89.

Hubel, D.H., and Wiesel, T.N. (1977) Functional architecture of macaque monkey cortex. *Proc. R. Soc. Lond. B.*, 198: 1–59.

Jankowska, E., Rastad, J. and Westman, J. (1976) Intracellular application of horseradish peroxidase and its light and electron microscopical appearance of spinocervical tract cells. *Brain Res.*, 105: 557–562.

Jones, E.G. (1975) Varieties and distribution of non-pyramidal cells in the somatic sensory cortex of the squirrel monkey. *J. Comp. Neurol.*, 160: 205–268.

Jones, E.G. (1984). History of cortical cytology. In: A. Peters and E.G. Jones (Eds.), *Cerebral cortex.* Vol. 1. *Cellular Components of the Cerebral Cortex*, Plenum Press, New York, pp. 1–32.

Jones, E.G. (1993) GABAergic neurones and their role in cortical plasticity in primates. *Cereb. Cortex*, 3: 361–372.

Jones, E.G. (2000) Microcolumns in the cerebral cortex. *Proc. Natl. Acad. Sci. USA*, 97: 5019–5021.

Jones, E.G. and Hendry, S.H.C. (1986) Co-localization of GABA and neuropeptides in neocortical neurons. *Trends Neurosci.*, 10: 71–76.

Jones, E.G.and Powell, T.P.S. (1969) Synapses on the axon hillocks and initial segments of pyramidal cell axons in the cerebral cortex. *J. Cell Sci.*, 5: 495–507.

Jones, E.G. and Powell, T.P.S. (1970) Electron microscopy of the somatic sensory cortex of the cat. I. Cell types and synaptic organization. *Philos. Trans. R. Soc. London Ser. B.*, 257: 1–11.

Jones, E.G. , Hendry, S.H.C, DeFelipe, J. and Benson, D.L. (1994) GABA neurons and their role in activity-dependent plasticity of adult primate visual cortex. In: A. Peters and K.S. Rockland (Eds.), *Cerebral Cortex,* Vol. 10, *Primary Visual Cortex in Primates*, Plenum Press, New York, pp. 61–140.

Kawaguchi, Y. and Kubota, Y. (1997) GABAergic cell subtypes and their synaptic connections in rat frontal cortex. *Cereb. Cortex*, 7: 476–486.

Katsumaru, H., Kosaka, T., Heizmann, C.W. and Hama, K. (1988) Immunocytochemical study of GABAergic neurons containing the calcium-binding protein parvalbumin in the rat hippocampus. *Exp. Brain Res.*, 72: 347–362.

Kimura, F. and Baughman, R.W. (1997) GABAergic transcallosal neurons in developing rat neocortex. *Eur. J. Neurosci.*, 9: 1137–1143.

Kisvárday, Z.F. (1992) GABAergic networks of basket cells in the visual cortex. *Prog. Brain Res.*, 90: 385–405.

Kisvárday, Z.F., Martin, K.A.C., Whitteridge, D. and Somogyi, P. (1985) Synaptyc connections of intracellularly filled clutch cells: a type of small basket cell in the visual cortex of the cat. Neuroscience. *J. Comp. Neurol.*, 241: 111–137.

Kisvárday, Z.F., Cowey, A. and Somogyi, P. (1986) Synaptyc relationships of a type of GABA-immunoreactive neuron (clutch cell), spiny stellate cells and lateral geniculate nucleus afferents in layer IVC of the monkey striate cortex. *Neuroscience*, 19: 741–761.

Kisvárday, Z.F., Gulyas, A.I., Beroukas, D., North, J.B., Chubb, I.W. and Somogyi, P. (1990) Syanpses, axonal and dendritic patterns of GABA-immunoreactive neurons in human cerebral cortex. *Brain*, 113: 793–812.

Krimer, L.S. and Goldman-Rakic, P.S. (2001) Prefrontal microcircuits: membrane properties and excitatory input of local, medium, and wide arbor interneurons. *J. Neurosci.*, 21: 3788–3796.

Lewis, D.A. and Lund, J.S. (1990) Heterogeneity of chandelier neurons in monkey neocortex: corticotropin-releasing factor- and parvalbumin-immunoreactive populations. *J. Comp. Neurol.*, 293: 599–615.

Lorente de Nó, R. (1922). La corteza cerebral del ratón. (Primera contribución-La corteza acústica). *Trab. Lab. Invest. Biol. Madrid*, 20: 41–78 (Translated by Fairén, A., Regidor, J. and Kruger, L. *Somatosens. Mot. Res.*, 9: 3–36, 1992).

Lorente de Nó, R. (1938) Architectonics and structure of the cerebral cortex. In: Physiology of the nervous system. In: J.F. Fulton (Ed.). Oxford University Press, New York, pp. 291–330.

Lund, J.S. (1973) Organization of neurons in the visual cortex, area 17, of the monkey *Macaca mulatta*. *J. Comp. Neurol.*, 147: 455–496.

Lund, J.S. (1984) Spiny stellate neurons. In: A. Peters and E.G. Jones (Eds.), *Cerebral Cortex*. Vol. 1. *Cellular Components of the Cerebral Cortex*, Plenum Press, New York, pp. 255–308.

Lund, J.S. (1990) Excitatory and inhibitory circuiting and laminar mapping strategies in the primary visual cortex of the monkey. In: G.M. Edelman, W.E. Gall and W.M. Cowan (Eds.), *Signal and Sense: Local and Global Order in Perceptual Maps*, Wiley-Liss, New York, pp. 51–82.

Lund, J.S. and Lewis, D.A. (1993) Local circuit neurons of developing and mature macaque prefrontal cortex: Golgi and immunocytochemical characteristics. *J. Comp. Neurol.*, 328: 282–312.

Lund, J.S., Henry, G.H., McQueen, C.L. and Harvey, A.R. (1979) Anatomical organization of the visual cortex of the cat: A comparison with area 17 of the macaque monkey. *J. Comp. Neurol.*, 184: 559–618.

Marin-Padilla, M. (1969) Origin of the pericellular baskets of the pyramidal cells of the human motor cortex: a Golgi study. *Brain Res.*, 14 : 633–646.

Marin-Padilla, M (1987) The chandelier cell of the human visual cortex: a Golgi study. *J. Comp. Neurol.*, 256: 61–70.

Marin-Padilla, M. (1998) Cajal-Retzius cells and the development of the neocortex. *Trends Neurosci.*, 21: 64–71.

McBain, C.J. and Fisahn, A. (2001) Interneurons unbound. *Nature Rev. Neuronsci.*, 2: 11–23.

Meskenaite, V. (1997) Calretinin-immunoreactive local circuit neurons in area 17 of the cynomolgus monkey, Macaca fascicularis. *J. Comp. Neurol.*, 379: 113–132.

Meyer, G., Goffinet, A.M. and Fairén, A. (1999) What is a Cajal-Retzius cell? A reassessment of a classical cell type based on recent observations in the developing neocortex. *Cereb. Cortex*, 9: 765–775.

Morrison, J.H., Magistretti, P.J., Benoit, R. and Bloom, F.E. (1984) The distribution and morphological characteristics of the intra-cortical VIP-positive cell: an immunohistochemical analysis. *Brain Res.*, 292: 269–282.

Morrison, J.H., Hof, P.R. and Huntley, G.W. (1998) Neurochemical organization of the primate visual cortex. In: F.E. Bloom, A. Björklund and T. Hökfelt (Eds.), *Handbook of Chemical Neuroanatomy*. Vol. 14: *The Primate Nervous System*, Part II, Elsevier, Amsterdam, pp. 299–433.

Mountcastle, V.B. (1957) Modality and topographic properties of single neurons of cat's somatic sensory cortex. *J. Neurophysiol.*, 20: 408–434.

Mountcastle, V.B. (1978) An organizing principle for cerebral function: the unit module and the distributed system. In: V.B. Mountcastle and G.M. Edelman (Eds.), *The mindful brain*, MIT Press, Cambridge, pp. 7–50.

Nadarajah, B., Thomaidou, D., Evans, W.H. and Parnavelas, J.G. (1996) Gap junctions in the adult cerebral cortex: regional differences in their distribution and cellular expression of connexins. *J. Comp. Neurol.*, 376: 326–342.

Nieuwenhuys, R. (1994) The neocortex. An overview of its evolutionary development, structural organization and synaptology. *Anat. Embryol.*, 190: 307–337.

Nimchinsky, E.A., Gilissen, E., Allman, J.M., Perl, D.P., Erwin, J.M. and Hof, P.R. (1999) A neuronal morphologic type unique to humans and great apes. *Proc. Natl. Acad. Sci. USA*, 96: 5268–5273.

Palay, S.L. (1956) Synapses in the central nervous system. *J. Biophys. Biochem. Cytol., Suppl.*, 2: 193–202.

Palade, G.E. and Palay, S.L. (1954) Electron microscope observations of interneuronal and neuromuscular synapses. *Anat. Rec.*, 118: 335–336.

Peters, A. (1984) Bipolar cells. In: A. Peters and E.G. Jones (Eds.), *Cerebral Cortex*. Vol. 1. *Cellular Components of the Cerebral Cortex*, Plenum Press, New York, pp. 381–407.

Peters, A. (1987) Synaptic specificity in the cerebral cortex. In: G.M. Edelman, W.E. Gall and W.M. Cowan (Eds.), *Synaptic Function*, Wiley, New York, pp. 373–397.

Peters, A. and Fairén, A. (1978) Smooth and sparsely-spined stellate cells in the visual cortex of the rat: a study using a combined Golgi-electron microscope technique. *J. Comp. Neurol.*, 181: 129–172.

Peters, A. and Kaiserman-Abramof, I.R. (1969) The small pyramidal neuron of the rat cerebral cortex. the synapses upon dendritic spines. *Z. Zellforsch.*, 100: 487–506.

Peters, A. and Kaiserman-Abramof, I.R. (1970) The small pyramidal neuron of the rat cerebral cortex: the perikaryon, dendrites and spines. *Am. J. Anat.*, 127: 321–356.

Peters, A. and Proskauer, C.C. (1980) Synaptic relationships between a multipolar stellate cell and a pyramidal neuron in the rat visual cortex. A combined Golgi-electron microscope study. *J. Neurocytol.*, 9: 163–183.

Peters, A. and Regidor, J. (1981) A reassessment of the forms of nonpyramidal neurons in area 17 of cat visual cortex. *J. Comp. Neurol.*, 203: 685–716.

Peters, A. and Sethares, C. (1996) Myelinated axons and the pyramidal cell modules in the monkey primary visual cortex. *J. Comp. Neurol.*, 365: 232–255.

Peters, A. and Sethares, C. (1997) The organization of double bouquet cells in monkey striate cortex. *J. Neurocytol.*, 26: 779–797.

Peters, A., Palay, S.L. and Webster, H. deF. (1970). *The Fine Structure of the Nervous System. The Cells and Their Processes.* Harper and Row, New York.

Peters, A., Palay, S.L. and Webster, H. deF. (1976). *The fine structure of the Nervous System. The Neurons and Supporting Cells.* Oxford University Press, New York.

Peters, A., Payne, B.R. and Josephson, K. (1990) Transcallosal non-pyramidal cell projections from visual cortex in the cat. *J. Comp. Neurol.*, 302: 124–142.

Peters, A., Proskauer, C.C. and Ribak, C.E. (1982) Chandelier cells in rat visual cortex. *J. Comp. Neurol.*, 206: 397–416.

Peters, A., Palay, S.L. and Webster, H. deF. (1991). *The Fine Structure of the Nervous System. Neurons and Their Supporting Cells.* Oxford University Press, New York.

Powell, T.P.S. and Mountcastle, V.B. (1959) Some aspects of the functional organization of the cortex of the postcentral gyrus of the monkey: a correlation of findings obtained in a single unit analysis with cytoarchitecture. *Bull. Johns Hopkins Hosp.*, 105: 133–162.

Preuss, T.M. (2000) Taking the measure of diversity: comparative alternatives to the model-animal paradigm in cortical neuroscience. *Brain Behav. Evol.*, 55: 287–299.

Prieto, J.J., Peterson, B.A. and Winer, J.A. (1994) Morphology and spatial distribution of GABAergic neurons in cat primary auditory cortex (AI). *J. Comp. Neurol.*, 344: 349–382.

Reyes, A., Lujan, R., Rozov, A., Burnashev, N., Somogyi, P. and Sakmann, B. (1998) Target-cell-specific facilitation and depression in neocortical circuits. *Nature Neurosci.*, 1: 279–285.

Ribak, C.E. (1978) Aspinous and sparsely-spinous stellate neurons in the visual cortex of rats contain glutamic acid decarboxylase. *J. Neurocytol.*, 7: 461–478.

Robertson, J.D. (1953) Ultrastructure of two invertebrate synapses. *Proc. Soc. Exp. Biol. Med.*, 82: 219–223.

Robertson, J.D. (1987) The early days of electron microscopy of nerve tissue and membranes. *Int. Rev. Cytol.*, 100: 129–201.

Rusakov, D.A., Kullmann, D.M. and Stewart, M.G. (1999) Hippocampal synapses: do they talk to their neighbours? *Trends Neurosci.*, 22: 382–388.

Sawatari, A. and Callaway, E.M. (2000) Diversity and cell type specificity of local excitatory connections to neurons in layer 3B of monkey primary visual cortex. *Neuron*, 25: 459–471.

Scheibel, M.E. and Scheibel, A.B. (1970) The rapid Golgi method: Indian summer or renaissance? In: W.J.H. Nauta and S.O.E. Ebbesson (Eds.), *Contemporary Research Methods in Neuroanatomy*, Springer, New York, pp. 1–11.

Schmechel, D.E., Vickrey, B.G., Fitzpatrick, D. and Elde, R.P. (1984) GABAergic neurons of mammalian cerebral cortex: widespread subclass defined by somatostatin content. *Neurosci. Lett.*, 47: 227–232.

Sholl, D.A (1956) *The Organization of the Cerebral Cortex.* Methuen, London.

Sloper, J.J. (1972). Gap junctions between dendrites in the primate cortex. *Brain Res.*, 44: 641–646.

Sloper, J.J. and Powell, T.P.S. (1978) Gap junctions between dendrites and somata of neurons in the primate sensori-motor cortex. *Proc. R. Soc. Lond. B.*, 203: 39–47.

Somogyi, P. (1990) Synaptic connections of neurones identified by Golgi impregnation: characterization by immunocytochemical, enzyme histochemical, and degeneration methods. *J. Electron. Microsc. Tech.*, 15: 332–351.

Somogyi, P. and Cowey, A. (1981) Combined Golgi and electron microscopic study on the synapses formed by double bouquet cells in the visual cortex of the cat and monkey. *J. Comp. Neurol.*, 195: 547–566.

Somogyi, P., Freund, T.F. and Cowey, A. (1982) The axo-axonic interneuron in the cerebral cortex of the rat, cat and monkey. *Neuroscience*, 7: 2577–2607.

Somogyi, P., Kisvárday, Z.F., Martin, K.A.C. and Whitteridge, D. (1983) Synaptic connections of morphologically identified and physiologically characterized large basket cells in the striate cortex of cat. *Neuroscience*, 10: 261–294.

Somogyi, P., Hodgson, A., Smith, A.D., Nunzi, M.G., Gorio, A. and Wu, J.-Y. (1984) Different populations of GABAergic neurons in the visual cortex and hippocampus of cat contain somatostatin- or cholecystokinin-immunoreactive material. *J. Neurosci.*, 4: 2590–2603.

Somogyi, P., Freund, T.F., Hodgson, A.J., Somogyi, J., Beroukas, D. and Chubb, I.W. (1985). Identified axo-axonic cells are immunoreactive for GABA in the hippocampus and visual cortex of cats. *Brain Res.*, 332: 143–149.

Somogyi, P., Tamás, G., Lujan, R. and Buhl, E.H. (1998) Salient features of synaptic organisation in the cerebral cortex. *Brain Res. Rev.*, 26: 113–135.

Staiger, J.F., Freund, T.F. and Zilles, K. (1997) Interneurons immunoreactive for vasoactive intestinal polypeptide (VIP) are extensively innervated by parvalbumin-containing boutons in rat primary somatosensory cortex. *Eur. J. Neurosci.*, 9: 2259–2268.

Stell, W.K. (1965). Correlation of retinal cytoarchitecture and ultrastructure in Golgi preparations. *Anat. Rec.*, 153: 389–397.

Szabadics, J., Lorincz, A. and Tamás, G. (2001) β and γ frequency synchronization by dendritic GABAergic synapses and gap junctions in a network of cortical interneurons. *J. Neurosci.*, 2: 5824–5831.

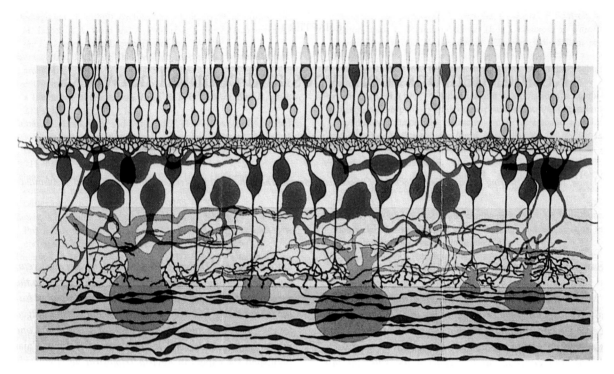

Fig. 1. The first published lithograph of Golgi-impregnated retina, reproduced from Ferrucio Tartuferi's 1887 paper on *Sull'anatomia della retina*, which was published in both *Internationale Monatsschrift für Anatomie und Physiologie* and *Archivio per le Scienze Mediche* (the source of this figure). The retina has a well-defined laminar structure with three somatic layers (outer nuclear layer, inner nuclear layer and ganglion cell layer) separated by two dendritic layers (outer plexiform layer and inner plexiform layer). The five major classes of retinal neurons are readily apparent in Tartuferi's drawing: there is a vertical pathway connecting photoreceptors to bipolar cells (*black*), and bipolar cells to ganglion cells (*blue*). In addition, there are two classes of laterally extending neurons (*red*): the horizontal cells branch in the outer plexiform layer while the amacrine cells branch in the inner plexiform layer.

Tartuferi's findings in the introduction to his 1893 monograph: "*Tartuferi was the first to demonstrate the terminal disposition of the ascendant and descendent processes of the tufted bipolar cells, and was the first to demonstrate the true morphology of several amacrine cells and horizontal cells, the presence of an axon in certain horizontal cells, and, finally, the structural details of the plexiform layers*" (Rodieck, 1973).

Although the neurons in the Golgi-impregnated retinas prepared by Tartuferi and Cajal probably appeared rather similar, the neuronal organization of the retina was interpreted very differently by Tartuferi (who was Camillo Golgi's student) and by Cajal (who would become Golgi's great antagonist). In particular, Tartuferi (1887) considered that the dendrites of bipolar cells made extensive anastomoses among themselves and with both the axon terminals of photoreceptors and the

dendrites of horizontal cells, thus forming an outer retinal network (*rete sottoepiteliale*) in which all the neurons had cytoplasmic continuity. In addition, Tartuferi (1887) considered that the axon terminals of bipolar cells formed an inner retinal network (*rete dei fiocchetti*), but he could not tell whether the processes of amacrine cells anastomosed with the bipolar cell terminals. Tartuferi's views were thus in accord with the reticular theory propounded by the Golgi School.

By contrast, Cajal's contemporary studies on the bird retina indicated that discrete retinal neurons were connected by *contiguity* rather than *continuity* (Fig. 2), and Cajal emphasized the importance of these conclusions by placing them at the beginning of his 25-point summary in *La Rétine des Vertébrés*: "1. *The nerve cells, the glial cells, the cones, and the rods of all vertebrate retinas are discrete cells, the true* neurons *of*

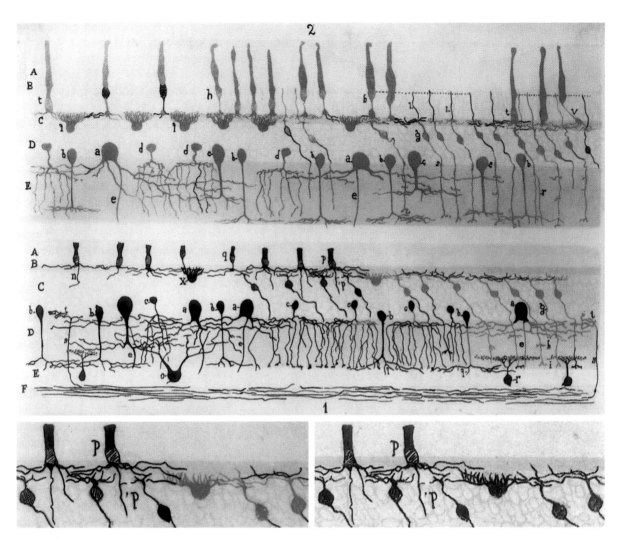

Fig. 2. Lithograph of Golgi-impregnated neurons in the duck and sparrow retinas, reproduced from Santiago Ramon y Cajal's first paper on the retina published in *Revista Trimestral de Histología Normal y Patológica* (Cajal, 1888b). The printing has faded and the paper has discolored in this rare surviving copy held in the *Museo Cajal*, but the lettering and many of the cells appear to have been re-inked by hand, particularly when viewed at higher magnification (lower left). The black pen strokes correspond exactly to those in *Trabajos Escogidos* ('Selected Works') reprinted in 1924 (lower right), suggesting that the printing had already faded by then and that the original was re-inked for the purpose of reproduction. In his autobiography, Cajal (1937) describes the fascinating background of the *Revista*: "A fever for publication devoured me. In order to make known my thoughts, I made use chiefly of a certain professional medical review, the *Gaceta Médica Catalana*. The tide of ideas and impatience for publication rising rapidly, however, this outlet became too narrow for me. I was much annoyed by the slowness of the press and the lateness of the dates of appearance. To extricate myself once and for all from such fetters, I decided to publish upon my own account a new review, the *Revista Trimestral de Histología Normal y Patológica*. The first number saw the light in May 1888, and the second appeared in the month of August of the same year. Naturally, all the articles, six in number, sprang from my own pen. From my hands emerged also the six lithographic plates which were included. Financial considerations obliged me not to print more than sixty copies altogether at the time and these were distributed almost entirely among foreign scientists. Needless to say the vortex of publication entirely swallowed up my income." Reproduced with permission of *Instituto Cajal, Consejo Superior de Investigaciones Científicas*, Madrid.

Waldeyer. 2. The transmission of neural signals takes place by means of articulation between the processes of the different retinal cells. The contacts are sometimes established between the processes of two opposed cells, but usually the links are extended to a greater number of cells. For example, the dendrites of a cone bipolar cell come into contact with several cone pedicles, each of which may make contact with dendrites arising from several bipolar cells" (Rodieck, 1973).

Cajal therefore recognized that there was both convergence and divergence in the vertical pathway from photoreceptors to bipolar cells to ganglion cells. An exception was provided by the central fovea of lizards and birds: each foveal cone appeared to contact a single bipolar cell, which in turn contacted a narrow-field ganglion cell, thereby preserving the spatial grain of the photoreceptor mosaic (Fig. 3). Although Cajal believed that the human fovea is constructed in accord with this plan, 50 years passed before Stephen Polyak (1941) provided the definitive description of the midget system in the primate retina, using the Golgi-impregnation technique refined by Cajal.

Although Cajal (1954) was very disparaging about the flimsy intellectual underpinnings of the reticular theory, he remarked on "*the formidable competition offered me by Dogiel, the great Russian histologist*" (Cajal, 1937). Alexander Dogiel was the first scientist to systematically apply the methylene blue method of Paul Ehrlich to the retina, leading to a succession of papers which were published in the same period as the bulk of Cajal's Golgi-impregnation studies (Dogiel, 1888, 1891, 1895). Both the Golgi and the Ehrlich methods capriciously

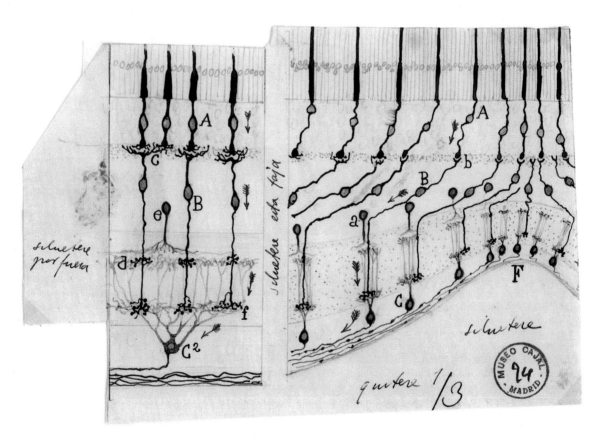

Fig. 3. An original drawing by Cajal of the sparrow retina, contrasting the organization of the neuronal pathways in central and peripheral retina. In the fovea (*F*), midget bipolar cells (*B*) provide a private line from each cone (*A*) to a ganglion cell (*C*) whereas, outside the fovea, several cones converge on each bipolar cell and several bipolar cells converge on each ganglion cell (*C2*). Reproduced with permission of *Instituto Cajal, Consejo Superior de Investigaciones Científicas*, Madrid.

stain individual nerve cells but, whereas the Golgi method was applied to fixed tissue, the Ehrlich method was applied vitally to fresh tissue.

Dogiel noted that the methylene blue method sometimes stained homogeneous arrays of neurons, as shown here for horizontal cells and ganglion cells in the human retina (Fig. 4); interestingly, Cajal (1893) illustrated a similar array of horizontal cells in methylene blue stained ox retina. Dogiel believed that the labeled cells were connected by anastomoses but, in contrast to Tartuferi, he

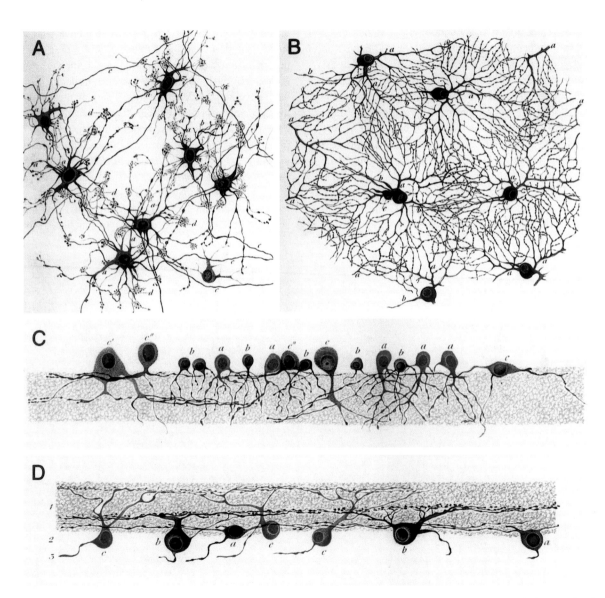

Fig. 4. Lithographs of methylene-blue stained human retina, reproduced from a paper by Alexander Dogiel published in *Archiv für Mikroskopische Anatomie* in 1891. **A**, Local array of horizontal cells stained in a wholemount preparation, showing the dendrites (*a*, *b*), axons (*c*) and receptor terminals (*d*). **B**, Local array of Type II ganglion cells stained in a wholemount preparation, showing the dendrites (*a*) and axons (*b*). **C**, Composite drawing of the neurons in the inner nuclear layer, showing large and small amacrine cells (*a*, *b*) and three types of displaced ganglion cells (*c*, *c'*, *c''*). **D**, Composite drawing of Type I (*a*), Type II (*b*) and Type III (*c*) ganglion cells, showing the stratified dendrites forming three syncitial networks in the inner plexiform layer (*Innere reticuläre Schicht*).

proposed that the outer and inner plexiform layers were made up of many neurosyncitia, each arising from a different type of neuron. For example, the three types of retinal ganglion cells that Dogiel identified would form three syncitial networks, stacked one above the other.

Cajal (1896) took great care to refute Dogiel's conclusions and, by the time Cajal finished his 'program of neuronal morphology' in 1902, the reticulum had given way to the neuron, a term coined by Wilhelm von Waldeyer-Hartz in 1891. Cajal resented the fact that the neuron doctrine in general was often attributed to Waldeyer, as he made clear forty years later in his valedictory review, *¿Neuronismo o reticularismo?* Cajal (1954) writes: "*Professor Waldeyer, to whom poorly informed persons attribute the neuron theory, supported it with the prestige of his authority but did not contribute a single personal observation. He limited himself to a short, brilliant exposition (1891) of the objective proofs, adduced by His, Kölliker, Retzius, Van Gehuchten and myself, and he invented the fortunate term of* neuron."

From 1903 onwards, Cajal turned his attention to reduced silver nitrate methods that delicately stain the neurofilaments, which form a cytoplasmic scaffold throughout the neuron. Interestingly, the neurofibrillar methods developed independently by Cajal and Max Bielschowsky weakened the position of the neuron doctrine when some scientists, led by Stephan von Apáthy, claimed that the neurofibrils formed an intercellular network. This particularly appeared to be the case for the neurofibrillar-stained horizontal cells in the retina (Embden, 1901; Bielschowsky and Pollack, 1904), whose overlapping dendrites form a tangled meshwork in the outer plexiform layer (Fig. 5). However, Cajal was quite clear in his own observations, stating that "*neither in the cells of the retina, nor in the sympathetic cells, nor yet in the sensory cells of the leech is it possible to perceive the slightest indication that the neurofibrils pass from one cell to another*" (Cajal, 1937).

Cajal could not have known that retinal horizontal cells are connected by extensive gap junctions, whose

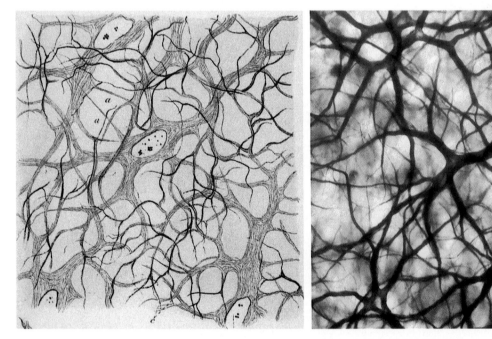

Fig. 5. Horizontal cells in the rabbit retina stained by reduced silver methods, as shown in a drawing of a transverse section (Cajal, 1904a,b) and in a micrograph of a wholemount preparation (courtesy of Brian Boycott and Leo Peichl). Neurofibrillar methods selectively stain the A-type horizontal cells, which do not have an axon, and the processes that Cajal considered axons (*a*) are incompletely stained dendrites. Cajal's lithograph appeared in two papers published in 1904: the original Spanish paper was published in *Trabajos del Laboratorio de Investigaciones Biológicas de la Universidad de Madrid* and the German translation was published in *Internationale Monatsschrift für Anatomie und Physiologie* (the source of this figure). Lithograph reproduced with permission of *Instituto Cajal, Consejo Superior de Investigaciones Científicas*, Madrid.

presence cannot be deduced from silver chromate or reduced silver preparations. With the advent of electron microscopy, Yamada and Ishikawa (1965) discovered that fish horizontal cells of the same morphological type are joined by fused membrane structures, which would later be termed 'gap junctions' (Goodenough and Revel, 1970). They noted that such structures are a device for electrical transmission of stimuli, indicating that horizontal cells are *"morphologically separate but functionally a single unit"*. A few years later, the intracellular injection of Procion Yellow or Lucifer Yellow revealed dye coupling between neighboring horizontal cells (Kaneko, 1971; Stewart, 1978) and this confirmed electrophysiological evidence that the horizontal cells form a functional neuro-syncitium, with receptive fields that are much larger than the dendritic field of a single neuron (Naka and Rushton, 1967).

Neuronal diversity in the retina

"For all those who are fascinated by the bewitchment of the infinitely small, there wait in the bosom of the living being millions of palpitating cells which, for the surren-der of their secret, and with the halo of fame, demand only a clear and persistent intelligence to contemplate, admire, and understand them." (Cajal, 1937)

Cajal's use of bird tissue in his early Golgi-impregna-tion experiments was fortuitous as the bird retina is very thick, showing the lamination of the inner plexiform layer to advantage. Thus, Cajal was able to perceive clearly that the axon terminals of different types of bipo-lar cells stratified at different levels, where they made contact with the stratified dendrites of different types of ganglion cells. In the mammalian retina, Cajal (1937) illustrated four types of cone bipolar cells terminating in strata 1–4 of the inner plexiform layer, and a single type of rod bipolar cell terminating in stratum 5, adjacent to the ganglion cell layer. Cajal's recognition that these neu-ronal pathways formed separate 'channels' provided the foundation for modern concepts of parallel processing in the visual system. We now know that there are about five types of cone bipolar cells terminating in strata 1 and 2 which convey Off-signals, and another five types terminating in strata 3 and 4 which convey On-signals (Boycott and Wässle, 1999).

Cajal's other outstanding contribution to retinal neuroscience was the discovery of the remarkable morphological diversity of both the ganglion cells and the interneurons of the inner retina, which Cajal (1893) termed 'amacrine' cells, from the Greek *a-makrós-inos* meaning 'without-long-fiber'. Cajal described three main categories of amacrine cells: the 'diffuse' cells were sub-divided into small and large varieties, and the 'stratified' and 'bistratified' cells were first subdivided according to their level of branching, and then by differences in their size and dendritic morphology. Cajal's Golgi-impreg-nated retinas were usually cut in vertical sections, making it impossible to trace the full extent of medium- and wide-field neurons. Thus, Cajal's original reports of the great neuronal diversity in the inner retina were not substantiated until the 1970s, when Golgi-impregnation methods for staining wholemounted retinas were devel-oped by several researchers including Brian Boycott and Helga Kolb (1973).

In the wholemount studies, the labeled neurons were sorted into separate types based on their dendritic branching pattern, stratification level and dendritic-field size. Kolb et al., (1981) identified 22 different types of amacrine cells in the cat retina, and subsequent studies have identified as many as 26 types in the primate retina (Mariani, 1990; Kolb et al., 1992) and 70 types in the teleost retina (Wagner and Wagner, 1988). Moreover, Golgi-impregnation is rather capricious and some types were represented by only one or a few labeled cells; apart from the problems of characterizing a neuronal type with so few cells, probability alone indicates that some other types of amacrine cells would be missing from the sample. Because of the qualitative nature of these Golgi-impregnation studies, the extraordinary neuronal diversity that they revealed was not accepted widely until other means were found to validate individual types of amacrine cells, usually by methods that specifically stained a whole population of cells.

The concept of neuronal type that underlies the Golgi-impregnation studies was explicitly addressed by Peter Sterling (1983) in his meticulous studies on the micro-circuitry of the cat retina. He noted that *"a 'type' has come to be defined by the regular association of particu-lar morphological, cytological, connectional, chemical, and physiological features…. Each type, so defined, turns out to have a characteristic stoichiometry and distribution in the retinal mosaic, thus further supporting the idea that the type is fundamental."* Bob Rodieck developed these ideas more formally, emphasizing that the demonstration of 'natural' types is dependent on the

248

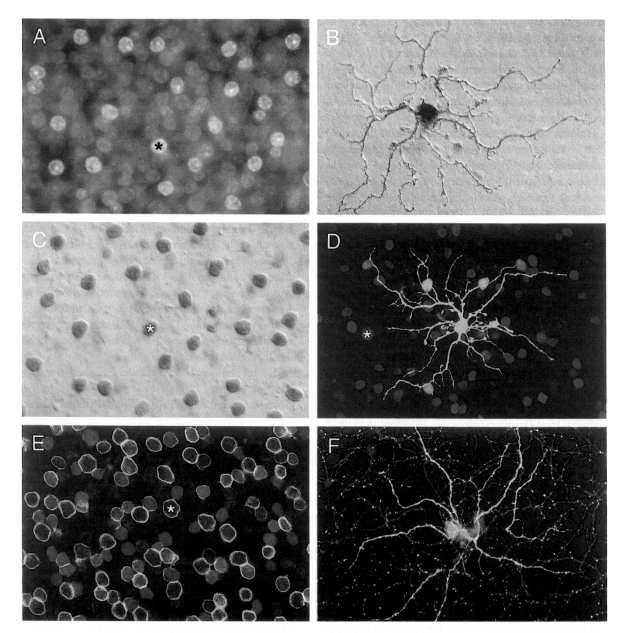

Fig. 6. The mosaic of AII amacrine cells in the rabbit retina as visualized by different methods in wholemounts; representative AII cells are marked with an asterisk. **A**, The AII cells can be identified in isolated living retina that has been labeled *in vivo* with Nuclear Yellow; under ultraviolet excitation, the nuclei of the AII cells fluoresce bright gold whereas the nuclei of several other types of amacrine cells fluoresce bright blue. **B**, Intracellular injection of an AII amacrine cell with Lucifer Yellow reveals its characteristic bistratified morphology; photo-oxidation of the fluorescent dye to an opaque reaction product delineates both the proximal lobular appendages and the distal arboreal dendrites. **C**, Intracellular injection of an AII amacrine cell with a gap-junction permeable tracer, Neurobiotin, reveals that the AII cells are homologously coupled with each other and heterologously coupled to On cone bipolar cells, whose smaller somata lie deeper in the inner nuclear layer. **D**, About 60% of the amacrine cells are glycine-immunoreactive (*red*), including the population of AII cells labeled by tracer coupling following Neurobiotin injection of the central cell (*green*). **E**, Although the AII cells are amongst the most weakly labeled of the glycine-immunopositive amacrine cells (*red*), they strongly express the glycine transporter GLYT1 (*cyan*), indicating that they are functionally glycinergic. **F**, The overlapping arboreal dendrites of a Neurobiotin-injected AII cell (*green*) and neighboring calretinin-immunoreactive AII cells (*magenta*) are studded with puncta (*white*) that are immunoreactive for the gap-junction protein, connexin 36. (**A** & **B** after Vaney et al., 1991; **C** after Hampson et al., 1992; **D** after Wright et al., 1997; **E** after Vaney et al., 1998; **F** after Mills et al., 2001)

Weiler and Ball, 1984) but these findings are now considered unremarkable because virtually all amacrine cells contain elevated levels of GABA or glycine (Marc et al., 1995; Crook and Pow, 1997). Nevertheless, there are two particularly interesting cases where the colocalization of neurotransmitters has foreshadowed unexpected complexity in the functions of amacrine cells.

In the first case, a distinct type of amacrine cell in the chicken retina was shown to contain three neuropeptides, namely enkephalin, neurotensin and somatostatin (Watt and Florack, 1994); these 'ENSLI' amacrine cells become inactivated at a critical light intensity, suggesting that they may play a complementary role to the dopaminergic amacrine cells in light adaptation (Morgan et al., 1994). In the second case, the starburst amacrine cells in the rabbit retina were shown to contain both acetylcholine and GABA (Brecha et al., 1988; Vaney and Young, 1988), which was the first instance where two 'fast-acting' transmitters – one excitatory and the other inhibitory—were colocalized in identified neurons. Vaney et al., (1989) proposed that the starburst cells may provide asymmetric excitatory and/or asymmetric inhibitory inputs to direction-selective ganglion cells and, currently, this is a very active area of retinal research (He and Masland, 1997; Taylor et al., 2000; Borg-Graham, 2001; Vaney et al., 2001; Yoshida et al., 2001).

In general, immunocytochemistry has not been useful for selectively labeling individual populations of retinal ganglion cells, although a variety of neuropeptides have been localized in ganglion cells of different vertebrate classes (Brecha et al., 1987; Hutsler et al., 1993). Given that all ganglion cells receive excitatory inputs from glutamatergic bipolar cells and inhibitory inputs from GABAergic and glycinergic amacrine cells, and that they all probably make glutamatergic synapses in the brain, there is little reason to expect that the ganglion cells would show much heterogeneity in their neurochemistry. The same argument also seemed to hold for either the On-types or Off-types of bipolar cells, notwithstanding the early studies showing spectacular PKC-immunolabeling of the rod bipolar cells (Negishi et al., 1988; Young and Vaney, 1991). However, different types of cone bipolar cells have since been shown to express an unexpected diversity of cellular markers, which has been critical for distinguishing bipolar cells that are morphologically similar (Kouyama and Marshak, 1992; Milam et al., 1993; Grünert et al., 1994; Rauen and Kanner, 1994; Jeon and Masland, 1995; Brown and Masland, 1999; Boycott and Wässle, 1999).

The colocalization of neurotransmitters and neuroactive substances in retinal neurons raised the exciting possibility that each cell type may be identified by a unique neurochemical signature (Lam et al., 1985), comparable to the chemical coding of enteric neurons (Costa et al., 1986). The signature hypothesis has been tested most rigorously by Robert Marc and his colleagues, who used postembedding immunocytochemistry and pattern recognition techniques to analyze quantitatively the amino acid content of all cells in serial plastic sections of goldfish, monkey and cat retinas (Marc et al., 1995, 1998; Kalloniatis et al., 1996). This analysis partitioned virtually all of the retinal neurons into as many as 15 'theme' classes that had statistically separable amino-acid signatures. Although the amacrine cells in monkey retina could be divided into four GABA-dominated classes and another four glycine-dominated classes (Kalloniatis et al., 1996), this falls far short of accommodating the known morphological diversity of the amacrine cells. Moreover, the restricted number of glutamate-dominated theme classes provides an even poorer match to the neuronal diversity of the bipolar cells and the retinal ganglion cells. However, if the quantitative immunocytochemical analysis could be extended to include neuropeptides and the dozens of enzymes involved in neurotransmission, then it is possible that the number of theme classes extracted might approach the number of morphological types of retinal neurons.

Tracer-coupling of retinal neurons

"*When chance permits an investigator to create a new or selective staining method or to perfect in a fortunate way one already known, histology sensibly extends its horizon. The harvesting of new and significant facts, the cataloguing of forms and structures, is performed easily and refreshingly as if one reaped at will in a wheat-field sown by others.*" (Cajal, 1937)

The AII amacrine cells are third-order neurons in the rod-signal pathway and their synaptic connections have been studied in detail (Famiglietti and Kolb, 1975; Sterling et al., 1988). Although the AII amacrine cells make extensive gap junctions, both with each other and with On cone bipolar cells, they show no evidence of dye coupling when injected with Lucifer Yellow (Vaney, 1985). In fact, the only neurons in the mammalian retina that show dye coupling are the A-type horizontal cells (Dacheux and Raviola, 1982), even though gap junctions are found throughout the retina. A quite different picture emerges when the AII amacrine cells are injected with small cationic tracers such as biocytin or Neurobiotin: they show a complex pattern of tracer coupling that reflects their gap-junction connectivity (Vaney, 1991). Moreover, the size of the tracer-coupled network of AII cells closely matches the receptive-field size of individual AII cells, and both increase with background light intensity indicating that the permeability of the homologous gap junctions is modulated dynamically, perhaps under dopaminergic control (Hampson et al., 1992; Bloomfield et al., 1997).

Tracer coupling has proved to be a powerful tool for selectively labeling local arrays of many types of amacrine cells, both by homologous coupling following injection of a single cell and by heterologous coupling following injection of a ganglion cell or a different type of amacrine cell (Vaney, 1991, 1994a, 1999). In fact, more types of amacrine cells can be selectively labeled by tracer coupling than by immunolabeling with presently available antisera. The selectivity of the coupling cannot be explained by the vertical stratification of different types of neurons. In the rabbit retina, for example, the S1 and S2 amacrine cells have similar dendritic morphologies and form a dense plexus in the inner stratum of the inner plexiform layer (Vaney, 1986) but it appears that the S1 cells are not heterologously coupled to the S2 cells, although each type shows homologous tracer coupling (Vaney, 1994a).

Biotinylated tracers do not mask the antigenicity of intracellular epitopes in the coupled cells and, therefore, a single preparation can be used to characterize the dendritic morphology, cellular array and neurotransmitter content of a cell type (Wright et al., 1997; Wright and Vaney, 1999). These studies have reinforced earlier evidence that different types of amacrine cells express characteristic levels of inhibitory transmitters (Pourcho and Goebel, 1985, 1987); for example, the DAPI-3 amacrine cells consistently show the strongest glycine immunoreactivity in the rabbit retina whereas the AII amacrine cells are amongst the most weakly labeled of the glycine-immunopositive cells (Wright et al., 1997).

Many types of retinal ganglion cells show diverse patterns of tracer coupling, with the simplest pattern represented by the homologous coupling shown by On-Off direction-selective (DS) ganglion cells in the rabbit retina (Fig. 7). Neighboring DS ganglion cells with a common preferred direction have regularly spaced somata and highly territorial dendritic fields, whereas DS ganglion cells with different preferred directions may have closely spaced somata and overlapping dendritic fields (Vaney, 1994b; Amthor and Oyster, 1995). It is arguable, therefore, that the On-Off DS ganglion cells comprise four natural types (superior, inferior, nasal and temporal preferred directions), in the same way that the alpha ganglion cells comprise two natural types (On- and Off-center), with each type independently mapping the visual space (Rodieck and Brening, 1983).

Many other types of retinal ganglion cells show heterologous tracer coupling, with the tracer diffusing from an injected ganglion cell to one or a few types of amacrine cells but, surprisingly, the tracer rarely diffuses from an injected amacrine cell to a ganglion cell. The only documented case involves a type of interstitial amacrine cell in the macaque retina (Stafford and Dacey, 1997) and it is interesting that the homologous cells in the rabbit retina show a similar pattern of tracer coupling. Other studies have shown that the coupling pattern of the parasol ganglion cells in monkey retina is very similar to that of the alpha ganglion cells in diverse mammalian retinas, with the cells showing both homologous coupling to neighboring ganglion cells and heterologous coupling to at least two types of wide-field unistratified amacrine cells, whose somata are located in the inner nuclear, inner plexiform and ganglion cell layers (Vaney, 1991; Dacey and Brace, 1992; Penn et al., 1994).

The clear evidence from tracer-coupling studies that many types of retinal neurons form homologously coupled networks has much in common with Dogiel's model of the retina, in which each type of neuron was presumed to form a syncitial sheet. However, this does not challenge Cajal's fundamental conclusion that the retina is composed of discrete cells that communicate by contact. Cajal (1937) took care to distinguish the objective nature of his observations from the subjective nature of his interpretations and he prophetically speculated how new observations might challenge his conception of the neuron doctrine: "*Let us imagine that there is discovered an exquisitely selective method of coloration, through which there is revealed an extremely delicate system of anastomotic fibres, absolutely invisible with existing procedures.... Once*

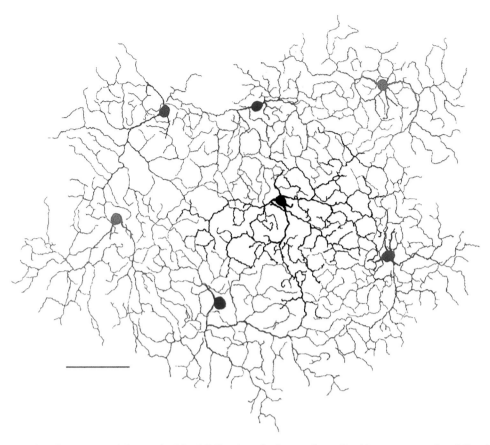

Fig. 7. Reconstruction of a tracer-coupled network of On-Off direction-selective ganglion cells with a common preferred direction, showing the dendritic arborization in the On sublamina of the inner plexiform layer. The Neurobiotin-injected cell is printed in black and the tracer-coupled cells are printed in color. The dendritic fields of neighboring cells are highly territorial, providing complete coverage of the retina with almost no overlap. Scale bar = 100 μm.

more the provisional character of our theoretical interpretations and the unavoidable need of revising and perfecting them in accordance with new discoveries would be made apparent."

Epilogue

Santiago Ramón y Cajal noted in his autobiography that: *"The retina has always shown itself generous with me."* This modest sentiment would have struck a chord with other great retinal anatomists such as Stephen Polyak and Brian Boycott, who are rightly regarded as Cajal's scientific heirs. Those of us who are privileged to study the structure and function of the retina with modern techniques can confirm that the generosity of the retina continues to this day.

Acknowledgments

I thank Rowan Tweedale for editing the manuscript and Maria Angustias Pérez-de-Tudela, Guy Elston, Leo Peichl, Heinz Wässle, Uli Siebeck and Piero Giorgi for their assistance in accessing historic publications. D.I.V. is supported by the National Health and Medical Research Council of Australia.

References

Agardh, E., Bruun, A., Ehinger, B. and Storm-Mathisen, J. (1986) GABA immunoreactivity in the retina. *Invest. Ophthalmol. Vis. Sci.*, 27: 674–678.

Amthor, F.R. and Oyster, C.W. (1995) Spatial organization of retinal information about the direction of image motion. *Proc. Natl. Acad. Sci. USA*, 92: 4002–4005.

Bielschowsky, M. and Pollack, B. (1904) Zur Kenntnis der Innervation des Säugethierauges. *Neurol. Zentbl.*, 23: 387–394.

Bloomfield, S.A., Xin, D. and Osborne, T. (1997) Light-induced modulation of coupling between AII amacrine cells in the rabbit retina. *Vis Neurosci.*, 14: 565–576.

Borg-Graham, L.J. (2001) The computation of directional selectivity in the retina occurs presynaptic to the ganglion cell. *Nature Neurosci.*, 4: 176–183.

Boycott, B.B. and Kolb, H. (1973) The horizontal cells of the rhesus monkey retina. *J. Comp. Neurol.*, 148: 115–140.

Boycott, B.B. and Wässle, H. (1974) The morphological types of ganglion cells of the domestic cat's retina. *J. Physiol.*, 240: 397–419.

Boycott, B. and Wässle, H. (1999) Parallel processing in the mammalian retina: the Proctor Lecture. *Invest. Ophthalmol. Vis. Sci.*, 40: 1313–1327.

Brandon, C., Lam, D.M.-K. and Wu, J.-Y. (1979) The γ-aminobutyric acid system in rabbit retina: localization by immunocytochemistry and autoradiography. *Proc. Natl. Acad. Sci. USA*, 76: 3557–3561.

Brecha, N., Karten, H.J. and Laverack, C. (1979) Enkephalin-containing amacrine cells in the avian retina: immunohistochemical localization. *Proc. Natl. Acad. Sci. USA*, 76: 3010–3014.

Brecha, N.C., Eldred, W., Kuljis, R.O. and Karten, H.J. (1984a) Identification and localization of biologically active peptides in the vertebrate retina. *Prog. Retinal Res.*, 3: 185–226.

Brecha, N.C., Oyster, C.W. and Takahashi, E.S. (1984b) Identification and characterization of tyrosine hydroxylase immunoreactive amacrine cells. *Invest. Ophthalmol. Vis. Sci.*, 25: 66–70.

Brecha, N., Johnson, D., Bolz, J., Sharma, S., Parnavelas, J.G. and Lieberman, A.R. (1987) Substance P-immunoreactive retinal ganglion cells and their central axon terminals in the rabbit. *Nature*, 327: 155–158.

Brecha, N., Johnson, D., Peichl, L. and Wässle, H. (1988) Cholinergic amacrine cells of the rabbit retina contain glutamate decarboxylase and gamma-aminobutyrate immunoreactivity. *Proc. Natl. Acad. Sci. USA*, 85: 6187–6191.

Brown, S.P. and Masland, R.H. (1999) Costratification of a population of bipolar cells with the direction- selective circuitry of the rabbit retina. *J. Comp. Neurol.*, 408: 97–106.

Cajal, S.R. (1888a) Estructura de los centros nerviosos de las aves. *Rev. Trimest. Histol. Norm. Patol.*, May.

Cajal, S.R. (1888b) Morfología y conexiones de los elementos de la retina de las aves. *Rev. Trimest. Histol. Norm. Patol.*, May. Reprinted in 1924, *Trabajos Escogidos*, Jiménez y Molina, Madrid, pp. 355–362.

Cajal, S.R. (1888c) Sobre las fibras nerviosas de la capa molecular del cerebelo. *Rev. Trimest. Histol. Norm. Patol.*, August.

Cajal, S.R. (1888d) Estructura de la retina de las aves. *Rev. Trimest. Histol. Norm. Patol.*, August.

Cajal, S.R. (1893) La rétine des vertébrés. *La Cellule*, 9: 119–257. English translation in Rodieck (1973).

Cajal, S.R. (1896) Nouvelles contributions à l'étude histologique de la rétine et à la question des anastomoses des prolongements protoplasmiques. *J. Anat. Physiol. Paris*, 32: 481–543.

Cajal, S.R. (1904a) El retículo neurofibrillar en la retina. *Trab. Lab. Invest. Biol. Univ. Madrid*, 3: 185–211.

Cajal, S.R. (1904b) Das Neurofibrillennetz der Retina. *Int. Monatsschr. Anat. Physiol.*, 21: 369–396.

Cajal, S.R. (1933) Les problèmes histophysiologiques de la rétine. XIV Conc. Ophthal. Hispan. 2: 11–19.

Cajal, S.R. (1937) *Recollections of My Life*. American Philosophical Society, Philadelphia. Reprinted in 1966, MIT Press, Cambridge Mass., pp. 1–638.

Cajal, S.R. (1954) *Neuron Theory or Reticular Theory: Objective Evidence of the Anatomical Unity of Nerve Cells*. Consejo Superior de Investigaciones Cientificas, Madrid, pp. 1–144.

Cohen, E. and Sterling, P. (1990) Demonstration of cell types among cone bipolar neurons of cat retina. *Phil. Trans. R. Soc. Lond. B*, 330: 305–321.

Costa, M., Furness, J.B. and Gibbins, I.L. (1986) Chemical coding of enteric neurons. *Prog. Brain Res.*, 68: 217–239.

Crook, D.K. and Pow, D.V. (1997) Analysis of the distribution of glycine and GABA in amacrine cells of the developing rabbit retina: a comparison with the ontogeny of a functional GABA transport system in retinal neurons. *Vis. Neurosci.*, 14: 751–763.

Dacey, D.M. (1990) The dopaminergic amacrine cell. *J. Comp. Neurol.*, 301: 461–489.

Dacey, D.M. and Brace, S. (1992) A coupled network for parasol but not midget ganglion cells in the primate retina. *Vis. Neurosci.*, 9: 279–290.

Dacheux, R.F. and Raviola, E. (1982) Horizontal cells in the retina of the rabbit. *J. Neurosci.*, 2: 1486–1493.

Darwin, C.R. (1860) In: F. Darwin (Ed.), *The Autobiography of Charles Darwin and Selected Letters*, Murray, London.

Dogiel, A.S. (1888) Ueber das Verhalten der nervösen Elemente in der Retina der Ganoiden, Reptilien, Vögel und Säugetiere. *Anat. Anz.*, 3: 133–143.

Dogiel, A.S. (1891) Ueber die nervösen Elemente in der Retina des Menschen. *Arch. Mikrosk. Anat.*, 38: 317–344.

Dogiel, A.S. (1895) Ein besonderer Typus von Nervenzellen in der mittleren gangliösen Schicht der Vogel-Retina. *Anat. Anz.*, 10: 750–760.

Ehinger, B. (1966) Adrenergic retinal neurons. *Z. Zellforsch.*, 71: 146–152.

Embden, G. (1901) Primitivfibrillenverlauf in der Netzhaut. *Arch. Mikrosk. Anat.*, 57: 570–593.

Famiglietti, E.V. and Kolb, H. (1975) A bistratified amacrine cell and synaptic circuitry in the inner plexiform layer of the retina. *Brain Res*, 84: 293–300.

Gábriel, R. and Straznicky, C. (1992) Immunocytochemical localization of parvalbumin and neurofilament triplet protein immunoreactivity in the cat retina: colocalization in a subpopulation of AII amacrine cells. *Brain Res.*, 595: 133–136.

Gallego, A. (1983) Advances in the knowledge of the organization of the outer plexiform layer of the retina since Cajal. In: S. Grisiolía, C. Guerri, F. Samson, N. Norton and F. Reinoso-Suárez (Eds.), *Ramón y Cajal's Contribution to the Neurosciences*, Elsevier, Amsterdam, pp. 183–200.

Gerlach, J. (1872) Von dem Rückenmark. In: S. Stricker (Ed.), *Handbuch der Lehre von den Geweben des Menschen und der Thiere*, Vol. 2, Engelmann, Leipzig, pp. 1–665.

Goodenough, D.A. and Revel, J.P. (1970) A fine structural analysis of intercellular junctions in the mouse liver. *J. Cell Biol.*, 45: 272–290.

Grünert, U., Martin, P.R. and Wässle, H. (1994) Immunocytochemical analysis of bipolar cells in the macaque monkey retina. *J. Comp. Neurol.*, 348: 607–627.

Häggendal, J. and Malmfors, T. (1965) Identification and cellular localization of the catecholamines in the retina and choroid of the rabbit. *Acta Physiol. Scand.*, 64: 58–66.

Hampson, E.C.G.M., Vaney, D.I. and Weiler, R. (1992) Dopaminergic modulation of gap junction permeability between amacrine cells in mammalian retina. *J. Neurosci.*, 12: 4911–4922.

He, S. and Masland, R.H. (1997) Retinal direction selectivity after targeted laser ablation of starburst amacrine cells. *Nature*, 389: 378–382.

Hutsler, J.J., White, C.A. and Chalupa, L.M. (1993) Neuropeptide Y immunoreactivity identifies a group of gamma-type retinal ganglion cells in the cat. *J. Comp. Neurol.*, 336: 468–480.

Jeon, C.J. and Masland, R.H. (1995) A population of wide-field bipolar cells in the rabbit's retina. *J. Comp. Neurol.*, 360: 403–412.

Kalloniatis, M., Marc, R.E. and Murry, R.F. (1996) Amino acid signatures in the primate retina. *J. Neurosci.*, 16: 6807–6829.

Kaneko, A. (1971) Electrical connexions between horizontal cells in the dogfish retina. *J. Physiol.*, 213: 95–105.

Karten, H.J. and Brecha, N. (1980) Localisation of substance P immunoreactivity in amacrine cells of the retina. *Nature*, 283: 87–88.

Kolb, H., Nelson, R. and Mariani, A. (1981) Amacrine cells, bipolar cells and ganglion cells of the cat retina: a Golgi study. *Vision Res.*, 21: 1081–1114.

Kolb, H., Linberg, K.A. and Fisher, S.K. (1992) Neurons of the human retina: a Golgi study. *J. Comp. Neurol.*, 318: 147–187.

Kouyama, N. and Marshak, D.W. (1992) Bipolar cells specific for blue cones in the macaque retina. *J. Neurosci.*, 12: 1233–1252.

Lam, D.M.-K., Su, Y.-Y.T., Swain, L., Marc, R.E., Brandon, C. and Wu, J.-Y. (1979) Immunocytochemical localization of L-glutamic acid decarboxylase in the goldfish retina. *Nature*, 278: 565–567.

Lam, D.M.-K., Li, H.-B., Su, Y.-Y.T. and Watt, C.B. (1985) The signature hypothesis: co-localizations of neuroactive substances as anatomical probes for circuitry analyses. *Vision Res.*, 25: 1353–1364.

MacNeil, M.A. and Masland, R.H. (1998) Extreme diversity among amacrine cells: implications for function. *Neuron*, 20: 971–982.

MacNeil, M.A., Heussy, J.K., Dacheux, R.F., Raviola, E. and Masland, R.H. (1999) The shapes and numbers of amacrine cells: matching of photofilled with Golgi-stained cells in the rabbit retina and comparison with other mammalian species. *J. Comp. Neurol.*, 413: 305–326.

Marc, R.E., Murry, R.F. and Basinger, S.F. (1995) Pattern recognition of amino acid signatures in retinal neurons. *J. Neurosci.*, 15: 5106–5129.

Marc, R.E., Murry, R.F., Fisher, S.K., Linberg, K.A., Lewis, G.P. and Kalloniatis, M. (1998) Amino acid signatures in the normal cat retina. *Invest. Ophthalmol. Vis. Sci.*, 39: 1685–1693.

Mariani, A.P. (1990) Amacrine cells of the rhesus monkey retina. *J. Comp. Neurol.*, 301: 382–400.

McGuire, B.A., Stevens, J.K. and Sterling, P. (1984) Microcircuitry of bipolar cells in cat retina. *J. Neurosci.*, 4: 2920–2938.

Milam, A.H., Dacey, D.M. and Dizhoor, A.M. (1993) Recoverin immunoreactivity in mammalian cone bipolar cells. *Vis. Neurosci.*, 10: 1–12.

Mills, S.L., O'Brien, J.J., Li, W., O'Brien, J. and Massey, S.C. (2001) Rod pathways in the mammalian retina use connexin 36. *J. Comp. Neurol.*, 436: 336–350.

Morgan, I.G., Wellard, J.W. and Boelen, M.K. (1994) A role for the enkephalin-immunoreactive amacrine cells of the chicken retina in adaptation to light and dark. *Neurosci. Lett.*, 174: 64–66.

Mosinger, J.L., Yazulla, S. and Studholme, K.M. (1986) GABA-like immunoreactivity in the vertebrate retina: a species comparison. *Exp. Eye Res.*, 42: 631–644.

Naka, K.-I. and Rushton, W.A.H. (1967) The generation and spread of S-potentials in fish (Cyprinidae). *J. Physiol.*, 192: 437–461.

Negishi, K., Kato, S. and Teranishi, T. (1988) Dopamine cells and rod bipolar cells contain protein kinase C-like immunoreactivity in some vertebrate retinas. *Neurosci. Lett.*, 94: 247–252.

Pasteels, B., Rogers, J., Blachier, F. and Pochet, R. (1990) Calbindin and calretinin localization in retina from different species. *Vis. Neurosci.*, 5: 1–16.

Penn, A.A., Wong, R.O. and Shatz, C.J. (1994) Neuronal coupling in the developing mammalian retina. *J. Neurosci.*, 14: 3805–3815.

Piccolino, M. (1988) Cajal and the retina: a 100-year retrospective. *Trends Neurosci.*, 11: 521–525.

Polyak, S.L. (1941) *The Retina*. University of Chicago Press, Chicago, pp. 1–607.

Pourcho, R.G. and Goebel, D.J. (1985) A combined Golgi and autoradiographic study of (^{3}H)glycine-accumulating amacrine cells in the cat retina. *J. Comp. Neurol.*, 233: 473–480.

Pourcho, R.G. and Goebel, D.J. (1987) Visualization of endogenous glycine in cat retina: an immunocytochemical study with Fab fragments. *J. Neurosci.*, 7: 1189–1197.

Pow, D.V. and Crook, D.K. (1993) Extremely high titre polyclonal antisera against small neurotransmitter molecules: rapid production, characterisation and use in light- and electron-microscopic immunocytochemistry. *J. Neurosci. Methods*, 48: 51–63.

Pow, D.V., Wright, L.L. and Vaney, D.I. (1995) The immunocytochemical detection of amino-acid neurotransmitters in paraformaldehyde-fixed tissues. *J. Neurosci. Methods*, 56: 115–123.

Rauen, T. and Kanner, B.I. (1994) Localization of the glutamate transporter GLT-1 in rat and macaque monkey retinae. *Neurosci. Lett.*, 169: 137–140.

Rodieck, R.W. (1973) *The Vertebrate Retina: Principles of Structure and Function*. Freeman, San Francisco, pp. 1–1044.

Rodieck, R.W. (1998) *The First Steps in Seeing*. Sinauer, Sunderland MA, pp. 1–562.

Rodieck, R.W. and Brening, R.K. (1983) Retinal ganglion cells: properties, types, genera, pathways and trans-species comparisons. *Brain Behav. Evol.*, 23: 121–164.

Sandell, J.H. and Masland, R.H. (1989) Shape and distribution of an unusual retinal neuron. *J. Comp. Neurol.*, 280: 489–497.

Stafford, D.K. and Dacey, D.M. (1997) Physiology of the A1 amacrine: a spiking, axon-bearing interneuron of the macaque monkey retina. *Vis. Neurosci.*, 14: 507–522.

Sterling, P. (1983) Microcircuitry of the cat retina. *Ann. Rev. Neurosci.*, 6: 149–185.

Sterling, P., Freed, M.A. and Smith, R.G. (1988) Architecture of rod and cone circuits to the on-beta ganglion cell. *J. Neurosci.*, 8: 623–642.

Stewart, W.W. (1978) Functional connections between cells as revealed by dye-coupling with a highly fluorescent naphthalimide tracer. *Cell*, 14: 741–759.

Strettoi, E. and Masland, R.H. (1996) The number of unidentified amacrine cells in the mammalian retina. *Proc. Natl. Acad. Sci. USA*, 93: 14906–14911.

Tartuferi, F. (1887) Sull'anatomia della retina. *Arch. Scienze Mediche*, 11: 335–358.

Tauchi, M. and Masland, R.H. (1984) The shape and arrangement of the cholinergic neurons in the rabbit retina. *Proc. R. Soc. Lond. B*, 223: 101–119.

Tauchi, M., Madigan, N.K. and Masland, R.H. (1990) Shapes and distributions of the catecholamine-accumulating neurons in the rabbit retina. *J. Comp. Neurol.*, 293: 178–189.

Taylor, W.R., He, S., Levick, W.R. and Vaney, D.I. (2000) Dendritic computation of direction selectivity by retinal ganglion cells. *Science*, 289: 2347–2350.

Vaney, D.I. (1984) 'Coronate' amacrine cells in the rabbit retina have the 'starburst' dendritic morphology. *Proc. R. Soc. Lond. B*, 220: 501–508.

Vaney, D.I. (1985) The morphology and topographic distribution of AII amacrine cells in the cat retina. *Proc. R. Soc. Lond. B*, 224: 475–488.

Vaney, D.I. (1986) Morphological identification of serotonin-accumulating neurons in the living retina. *Science*, 233: 444–446.

Vaney, D.I. (1990) The mosaic of amacrine cells in the mammalian retina. *Prog. Retinal Res.*, 9: 49–100.

Vaney, D.I. (1991) Many diverse types of retinal neurons show tracer coupling when injected with biocytin or Neurobiotin. *Neurosci. Lett.*, 125: 187–190.

Vaney, D.I. (1994a) Patterns of neuronal coupling in the retina. *Prog. Retinal Eye Res.*, 13: 301–355.

Vaney, D.I. (1994b) Territorial organization of direction-selective ganglion cells in rabbit retina. *J. Neurosci.*, 14: 6301–6316.

Vaney, D.I. (1999) Neuronal coupling in the central nervous system: lessons from the retina, *Gap Junction-Mediated Intercellular Signalling in Health and Disease (Novartis Foundation Symposium 219)*, Wiley, Chichester, pp. 113–133.

Vaney, D.I. and Young, H.M. (1988) GABA-like immunoreactivity in cholinergic amacrine cells of the rabbit retina. *Brain Res.*, 438: 369–373.

Vaney, D.I., Peichl, L. and Boycott, B.B. (1981) Matching populations of amacrine cells in the inner nuclear and ganglion cell layers of the rabbit retina. *J. Comp. Neurol.*, 199: 373–391.

Vaney, D.I., Collin, S.P. and Young, H.M. (1989) Dendritic relationships between cholinergic amacrine cells and direction-selective retinal ganglion cells. In: R. Weiler and N.N. Osborne (Eds.), *Neurobiology of the Inner Retina*, Springer, Berlin, pp. 157–168.

Vaney, D.I., Gynther, I.C. and Young, H.M. (1991) Rod-signal interneurons in the rabbit retina: 2. AII amacrine cells. *J. Comp. Neurol.*, 310: 154–169.

Vaney, D.I., Nelson, J.C. and Pow, D.V. (1998) Neurotransmitter coupling through gap junctions in the retina. *J. Neurosci.*, 18: 10594–10602.

Vaney, D.I., He, S., Taylor, W.R. and Levick, W.R. (2001) Direction-selective ganglion cells in the retina. In: J.M. Zanker and J. Zeil (Eds.), *Motion Vision: Computational, Neural, and Ecological Constraints*, Springer, Berlin, pp. 13–55.

Wagner, H.J. and Wagner, E. (1988) Amacrine cells in the retina of a teleost fish, the roach (*Rutilus rutilus*): a Golgi study on differentiation and layering. *Phil. Trans. R. Soc. Lond. B*, 321: 263–324.

Waldeyer, W. (1891) Ueber einege neuere Forschungen im Gebiete der Anatomie des Centralnervensystems. *Deutsche Med. Wochenschr.*, 17: 1213–1218, 1244–1246, 1267–1269, 1287–1289, 1331–1332, 1352–1356.

Wässle, H., Peichl, L. and Boycott, B.B. (1978) Topography of horizontal cells in the retina of the domestic cat. *Proc. R. Soc. Lond. B*, 203: 269–291.

Wässle, H., Peichl, L. and Boycott, B.B. (1981a) Morphology and topography of on- and off-alpha cells in the cat retina. *Proc. R. Soc. Lond. B*, 212: 157–175.

Wässle, H., Boycott, B.B. and Illing, R.B. (1981b) Morphology and mosaic of on- and off-beta cells in the cat retina and some functional considerations. *Proc. R. Soc. Lond. B*, 212: 177–195.

Wässle, H., Peichl, L. and Boycott, B.B. (1981c) Dendritic territories of cat retinal ganglion cells. *Nature*, 292: 344–345.

Watanabe, M. and Rodieck, R.W. (1989) Parasol and midget ganglion cells of the primate retina. *J. Comp. Neurol.*, 289: 434–454.

Watt, C.B. and Florack, V.J. (1994) A triple-label analysis demonstrating that enkephalin-, somatostatin- and neurotensin-like immunoreactivities are expressed by a single population of amacrine cells in the chicken retina. *Brain Res.*, 634: 310–316.

Watt, C.B., Su, Y.-Y.T. and Lam, D.M.-K. (1984) Interactions between enkephalin and GABA in avian retina. *Nature*, 311: 761–763.

Weiler, R. and Ball, A.K. (1984) Co-localization of neurotensin-like immunoreactivity and ^{3}H-glycine uptake system in sustained amacrine cells of turtle retina. *Nature*, 311: 759–761.

Witkovsky, P. and Dearry, A. (1992) Functional roles of dopamine in the vertebrate retina. *Prog. Retinal Res.*, 11: 247–292.

Wright, L.L. and Vaney, D.I. (1999) The fountain amacrine cells of the rabbit retina. *Vis. Neurosci.*, 16: 1145–1156.

Wright, L.L., Macqueen, C.L., Elston, G.N., Young, H.M., Pow, D.V. and Vaney, D.I. (1997) The DAPI-3 amacrine cells of the rabbit retina. *Vis. Neurosci.*, 14: 473–492.

Yamada, E. and Ishikawa, T. (1965) The fine structure of the horizontal cells in some vertebrate retinae. *Cold Spring Harb. Symp. Quant. Biol.*, 30: 383–392.

Yoshida, K., Watanabe, D., Ishikane, H., Tachibana, M., Pastan, I. and Nakanishi, S. (2001) A key role of starburst amacrine cells in originating retinal directional selectivity and optokinetic eye movement. *Neuron*, 30: 771–780.

Young, H.M. and Vaney, D.I. (1991) Rod-signal interneurons in the rabbit retina: 1. Rod bipolar cells. *J. Comp. Neurol.*, 310: 139–153.

E.C. Azmitia, J. DeFelipe, E.G. Jones, P. Rakic and C.E. Ribak (Eds.)
Progress in Brain Research, Vol. 136

CHAPTER 19

Cajal and glial cells

Luis M. Garcia-Segura*

Instituto Cajal (CSIC), Avenida del Doctor Arce 37, 28002 Madrid, Spain

Introduction—Cajal and glia: an unexplored story

The scientific contributions of Cajal may be placed, without doubt, among the best highlights of the biological sciences of the end of the 19th and the beginning of the 20th centuries. In addition to its own scientific value, Cajal's writing is still an enjoyable read. We may find many sources of delight when reading his scientific books and papers. His beautiful drawings, which remain as true masterpieces of art, and his marvelous literary style are also part of the pleasure conveyed to neurobiologists of our time when reading Cajal's original work. Cajal, who spent many hours in his laboratory, mastered and improved the scientific technology of his time. He was a fruitful thinker full of curiosity and, if this were not enough, he also revealed himself as a gifted artist. Among the many possible approaches to Cajal's work, we present here an almost unexplored trail: the contribution of Cajal to our present knowledge of glia.

There is no doubt that the name of Cajal is associated with the morphology of neurons and neuronal circuits. However, in very arduous work that included many technical and theoretical difficulties, Cajal and his colleagues were able to start deciphering the glia mystery. Cajal developed new tools that were used by himself and by other members of his laboratory to identify and classify glial cells. This was not an easy task, and reading the papers on glia by Cajal and his colleagues, we can appreciate how difficult it was to identify oligodendroglia and

microglia, and the problem of placing the glial cells in the conceptual picture of the brain. The interpretation of the role of glia by the Cajal school was not free from intellectual debate among his members and, as with all human achievements, it was not free from personal feelings. The fascinating contribution of the Cajal school to the neurobiology of glia remains to be written. The following notes are no more than a brief introduction to the story of this impressive scientific achievement.

Not only neurons

In 1888 Cajal published his first papers on the structure of the cerebellum and the avian brain, studies that represent the starting point of his fructiferous scientific career. Before these studies, Cajal was attracted by several different issues. His doctoral dissertation, of 1877, was entitled *Patogenia de la inflamación* (Pathogenesis of inflammation), and his first paper, published in 1880, dealt with experimental studies of inflammation and the migration of leucocytes. Although his second paper, published in 1881, was on the branching of nerve endings in striatal muscles, his subsequent studies, in 1884 and 1885, were devoted to microbiology and then, in 1886 and 1887, to the histological characteristics of different tissues. Cajal took more than a decade from finishing his doctoral thesis to discover the wonders of the histological structure of the central nervous system and his personal path in scientific research. However, as soon as he entered the field of neuroscience he started the study of glia. For instance, in a description of the histological structure of the spinal cord, published as early as 1889,

---
*Corresponding author: Tel.: +34-915854729;
Fax: +34-915854754; E-mail: lmgs@cajal.csic.es

he presented a detailed description of ependymal cells and radial glia, discussing the embryonic origin of neuroglia supporting the concept of the glial cells as individual units in contrast with other reticular theories of his time (Cajal, 1889a; see also Cajal, 1899a).

Glia cells appeared in several publications by Cajal between 1888 and 1896. However, it was not until 1896 when Cajal published a paper completely devoted to glia. It was in the first volume of his journal *Revista Trimestral Micrográfica*, where he published a short note on the spatial relationship of neurons and glia (Ramón y Cajal, 1896). This is a beautiful study, based on Nissl staining of the rabbit cerebellum and other brain areas, describing several details of the distribution of glial cells around the cell body and the axon of neurons. Although glial cells were mentioned by Cajal in several of his previous studies, this was his first paper in which glial cells were the main player. We should realize that, by this time, Cajal had already put forward many of his ideas about the function of neurons and the organization of neuronal networks. In contrast, no solid functional hypothesis was established for glial cells. Cajal concluded that the specific location of glial cells around neurons was not an arbitrary phenomenon. The peculiar *Crown* of glial cells around neurons had to be related to their function, but their exact role was still a mystery.

Cajal decided to discover that mystery, and it took him just one more year to publish his first paper on the function of glial cells. The second volume of his journal *Revista Trimestral Micrográfica* contains two important theoretical papers by Cajal. The first one (Ramón y Cajal, 1897a) was a summary of his theories on the laws governing the morphology and function of neurons. In the second paper, entitled: *Something on the physiological function of neuroglia* (Cajal, 1897b), Cajal exposed his first theory on the role of these cells. Using material from this paper, he further developed this subject in his book on the histology of the nervous system (Cajal, 1899a). The basic ideas presented in his paper of 1897 and in his book of 1899 were the same.

The insulating theory

For Cajal, the main role of glial cells was to insulate neurons to avoid wrong contacts among them and to preserve the function of neuronal circuits. This is his theory of the insulating role of the neuroglia. First we must mention that at that time the distinction among the different types of glial cells, as we know them today, was still emerging. Thus, Cajal made a distinction among myelin and neuroglia in the gray and white matter. Neuroglia for Cajal represented what we call today astroglia. Cells responsible for myelin formation in the central nervous system were still uncharacterized. For Cajal, the processes of neuroglia in the gray matter represented a medium that resisted the passage of nerve impulses, preventing contacts among dendrites and non-myelinated fibers. When Cajal mentioned the processes of neuroglia he was mainly referring to the processes of astrocytes, as the inspection of many of his drawings demonstrate (Fig. 1). Cajal considered that myelin was an improvement in the insulating function of glial cells. For this reason, the presence of neuroglia in the white matter was a puzzle for Cajal. Since axons in the white matter were already insulated by myelin, why was the presence of neuroglia necessary? In addition to the fact that the link between oligodendrocytes and myelin in the central nervous system was still undiscovered, the presence of astrocytes in the white matter was difficult to explain based on his insulating theory.

Although the insulating theory of Cajal on glia was limited, and even though we now know many other metabolic (Magistretti and Pellerin, 2000) and signaling (Araque et al., 1999; 2001) functions of glial cells, his basic idea on glia function is still valid. Recent studies in different areas of the brain have shown that the glial covering of neuronal surfaces may regulate the formation of synaptic connections and that the processes of astrocytes and microglia participate in the plasticity of synaptic inputs (Garcia-Segura et al., 1994; Schiefer et al., 1999; Theodosis and Poulain, 1999).

Cajal recognized that the idea of the insulating role of neuroglia was developed by his brother Pedro. However he supported the theory with his own findings, presented in a medical meeting in Valencia in 1891 (Cajal, 1891), as well as by further studies from his collaborators Claudio Sala y Pons (1894) and Terrazas (1897). It is of interest that the first paper quoted by Cajal in support of his theory was his own communication for the meeting in Valencia, three years before the doctoral dissertation of Sala y Pons on glial cells was published (Sala y Pons, 1894). Thus, although many of the consecutive studies from the laboratory of Cajal on glia were published under

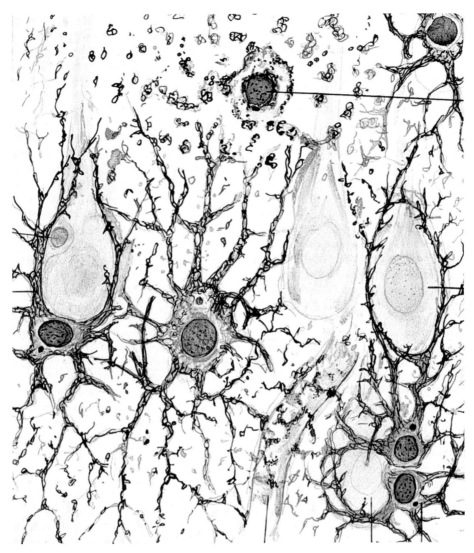

Fig. 1. Neuroglia from the hippocampal formation (stratum radiatum of the Ammon horn) of a human brain. In this drawing Cajal shows astrocytic processes embracing pyramidal neurons as well as astrocytic processes in contact with blood vessels. Reproduced with permission from an original drawing conserved in the Legado Cajal.

the name of his collaborators, we have to conclude that Cajal himself showed an early interest in glial cells.

The neurotrophic hypothesis

Cajal's interest with glial cells never declined. It is true that he devoted much more effort to the study of neurons and that the main contributions to understanding glia by Cajal's laboratory were published by his collaborators.

If we go through the volumes of the journals originally founded and edited by Cajal, we will encounter many relevant papers on glial cells authored by scientists directly related to Cajal or by members of his laboratory. Names such as Sala y Pons, Terrazas, Achúcarro, Lafora, Del Río-Hortega, Ramón y Fañanas, Sánchez y Sánchez, De Castro, Serra, Somoza, Rodríguez-Pérez, represent an impressive list, for that time, of scientists contributing to the glia field. Among these advances we have to mention the studies by Tello on regeneration (Tello, 1911), particularly because this work led Cajal to postulate a second theory for the function of glial cells: the secretion of trophic factors to support neuronal growth.

Tello was ahead of his time when he addressed the question of the differences in the regeneration of central and peripheral axons. He considered that Schwann cells may be the cause of these differences and he tested this hypothesis with a revolutionary experiment: he transplanted Schwann cells in the brain to determine the effect on the regeneration of central axons. Tello observed that Schwann cell transplants induced the growth of central axons. This experiment was reviewed and commented by Cajal in his book on the degeneration and regeneration of central nervous system (Cajal, 1914). Cajal postulated that Schwann cells release a trophic factor for neurons, an hypothesis proposed by Tello. Interestingly, Cajal did not consider Schwann cells as glia. However, his hypothesis on Schwann cells represents the most advanced idea that Cajal ever formulated for glia function. For a modern neurobiologist, it is impressive to read the papers by Tello and Cajal on central axon regeneration, made many years before the discovery of the first neurotrophin by Rita Levi-Montalcini and also many years before the rediscovery of the ability of Schwann cells to support central axonal growth.

A sustained effort for the study of glia

That Cajal did not wish to co-author the many papers on glia published by members of his laboratory does not reflect a lack of interest on the subject. We should remember that co-authorship of papers was then not so popular as today. Scientific research and discovery was considered to be the result of a personal inquiry rather than the result of the work of an organized scientific team. Apparently at that time the director of a laboratory did not coauthor the papers of his students. Cajal himself profusely contributed to the field of glia and many of his papers mentioned these cells. As a case in point, he was unable to correctly identify microglia which he identified as small neurons in a study on the structure of the human cerebral cortex (Cajal, 1899b), but later rectified his initial observations (Cajal, 1925). Among his more important studies on glia, we should mention an extensive study on the neuroglia in human brain that was published in 1913 in *Trabajos del Laboratorio de Investigaciones Biológicas de la Universidad de Madrid* (Cajal, 1913).

This paper describes many cytological and histological features of astrocytes and their relationships with neurons and blood vessels. The ectodermal origin of astrocytes as well as their capacity for proliferation in the adult brain are recognized. The descriptions of Cajal were based on his own observations as well as in the material previously published by other members of his laboratory. Interestingly, in this study there is a description of oligodendrocytes, under the name of the third element of the nervous centers or small adendritic cells. Cajal, who probably included microglia among adendritic cells, considered that these cells had a mesodermal origin and pointed to its possible homology with Schwann cells. It was his collaborator Del Río-Hortega who made some years later a complete description of the morphology of microglia (Del Río-Hortega, 1920) and of oligodendrocytes (Del Río-Hortega, 1928) and correctly interpreted their function as well as their embryonic origin.

Between 1913 and 1916, there were many other essential contributions made by Cajal and colleagues on glial cells. We found several papers by Achúcarro, such as his impressive study on the gliotectonics of the cerebral cortex (Achúcarro, 1914), Lafora, Del Río-Hortega, Sánchez y Sánchez and Ramón y Fañanas, among others. The year of 1916 probably marked the main peak in the production of papers on glia from Cajal's laboratory. For instance, eight of the 13 papers that composed volume 14 of *Trabajos del Laboratorio de Invstigaciones Biológicas de la Universidad de Madrid* published in 1916, are on glial cells, including a technical paper by Cajal on the staining of neuroglia (Cajal, 1916) in which Cajai made use of microphotographs to illustrate astrocytes stained with his method.

The peak in glia research made by Cajal's laboratory coincided with one of the most dramatic situations in European history: the First World War. Fortunately, Spain was a neutral country and Cajal and his collaborators were able to pursue research in Madrid without the restrictions imposed by the devastating war that desolated Europe. However, the war seriously restricted the diffusion of scientific publications. Obviously, this was not the best moment for the publication of the new discoveries made by Cajal's laboratory on glial cells. War conditions hampered the distribution of Cajal's publications among scientists working in Germany, France, Italy and other European countries. And of course these same scientists were at that moment involved in other more urgent tasks.

The last years: glia are the main player

In the years following the First World War, glia progressively attracted more attention from Cajal's laboratory. Cajal's collaborators, De Castro, Del Río-Hortega, Somoza and Rodríguez-Pérez were among the main contributors to the understanding of glia at that time. The production of papers on glial cells by Cajal's laboratory reached a second peak in 1920. Fernando de Castro published in this year two beautiful and detailed studies on the astroglia in the olfactory bulb (De Castro, 1920a,b). De Castro described many new aspects of the morphology and distribution of astrocytes as well as the process of gliogenesis. Based on the relationship of astrocytic processes with blood vessels, De Castro proposed that astrocytes could act as endocrine cells, releasing hormones into the circulation (De Castro, 1920a,b). This hypothesis, not yet confirmed, was advanced for its time, considering that the study of endocrinology was at an early stage. It is also interesting that a role of astroglia in the regulation of neuroendocrine events has recently received experimental support (Garcia-Segura et al., 1996; Melcangi et al., 1997; Ojeda et al., 2000).

The year of 1920 also saw the discrepancy between Cajal (Cajal, 1920) and Del Río-Hortega (1920) regarding the interpretation of adendritic cells. It was the opinion of Del Río-Hortega that Cajal was deceived by adendritic cells due to a technical artifact. Del Río-Hortega said that these cells had processes that Cajal was unable to see by a limitation of his method of staining. Cajal's reply was in the same journal issue. Even with processes, Cajal argued, these cells would represent a unique population, because these questionable processes were not stained with the same methods that revealed the cell processes of other glial cells. A pure scientific debate or an obscure query among master and disciple? It is hard to give a reliable answer to this question today. We may only guess that, with all probability, both aspects were mixed in the debate. However, it is clear that Del Río-Hortega was correct in his assumption, as we know that oligodendrocytes have cell processes. Another aspect that is now obvious is that the personal relation between Del Río-Hortega and Cajal will from then suffer a dramatic deterioration.

In his last years Cajal was very well aware of the importance of glial cell function in the damaged brain. In 1925, he published an outstanding paper describing reactive astroglia and microglia in the human brain (Cajal, 1925). As additional proof of the importance that Cajal gave to glial cells at that time is that he prepared a French version of his Spanish papers of 1913 and that he published then in the volume corresponding to the years 1931–1932 of his journal *Trabajos del Laboratorio de Investigaciones Biológicas de la Universidad de Madrid*. Probably, Cajal considered that these studies, published just before the declaration of the First World War had not reached a wide audience. Furthermore, Cajal continued to support the work of his collaborators on glia. Not only Del Río-Hortega, who having established his own laboratory continued the work initiated by Cajal on glia. The other collaborators of Cajal, such as Rodríguez-Pérez, Sánchez y Sánchez and Sanz-Ibáñez, pursued in the subsequent years work on glia with new original descriptions and modern experimental approaches.

In conclusion, it may have been an inevitable consequence of the revolution initiated by Cajal in the study of neurons that his contribution to the understanding of glia remained hidden in second place. However, reading the papers on glia by Cajal and his collaborators, it is impossible to refrain from the admiration of their pioneering exploration into such a difficult field. The exceptional quality and novelty of the studies made by Cajal and his school on glia will remain forever among the most remarkable and outstanding contributions to the history of neuroscience.

Acknowledgments

I want to thank Drs. Julian Taylor and Javier de Felipe for a critical reading of the manuscript.

References

Achúcarro, N. (1914) Contribución al estudio gliotectónico de la corteza cerebral. El asta de Ammon y la fascia dentata. *Trab. Lab. Inv. Biol. Univ. Madrid*, 12: 229–272.

Araque, A., Purpura, V., Sanzgiri, R.P. and Haydon, P.G. (1999) Tripartite synapses: glia, the unacknowledged partner. *Trends Neurosci.*, 22: 208–215.

Araque, A., Carmignoto, G. and Haydon, P.G. (2001) Dynamic signaling between astrocytes and neurons. *Annu. Rev. Physiol.*, 63: 795–813.

Cajal, S.R. (1889) Contribución al estudio de la estructura de la médula espinal. *Revista Trimestral de Histología Normal y Patológica*, 1: 79–106.

Cajal, S.R. (1891) Significación fisiológica de las expansiones protoplásmicas y nerviosas de las células de la sustancia gris.

Revista de Ciencias Médicas de Barcelona, 17: 671–679 and 715–723.

Cajal, S.R. (1896) Sobre la relación de las células nerviosas con las neuróglicas. *Revista Trimestral Micrográfica*, 1: 123–126.

Cajal, S.R. (1897a) Leyes de la morfología y dinamismo de las células nerviosas. *Revista Trimestral Micrográfica*, 2: 1–12.

Cajal, S.R. (1897b) Algo sobre la significatión fisiológica de la neuroglia. *Revista Trimestral Micrográfica*, 2: 33–47.

Cajal, S.R. (1899a) Textura del Sistema Nervioso del Hombre y los Vertebrados. Vol. I. Nicolás Moya, Madrid. [English translation by Pasik, P. And Pasik, T. (1999) *Texture of the Nervous System of Man and Vertebrates*. Vol. 1. Springer, Barcelona.]

Cajal, S.R. (1899b) Estudios sobre la corteza cerebral humana. II. Estructura de la corteza motriz del hombre y mamíferos superiores. *Revista Trimestral Micrográfica*, 4: 117–200.

Cajal, S.R. (1913) Contribución al conocimiento de la neuroglia del cerebro humano. *Trab. Lab. Inv. Biol. Univ. Madrid*, 11: 255–315.

Cajal, S.R. (1914) Estudios sobre la degeneración y regeneración del sistema nervioso. Vol. 2. Degeneración y regeneración de los centros nerviosos. Nicolás Moya. Madrid.

Cajal, S.R. (1916) El proceder del oro-sublimado para la coloración de la neuroglia. *Trab. Lab. Inv. Biol. Univ. Madrid*, 12: 155–162.

Cajal, S.R. (1920) Algunas consideraciones sobre la mesoglía de Roberston y Río-Hortega. *Trab. Lab. Inv. Biol. Univ. Madrid*, 18: 109–127.

Cajal, S.R. (1925) Contribution á la connaissance de la néuroglie cérébrale et cérébelleuse dans la paralysie générale progressive. Avec quelques indications techniques sur l' imprégnation argentique du tissu nerveux pathologique. *Trab. Lab. Inv. Biol. Univ. Madrid*, 23: 157–216.

De Castro, F. (1920a) Estudios sobre la neuróglia de la corteza cerebral del hombre y de los animates. I. La arquitectura neuróglica y vascular del bulbo olfativo. *Trab. Lab. Inv. Biol. Univ. Madrid*, 18: 1–35.

De Castro, F. (1920b) Algunas observaciones sobre la histogénesis de la neuroglia en el bulbo olfativo. *Trab. Lab. Inv. Biol. Univ. Madrid*, 18: 83–108.

Del Río-Hortega, P. (1920) La microglía y su transformación en células en bastoncito y cuerpos gránulo-adiposos. *Trab. Lab. Inv. Biol. Univ. Madrid*, 18: 37–82.

Del Río-Hortega, P. (1928) Tercera aportación al conocimiento morfológico e interpretación funcional de la oligodendroglía. *Memorias de la Sociedad Española de Historia Natural*, 14: 5–122.

Garcia-Segura, L.M., Chowen, J.A., Parducz, A. and Naftolin, F. (1994) Gonadal hormones as promoters of structural synaptic plasticity: cellular mechanisms. *Prog. Neurobiol.*, 44: 279–307.

Garcia-Segura, L.M., Chowen, J.A. and Naftolin, F. (1996) Endocrine glia: roles of glial cells in the brain actions of steroid and thyroid hormones and in the regulation of hormone secretion. *Front. Neuroendocrinol.*, 17: 180–211.

Magistretti, P.J. and Pellerin, L. (2000) The astrocyte-mediated coupling between synaptic activity and energy metabolism operates through volume transmission. *Prog. Brain Res.*, 125: 229–240.

Melcangi, R.C., Galbiati, M., Messi, E., Magnaghi, V., Cavarretta, I., Riva, M.A. and Zanisi, M. (1997) Astrocyte-neuron interactions *in vitro*: role of growth factors and steroids on LHRH dynamics. *Brain Res. Bull.*, 44: 465–469.

Ojeda, S.R., Ma, Y.J., Lee, B.J. and Prevot, V. (2000) Glia-to-neuron signaling and the neuroendocrine control of female puberty. *Recent Prog. Horm. Res.*, 55: 197–223.

Sala y Pons, C. (1894) La neuroglia de los vertebrados. Estudio de histología comparada. *Imprenta Casa Provincial de Caridad. Barecelona*, pp. 1–44.

Schiefer, J., Kampe, K., Dodt, H.U., Zieglgansberger, W. and Kreutzberg, G.W. (1999) Microglial motility in the rat facial nucleus following peripheral axotomy. *J. Neurocytol.*, 28: 439–453.

Tello, F. (1911) La influencia del neurotrofismo en la regeneración de los centros nerviosos. *Trab. Lab. Inv. Biol. Univ. Madrid*, 9: 123–159.

Terrazas, R. (1897) Notas sobre la neuroglia del cerebelo y el crecimiento de los elementos nerviosos. *Revista Trimestral Micrográfica*, 2: 49–66.

Theodosis, D.T. and Poulain, D.A. (1999) Contribution of astrocytes to activity-dependent structural plasticity in the adult brain. *Adv. Exp. Med. Biol.*, 468: 175–182.

Mechanisms of neuronal birth, growth and death

E.C. Azmitia, J. DeFelipe, E.G. Jones, P. Rakic and C.E. Ribak (Eds.)
Progress in Brain Research, Vol. 136

CHAPTER 20

Mechanisms of neuronal birth, growth and death (an overview)

Patricia Whitaker-Azmitia*

Department of Psychology, State University of New York, Stony Brook, NY 11794-2500, USA

In order to further his studies of the nervous system, Santiago Ramón y Cajal often used the approach he referred to as "the ontogenetic or embryologic method"—simply stated, to understand the structures of the mature brain, one can study all the steps along the way which led to those structures. As a result of this approach, Cajal has left us with many detailed and exquisite studies of brain development, which laid the foundation for so much research still being done today. This symposium therefore, presents key aspects of today's research on neuronal birth, growth and death, and how today's studies depend on the original findings of Cajal. As stated by Victor Hamburger *"Indeed, it is very difficult to be original in (ideas about) neurogenesis, with Cajal overlooking one's shoulder"*.

The "Mechanisms of Neuronal Birth, Growth and Death" section starts with detailed descriptions of what we now know of cortical development, as described by the scientist whose name is synonymous with cortical development—Pasko Rakic. Dr. Rakic's chapter describes the hundred years of research from Cajal's earliest interpretations of Golgi staining in immature brains to his own most recent work on the genes controlling development. These are genes involved in all stages of development—proliferation and death (Caspases, Bax, JNK), migration (ion channels), and differentiation (Notch signaling). Much of Cajal's writing on development uses vivid visual imagery of living and moving cells. For example, Cajal used terms for migrating cells as *"climbing"* and of growth cones as *"sniffing out"* their targets and having *"rapid ameboid movements"*.

This rich imagery of Cajal's is brought to life in the videomicrography and computer animations presented by Dr. Rakic.

Next, a chapter is presented on the most recent findings on cells which were favorites of Cajal's—his *"special cells of the molecular layer"*—the Cajal-Retzius cell, as discussed by Alfonso Fairén (Alicante, Spain). Cajal described these cells as occurring in the marginal zone of the developing cortex and having horizontal projections of unknown polarity. Today, these cells are known to produce reelin. As reelin is considered essential for radial neuroblast migration, we now know much of the role of Cajal-Retzius (CR) cells. Cajal thought CR cells matured in the same place, but lost some of the fine processes. However, Dr. Fairén suggests that there are two different types of reelin positive CR cells in humans—both exist for a time, but only one form lasts into adulthood, where it may function as an interneuron. Dr. Fairén also presents an excellent synopsis of his own work on other marginal zone pioneer neurons and on the marginal zone as a highly fluid region, to which cells migrate, assemble and form patterns of aggregation.

As stated by Cajal *"The morphology of nerve cells does not correspond to an unchanging and inevitable pattern laid down by heredity. It depends entirely on environmental, physical and chemical circumstances"*. Thus, a concern of Cajal's became determining if there was a finite point at which development ended and degeneration started and if there were selective factors for each. He concluded that there were likely to be many factors for each process, and that they may co-exist in the brain. The final three presentations in this section address these questions.

*Corresponding author: Tel.: 631 632 9899;
E-mail: pwhitaker@notes.cc.sunysb.edu

264

Shuichi Ueda (Mibu, Japan) presents work on a factor which has become of increasing interest in recent years—the role of free radicals in oxidative stress-induced neurodegeneration. Using an animal model of Parkinson's disease, the zitter rat, Dr. Ueda shows that oxidative stress can selectively damage dopaminergic neurons. Furthermore, his studies show that free radical scavengers such as melatonin can prevent the degeneration and that healthy dopamine neurons transplanted into a zitter rat undergo degeneration. These findings have important implications for proposing treatments for Parkinson's disease.

The work of Manuel Nieto Sampedro (Madrid, Spain) addresses the often-quoted belief of Cajal's, that spontaneous regeneration of a damaged CNS is not possible. Cajal felt that neuroregeneration was not possible in the CNS, in large part due to the hostile environment produced by reactive astroglial cells. Conversely, regrowth of damaged axons in the PNS was made possible by the support of Schwann cells. These observations have been extended and refined over many years of research by Dr. Nieto-Sampedro, with very promising results. Firstly, he and his group have studied the astroglial response to CNS injury and identified two factors which must be controlled in order to prevent inhibitory activities of these cells—a new neurite inhibitory factor produced by astroglial cells, and an endogenous astroblast antimitotic

factor. Secondly, and perhaps more excitingly, this groups reports on a new form of CNS macroglial cell, which has Schwann-cell like growth-promoting properties. The investigators have named these cells "aldynoglia" meaning to "make grow". Dr. Nieto-Sampedro ends his discussion by quite justifiably stating that his findings would have made Cajal very happy.

This section of papers ends with work of Dr. Charles Ribak (Irvine, USA) which shows the importance of plasticity and neurogenesis in disease states. Cajal was the first to suggest the synaptic circuitry of the hippocampus, which is now so well known. However, as pointed out by Dr. Ribak, Cajal apparently never studied this circuitry in a damaged brain, in particular a brain damaged by epilepsy. Had he done so, he may have observed several neuroplasticity changes. In Dr. Ribak's chapter, the principal finding is that repeated stimulation, such as in epileptiform activity, causes increased neurogenesis of granule cells. As well, these cells change their circuitry, such that mossy fibers sprout axons into the inner molecular layer and their collateral axons in the hilus begin to make connections with newly formed hilar basal dendrites. Interestingly, these hilar basal dendrites are a transient feature for granule cells in development. These changes in the epileptic animal contribute to the formation of new recurrent excitatory circuitry.

E.C. Azmitia, J. DeFelipe, E.G. Jones, P. Rakic and C.E. Ribak (Eds.)
Progress in Brain Research, Vol. 136
© 2002 Elsevier Science B.V. All rights reserved

CHAPTER 21

Evolving concepts of cortical radial and areal specification

Pasko Rakic*

Department of Neurobiology, Yale University School of Medicine, P.O. Box 208001, New Haven, CT 06520-8001, USA

Absract: The fundamental principles of cortical organization and its development, postulated by Santiago Ramón y Cajal at the turn of the century, based on his exquisite observations and ingenious interpretation of neuronal assemblies impregnated with the Golgi method, are being expanded with the application of advanced methods of anatomy, molecular biology and genetics. In this chapter, I will focus on the concept of columnar organization and areal specifications of the cerebral cortex that has served as a useful framework for understanding its development as well as its function as an evolving organ of thought.

Introduction

A consistent feature of the cerebral cortex in all species, including human, is the organization of its neurons into horizontal and vertical arrays, which form anatomically and physiologically distinct laminar and columnar compartments. This radial pattern of cortical deployment can already be depicted in Cajal's early rendering of cortical circuits (e.g. Cajal, 1881). Over the past 100 years, introduction of ever more sophisticated methods of analysis produced new data and ideas that formed our present understanding of the development, evolution and function of this particular organizational feature of the cerebral cortex. In the most general sense, the concept of columnar organization is based upon the observation of an array of an iterative pattern of neuronal grouping (described interchangeably as columns or modules) that extend radially (perpendicular to the pial surface) across cellular layers II to VI (Mountcastle, 1997). The neurons within a given column are stereotypically interconnected in the vertical dimension, share extrinsic connectivity,

and hence, act as basic units subserving a set of common functions. This concept has gradually evolved through the discoveries of functional columns subserving various attributes of somatic sensation (Mountcastle, 1957), vision (Hubel et al., 1977) and cognition (Goldman-Rakic, 1987). The columns are assembled into modular compartments or areas dedicated to processing a particular function (Mountcastle, 1997; Kinsbourne, 1998). Throughout evolution the neocortex has shown expansion in surface area, the larger the area and the cortical surface in a given species, the larger the number of participating columnar units (Rakic, 1988, 1995b). Thus, radial organization is directly relevant to the areal expansion and regional specialization of the cerebral cortex during evolution.

This chapter is primarily based on studies of neocortical development in the mouse, macaque and human brain carried out in my laboratory over the past three decades. Although the basic principles of cortical development in these three mammalian species are very similar, we believed that even small differences in sequences and timing might provide some critical clues, as to how the cerebral neocortex has evolved. Since the functions of neurotransmitters, receptors and ion channels have not changed substantially over the phylogenetic scale, the secret to the success of the human species may be

---

*Corresponding author: Tel.: (203) 785-4330;
Fax: (203) 785-5263; E-mail: pasko.rakic@yale.edu

primarily due to an increased number of cortical neurons, more elaborate patterns of their connections, and functional sub-specialization of cortical areas. This review focuses on the early developmental events leading to formation of the cellular constituents of the cortical plate. Elucidation of these issues is an essential prerequisite for understanding the subsequent formation of neuronal connections and synaptic architecture that underlie our cognitive capacity.

Cell proliferation and migration

Most cortical neurons originate near the surface of the embryonic cerebral ventricle and, after their last division, migrate to their final positions in the cortical plate that develops at the outer territories of the cerebral wall, below the pial surface. The presence of large numbers of mitotic figures near the lumen of the cerebral cavity of the embryonic human cerebrum and their paucity in the cortical plate itself, led to the initial suggestion that cortical neurons are produced in the germinal matrix situated at the ventricular surface (His, 1904). This hypothesis of the dynamic relocation of postmitotic cells was substantiated by the application of modern methods for labeling dividing cells in mice (Angevine and Sidman, 1961), monkeys (Rakic, 1974), and human (Rakic and Sidman, 1968). The germinal, ventricular zone in these mammals is organized as a pseudostratified epithelium in which neuronal stem cells initially divide symmetrically to produce a species specific number of cortical founder cells. The nucleus of each stem cell moves away from the ventricle to replicate its DNA and then moves back to the ventricular surface where the cell divides (Rakic and Sidman, 1973). At one point in time, which in the mouse, monkey and human occurs at a different embryonic age, some stem cells switch the mode of their division from the symmetrical to the asymmetrical, producing one neuron, that migrates away to the cortical plate and one stem cell that remains at the ventricular surface (Rakic, 1988, 1995b).

Because the size of a migratory neuron in the mouse and human embryo is approximately the same, the negotiation of the tortuous, several thousand microns long pathway in the convoluted primate brain poses a much larger navigational problem for the young human neuron. Indeed, the peak of neuronal migration in primates, including humans, during the midgestational period

coincides with the rapid increase in the width of the cerebral wall and formation of the sulci and gyri (Rakic, 1978). The stream of migratory neurons is so dramatic that the phenomenon of migration was originally inferred from an observation made on histological sections of the human cerebrum by Wilhelm His (1874). He was also the first to suggest that elongated neuroepithelial cells may play a role in orienting migrating neuroblasts, the concept of which appealed to Cajal (Cajal, 1881). Using the silver impregnation method developed by Camilio Golgi (1974), several investigators including Magini (1888), Cajal (1890, 1911), Lenoshek (1895) and Retzius (1884) all classified these "epithelial" cells as glial. They pointed out specific morphological characteristics, including the presence of lamellate expansions that distinguishes them from neural cells (Fig. 1), However, the available methods at the time did not allow definitive phenotypic distinction between various classes of cells and there was relatively little advancement in this field until the 1970s when a combination of powerful electron microscopic, ^{3}H-thymidine (^{3}H-TdR) autoradiographic and immuncytochemical

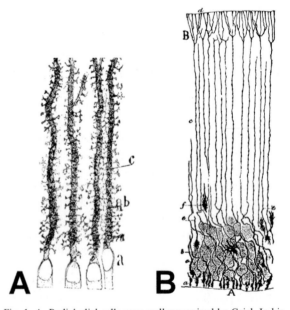

Fig. 1. **A**. Radial glial cells were well recognized by Cajal. In his drawings he emphasized epithelial cells, that in many species display characteristic lamellate expansions. **B**. Epithelial (radial glial) cells in neonatal rabbit are spanning the entire cerebral wall. However, at this stage, there are numerous transitional forms into more mature neuroglial cells. Golgi impregnation method. After Cajal (1909, Vol. 2, p. 859).

methods allowed identification of cell classes and analysis of dynamic spatial and temporal resolution of developmental events both *in vivo* and *in vitro*. (reviewed by Cameron and Rakic, 1994; Rakic, 1997).

The use of a combination of Golgi impregnation and reconstruction from electron microscopic (EM) serial sections in the early 1970s revealed that postmitotic neurons migrate across the wide intermediate zone of the monkey telencephalon by following elongated shafts of non-neural elements called radial glial cells (Fig. 2 and Rakic, 1972). These transient glial cells initially described by the Golgi method (Retzius, 1884; Magini, 1888; Cajal, 1890) stretch their outward process across the entire fetal cerebral wall from the onset of

corticogenesis and become increasingly longer, as the wall of the fetal cerebrum grows in width during midgestation in primates (Schmechel and Rakic, 1979a). Subsequent immunohistochemical identification of glial acidic fibrillary protein (GFAP) revealed that neuronal and radial glial cell lineages in primates, including the human, can be identified from the onset of corticogenesis (Choi and Lapham, 1978; Levitt and Rakic, 1980; Levitt et al., 1981, 1983; Choi, 1986). This enables direct physical continuity between the maps at the ventricular surface and the increasingly distant cortical plate (Fig. 3). This glial scaffolding becomes most prominent during midgestation when many of the radial glial cells in monkey temporarily stop dividing while serving as

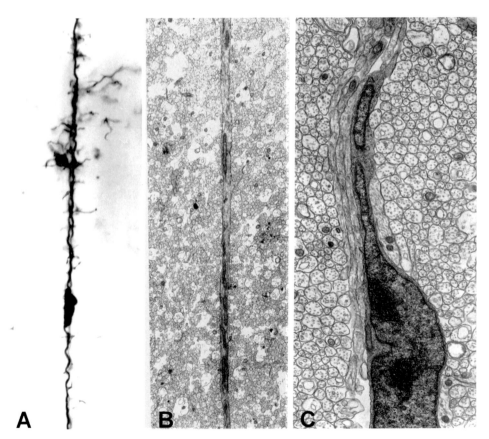

Fig. 2. Morphology of radial glial and neuronal cells in primates has been extrapolated from the Golgi images in the fetal cerebral vesicles in the early 1970's. **A**. An example of a Golgi impregnated radial glial fiber that is closely associated with a migrating neuron. The exceptionally elongated process of the radial glial cells in primates is also decorated with numerous lamellate expansions. **B**. Electron micrograph that reveals a distinct profile of radial glial fibers running through the embryonic intermediate zone (prospective white matter) which, at this late stage of coticoneurogenesis, is already packed with numerous axons from the previously generated neurons. **C**. A young neuron migrating along radial glial fiber shows a distinct ultrastructural characteristic of its cytoplasm that is discriminable from the lighter stained profiles of the radial glial fiber.

268

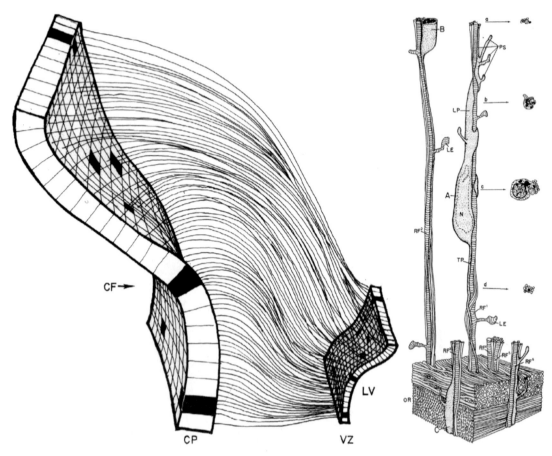

Fig. 3. Schematic three-dimensional reconstruction of the portion of the medial cerebral wall at the level of the incipient calcarine fissure (CF) in the 80-day-old monkey fetus. The reconstruction illustrates how the corresponding points in the ventricular zone (VZ) are connected by radial the elongated radial glial fibers which span the full thickness of the cerebral wall to the increasingly distant cortical plate (CP) situated below the convoluted pial surface. We have suggested that these elongated fibers provide scaffolding that enables precise translation of the positional information from the ventricular surface to the cortical plate (From Rakic, 1978).

scaffolding for migrating neurons (Schmechel and Rakic, 1979b). In rodents, the radial glia differentiates at much later stages and develops GFAP positivity only after birth. Thus, it is possible that this more prominent and sturdier glial scaffolding may be essential for migration and allocation of neurons in larger, more convoluted cerebrums. Recent studies indicate that specification of neuronal and glial cell lineages in mice occurs at much later developmental stages than in primates, and the uncommitted bipolar cells asymmetrically divide to give origin to neurons which subsequently migrate as bipolar neuroblasts along the radial process of cells remaining at the ventricular surface (Noctor et al., 2001). Alternatively, it was proposed that a cell with a radial

process becomes a neuron and translocates its nucleus within its own radial process, while the round stem cell remains near the ventricular surface (Miyata et al., 2001). Although these two studies suggest mutually contradicting models in regard to which of the daughter cells becomes a neuron and which remains a stem cell, they both indicate a significant difference between rodent and primate corticoneurogenesis in this important respect. There seems to be a difference in cell behavior of the ventricular zone which increases at later stages of corticogenesis (Harfuss et al., 2001). Indeed in human, at the very early stages of corticogenesis, when the migratory pathway is as short as in the rodent, migratory cells display a similar nuclear displacement and a short radial process (Sidman and Rakic, 1973). However, as the cerebral wall in primates expands enormously in size, a more differentiated and prominent radial glial scaffolding becomes readily apparent (Schmechel and Rakic, 1979a; Levitt and Rakic, 1980, 1981; Levitt et al., 1983). For example, at later stages of corticogenesis, the radial glial cells in monkey occipital lobe may be as long as 2500 μm while the leading process of bipolar migratory neurons 50–200 μm in length, similar in size to those in mice (Rakic, 1972).

Both EM and immunocytochemical analyses revealed that a cohort of postmitotic cells originating in the proliferative mosaic follow a radial pathway consisting of single or, more often, multiple glial fibers, which span the developing cerebral wall (Figs. 1 and 2, from Experientia). While moving across the intermediate zone, migrating neurons may be in contact with a myriad of axonal and dendritic processes, but nevertheless, remain preferentially attached to the surface of glial fibers. Furthermore, unlike the straight and short migratory pathway in rodents, in the large gyrencephalic primate brain, the migratory pathway became not only much longer, but also increasingly curved (Fig. 3 and Rakic, 1978). Nevertheless, bipolar migratory neurons follow this convoluted pathway rather than moving in a straight fashion (Rakic, 1978).

Molecular mechanisms of neuronal migration

The methods used at the turn of the century were not capable of unraveling the cellular and molecular mechanisms of pathway selection and locomotion of migrating cells. The EM-observation of a close neuron-glial relationship described above, has indicated the presence of a differential binding affinity and suggested the existence of a 'gliophilic' mode of migration that may be mediated by heterotypic adhesion molecules present on apposing neuronal and glial cell surfaces (Rakic, 1985; Rakic et al., 1994). The postmitotic cells which did not obey glial constraints and appear to move along axonal tracts (e.g., red bipolar cell in Fig. 3) were considered 'neurophilic' (Rakic, 1985). In the past three decades radial glial guided migration has been observed in a variety of mammalian species, including human (e.g. Sidman and Rakic, 1973; Kadhim et al., 1988; Hatten and Mason, 1990; Misson et al., 1991; O'Rourke et al., 1992, 1995).

The inference of differential adhesion between migrating neurons and radial glial fibers suggests the possibility that, at least with single pair binding, complementary molecules account for this guidance (Rakic, 1981). However, in reality, several classes of putative recognition and adhesion molecules that may be involved in this phenomenon have been identified (e.g., Cameron and Rakic, 1994; Edelman, 1983; Hatten and Mason, 1986, 1990; Fishell and Hatten, 1991; Schachner et al., 1985; Anton et al., 1996, 1997, 1999). It is possible that a different set of surface molecules is involved in recognition, adhesion and cessation of neuronal cell migration (Rakic et al., 1994; Komuro and Rakic, 1998) (Fig. 4). These potential recognition molecules are expressed selectively and transiently in the leading process of postmitotic neurons at the surface adjacent to the radial glial fibers. For example, we have identified antibodies (D4 and NJPA1) that recognize a polypeptide forming plasmalemmal junctions situated between migrating neurons and adjacent radial glial fibers (Cameron and Rakic, 1994; Cameron et al., 1996). When applied to the embryonic cerebral wall, this antibody causes withdrawal of the leading process, changes in microtubular organization and, finally, detachment of neurons from their radial glial shafts (Anton et al., 1996).

Progress has also been made in understanding the mechanism of nuclear and somatic translocation within the growing leading processes. It has been postulated that the signals controlling the cellular machinery may be involved in initiation and cessation of this movement (Rakic, 1981). However, only recently, the mechanism of the actual physical displacement of cell perikarya has begun to be explored experimentally (reviewed in Rakic and Komuro, 1995; Komuro and Rakic, 1998). Using a living slice and explant preparations of the developing cerebellar tissue to measure the effect of various substances on the rate of cell migration, we found that a voltage gated, N-type Ca^{++} channel (Komuro and Rakic, 1992) and a ligand gated, NMDA channel (Komuro and Rakic, 1993) are particularly active. The composition of the receptor/channel complexes on the surface of migrating neurons is different from the composition they have after reaching their final destination (Farrant et al., 1994), but they can regulate Ca^{2+} levels in the migrating neurons in the absence of any synaptic contacts (Rossi and Slater, 1993). Similar studies conducted in the telencephalon indicate that this mechanism may also be operational during neuronal migration to the cerebral

270

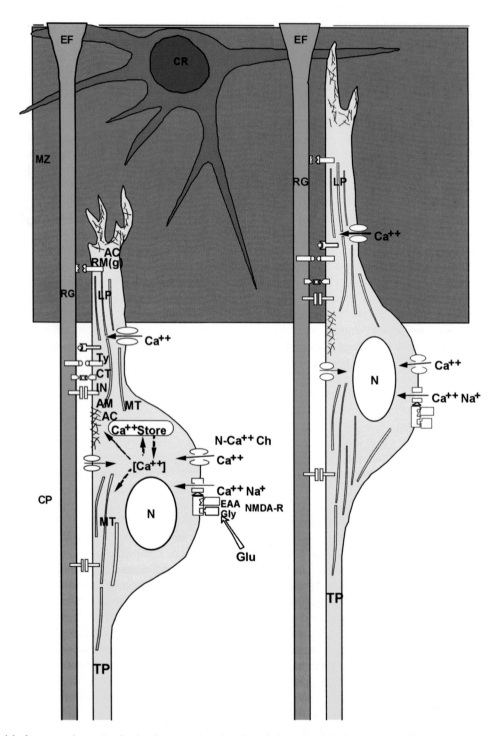

Fig. 4. Model of a proposed cascade of molecular events that takes place during migration of postmitotic cells across the developing cerebral wall. Migrating cells extend a leading process (LP) that selectively follows the contours of the radial glial fiber (RG) as it spans the expanding cerebral wall. The cytoskeleton within the LP and trailing process (TP) contain prominent assemblies of microtubules (MT) and actin-like contractile proteins (AC) that are involved in elongation of the leading process (LP) and translocation of the nucleus (N) and the surrounding

cortex (Behar et al., 1999; Hirai et al., 1999). Furthermore, we have observed that the amplitude and frequency components of Ca^{2+} fluctuations are positively correlated with the rate of migrating granule cells in cerebellar microexplant cultures. Also, the blockade of calcium influx across the plasma membrane results in a reversible retardation of cell movement (Komuro and Rakic, 1998). These results indicate that the combination of amplitude and frequency components of intracellular Ca^{2+} fluctuations may provide an intracellular signal controlling the rate of neuronal cell migration (Fig. 4).

To further explore the cellular machinery underlying translocation of the nucleus during neuronal migration, we determined the polarity of microtubule assemblies situated within the leading and trailing processes of migrating cerebellar granule cells *in situ* (Rakic et al., 1996). Our analysis reveals that the positive ends of the newly assembled microtubules situated in the leading process are uniformly facing the growing tip, while their disintegrating negative ends face the nucleus. In the trailing process, by contrast, microtubule arrays are of mixed polarity. These results suggest that the extension of the leading process and translocation of the nucleus and surrounding cytoplasm within the membrane envelope may be orchestrated by a synchronized polymerization and disintegration of the microtubule that creates a rearrangement of the cytoskeletal scaffolding (Rakic et al., 1996). Caged by the cytoskeletal network, the nucleus could not move without rearrangement of the microtubules. The rate of assembling the microtubule polymer depends on the concentration of cytosolic Ca^{2+}, which is delivered through specific voltage and ligand gated channels (Fig. 4). Thus, a rapid, coordinated depolymerization of microtubule sheets alternating with a phase of relative stability at their negative ends, as observed during locomotion of non-neuronal cells (Kirshner and Mitchison, 1986), may underlie the alternation of movement and stationary periods observed during nuclear displacement in migrating neurons. Our hypothesis that the somatic translocation of the

migrating cell may, at least in part, depend on the dynamics of polymerization and depolymerization of the microtubule protein in the cytoplasm of the leading and trailing processes is consistent with the finding that the slow extension of the leading process of migrating neurons precedes the phase of more rapid nuclear displacement (Hatten and Mason, 1990; Komuro and Rakic, 1995, 1998; Ang et al., 2002). In addition, this is harmonious with the finding that disruption of the microtubule structure results in collapse of the migrating cell body and cessation of nuclear translocation (Rivas and Hatten, 1995). However, it should be underscored that the proposed role of microtubules in nuclear displacement during neuronal migration does not exclude the synergistic action of actin-like contractile proteins, which may also participate in this event (Rakic, 1985).

After passing between previously generated neurons already settled in the deeper strata of the cortical plate, the leading process enters the territory of the marginal zone (MZ) while the movement of the nucleus abruptly stops at the CP/MZ border (Fig. 4). When migrating cells are prevented from detaching from the glial fibers at the interface between the cortical plate and marginal zone, subsequently arriving neurons cannot bypass their predecessors and accumulate beneath the previously generated neurons, forming an outside-to-inside gradient of neurogenesis (Anton et al., 1996). A similar outside-to-inside sequence has been observed in the cortex of the *reeler* mouse (Caviness and Rakic, 1978), although in this case, a deficit of a different molecule is likely to be involved (Ogawa et al., 1995; Rakic and Caviness, 1995). These studies suggest that cessation of migration may be regulated by a different class of molecules that are involved in the disintegration of neuron glia attachment.

Radial unit hypothesis of cortical development

The concept of radial deployment of neurons is central to our understanding of how the neocortex expands during

cytoplasm. The leading process enters the cortical plate (CP) and marginal zone (MZ), but the nucleus stops at the CP/MZ interface (gray area). Various intracellular, membrane bound and extracellular matrix molecules provide signals or are directly engaged in selection of the migratory pathway, rate of cell movement, and finally in the cessation of migration at the CP/MZ borderline. Further explanation in text. Abbreviations: AC, actin-like filaments; AM, homotypic adhesion molecule; CR, Cajal-Retzius cell; CT, catenin; EAA, excitatory amino acids; EF, endfoot of radial glial fiber; Glu, glutamate; Gly, glycine; I, integrine; LP, leading process; MT, microtubule; N, cell nucleus; RM(g) gliophilic recognition molecule; RM(n) neurophilic recognition molecule.

evolution as a sheet of cells of uniform thickness, rather than enlarging as a globe as observed in the subcortical nuclei of the neostriatum. Although the exact relationship between the functional columns in the adult cortex and embryonic columns is not clear, the deployment of migrating neurons into radial columns during evolution can be explained in the context of the *radial unit hypothesis* (Rakic, 1988). According to this model, the embryonic cortical plate consists of vertically oriented cohorts of neurons generated at the same site in the proliferative ventricular zone of the embryonic cerebral vesicle (Rakic, 1976). Each radial unit is formed by several clones (polyclones) that migrate to the cortex following glial fascicles spanning the cerebral wall from the ventricular to pial surfaces. In the cortical plate, later generated cells bypass earlier generated ones and settle in an inside-out gradient of neurogenesis (Fig. 5). Thus, the two-dimensional positional information of the proliferative units in the ventricular zone is transformed into a three-dimensional cortical architecture: the X and Y axis of cells is provided by the site of cell origin whereas the Z axis is provided by the time of their origin (Rakic, 1988).

The hypothesis that cells in a given radial column may be clonally related became possible to test experimentally after the introduction of the retrieval gene transfer method for *in vivo* analysis of cell lineages in the mammalian brain (Sanes, 1989). The use of the retroviral gene transfer method in the embryonic primate brain showed that even in the large and highly convoluted cerebrum, radial deployment of many clones is remarkably preserved (Kornack and Rakic, 1995). Use of the same methods in slice preparation of the human fetal cerebrum indicates that the same holds for the human cortex (Letinic et al., 2002). Although, the clonal relationship of labeled cells using this approach was originally based on the law of probability, cell distribution strongly suggested that most progenitors originating in the same site at the ventricular surface remain radially deployed during migration and settle in a columnar fashion in the cortex (Luskin et al., 1988). A number of studies in chimeric and transgenic mice have provided more direct evidence that the majority of postmitotic, clonally related neurons move and remain radially distributed within the cortex (Tan et al., 1988; Nakatsuji et al., 1991; Parnaveals et al., 1991; Tan and Breen, 1993; Soriano et al., 1995; reviewed in Rakic, 1995a).

In addition to those radially deployed clones, certain populations of clonally related cortical cells do not obey strict radial constraints, although lateral dispersion of postmitotic neurons was observed in the early Golgi studies. For example, I drew horizontally oriented migrating cells in the original corticogenesis scheme that was reproduced as Figure 1 in the Boulder Committee Report (1970) and we have reconstructed nonradially moving cells from EM serial sections (Rakic et al., 1974). However, tangential migration attracted renewed attention after the use of the retroviral gene transfer method which revealed widespread dispersion of clonally related cortical cells in the mouse (Ware et al., 1999), and the discovery that in rodents most, if not all, of the GABAergic interneurons (representing 30% of all cortical neurons) originate in the ganglionic eminence (e.g. deCarlos et al., 1996; Anreson et al., 1999; Lavadis et al., 1999; Powell et al., 2001; Letinic et al., 2002). In the ferret telencephalon only about 15% of neurons appear to migrate nonradially (O'Rourke et al., 1992), while the percentage is much smaller in the macaque monkey (Kornack and Rakic, 1995). Recent studies indicate that in human less than 40% of GABAergic cells or 10% of total cortical neurons originate from the ganglionic eminence and move to the epencephalon tangentially (Letinic et al., 2002). It should be emphasized that even cells that disperse widely in the fetal cerebrum eventually migrate radially along glial shafts, in full harmony with the radial unit hypothesis (Reed and Walsh, 1995; Ware et al., 1999, Letinic et al., 2002).

The radial unit hypothesis can provide an explanation for how a large expansion of the cortical surface without a significant increase in thickness could have occurred during both ontogenetic development (Rakic, 1988) as well as during evolution of the mammalian species (Rakic, 1995b). A relatively small change in the timing of developmental cellular events could have large functional consequences. For example, a minor increase in the length of cell cycles or the number of cell divisions in the ventricular zone can result in a large increase in the number of founder cells that form proliferative units (Rakic, 1988; Rakic and Kornack, 2001). Since initial proliferation in the ventricular zone proceeds exponentially by the prevalence of symmetrical divisions, an additional round of mitotic cycles during this phase doubles the number of proliferative units and, consequently, the number of radial columns (Rakic, 1995b). According to this model, fewer than four extra rounds of cell divisions can account for the 10-fold difference in size of the cortical surface between monkeys and human (Fig. 4 in Rakic, 1995b). In contrast, the 1000-fold difference between the size of the

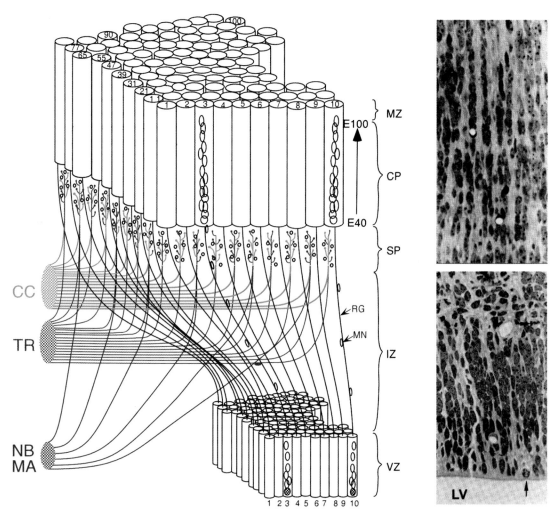

Fig. 5. Left: A three-dimensional illustration of the basic developmental events and types of cell–cell interactions occurring during the early stages of corticogenesis. This cartoon emphasizes radial migration, a predominant mode of neuronal movement which, in primates, underlies the elaborate columnar organization of the neocortex. After their last division, cohorts of migrating neurons (MN) traverse the intermediate zone (IZ) and the subplate zone (SP), where they initially interact with 'waiting' afferents arriving sequentially from the nucleus basalis (NB), monoamine subcortical centers (MA) and later from thalamic radiation (TR), and from several ipsilateral and contralateral corticocortical bundles (CC). After the newly generated neurons bypass the earlier generated ones situated in the deep cortical layers, they settle at the interface between the developing cortical plate (CP) and the marginal zone (MZ) and, eventually, form a radial stack of cells that share a common site of origin but are generated at different times. For example, neurons produced between embryonic day E40 and E100 in radial unit 3 follow the same radial glial fascicle and form ontogenetic column 3. Although some cells, presumably neurophilic in the nature of their surface affinities, may detach from the cohort and move laterally, guided by an axonal bundle (e.g. horizontally oriented, black cell leaving radial unit 3), most postmitotic cells are gliophilic, e.g. they have an affinity for the glial surface and strictly obey constraints imposed by transient radial glial scaffolding (RG). This cellular arrangement preserves the relationships between the proliferative mosaic of the ventricular zone (VZ) and the corresponding protomap within the SP and CP, even though the cortical surface in primates shifts during formation of cerebral convolutions. Right bottom: Photomicrograph of an array of proliferative units within the ventricular zone of monkey embryo showing mitotic figures located at the ventricular surface (arrow). Right top: Cortical plate in the occipital lobe of the same animal, showing radial columns composed of neurons that have originated from the set of proliferative units illustrated at the bottom figure. (Based on Rakic, 1988)

cerebral cortex in mouse and human can be achieved by less than 7 extra symmetrical divisions in the ventricular zone before the onset of corticogenesis.

After the number of founder cells that will form individual radial units is set and corticogenesis has begun, many progenitor cells start to divide asymmetrically. Therefore, during this phase of development, an extra round of cell divisions would have a negligible effect on the thickness of the cortex (See Fig. 4 in Rakic, 1995a). According to this model, one can predict that an approximate additional duration of two weeks of corticogenesis in human than in the macaque should enlarge the cortical thickness by only 10–20%, which is actually observed (Rakic, 1995b). In contrast, even a small delay of onset of the second phase of corticogenesis results in a larger cortical surface on the order of magnitude due to the increasing number of proliferative units at the ventricular zone (Rakic, 1995b).

Excessive proliferation, as well as diminished-programmed cell death (apoptosis) could also affect the number of neurons in the radial columns. An instructive example in this category is the abnormal development of the cerebral cortex in transgenic mice, which was obtained using homologous recombination deficient in caspase 3 and 9 protease that is essential for the normal process of programmed cell death (apoptosis) (Kuida et al., 1996, 1998). In mice lacking both copies of these genes, apoptosis is reduced in the proliferative ventricular zone of the cerebral ventricular zone at early stages, during production of the founder progenitor cells. Thus, the affected mouse has a larger number of both founder cells and radial glial cells (Fig. 6 and Haydar et al., 1999). The main finding, relevant to the subject of this present article, is that in accord with the radial unit hypothesis, a larger-than-normal number of founder cells resulted in a cortex with an increased surface area and the formation of convolutions. By this single gene mutation, a lyssencephalic mouse cortex can be transformed into a gyrencephalic cerebrum. This illustrates the remarkable power of molecular and developmental neurobiology—here we used a gene identified in a roundworm that may help to understand some aspect of cortical expansion during primate evolution.

Protomap hypothesis of cytoarchitectonic diversity

The evolution of the cerebral cortex involves not only expansion in surface but also increase in the number of cytoarchitectonic areas that include duplication of sensory representations (Allman and Kaas, 1971). A major challenge to developmental neurobiology in the past 100 years is how individual and species-specific cytoarchitectonic areas have emerged from the initial, seemingly uniform ventricular zone and cortical plate. Both intrinsic and extrinsic factors have been suggested. Traditionally, it was thought that all cortical neurons are equipotential (tabula rasa model) and that laminar and areal differences are induced by extrinsic influences exerted via thalamic afferents (Creutzfelt, 1976). Indeed, the structural and functional homogeneity of the cortex emphasized by Lashley and his followers in the middle of the twentieth century (e.g., Lashley and Clark, 1946) appears to be supported by the ostensible similarity in the laminar pattern of cell distribution in various cortical areas and by the acknowledged resemblance of their synaptic circuitry (Eccles, 1984; Rakic and Singer, 1988; Szentagothai, 1987; Montcastle, 1996). This hypothesis is also in harmony with the overwhelming evidence that development of many features of cortical organization is highly dependent on interaction with thalamic afferents (Rakic, 1976a, 1981; Hubel et al., 1977; Frost and Metin, 1985; Sur et al., 1988).

More recently, it was postulated that cells of the embryonic cerebral vesicle themselves may be a target of evolution and have intrinsic programs for basic species-specific cortical regionalization (protomap model) (Rakic, 1988). This hypothesis, based on experimental manipulations of cortical input in primate embryos, indicates that some region-specific cytoarchitectonic features develop independently of input (Kuljis and Rakic, 1991; Rakic et al., 1991; Rakic and Lidow, 1995). The word 'proto' emphasized the malleable feature of this primordial map in which intrinsic cues, generated within cortical neurons, attract appropriate input and cooperatively create a final area-specific, three-dimensional organization.

The initial indication that developmental events in the ventricular zone foreshadow prospective regional differences in the overlaying cerebral mantle comes from ^{3}H-thymidine labeling of dividing cells, which shows that the ventricular region subjacent to area 17 produces more neurons per radial unit (Rakic, 1976b) than the region subjacent to area 18 (Dehay et al., 1993). Therefore, certain region-specific differences in production of the ventricular zone can be detected even before neurons arrive at the cortex and become exposed to input from the periphery via the thalamic afferents (Kennedy and Dehay, 1993; Algan and Rakic, 1997). The development

Wild-type

Casp-9 KO

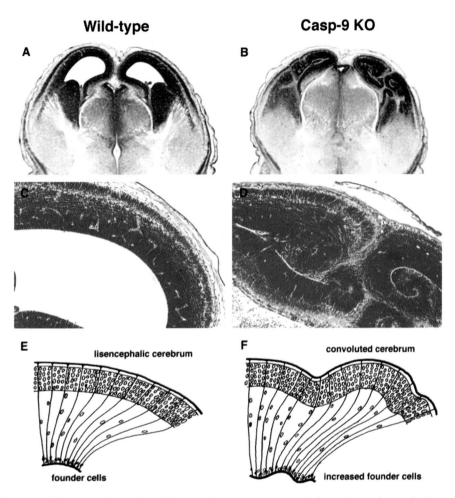

Fig. 6. Deletion of apoptotic killer gene (Caspase-3 and 9) results in substantial changes in forebrain morphogenesis. By preventing selected apoptotic deaths in the early forebrain progenitor lineage, caspase deletion causes an increase in forebrain founder cells. (A and B) Nissl-stained coronal brain sections at E17. The third ventricle (III) is labeled for orientation. Compared to the wild-type littermate (A), the section from the $casp-3^{-/-}$ individual illustrates the thicker cerebral wall and enlarged ventricular epithelium in these animals. (C and D) Sagittal Nissl-stained brain sections from wild-type (C) and Casp-3 deficient individuals at postnatal day 16 illustrate heterotopic cell masses (asterisk) and sulci-like indentations (arrow) of the cortical wall causing an increase in surface area of the mutant cortex. Instead of a smooth cerebrum (E), this increase in forebrain progenitors leads to a larger expansion of the cerebral wall (F) and a convoluted cerebrum of larger surface area. (Based on Kuida et al., 1996, 1998; Haydar et al., 1999).

of correct topological connections in anophthalmic mice and in early-enucleated animals indicates that a basic map can form in the absence of information from the periphery (Kaiserman-Abramoff et al., 1983; Olivaria and Van Sluyters, 1984; Rakic, 1988). Likewise, from early embryonic stages, the monkey primary visual cortex acquires a normal pattern of cytochrome oxidase (Kennedy et al., 1988; Rakic, 1988; Kuljis and Rakic, 1990), major neurotransmitter receptors (Rakic and Lidow, 1995), and synaptic architecture (Bourgeois and

Rakic, 1997) in the absence of any retinal input via the thalamus.

In the early 1990's, *in vivo* and *in vitro* studies began to show high specificity of the growing thalamic axons for selective regions of the embryonic cerebral cortex (Boltz et al., 1992; Agmon et al., 1995). More direct support has accumulated for the intrinsic specification of cortical maps with reports that a number of genes and morphoregulatory molecules are expressed in discrete gradients and cortical regions before or independently of the incoming input (Barbe, and Levitt, 1991: Arimatsu et al., 1992: Simeone et al., 1992; Cohen-Tanudji et al., 1994; Levitt, 1994; Gitton et al., 1999; Fukuchi-Shimogori and Grove, 2001; Sestan et al., 2001). The protomap hypothesis gained strong support from evidence that abolition of thalamic input by genetic manipulation does not prevent cortical parcellation (Myjashita-Lyn, 1999; Mallamaci et al., 2000; Bishop et al., 2000). The study by Fukuchi-Shimogori and Grove (2001) is particularly convincing as it reveals that change across the cerebral wall in the strength of molecular gradients of a single growth factor may have a dramatic effect on the organization of the cortical map. They used *in utero* microelectroporation-mediated gene transfer to alter the expression level and sites of FGF8 production in the developing neocortex before onset of the formation of thalamo-cortical connectivity. The surviving mice displayed a dramatic reorganization of the cortical map including a shift of the boundaries among the frontal, parietal and occipital areas with no visible disturbance of the remaining brain. Remarkably, introduction of an extra source of FGF8 into the occipital pole produced an extra barrel field situated in the occipital lobe. It is especially intriguing that ectopic barrel fields have a reverse (mirror image) representation of the whiskers, as occurs when an area becomes duplicated during evolution (Allman and Kass, 1972).

Although input from the thalamus appears to have little influence on the initial regionalization of the cortex, it is essential for its proper maturation (Rakic, 1988; Rakic et al., 1991). Since the embryonic cerebral wall exhibits gradients of morphoregulatory molecules, as well as more specific area-specific molecular differences, the precise position of interareal borders, the overall size of each cytoarchitectonic area, and the details of their cellular and synaptic characteristics in the adult cerebral cortex is only achieved through a cascade of reciprocal interactions between cortical neurons and the cues they receive from afferents arriving from a variety of extracortical sources (Rakic, 1988). Such afferents may serve to coordinate and adjust the ratio of various cell classes with the subcortical structures, as has been shown in the primary visual system (Messier et al., 1997). For example, the experimental manipulation of geniculocortical input to the visual cortex indicates that the size of a given cytoarchitectonic area can be regulated by afferents originating from subcortical structures (Rakic et al., 1991; Kennedy and Dehay, 1993; Rakic and Lidow, 1995).

Since the overall size of the cerebrum in the experimental animals was reduced, it is likely that many other competing signaling pathways are also involved. It is important to search for the additional genes and morphoregulatory molecules that may be involved in cortical specification and development in rodent, and possibly primate, models of cortical dysgenesis that mimic specific genetic or acquired cortical disorders (Rubenstein and Rakic, 1999).

In summary, our understanding of the radial and areal specification of the cerebral cortex during individual ontogenetic development and evolution has evolved considerably from the foundations laid by Cajal and his contemporaries over 100 years ago. The fact that it is now possible to study migrating cells *in vivo* or to rearrange and even duplicate at will the sensory representations of the periphery in the cerebral cortex presents an unprecedented opportunity to study how these maps develop at the cellular and molecular level.

Acknowledgments

This work was supported over the years by grants from the US Public Health Service. I am indebted to the present and past members of my laboratory for their contribution and incisive discussion on this subject.

References

Agmon, A.A., Yang, L.T., Jones, G.E. and O'Dowd, D.K. (1995) Topological precision in the thalamic projection to the neonatal mouse. *J. Neurosci.*, 13: 5365–5382.

Algan, O. and Rakic, P. (1997) Radiation-induced area- and lamina-specific deletion of neurons in the primate visual cortex. *J. Comp. Neurol.*, 381: 335–352.

Allman, J.M. and Kass, J.H. (1971) A representation of the visual field in the caudal third of the middle temporal gyrus of the owl monkey (*Aotus trivirgatus*). *Brain Res.*, 31: 85–105.

Anderson, S., Mione, M., Yun, K. and Rubenstein, J.L.R. (1999) Differential origins of neocortical projection and local circuit neurons: Role of Dlx Genes in neocortical interneuronogenesis. *Cereb. Cortex*, 9: 646–654.

Ang, E.S.B.C., Jr., Haydar, T.F., Gluncic, V. and Rakic, P. (2002) Early coordinates of cortical specification, *submitted*.

Angevine, J.B., Jr. and Sidman, R.L. (1961) Autoradiographic study of cell migration during histogenesis of cerebral cortex in the mouse. *Nature*, 192: 766–768.

Anton, E.S., Marchionni, M.A., Lee, K.-F. and Rakic, P. (1997) Role of GGF/ neuregulin signaling in interactions between migrating neurons and radial glia in the developing cerebral cortex. *Development*, 124: 3501–3510.

Anton, E.S., Kreidberg, J. and Rakic, P. (1999) Distinct functions of α_3 and α_v integrin receptors in neuronal migration and laminar organization of the cerebral cortex. *Neuron*, 22: 227–289.

Anton, E.S., Matthew, W.D. and Rakic, P. (1996) A regionally distributed radial glial antigen: a candidate for signaling an end to neuronal migration. *Abst. Soc. Neurosci.*, 22: 1206.

Anton, S.A., Cameron, R.S. and Rakic, P. (1996) Role of neuron-glial junctional proteins in the maintenance and termination of neuronal migration across the embryonic cerebral wall. *J. Neurosci.*, 16: 2283–2293.

Arimatsu, Y., Miyamoto, M., Nihonmatsu, I., Hirata, K., Urataini, Y., Hatanka, Y. and Takiguchi-Hoyash, K. (1992) Early regional specification for a molecular neuronal phenotype in the rat neocortex. *Proc. Nat. Acad. Sci. USA*, 89: 8879–8883.

Barbe, M.F. and Levitt, P. (1992) Attraction of specific thalamic input by cerebral grafts depends on the molecular identity of the implant. *Proc. Nat. Acad. Sci. USA*, 89: 3706–3710.

Behar, T.N., Scott, C.A., Greene, C.L., Wen, X., Smith, S.V., Maric, D., Liu, Q.Y., Colton, C.A. and Baker, J.L. (1999) Glutamate acting at NMDA receptors stimulates embryonic cortical neuronal migration. *J. Neurosci.*, 19: 4449–4461.

Bishop, K.M., Gourdeau, G. and O'Leary, D.D.M. (2000) Regulation of area identity in the mammalian neocoretex by *Emx2* and Pax6. *Science*, 288: 344–349.

Bolz, J., Novak, N. and Staiger, V. (1992) Formation of specific afferent connections in organotypic slice cultures from rat visual cortex co-cultured with lateral geniculate nucleus. *J. Neurosci.*, 12: 3054–3070.

Bouergois, J.-P. and Rakic, P. (1996) Synaptoarchitecture of the occipital cortex in macaque monkey devoid of retinal input from early embryonic stages. *Euro. J. Neurosci.*, 8: 942–950.

Boulder Committee (1970) Embryonic vertebrate central nervous system. Revised terminology. *Anatomical Record*, 166: 257–261.

Buffone, A., Kim, H.J., Puelles, L., Proteus, M.H., Frohman, M.A., Martin, G.R. and Rubinstein, J.L.R. (1993) The mouse DLX-2 (Tes-1) Gbx-2 and Wnt-3 in the embryonic day 12.5 mouse forebrain defines potential transverse and longitudinal segmental boundaries. *Mech. Dev.*, 40: 129–140.

Cajal, S.R. (1881) Sur la structure de l'ecorce cerebrale de quelques mammiferes. *La Cellule*, 7: 125–176.

Cajal, S.R. (1890) Sur l'origine et les ramifications des fibres nerveuses de la moelle embryonnaire. *Anat. Anz.*, 5: 85–95 and 111–119.

Cajal, S.R. (1909) *Histologie du Système Nerveux de l'Homme et des Vertébrés*. Vol. 1, Paris: A. Maloine (Reprinted in 1952 by Consejo Superior de Investigaciones Cientificas, Instituto Ramón y Cajal, Madrid).

Cameron, R.S. and Rakic, P. (1994) Polypeptides that comprise the plasmalemal microdomain between migrating neuronal and glial cells. *J. Neurosci.*, 14: 3139–3155.

Cameron, R.S., Ruffin, J.W., Cho, N.K., Cameron, L.P. and Rakic, P. (1997) Developmental expression, pattern of distribution, and effect on cell aggregation implicate a neuron-glial junctional domain polypeptide in neuronal migration. *J. Comp. Neurol.*, 387: 467–488.

Caviness, V.S., Jr. and Rakic, P. (1978) Mechanisms of cortical development: a view from mutations in mice. *Ann. Rev. Neurosci.*, 1: 297–326.

Choi, B.H. (1986) Glial fibrillary acid protein in radial glia of early human fetal cerebrum: a light and electron microscopic immunocytochemical study. *J. Neuropath. Exp. Neurol.*, 45: 408–418.

Choi, B.H. and Lapham, L.W. (1978) Radial glia in the human fetal cerebrum: a combined Golgi, immunofluorescent and electron microscopic study. *Brain Res.*, 148: 295–311.

Cohen-Tannoudji, M., Babinet, C. and Wassef, M. (1994) Early intrinsic regional specification of the mouse somatosensory cortex. *Nature*, 368: 460–463.

Creutzfeldt, O.D. (1977) Generality of the functional structure of the neocortex. *Naturwissenschaften*, 64: 507–517.

de Carlos, J. A., López-Mascaraque, L. and Valverde, F. (1996) Dynamics of cell migration from the lateral ganglionic eminence in the rat. *J. Neurosci.*, 16: 6146–6156.

Dehay, C., Giroud, P., Berland, M., Smart, I. and Kennedy, H. (1993) Modulation of the cell cycle contributes to the parcellation of the primate visual cortex. *Nature*, 366: 464–466.

Eccles, J.C. (1984) The cerebral neocortex: a theory of its operation. In: E.G. Jones, and A. Peters, (Eds.), *Cerebral Cortex*, Vol. II. Plenum Press, New York, pp. 1–36.

Edelman, G.M. (1983) Cell adhesion molecules. *Science*, 219: 450–457.

Farrant, M., Feldmeyer, D., Takahashi, T. and Cull-Candy, S.G. (1994) NMDA-receptor channel diversity in the developing cerebellum. *Nature*, 368: 335–339.

Ferri, R.T. and Levitt, P. (1993) Cerebral cortical progenitors are fated to produce region-specific neuronal populations. *Cerebral Cortex*, 3(3): 187–198.

Fishell, G. and Hatten, M.E. (1991) Astrotactin provides a receptor system for CNS neuronal migration. *Development*, 113: 755–765.

Frost, D.O. and Metin, C. (1985) Introduction of functional retinal projections to the somatosensory system. *Nature*, 317: 162–164.

Fukuchi-Shimogori, T. and Grove, E.A. (2000) Neocortex Patterning by the secreted signaling molecule FGF8. *Science*, 294: 1071–1074.

Gitton, Y., Cohn-Tannoudji, M., and Wassef, M. (1999) Specification of somatosensory area identity in cortical explants. *J. Neurosci.*, 19: 4889–4898.

Goldman-Rakic, P.S. (1987) Circuitry of primate prefrontal cortex and regulation of behavior by representational memory. In: F. Plum (Ed.), *Handbook of Physiology, The Nervous System, Higher Functions of the Brain*, Section I, Vol. V., Part 1, Chapter 9, Am. Physiol. Soc., Bethesda, Md., pp. 373–417.

Golgi, C. (1874) Sulla fina anatomia del cervelleto umano. In: *Opera Omnia. Hoepli.*, Milan, Italy.

Harfuss, E., Galli, R., Henis, N. and Gotz, M. (2001) Characterization of CBS precursor subtypes and radial glia. *Dev. Biol.*, 226: 15–30.

Hatten, M.E. and Mason, C.A. (1986) Neuron-astroglia interactions *in vitro* and *in vivo*. *Trends in Neurosci.*, 9: 168–174.

Hatten, M.E. and Mason, C.A. (1990) Mechanism of glial-guided neuronal migration *in vitro* and *in vivo*. *Experientia*, 46: 907–916.

Haydar, T.F., Kuan, C.-Y., Flavell, R.A. and Rakic, P. (1999) The role of cell death in regulating the size and shape of the mammalian forebrain. *Cereb. Cortex*, 9: 621–626.

Hirai, K., Yoshioka, H., Kihara, M., Hasegawa, K., Sakamoto, T., Sawada, T. and Fushiki, S. (1999) Inhibition of neuronal migration by blocking NMDA receptors in the embryonic rat cerebral cortex: a tissue culture study. *Dev. Brain Res.*, 114: 63–67.

His, W. (1874) *Unserer Koperform und das Physiologishe Problem inrer Enstehung.* Engelman, Leipzig.

His, W. (1904) *Die Entwickelung des menschlichen Gehirns*, Hirzel, Leipzig.

Hubel, D.H., Wiesel, T.N. and LeVay, S. (1977) Plasticity of ocular dominance columns in monkey striate cortex. *Phil. Trans. Roy. Soc. Lond. Serv.*, B, 278: 377–409.

Kadhim, H.J., Gadisseux, J.-F. and Evrard, P. (1988) Topographical and cytological evolution of the glial phase during prenatal development of the human brain: histochemical and electron microscopic study. *J. Neuropath. Exp. Neurol.*, 47: 166–188.

Kaiserman-Abramoff, I., Graybiel, A. and Nauta, W.H. (1983) Thalamic projection to area 17 in a congenitally anophthalmic mouse strain. *Neurosci.*, 5: 41–52.

Kennedy, H. and DeHay, C. (1993) Cortical specification of mice and men. *Cereb. Cortex*, 3: 171–186.

Kennedy, H., Dehay, C. and Horsburgh, G. (1990) Striate cortex periodicity. *Nature*, 384: 494.

Kinsbourne, M. (1998) Unity of diversity in the human brain: evidence from injury. *Daedalus*, 127: 233–256.

Kirschner, M. and Mitchison, T. (1986) Beyond self-assembly: from microtubules to morphogenesis. *Cell*, 45: 329–342.

Komuro, H. and Rakic, P. (1992) Specific role of N-type calcium channels in neuronal migration. *Science*, 257: 806–809.

Komuro, H. and Rakic, P. (1993) Modulation of neuronal migration by NMDA receptors. *Science*, 260: 95–97.

Komuro, H. and Rakic, P. (1998) Orchestration of neuronal migration by the activity of ion channels, neurotransmitter receptors and intracellular Ca^{+2} fluctuations. *J. Neurobio.*, 37: 110–130.

Kornack, D.R. and Rakic, P. (1995) Radial and horizontal deployment of clonally related cells in the primate neocortex: Relationship to distinct mitotic lineages. *Neuron*, 15: 311–321.

Kuida, K., Haydar, T., Kuan C.-Y., Yong, G., Taya, C., Karasuyama, A., Su, S.-H., Rakic, P. and Flavell, R.A. (1998) Reduced apoptosis and cytochrome c-mediated caspase activation in mice lacking Caspase-9. *Cell*, 94: 325–33.

Kuida, K., Zheng, T.S., Na, S., Kuang, C., Yang, D., Karasuyama, H., Rakic, P. and Flavell, R. (1996) Decreased apoptosis in the brain and premature lethality in CPP32-deficient mice. *Nature*, 384: 368–372.

Kuljis, R.O. and Rakic, P. (1990) Hypercolumns in the monkey visual cortex can develop in the absence of cues from photoreceptors. *Proc. Natl. Acad. Sci. USA*, 87: 5303–5306.

Lashley, K.S. and Clark, G. (1946) The cytoarchitecture of the cerebral cortex of Ateles: a critical examination of cytoarchitectonic studies. *J. Comp. Neurol.*, 85: 223–305.

Lavdas, A.A., Grigoriou, M., Pachnis, V. and Parnavelas, J.G. (1999) The medial ganglionic eminence gives rise to a population of early neurons in the developing cerebral cortex. *J. Neurosci.*, 19: 7881–7888.

Letinic, K. and Rakic, P. (2001) Telencephalic origin of human thalamic GABAergic neurons *Nature Neurosci.*, 4: 931–936.

Letinic, K., Zoncu, R. and Rakic, P. (2002) Novel origin of GABAegic neurons in the human neocortex. *Nature*, in press.

Levitt, P. (1994) Experimental approaches that reveal principles of cerebral cortical development. In: M. Gazzaniga (Ed.), *The Cognitive Neurosciences.* MIT Press, Cambridge, MA, pp. 147–163.

Levitt, P. and Rakic, P. (1980) Immunoperoxidase localization of glial fibrillary acid protein in radial glial cells and astrocytes of the developing rhesus monkey brain. *J. Comp. Neurol.*, 193: 815–840.

Levitt, P., Cooper, M.L. and Rakic, P. (1983) Early divergence and changing proportions of neuronal and glial precursor cells in the primate cerebral ventricular zone. *Dev. Biology*, 96: 472–484.

Levitt, P., Cooper, M.L. and Rakic, P. (1981) Coexistence of neuronal and glial precursor cells in the cerebral ventricular zone of the fetal monkey: an ultrastructural immunoperoxidase analysis. *J. Neurosci.*, 1: 27–39.

Luskin, M.B., Pearlman, A.L. and Sanes, J.R. (1988) Cell lineage in the cerebral cortex of the mouse studied *in vivo* and *in vitro* with a recombinant retrovirus. *Neuron*, 1: 635–647.

Magini, G. (1888) Sur la nevroglie et les cellules nerveuses cerebrales chez les foetus. *Arch. Ital. Biol.*, 9: 59–60.

Mallamaci, A., Muzio, L., Chan, C.-H., Parnavelas, J. and Boncinelli, E. (2000) Area identity shifts in the early cerebral cortex of Emx2-/- mutant mice. *Nat. Neurosci.*, 7: 679–686.

McConnell, S.K. (1988) Development and decision-making in the mammalian cerebral cortex. *Brain Res. Rev.*, 13: 1–23.

Meissirel, C., Wikler, K.C., Chalupa, L.M. and Rakic, P. (1997) Early divergence of M and P visual subsystems in the embryonic primate brain. *Proc. Nat. Acad. Sci. USA*, 94: 5900–5905.

Misson, J.P., Austin, C.P., Takahashi, T., Cepko, C.L. and Caviness, V.S. (1991). The alignment of migrating neural cells in relation to the murine neopallial radial glial fiber system. *Cerebral Cortex*, 1: 221–229.

Miyashita-Lin, E.M., Hevner, R., Wassarman, K.M., Martinez, S. and Rubenstein, J.L.R. (1999) Early neocortical regionalization in the absence of thalamic innervation. *Science*, 285: 906–909.

Miyata, T., Kawaguchi, A., Okano, H. and Ogawa, M. (2001) Asymmetric inheritance of radial glial fibers by cortical neurons. *Neuron*, 31: 727–41.

Mountcastle, V.B. (1997) The columnar organization of the neocortex. *Brain*, 12: 701–722.

Mountcastle, V.B. (1957) Modality and topographic properties of single neurons of cat's somatic sensory cortex. *J. Neurophysiol.*, 20: 408–434.

Nakatsuji, M., Kadokawa, Y. and Suemori, H. (1991) Radial columnar patches in the chimeric cerebral cortex visualized by use of mouse embryonic stem cells expressing β-galactosidase. *Dev. Growth and Differ.*, 33: 571–578.

Noctor, S.C., Flint, A.C., Weissman, T.A., Dammerman, R.S. and Kriegstein, A.R. (2001) Neurons derived from radial glial cells establish radial units in neocortex. *Nature*, 409: 714–720.

O'Rourke, N.A., Dailey, M.E., Smith, S.J. and McConnell, S.K. (1992) Diverse migratory pathways in the developing cerebral cortex. *Science*, 258: 299–302.

O'Rourke, N.A., Dulivan, N.A., Smith, D.P., Kazanowski, S.E., Jacobs, A.A. and McConnell, S.K. (1995) Tangential migration in developing cerebral cortex. *Development*, 1212: 2165–2176.

Ogawa, M., Miyata, T., Nakajima, K., Yagyu, K., Selke, M., Ikenaka, K., Yamamoto, H. and Mikoshiba, K. (1995) The *reeler* gene-associated antigen on Cajal-Retzius neurons is a crucial molecule for laminar organization of cortical neurons. *Neuron*, 14: 1–20.

Olivaria, J. and Van Sluyters, R.C. (1984) Callosal connections of the posterior neocortex in normal-eyed, congenitally anophthalmic and neonatally enucleated mice. *J. Comp. Neurol.*, 230: 249–268.

Parnavelas, J.G., Barfield, J.A., Franke, E. and Luskin, M.B. (1991) Separate progenitor cells give rise to pyramidal and nonpyramidal neurons in the rat telencephalon. *Cereb. Cortex*, 1: 463–491.

Powel, E.M., Mara, W.M. and Levitt, P. (2000) Hepatocyte growth factior/scatter factor is mitogen for interneuron migrating from the ventral to dorsal telencephaon. *Neuron*, 30: 1–20.

Rakic, P. (1972) Mode of cell migration to the superficial layers of fetal monkey neocortex. *J. Comp. Neurol.*, 145: 61–84.

Rakic, P. (1974) Neurons in the monkey visual cortex: Systematic relation between time of origin and eventual disposition. *Science*, 183: 425–427.

Rakic, P. (1976) Prenatal genesis of connections subserving ocular dominance in the rhesus monkey. *Nature*, 261: 467–471.

Rakic, P. (1976) Differences in the time of origin and in eventual distribution of neurons in areas 17 and 18 of the visual cortex in the rhesus monkey. *Exp. Brain Res. Suppl.*, 1: 244–248.

Rakic, P. (1978) Neuronal migration and contact interaction in primate telencephalon. *Postgrad. Med., J.*, 54: 25–40.

Rakic, P. (1981) Neuron-glial interaction during brain development. *Trends Neurosci.*, 4: 184–187.

Rakic, P. (1985) Contact regulation of neuronal migration. In: G.M. Edelman, and J.-P. Thiery, (Eds.), *The Cell in Contact: Adhesions and Junctions as Morphogenetic Determinants*. Wiley and Sons, New York, pp. 67–91.

Rakic, P. (1986) Mechanism of ocular dominance segregation in the lateral geniculate nucleus: competitive elimination hypothesis. *Trends in Neuroscience*, 9: 11–15.

Rakic, P. (1988) Specification of cerebral cortical areas. *Science*, 241: 170–176.

Rakic, P. (1995a) Radial versus tangential migration of neuronal clones in the developing cerebral cortex. *Proc. Nat. Acad. Sci. USA*, 92: 11323–11327.

Rakic, P. (1995b) A small step for the cell—a giant leap for mankind: a hypothesis of neocortical expansion during evolution. *Trends in Neuroscience*, 18: 383–388.

Rakic, P. (1995) Radial glial cells: Scaffolding for brain construction. In: H. Ketterman, and B.R. Ransom (Eds.), *Neuroglial Cells*, Oxford University Press, New York, 746–762.

Rakic, P. (1997) Intra and extracellular control of neuronal migration: relevance to cortical malformations. In: A.M. Galaburda, and Y. Christen, (Eds.), *Normal and Abnormal Development of Cortex, Research and Perspectives in Neurosciences*, Springer, 81–89.

Rakic, P. (1999) Discriminating migrations. *Nature*, 400: 315–316.

Rakic, P. (2002) Neurobiologist's creationalism: making new cortical maps. *Science*, 294: 1011–1012.

Rakic, P., Cameron, R.S. and Komuro, H. (1994) Recognition, adhesion, transmembrane signaling, and cell motility in guided neuronal migration. *Current Opinion in Neurobiology*, 4: 63–69.

Rakic, P., Knyihar-Csillik, E. and Csillik, B. (1996) Polarity of microtubule assembly during neuronal migration. *Proc. Nat. Acad. Sci. USA*, 93: 9218–9222.

Rakic, P., Stensaas, L.J. and Sayre, E.P. (1974) Computer-aided three-dimensional reconstruction and quantitative analysis of cells from serial electronmicroscopic montages of fetal monkey brain. *Nature*, 250: 31–34.

Rakic, P., Suner, I. and Williams, R.W. (1991) Novel cytoarchitectonic areas induced experimentally within primate striate cortex. *Proc. Natl. Acad. Sci. USA*, 88: 2083–2987.

Rakic, P. and Kornack, R. D. (2001) Neocortical expansion and elaboration during primate evolution: A view from neuroembryology. In: D. Falk and K. Gibson (eds.), *Evolutionary Anatomy of Primate Cerebral Cortex*, Cambridge University Press, London, 30–56.

Rakic, P. and Lidow, M.S. (1995) Distribution and density of neurotransmitter receptors in the visual cortex devoid of retinal input from early embryonic stages. *J. Neurosci.*,15: 2561–2574.

Rakic, P. and Sidman, R.L. (1968) Supravital DNA synthesis in the developing human and mouse brain. *J. Neuropath. Exp. Neurol.*, 27: 246–276.

Rakic, P. and Singer, W. (1988) *Neurobiology of the Neocortex*. Wiley and Sons, New York, NY. 461pp.

Rakic, P. and Caviness, V.S., Jr. (1995) Cortical development: view from neurological mutants two decades later. *Neuron*, 14: 1101–1104.

Reid, C., Liang, I. and Walsh, C. (1995) Systematic widespread clonal organization in cerebral cortex. *Neuron*, 15: 299–310.

Reiner, O., Carrozzo, R., Shen, Y., Wehnert, M., Faustinella, F., Dobyns, W.B., Caskey, C.T., and Ledbetter, D.H. (1993) Isolation of a Miller-Dieker lissencephaly gene containing G protein b-subunit-like repeats. *Nature*, 364: 717–721.

Retzius, G. (1893) Studien uber Ependym und Neuroglia. *Biol. Untersuch.* Stockholm, N.S. 5: 9–26.

Rivas, R.J. and Hatten, M.B. (1995) Motility and cytoskeletal organization of migrating cerebellar granule neurons. *J. Neurosci.*, 15: 981–989.

Rossi, D., Slater, T.N. (1993) The developmental onset of NMDA receptor channel activity during neuronal migration. *Neuropharmacol.*, 32: 1239–1248.

Rubenstein, J.L.R. and Rakic, P. (1999) Genetic control of cortical development. *Cerebral Cortex*. 9: 521–523.

Sanes, J.R. (1989) Analyzing cell lineages with a recombinant retrovirus. *Trends in Neurosci.*, 12: 21–28.

Schachner, M., Faissner, A. and Fischer, G. (1985) Functional and structural aspects of the cell surface in mammalian nervous system development. In: G.M. Edelman, W.E. Gall and J.P. Thiery (Eds.), *The Cell in Contact: Adhesions and Junctions as Morphogenetic Determinants*, John Wiley & Sons, New York.

Schmechel, D.E. and Rakic, P. (1979a) Arrested proliferation of radial glial cells during midgestation in rhesus monkey. *Nature*, 227: 303–305.

Schmechel, D.E. and Rakic, P. (1979b) A Golgi study of radial glial cells in developing monkey telencephalon. *Anat. Embryol.*, 56: 115–152.

280

Sestan, N., Rakic, P. and Donoghue, M.J. (2001) Independent parcellation of the embryonic visual cortex and thalamus revealed by combinatorial Eph/ephrine gene expression. *Current Biology*. 11: 39–43.

Sidman, R.L. and Rakic, P. (1973) Neuronal migration with special reference to developing human brain: a review. *Brain Res.*, 62: 1–35.

Sidman, R.L. and Rakic, P. (1982) Development of the human central nervous system. In: W. Haymaker and R.D. Adams (Eds.), *Histology and Histopathology of the Nervous System.* Charles C Thomas, Springfield, IL, pp. 3–145.

Simeone, A., Acampora, D., Gulisano, M., Stornaiuolo, A., Boncinelli, E. (1992) Nested expression domains of four homeobox genes in developing rostral brain. *Nature*, 358: 687–690.

Soriano, E., Dumesnil, N., Auladell, C., Cohen-Tannoudji, M. and Sotelo, C. (1995) Molecular heterogeneity of progenitors and radial migration in the developing cerebral cortex revealed by transgene expression. *Proc. Natl. Acad. Sci. USA*, 92: 11676–11680.

Sur, M., Garraghty, P.E. and Roe, A.W. (1988) Experimentally induced visual projections in auditory thalamus and cortex. *Science*, 242: 1434–1441.

Szentagothai, J. (1987) The neuronal network of the cerebral cortex: A functional interpretation. *Prog. Brain Res.*, 201: 219–248.

Tan, S.-S. and Breen, S.J. (1993) Radial mosaicism and tangential cell dispersion both contribute to mouse neocortical development. *Nature*, 362: 638–640.

Tan, S.-S., Kalloniatis, M., Sturm, K., Tam, P.P.L., Reese, B.E. and Faulkner-Jones, B. (1998) Separate progenitors for radial and tangential cell dispersion during development of the cerebral neocortex. *Neuron*, 21: 295–304.

Volpe, J.J. (1987) *Neurology of the Newborn*, 2nd Ed., WB Saunders, Philadelphia.

Von Lenhossék, M. (1895) Centrosom and Sphäre in den Spinalganglienzellen des Frosches. *Arch. f. mirk. Anat.*, 46: 345–369.

Walsh, C. and Cepko, C.L. (1988) Clonally related cortical cells show several migration patterns. *Science*, 241: 1342–1345.

Ware, M.L., Tavazoie, S.F., Reid, C.B. and Walsh, C.A. (1999) Coexistence of widespread clones and large radial clones in early embryonic ferret cortex. *Cereb. Cortex*, 9: 636–645.

E.C. Azmitia, J. DeFelipe, E.G. Jones, P. Rakic and C.E. Ribak (Eds.)
Progress in Brain Research, Vol. 136

CHAPTER 22

The surface of the developing cerebral cortex: still *special cells* one century later

Alfonso Fairén[1,*], Javier Morante-Oria[1] and Carolina Frassoni[2]

[1]*Instituto de Neurociencias, Consejo Superior de Investigaciones Científicas and Universidad Miguel Hernández,*
Campus de San Juan, Apartado 18, 03550 San Juan de Alicante, Spain
[2]*Istituto Nazionale Neurologico C. Besta, 20133 Milan, Italy*

Abstract: The marginal zone of the developing cerebral cortex is formed by different types of neurons, some of which were described more than one century ago. It is the case of Cajal-Retzius cells, which are known to synthesize and secrete Reelin, an extracellular matrix glycoprotein critically involved in the radial migration and early cortical cytoarchitectonic organization. These cells do not emit projection axons, a characteristic that bespeaks against these cells being considered as pioneer neurons. The true pioneer neurons of the marginal zone are part of a distinct cell entity: these are cells that emit the earliest descending axonal projection from the cerebral cortex into the subpallium, even before than subplate neurons, the other population of pioneer neurons in the cortical anlage. Finally, the marginal zone is a territory where cohorts of undifferentiated cortical interneurons migrate into the upper layers of the cerebral cortex. Marginal zone neurons, including Cajal-Retzius cells, tend to distribute non-uniformly over the cortical surface. Such a mosaic structural configuration points towards more complexities regarding their possible functions during cortical development.

A brief historical introduction: Cajal and Retzius on Cajal-Retzius cells

The neurons we now call Cajal-Retzius cells were discovered more than one century ago. Cajal (1890, 1891) reported on unusual neurons in the superficial layer of the cerebral cortex seen in Golgi preparations of early postnatal rabbits. He called these neurons the "*special cells of the molecular layer*". They were fusiform cells with long horizontal processes, which sent vertical ascending branchlets to the pial surface (Fig. 1A).

Why these cells looked unusual (special) to Cajal is not entirely clear, but one of the peculiarities that struck this author were the characteristics of the processes. It was not clear, indeed, if they were axonal or dendritic in nature, and the controversy has endured until Verney and

Derer (1995) used specific markers for these neuronal compartments. This was of obvious importance to Cajal, who was looking at every neuron as a new case to test his hypothesis of the dynamic polarization of neurons (Cajal, 1909–11). Whatever the case, Cajal's writings reflect how these cells intrigued his imagination. Incidentally, it is noteworthy that his sketches of the developing cortex always had one *special cell* on the top (Fig. 2).

Retzius (1893) studied with the Golgi method fetuses of diverse species (rabbits, cats, dogs and humans) and described what he believed were the homologues of the neurons described by Cajal (1891). Accordingly, Retzius (1893, 1894) named them Cajal cells (*Cajal'schen Zellen*). Cajal obviously loved such a denomination (DeFelipe and Jones, 1988), and the term *Cajal'sche Zellen de Retzius* appeared even in Cajal's Histology textbook for medical students (Cajal, 1910, p. 577). In a further report, Retzius (1894) completed his observations of human fetal material, and described these cells with considerable morphological detail (for reproductions of

---
*Corresponding author: Tel.: +3496 591-9422;
Fax: +3496 591-9549; E-mail: fairen@umh.es

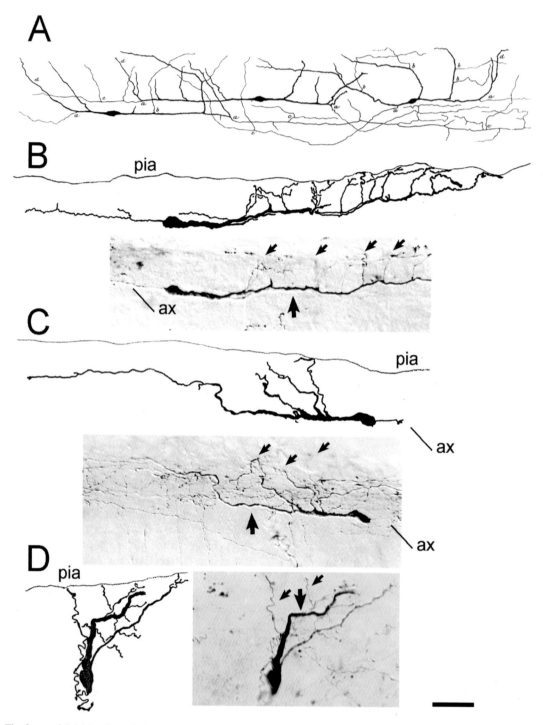

Fig. 1. The forms of Cajal-Retzius cells in postnatal lagomorphs and rodents. **A**. Drawing of the slender, horizontal special cells published in 1891 by Cajal. These are from 8-day-old rabbits stained with the Golgi method. According to Cajal, the cells were oriented antero-posteriorly. For Cajal (1891), *a* was the main axon, *b* were supernumerary axons and *c,* axon collaterals. **C–D** Cajal-Retzius cells in modern preparations. Biotinylated dextran-amine (BDA) was iontophoretically injected into the somatosensory cortex of rats ranging from postnatal day (P) 0 to P30

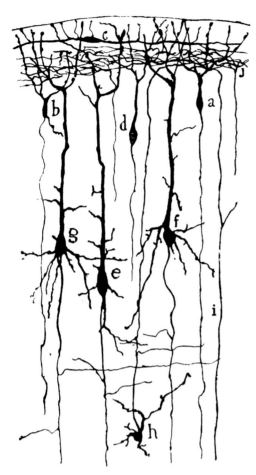

Fig. 2. This is a reproduction of Fig. 542 of Cajal's Histologie (Cajal, 1911). The drawing is from a 4-day-old mouse stained with the Golgi method. It is quite remarkable the resolute representation of an inside–out gradient of pyramidal cell maturation (cf. Cajal, 1891). For Cajal, *a, b* and *d* were pyramidal cells in an immature "*bipolar stage*" and cell *b* was referred as being slightly more mature by having a short basal dendrite (labeled as "*ascending dendrite*" probably by typographic mistake in Cajal's legend). *c* is a special cell. *e, f, g* are pyramidal cells and *h* is a Martinotti cell with its typical ascending axon. *i* is an afferent axon going to MZ, and *j* points to the terminal arborization of one such axon.

Retzius drawings, see Frotscher, 1997; Meyer et al., 1999). In spite of their morphological complexity and of their visible heterogeneity, all these cells showed some constant traits: the distinctive horizontal dendrites, a

collection of conspicuous branchlets ascending to the pial surface and a horizontal, dense axonal plexus beneath the cell. These cells are just what we call Cajal-Retzius cells. Nowadays, it is accepted that expression of the extracellular matrix glycoprotein Reelin is an essential trait of Cajal-Retzius cells of rodents, carnivores and primates (Ogawa et al., 1995; D'Arcangelo et al., 1995, 1997; Meyer et al., 1998, 1999, 2000b; Meyer and Goffinet, 1998; Alcántara et al., 1998; Zecevic et al., 1999; Zecevic and Rakic, 2001). The analysis of the *reelin*-null phenotype (*reeler* mouse) have revealed the fundamental role of this cells in radial migration of the cortical neurons and their correct organization in six cortical layers following an inside-out gradient. Reelin, secreted by Cajal-Retzius cells during cortical development, has been shown to act on target cells through the liporeceptors ApoER2 and VLDLR and the docking protein disabled-1, thus defining a Reelin signaling pathway (see e.g. Curran and D'Arcangelo, 1998; Rice and Curran, 2001 for excellent reviews).

Retzius did not succeed to stain *Cajal'sche Zellen* with the Golgi method in postnatal brains of humans. Cajal (1899, 1900) found the *special cells* in newborn children. On this occasion, the cells differed somewhat from those seen by Retzius in fetuses: while the long horizontal dendrites were still recognizable, the ascending processes to the pial surface were rare, and the cell bodies were encountered immediately below the pia. Cajal (1899a,b, 1911) interpreted these cells as the *adult form* of the *special cells*, being the result of the atrophy of the fine ascending processes characteristic of the Cajal-Retzius cells during the fetal period (see also, Marín-Padilla, 1984, 1998), i.e., the result of a transformation from a *fetal form* into an *adult form* (Fig. 3). The senior author of the present report has recently questioned such an interpretation (Meyer et al., 1999; cf. Meyer and González-Hernández, 1993; Meyer and Goffinet, 1998) and favored the alternative hypothesis that two successive cohorts of Reelin-expressing Cajal-Retzius cells might exist in humans. According to this interpretation, no transformation between a *fetal* and an *adult* form occurs during development and, additionally, only the postnatal cells would survive into adulthood. This interpretation is

(see Frassoni et al., 1995 for technical details). **B** and **C** are from one 4-day-old rat, and **D** from a 3-day-old rat. The cell in **D** may correspond to a transitional morphology (see Meyer et al., 1998). The pial border is indicated in the camera lucida drawings. Thick arrows point to the horizontal dendrites and the small arrows point to the ascending branchlets. According to current interpretations, the axon (ax) is unique. Scale bar: 50 μm, applies to **B–D**.

compatible with the results by Spreafico et al. (1995, 1999), who have explored with the TUNEL method the death of Cajal-Retzius cells in rats and in humans. Their results showed no TUNEL-positive cells that could be identified as Cajal-Retzius cells but, as suggested by these authors (Spreafico et al., 1995), these cells could die by other alternative mechanisms.

The morphology of the human postnatal Cajal-Retzius cells has been reexamined with great detail by Marín-Padilla (1984, 1998), who suggested these cells might play in the adult the role of a cortical interneuron (Marín-Padilla, 1998). Several arguments seem in favor of such an interpretation. On the one hand, the dendritic and axonal forms of these *Cajal cells*, so far only described with sufficient detail with the Golgi method (Fig. 3) resemble those of some cortical basket cells

(cf. Fairén et al., 1984). On the other hand, in rodents, certain subpopulations of layer I neurons express GABA and share with the ones described in man by Cajal and Marín-Padilla the immediate subpial localization of their somata (Imamoto et al., 1994). Moreover, they colocalize Reelin (Alcántara et al., 1998). In early developmental period, Reelin expression is a trait of Cajal-Retzius cells but, in the adult, Reelin is expressed by certain subsets of cortical interneurons (Pesold et al., 1999) that exclude basket or chandelier cells (cf. Fairén et al., 1984). The interpretation of the so-called "*adult*" forms of Cajal-Retzius cells as interneurons goes along with the novel name we proposed for these cells, that of *Cajal cells* (Meyer et al., 1999) and sets them apart from the Cajal-Retzius cells found during prenatal development of the human cerebral cortex. This proposal, which still awaits

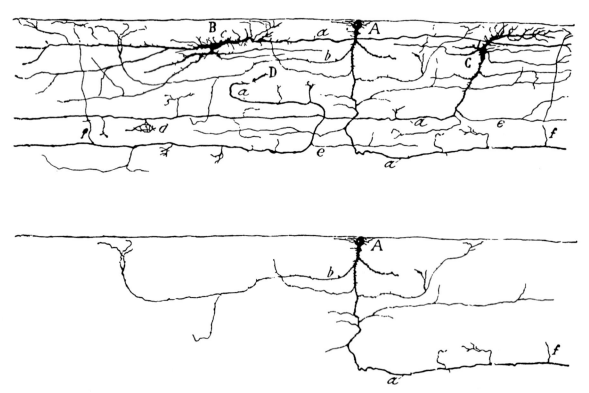

Fig. 3. On the top there is a reproduction of Fig. 341 of Cajal's Histologie (Cajal, 1911), a drawing from Golgi preparations of a month-old human. **A** is a "*cellule marginale ou piriforme*" considered by Cajal as paradigm of the adult form of the *special cells*. **B** resembles the cells illustrated by Retzius (1894). Cajal could consider **C** as a transition form between the *fetal* and the *adult* forms. In Cajal's legend, *a*, *d* and *e* are axons, *b* are horizontal dendrites, *c* are short dendrites, and **D** is the stained axon of an unstained cell body. *f* is not named in the original legend. The drawing in the bottom is the cell labeled as **A** by Cajal, freed of all the alien elements using *Photoshop*. The cell body is immediately subpial. From a descending process emanate horizontal axonal collaterals provided with short side-branches (see also *d* in the complete drawing) that resemble the ones shown by cortical basket cells in the (generally incomplete) Golgi stains.

experimental support in non-human primates, is intriguing as it may shed new perspectives to the old dispute whether Cajal-Retzius cells do die or become diluted in a growing volume of the developing brain (cf. Spreafico et al., 1999; Belichenko et al., 1995). The problem is far from being settled, however, and the suggestion above may not apply to pathological conditions. Recent data on cortical dysplasia in humans (Garbelli et al., 2001) has revealed (in one form of such a condition called architectural dysplasia) a significant increase in numbers of layer I cells akin to the adult forms just described; in these cases, the cells expressed Reelin but not GABA.

It must be stressed that the forms of Cajal-Retzius cells in *postnatal* lagomorphs (as described first by Cajal, 1981; see Fig. 1 of the present essay) and postnatal rodents (Derer and Derer, 1995; Meyer et al., 1999) resemble those of Cajal-Retzius cells in *fetal* carnivores and humans, and this addresses to differences in the respective calendars of cerebral development (cf. Kennedy and Dehay, 1993).

In addition, we will review recent observations indicating that, besides Cajal-Retzius cells, there are other additional cell types in the marginal zone (MZ) of fetal rodents. In particular, certain projecting neurons (the MZ pioneer neurons), apparently present also in other species, have been considered as immature forms of Cajal-Retzius cells in classical studies (e.g., Marín-Padilla, 1971, 1984).

Cajal-Retzius cells and other preplate neurons in rodents

Figure 1B–D brings to light the detailed morphological features of Cajal-Retzius cells of postnatal rodents just as they were seen and drawn in 1890 and 1891 by Cajal (Fig. 1A), but in this case the images are from modern preparations of postnatal rats. Local injections of biotinylated dextran-amine revealed in a Golgi-like fashion the horizontal branches, the single axon (in rodents, the axon is much simpler than in primates, and forms a sparse plexus located not below, but at the level of the horizontal dendrites) and overall, the ascending branchlets touching the pia that resemble the ones found in prenatal carnivores and primates by Retzius (cf. Derer and Derer, 1990). In *reeler* mice, Cajal-Retzius cells remain below the pia and do not form the ascending branchlets (Derer, 1985). What the functions of these subpial end-feet may

be is unknown yet, albeit their location suggests a functional relationship with the basement membrane (Hartmann et al., 1999; Fairén et al., 2000; Graus-Porta et al., 2001). Interestingly, some of these cells in the rat descend into deep layer I (Meyer et al., 1998, their Fig. 11D), just as also shown in Fig. 1D, while the subpial end-feet are retained. Cajal-Retzius cells may transform into cortical interneurons (Parnavelas and Edmunds, 1982; Edmunds and Parnavelas, 1983) and these apparently transitional pictures may be a representation of such a phenomenon. However, the cortical MZ contains, besides Cajal-Retzius cells, immature interneurons that originate from a subpallial origin, the medial ganglionic eminence (Lavdas et al., 1999; reviewed in Parnavelas, 2000). These future interneurons do not express Reelin (G. López-Bendito, R. Luján and A. Fairén, *unpublished data*). It is not known, yet indeed unlikely, that migrating interneurons may have such subpial end-feet.

It is reasonable to refer to all Reelin-expressing neurons in the prenatal preplate of rodents as Cajal-Retzius cells in spite of morphological differences with the postnatal cells depicted in Fig. 1. Prenatal Cajal-Retzius cells in rodents have the typical morphology of tangentially migrating neurons, i.e., they are fusiform cells provided with a thick leading process ending in a large growth cone (Lavdas et al., 1999) and do not display subpial end-feet. Thus, immature interneurons in the MZ may be mistakenly labeled as Cajal-Retzius cells unless it is explicitly proven that they do not express Reelin. On the other hand, Tomioka et al., (2000) have described a different population of migrating neurons in the MZ that, unlike the interneurons, has a neocortical origin and the cells migrate to the lateral olfactory tract where they act as guidepost cells (Sato et al., 1998).

Cajal-Retzius cells cover the whole surface of the rodent cortex from very early in corticogenesis (D'Arcangelo et al., 1995), which is compatible with the common belief that these cells originate in the neuroepithelium of the local ventricular zone. It has been proposed, however, that Cajal-Retzius cells may have a subpallial origin (Meyer and Goffinet, 1998; Meyer et al., 1998; Lavdas et al., 1999). In human (Brun, 1965; Gadisseux et al., 1992; Meyer and Wahle, 1999) and non-human primates (Zecevic and Rakic, 2001), the superficial part of the MZ contains a multitude of small cells that constitute a layer on its own, the so-called *subpial granule layer*. These cells have been postulated to originate in the paleocortical ventricle, in the "*retrobulbar area*"

(Gadisseux et al., 1992; Meyer and Wahle, 1999) and to invade the surface of the neocortex by subpial, tangential migration. Such a subpial layer would be the origin of Cajal-Retzius cells (Meyer and Goffinet, 1998). Recently, the senior author of this review referred the existence of a *subpial granule layer* in prenatal rats (Meyer et al., 1998, 2000a) and proposed a similar retrobulbar origin for their cells. In rodents, an alternative source is the medial ganglionic eminence that provides Cajal-Retzius cells and other types of neurons to the MZ (Lavdas et al., 1999; Morante-Oria et al., submitted).

Many recent writings refer to Cajal-Retzius cells as *pioneer Cajal-Retzius cells* (e.g., Ogawa 1995; Supèr et al., 1998; Jang et al., 2001). However, Cajal-Retzius cells do not emit pioneering axons (see above, and Meyer et al., 1999). The continued usage of the term "*pioneer Cajal-Retzius cell*" reflects the possibility that a classical concept of developmental neurobiology is beginning to fall into oblivion among students of cortical development and, if so, it is thought to be of interest to define the term precisely again. The name *pioneer neuron* refers to the property of a given cell of sending out a pioneering axon (Harrison, 1910). In the embryonic insect brain, axonal pathways are established by small sets of pioneering axons that are used for guidance and fasciculation by follower axons (Bate, 1976; Reichert and Boyan, 1997; Ludwig et al., 2001). Although pioneering axons have been less amenable to experimental analysis in the mammalian brain, it is accepted that such a class of axons exists during corticogenesis. The axons of subplate neurons pioneer the first axon pathway from the cerebral cortex (McConnell et al., 1989, 1994; Kim et al., 1991; DeCarlos et al., 1992). Recently, we have described a novel neuronal population that is seen, in views perpendicular to the cortical surface, to crowd the surface of the MZ in rat fetuses (Meyer et al., 1998, 1999; Soria and Fairén, 2000). These cells do not express Reelin and therefore are not, by definition, Cajal-Retzius cells. Their axons invade the lateral ganglionic eminence before a subplate is visible; later on, after the cortical plate and the subplate are present, the axons project to the subplate. MZ pioneer neurons and subplate neurons seem to have some molecular traits in common (Landry et al., 1998; Hevner et al., 2001). The fact that a numerically major subpopulation of cortical pioneer neurons remain at the cortical surface during early corticogenesis was unexpected in experiments tracing early projecting axons with

carbocyanines in fixed tissue (Molnar et al., 1998), where only a moderate amount of MZ cells were retrogradely labeled with these tracers. The most likely explanation for the discrepancy is that we used neurochemical markers selective for these MZ neurons that stained the whole populations. In the case of rats, these markers were the calcium binding proteins calbindin and calretinin (separate subsets of such pioneer neurons expressed each one of these proteins: Meyer et al., 1998; Soria and Fairén, 2000). These clearly are neurons in search of a function, and we have started this analysis in mice, where calcium-binding proteins are not markers of such neuronal populations. In our recent study, cells terminating their tangential migration in the MZ were labeled at their place of origin with fluorescent markers that permitted the subsequent electrophysiological analysis (Morante-Oria et al., submitted). Interestingly, MZ pioneer neurons showed early signs of functional maturity (see also, Soria et al., 1999), in contrast with the rather immature status detected in prenatal Cajal-Retzius cells, as compared to the same cells in postnatal stages (e.g., Zhou and Hablitz, 1996; Mienville, 1999; Mienville and Pesold, 1999; Martínez-Galán et al., 2001). Moreover, MZ pioneer neurons were found to originate in the medial ganglionic eminence (Morante-Oria et al., submitted), challenging the postulate that these neurons might generate in the neuroepithelium of the pallial ventricular zone (Meyer et al., 1998; Soria and Fairén, 2000).

Early neurons in the MZ sending out axonal projections into the subplate were seen much before. Marín-Padilla (1971, 1984, 1998) has described such cells forming part of the early neuronal network termed *primordial plexiform layer*, formed by descending connections from the MZ, by ascending axons from Martinotti cells and by extrinsic afferents arriving to the cortical surface (cf. Fig. 2 of the present essay, from Cajal, 1911).

The MZ is a fluid system where neurons migrate, assemble, and form distinct patterns of cell aggregations

By using flat-mount or whole-mount staining techniques we investigated the distribution of Cajal-Retzius and MZ pioneer neurons over the surface of the developing rat cerebral cortex. For this purpose, we used immunocytochemical and *in situ* hybridization methods to detect selective neurochemical markers such as Reelin, the calcium-binding proteins calbindin and calretinin, and medium-weight neurofilaments. We mounted these stained brains flat under coverslips and we observed large, unobstructed extensions of the cortical surface and major anatomical landmarks such as the territory of the lateral olfactory tract, or the middle cerebral artery. Neurofilament immunocytochemistry revealed that the overall distribution of neurons in the MZ is inhomogeneous (not shown). In rats, calretinin was a common marker for a subset of MZ pioneer neurons and Cajal-Retzius cells while calbindin stained a different subset of MZ pioneer neurons and also migrating interneurons (Vogt Weisenhorn et al., 1994; Anderson et al., 1997; Meyer et al., 1998). In flat mounts, we could distinguish pioneer neurons from other MZ neurons on account of their large size and their multipolar forms (Soria and Fairén, 2000). Moreover, pioneer neurons and Cajal-Retzius cells (Fig. 4) were located in different planes: as seen in this pair of

photomicrographs, the pioneer neurons in the rat tended to be deeper than Cajal-Retzius cells, and even became deeper along development.

Pioneer neurons distributed uniformly (i.e., the cell-to-cell distances were quite uniform) over most of the cortical surface but, surprisingly enough, they formed cellular aggregates in quite precise zones. The topographical distribution of the aggregates of each subpopulation of MZ pioneer neurons in the rat (i.e., the calbindin- *or* the calretinin-immunoreactive ones, see above) showed different time dependence. The calbindin-positive population formed clusters at the caudal and medial territories of the pallium already at E12, but clustering affected all these cells over the whole surface by E17. The calretinin-positive population formed clusters and honeycomb-like patterns in the temporal part of the developing pallium at E12, but the extension of the MZ showing such honeycomb-like patterns did not change much along further development.

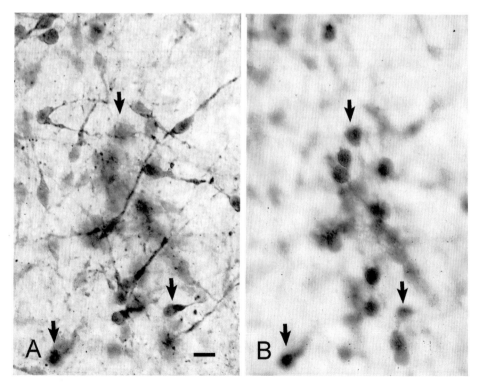

Fig. 4. The cortical surface as seen from above. This pair of photomicrographs shows two planes of focus of the same field to illustrate how two different populations of neurons reside at different levels of the MZ. **A**. On top are the Cajal-Retzius cells, characterized by their slender cell bodies. **B**. In this deeper plane of focus there is a cluster of MZ pioneer neurons. Immunostaining for calretinin. The arrows point to reference elements visible in both images. Scale bar: 25 μm. Taken from Soria and Fairén (2000), with permission.

Interestingly, the MZ neurons formed such aggregates and their axons formed fascicles, so that these two characters seemed to be mutually related. It was tempting to postulate that the distinct topography of the pioneer cell aggregates might be an anatomical manifestation of a tangential discontinuity in the pallium, i.e., of an early cortical parcelation. Recent studies have mapped the expression of specific genes that may define an early differentiation of the pallium into primordia of cortical areas (e.g., Bishop et al., 2000; Mallamaci et al., 2000). A direct correlation between the two sets of data (selective tangential distribution of MZ neurons vs. selective areal patterns of gene expression) seems implausible so far since these *in situ* hybridization studies lack cellular resolution. The recent finding that MZ pioneer neurons

may originate in the subpallial medial ganglionic eminence (Morante-Oria et al., 2002) raises the provocative suggestion that geometrical patterns of cell distribution might also reflect specific migration patterns beneath the brain surface.

Regarding Cajal-Retzius cells, we here report that they do not distribute themselves uniformly over the surface of the MZ. Figure 5 shows photomicrographs of rat whole-brain *in situ* hybridizations for *reelin*, subsequently observed as flat mounts. Already at the very early age of E12 (Fig. 5A and B), Cajal-Retzius cells form honeycomb-like aggregates that show little regional differences in the cortex. The honeycomb-like pattern persists along the bulk of the neurogenesis period and it is easier to document in temporal and occipital regions.

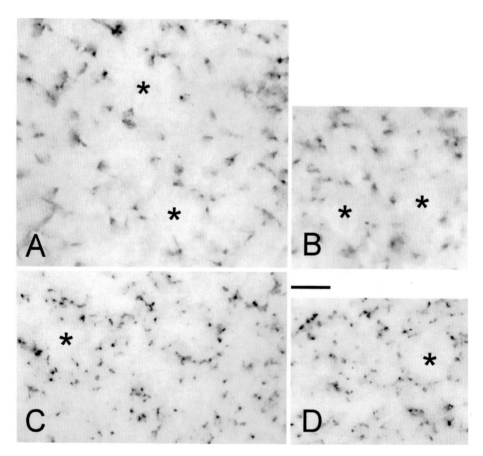

Fig. 5. The cortical surface as seen from above. *In situ* hybridization for *reelin* performed using a digoxigenin-labeled riboprobe on whole brains. The *reelin* cDNA (1.5 Kb) was provided by Dr. A. Goffinet. **A** is from the occipital region and **B** from the parietal region of the pallium of an E12 rat fetus. **C** is from the parietal region and **D** from the occipital region of the pallium of an E14 rat fetus. Cajal-Retzius cells group together is a honeycomb-like pattern. Asterisks label the hollow centers. Calibration bar: 50 μm.

Each one of the honeycomb-like units is best viewed as a hexagonal structure that shares their sides with the contiguous hexagonal ones.

We propose that MZ can be regarded as a fluid system where neurons migrate, assemble, and form distinct patterns of cell aggregations. Obviously, it is unavoidable to be intrigued about the functional significance of such a mosaic organization. Indeed, the idea of a geometrical organization with functional implications is not new (see e.g., Lorente de Nó, 1922). Cortical cytoarchitectonics could be determined by MZ neurons and, more specifically, by Cajal-Retzius cells, not just via molecular signaling, but also by the geometrical features conveyed by their mosaic cellular pattern. Such a configuration could be also reflect specific migration patterns or could subserve the channeling of extraparenchymal signals from the pial basal lamina. Whatever the case, it seems to reflect a fluid organization where the neurons navigate according to so far undisclosed paradigms or mechanisms.

It is clear that there is still much to figure out about the function of these cells and about cortical development in general. The correlation between these geometric anatomical patterns and the growing knowledge about the expression patterns of specific genes will shed light on these questions. The analysis of the available mutants will also be most helpful. A deeper knowledge of the functional consequences of this mosaic configuration of the cortical surface could give us some keys to understand cortical development. Doubtless, current data demonstrate that Cajal-Retzius cells are still "special cells" and they would intrigue today, even more than one century ago, Cajal's imagination.

Acknowledgments

We thank Dr. J.M. Luque for constructive criticisms during the preparation of this manuscript and Dr. A.M. Goffinet for providing us with *reelin* cDNA and Reelin antibodies. Supported by grant P97-0582-CO2-01 from the Spanish Ministerio de Ciencia y Tecnología and by the Italian Ministry of Health.

References

Alcántara, S., Ruiz, M., D'Arcangelo, G., Ezan, F., de Lecea, L., Curran, T., Sotelo, C. and Soriano E. (1998) Regional and cellular patterns of reelin mRNA expression in the forebrain of the developing and adult mouse. *J. Neurosci.*, 18: 7779–7799.

Anderson, S.A., Eisenstat, D.D., Shi, L. and Rubenstein, J.L. (1997) Interneuron migration from basal forebrain to neocortex: dependence on Dlx genes. *Science*, 278: 474–476.

Bate, C.M. (1976) Pioneer neurones in an insect embryo. *Nature*, 260: 54–56.

Belinchenko, P.V., Vogt Weisenhorn, D.M., Myklossy, J. and Celio M.R. (1995) Calretinin-positive Cajal-Retzius cells persist in the adult human neocortex. *NeuroReport*, 6: 1869–1874.

Bishop, K.M., Goudreau, G. and O'Leary, D.D. (2000) Regulation of area identity in the mammalian neocortex by Emx2 and Pax6. *Science*, 288: 344–349.

Brun, A. (1965) The subpial granular layer of the foetal cerebral cortex in man. Its ontogeny and significance in congenital cortical malformations. *Acta Pathol. Microbiol. Scand.*, 179 (Suppl.): 1–98.

Cajal, S.R. (1890) Textura de las circunvoluciones cerebrales de los mamíferos inferiores. Nota preventiva. *Gaceta Médica Catalana*, 30 November: 22–31. English translation in DeFelipe, J. and Jones, E.G. (1988) Cajal on the Cerebral Cortex, pp. 10–16.

Cajal, S.R. (1891) Sur la structure de l'écorce cérébrale de quelques mammifères. *La Cellule* 7: 123–176. English translation in DeFelipe, J. and Jones, E.G. (1988) Cajal on the Cerebral Cortex, pp. 23–54.

Cajal, S.R. (1899a) Estudios sobre la corteza cerebral humana. I. Corteza visual. *Revista Trimestral Micrográfica*, 4: 1–63. English translation in DeFelipe, J. and Jones, E.G. (1988) Cajal on the Cerebral Cortex, pp. 147–187.

Cajal, S.R. (1889b) Estudios sobre la corteza cerebral humana. II. Estructura de la corteza motriz del hombre y mamíferos superiores. *Revista Trimestral Micrográfica*, 4: 117–200. English translation in DeFelipe, J. and Jones, E.G. (1988) *Cajal on the Cerebral Cortex*, pp. 188–250.

Cajal, S.R. (1889b) Estudios sobre la corteza cerebral humana. II. Estructura de la corteza motriz del hombre y mamíferos superiores. *Revista Trimestral Micrográfica*, 4: 117–200. English translation in DeFelipe, J. and Jones, E.G. (1988) Cajal on the Cerebral Cortex, pp. 188–250.

Cajal, S.R. (1909–1911) Histologie du Système Nerveux de l'Homme et des Vertébrés (translated by L. Azoulay). A. Maloine, Paris.

Cajal, S.R. (1910) Manual de Histología Normal y de Técnica Micrográfica. Imprenta y Librería de Nicolás Moya, Madrid.

Curran, T. and D'Arcangelo, G. (1998) Role of reelin in the control of brain development. *Brain Res. Rev.*, 26: 285–294.

D'Arcangelo, G., Miao, G.G., Chen, S.C., Soares, H.D., Morgan, J.I. and Curran, T. (1995) A protein related to extracellular matrix proteins deleted in the mouse mutant reeler. *Nature*, 374: 719–723.

D'Arcangelo, G., Nakajima, K., Miyata, T., Ogawa, M., Mikoshiba, K. and Curran T. (1997) Reelin is a secreted glycoprotein recognized by the CR-50 monoclonal antibody. *J. Neurosci.*, 17: 23–31.

De Carlos, J.A. and O'Leary, D.D.M. (1992) Growth and targeting of subplate axons and establishment of major cortical pathways. *J. Neurosci.*, 12: 1194–1211.

DeFelipe, J. and Jones, E.G. (1988) Cajal on the Cerebral Cortex. Oxford University Press, New York, Oxford.

Derer, P. (1985) Comparative localization of Cajal-Retzius cells in the neocortex of normal and reeler mutant mice fetuses. *Neurosci. Lett.*, 54: 1–6.

Derer, P. and Derer, M. (1990) Cajal-Retzius cell ontogenesis and death in mouse brain visualized with horseradish peroxidase and electron microscopy. *Neuroscience*, 36: 839–856.

Edmunds, S.M. and Parnavelas, J.G. (1982) Retzius-Cajal cells: An ultrastructural study in the developing visual cortex of the rat. *J. Neurocytol.*, 11: 427–446.

Fairén, A., DeFelipe, J. and Regidor, J. (1984) Nonpyramidal neurons. General Account. In: A. Peters and E.G. Jones (Eds.) *Cerebral Cortex*, Vol. 1. *Cellular Components of the Cerebral Cortex*. Plenum Press, New York, London, pp. 201–253.

Fairén, A., Morante-Oria, J., Bellmunt, E., García-Verdugo, J.M., Gustafsson, E., Fässler, R. and Costell, M. (2000) Altered corticogenesis in perlecan deficient mice. *Eur. J. Neurosci.*, 12. Suppl., 11: 274.

Frassoni, C., Arcelli, P., Regondi, M.C., Selvaggio, M., De Biasi, S. and Spreafico, R. (1995) Branching pattern of corticothalamic projections from the somatosensory cortex during postnatal development in the rat. *Dev Brain Res.*, 90: 111–121.

Frotscher, M. (1997) Dual role of Cajal-Retzius cells and reelin in cortical development. *Cell Tissue Res.*, 290: 315–322.

Gadisseux J.F., Goffinet, A.M., Lyon, G. and Evrard, P. (1992) The human transient subpial granular layer: an optical, immunohistochemical, and ultrastructural analysis. *J. Comp. Neurol.*, 324: 94–114.

Garbelli, R., Frassoni, C., Ferrario, A., Tassi, L., Bramerio, M. and Spreafico, R. (2001) Cajal-Retzius cell density as marker of type of focal cortical dysplasia. *Neuroreport*, 12: 2767–2771.

Graus-Porta, D., Blaess, S., Senften, M., Littlewood-Evans, A., Damsky, C., Huang, Z., Orban, P., Klein, R., Schittny, J.C. and Müller, U. (2001) β1-class integrins regulate the development of laminae and folia in the cerebral and cerebellar cortex. *Neuron*, 31: 367–379.

Harrison, R.G. (1910) The outgrowth of the nerve fiber as a mode of protoplasmic movement. *J. Exp. Zool.*, 9: 787–848.

Hartmann, D., De Strooper, B. and Saftig, P. (1999) Presenilin-1 deficiency leads to loss of Cajal-Retzius neurons and cortical dysplasia similar to human type 2 lissencephaly. *Curr. Biol.*, 9: 719–727.

Hevner, R.F., Shi, L., Justice, N., Hsueh, Y., Sheng, M., Smiga, S., Bulfone, A., Goffinet, A.M., Campagnoni, A.T., and Rubenstein, J.L. (2001). Tbr1 regulates differentiation of the preplate and layer 6. *Neuron*, 29: 353–366.

Imamoto, K., Karasawa, N., Isomura, G. and Nagatsu, I. (1994) Cajal-Retzius neurons identified by GABA immunohistochemistry in layer I of the rat cerebral cortex. *Neurosci. Res.*, 20: 101–105.

Jang, M., Oliva, Jr., A.A., Lam, L. and Swann, J.W. (2001) GABAergic neurons that pioneer hippocampal area CA1 of the mouse: morphologic features and multiple fates. *J. Comp. Neurol.*, 439: 176–192.

Kennedy, H. and Dehay, C. (1993) Cortical specification of mice and men. *Cereb. Cortex*, 3: 171–186.

Kim, G.J., Shatz, C.J. and McConnell, S.K. (1991) Morphology of pioneer and follower growth cones in the developing cerebral cortex. *J. Neurobiol.*, 22: 629–642.

Landry, C.F., Pribyl, T.M., Ellison, J.A., Givogri, M.I., Kampf, K., Campagnoni, C.W. and Campagnoni, A.T. (1998). Embryonic expression of the myelin basic protein gene: identification of a promoter region that targets transgene expression to pioneer neurons. *J. Neurosci.*, 18: 7315–7327.

Lavdas, A.A., Grigoriou, M., Pachnis, V. and Parnavelas, J.G. (1999) The medial ganglionic eminence gives rise to a population of early neurons in the developing cerebral cortex. *J. Neurosci.*, 19: 7881–7888.

Lorente de Nó, R. (1922) La corteza cerebral del ratón (Primera contribución - La corteza acústica). English translation by Fairén, A., Regidor, J. and Kruger, L. *Somatosens. Mot. Res.*, 9: 3–36, 1992.

Ludwig, P., Williams, L., Nassel, D.R., Reichert. H. and Boyan, G. (2001) Primary commissure pioneer neurons in the brain of the grasshopper Schistocerca gregaria: development, ultrastructure, and neuropeptide expression. *J. Comp. Neurol.*, 430: 118–130.

Mallamaci, A., Muzio, L., Chan, C.H., Parnavelas, J. and Boncinelli, E. (2000) Area identity shifts in the early cerebral cortex of Emx2-/- mutant mice. *Nat. Neurosci.*, 3: 679–686.

Marín-Padilla, M. (1971). Early prenatal ontogenesis of the cerebral cortex (neocortex) of the cat (*Felis domestica*). A Golgi study. I. The primordial neocortical organization. *Z Anat. Entwicklungs.-gesch.*, 134: 117–145.

Marín-Padilla, M. (1984) Neurons of layer I. A developmental analysis. In: A. Peters and E.G. Jones (Eds.), *Cerebral Cortex*, Vol. 1. *Cellular Components of the Cerebral Cortex*. Plenum Press, New York, London, pp. 447–478.

Marín-Padilla, M. (1998) Cajal-Retzius cells and the development of the neocortex. *Trends Neurosci.*, 21: 64–71.

Martínez-Galán, J.R., López-Bendito, G., Luján, R., Shigemoto, R., Fairén, A. and Valdeolmillos, M. (2001) Cajal-Retzius cells in early postnatal mouse cortex selectively express functional metabotropic glutamate receptors. Eur. J. Neurosci., 13: 1147–1154.

McConnell, S.K., Ghosh, A. and Shatz, C.J. (1989) Subplate neurons pioneer the first axon pathway from the cerebral cortex. *Science*, 245: 978–982.

McConnell, S.K., Ghosh, A. and Shatz, C.J. (1994) Subplate pioneers and the formation of descending connections from cerebral cortex. *J. Neurosci.*, 14: 1892–1907.

Meyer, G. and Gonzalez-Hernandez, T. (1993) Developmental changes in layer I of the human neocortex during prenatal life: A DiI-tracing and AChE and NADPH-d histochemistry study. *J. Comp. Neurol.*, 338: 317–336.

Meyer, G. and Goffinet, A.M. (1998) Prenatal development of reelin-immunoreactive neurons in the human neocortex. *J. Comp. Neurol.*, 397: 29–40.

Meyer, G., Soria, J.M., Martínez-Galán, J.R., Martín-Clemente, B. and Fairén, A. (1998) Different origins and developmental histories of transient neurons in the marginal zone of the fetal and neonatal rat cortex. *J. Comp. Neurol.*, 397: 493–518.

Meyer, G., Goffinet, A.M. and Fairén, A. (1999) What is a Cajal-Retzius cell? A reassessment of a classical cell type based on recent observations in the developing neocortex. *Cereb. Cortex*, 9: 765–775.

Meyer, G. and Wahle, P. (1999) The paleocortical ventricle is the origin of reelin-expressing neurons in the marginal zone of the foetal human neocortex. *Eur. J. Neurosci.*, 11: 3937–3944.

Meyer, G., Castro, R., Soria, J.M. and Fairén, A. (2000a) The subpial granular layer in the developing cerebral cortex of rodents. *Results Probl. Cell. Differ.*, 30: 277–291.

Meyer, G., Schaaps, J.P., Moreau, L. and Goffinet, A.M. (2000b) Embryonic and early fetal development of the human neocortex. *J. Neurosci.*, 20: 1858–1868.

Mienville, J.M. (1999). Cajal-Retzius cell physiology: just in time to bridge the 20th century. *Cereb. Cortex*, 9: 776–782.

Mienville, J.M. and Pesold, C. (1999) Low resting potential and postnatal upregulation of NMDA receptors may cause Cajal-Retzius cell death. *J. Neurosci.*, 19: 1636–1646.

Molnar, Z., Adams, R. and Blakemore, C. (1998) Mechanisms underlying the early establishment of thalamocortical connections in the rat. *J. Neurosci.*, 18: 5723–5745.

Morante-Oria, J., Carleton, A., Kremer, E.J., Fairén, A. and Lledo, P.-M. (2002) A dual contribution of the medial ganglionic eminence during the development of the neocortex. Submitted.

Ogawa, M., Miyata, T., Nakajima, K., Yagyu, K., Seike, M., Ikenaka, K., Yamamoto, H. and Mikoshiba K. (1995) The reeler gene-associated antigen on Cajal-Retzius neurons is a crucial molecule for laminar organization of cortical neurons. *Neuron*, 14: 899–912.

Parnavelas, J.G. and Edmunds S.M. (1983) Further evidence that Retzius-Cajal cells transform to non-pyramidal neurons in the developing rat visual cortex. *J. Neurocytol.*, 12: 863–871.

Parnavelas, J.G. (2000) The origin and migration of cortical neurones: new vistas. *Trends Neurosci.*, 23: 126–131.

Pesold, C., Liu, W.S., Guidotti, A., Costa, E. and Caruncho, H.J. (1999) Cortical bitufted, horizontal, and Martinotti cells preferentially express and secrete reelin into perineuronal nets, nonsynaptically modulating gene expression. *Proc. Natl. Acad. Sci. U.S.A.*, 96: 3217–3222.

Reichert, H. and Boyan, G. (1997) Building a brain: developmental insights in insects. *Trends Neurosci.*, 20: 258–264.

Retzius, G. (1893) Die Cajal'schen Zellen der Grosshirnrinde beim Menschen und bei Säugetieren. *Biologische Untersuchungen, Neue Folge*, 5: 1–8.

Retzius, G. (1894) Weitere Beiträge zur Kenntniss der Cajal'schen Zellen der Grosshirnrinde des Menchen. *Biologische Untersuchungen, Neue Folge*, 6: 29–36.

Rice, D.S. and Curran, T. (2001) Role of the reelin signaling pathway in central nervous system development. *Annu. Rev. Neurosci.*, 24: 1005–1039.

Sato, Y., Hirata, T., Ogawa, M. and Fujisawa, H. (1998) Requirement for early-generated neurons recognized by monoclonal antibody lot1 in the formation of lateral olfactory tract. *J. Neurosci.*, 18: 7800–7810.

Soria, J.M., Martínez-Galan, J.R., Luján, R., Valdeolmillos, M. and Fairén, A. (1999) Functional NMDA and GABA$_A$ receptors in pioneer neurons of the cortical marginal zone. *Eur. J. Neurosci.*, 11: 3351–3354.

Soria, J.M. and Fairén, A. (2000) Cellular mosaics in the rat marginal zone define an early neocortical territorialization. *Cereb. Cortex*, 10: 400–412.

Spreafico, R., Frassoni, C., Arcelli, P., Selvaggio, M. and De Biasi, S. (1995) *In situ* labeling of apoptotic cell death in the cerebral cortex and thalamus of rats during development. *J. Comp. Neurol.*, 363: 281–295.

Spreafico, R., Arcelli, P., Frassoni, C., Canetti, P., Giaccone, G., Rizzuti, T., Mastrangelo, M. and Bentivoglio, M. (1999) Development of layer I of the human cerebral cortex after midgestation: architectonic findings, immunocytochemical identification of neurons and glia, and *in situ* labeling of apoptotic cells. *J. Comp. Neurol.*, 410: 126–142.

Supèr, H., Soriano, E. and Uylings, H.B. (1998) The functions of the preplate in development and evolution of the neocortex and hippocampus. *Brain Res. Rev.*, 27: 40–64.

Tomioka, N., Osumi, N., Sato, Y., Inoue, T., Nakamura, S., Fujisawa, H. and Hirata, T. (2000) Neocortical origin and tangential migration of guidepost neurons in the lateral olfactory tract. *J. Neurosci.*, 20: 5802–5812.

Verney, C. and Derer, P. (1995) Cajal-Retzius neurons in human cerebral cortex at midgestation show immunoreactivity for neurofilament and calcium-binding proteins. *J. Comp. Neurol.*, 359: 144–153.

Vogt Weisenhorn, D.M., Weruaga-Prieto, E. and Celio, M.R. (1994) Localization of calretinin in cells of layer I (Cajal-Retzius cells) of the developing cortex of the rat. *Dev Brain Res.*, 82: 293–297.

Zecevic, N., Milosevic, A., Rakic, S. and Marin-Padilla, M. (1999) Early development and composition of the human primordial plexiform layer: an immunohistochemical study. *J. Comp. Neurol.*, 412: 241–254.

Zecevic, N. and Rakic, P. (2001) Development of layer I neurons in the primate cerebral cortex. *J. Neurosci.*, 21: 5607–5619.

Zhou, F.M. and Hablitz, J.J. (1996). Postnatal development of membrane properties of layer I neurons in rat neocortex. *J. Neurosci.*, 16: 1131–1139.

E.C. Azmitia, J. DeFelipe, E.G. Jones, P. Rakic and C.E. Ribak (Eds.)
Progress in Brain Research, Vol. 136

CHAPTER 23

Vulnerability of monoaminergic neurons in the brainstem of the zitter rat in oxidative stress

Shuichi Ueda[1],*, Shinichi Sakakibara[1], Eriko Watanabe[1], Kanji Yoshimoto[2] and Noriyuki Koibuchi[3]

[1]*Department of Histology and Neurobiology, Dokkyo University School of Medicine, Mibu, Tochigi 321-0293, Japan.*
[2]*Department of Legal Medicine, Kyoto Prefectural University of Medicine, Kawaramachi Hirokoji, Kamikyo-ku, Kyoto 602-0841, Japan.*
[3]*Department of Physiology, Gunma University School of Medicine, Maebashi, Gunma 371-8511, Japan.*

Abstract: In the monograph of Santiago Ramon y Cajal, he provided a detailed description about the morphological changes in degeneration and regeneration of peripheral and central nervous systems following lesions. He discussed factors that may promote or inhibit axonal growth after peripheral and/or central nerve injury. Cajal with a brilliant insight anticipated the existence of several factors acting on degeneration and regeneration. Free radicals have been proposed to be one of such factors. These highly reactive oxygen species-derived free radicals play a pathogenetic role in neurological disorders, including ischemia, trauma, Alzheimer's disease and Parkinson's disease (PD). In this review we will discuss the similarities and differences between the morphological changes under oxidant stress and Cajal's drawings of degeneration and regeneration following the central injury. The monoaminergic neuron systems in the brainstem appear vulnerable to these free radicals, which have also been implicated in the selective degeneration of the nigrostriatal DA system. We analyzed the degeneration of fibers and the neuronal cell death of brainstem monoaminergic neuron systems in a mutant rat, which has abnormal metabolism of oxygen species in the brain. The degeneration of DA cell bodies and fibers was characterized by swollen varicosities and clustered fibers.

Introduction

Within the field of neurohistology, Santiago Ramón y Cajal stands out as a towering figure for his theory concerning the degeneration and regeneration of nervous tissue. In 1913/1914, Cajal published his evidence in a monograph. However, this work remained almost unknown outside his own country until it appeared in an English translation in 1928 as "Degeneration and Regeneration of the Nervous System". In this book, he provided a detailed description of the morphological changes in the degeneration and regeneration of the peripheral and central nervous systems following lesions.

*Corresponding author: Tel.: 81 282 87 2124 ext. 2110;
Fax: +81-282-86-1463; E-mail : shu-ueda@dokkyomed.ac.jp

Figure 1 shows an example of Cajal's drawings (Cajal, 1928). He has indicated the retraction balls and the hypertrophic segment in the central stump of a cerebral wound (Fig. 1). Toward the end of the book, he discussed factors that might promote or inhibit axonal growth following peripheral and/or central nerve injury. Cajal, with brilliant insight, anticipated the existence of several factors acting on degeneration and regeneration. However, given the analytical methods available in those days, he was not able to identify these factors. Nevertheless, many of today's discoveries can be traced back to his insights.

Free radicals and substantia nigra

Free radicals have been proposed as a neurodegenerative factor. Oxidation and reduction, or 'Redox' reaction,

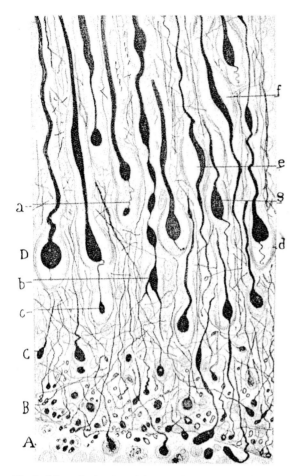

Fig. 1. Schematic drawing of degenerating axons by Cajal (From Cajal 1928).

involve the transfer of electrons and can generate by-products known as free radicals. Free radicals are atoms or molecules that contain an orbital with an unpaired electron. Some free radicals are highly reactive and are known to play a pathogenetic role in several kinds of neurological disorders, such as Parkinson's disease (Olanow, 1993). In the brain, either monoamine oxidase-type B (MAO-B)-induced-enzymatic oxidation or auto-oxidation of dopamine (DA) within the substantia nigra (SN) results in the production of hydrogen peroxide (H_2O_2), which is normally detoxified by glutathione peroxide or catalase, but an increase in the rate of dopamine turnover—or a deficiency in the clearance system—can result in an increase in the steady state concentration of H_2O_2. In the presence of a reactive iron species, H_2O_2 is catalyzed to form a hydroxyl radical

($OH^\bullet$) in accordance with the Fenton reaction. This hydroxyl radical ($OH^\bullet$) can damage a variety of critical biological molecules, including DNA, essential cellular proteins and membrane lipids (Fig. 2).

In the brain in Parkinson's disease, DA turnover is increased, H_2O_2 is increased, glutathione peroxidase and catalase are decreased, and reactive irons are increased (Table 1). These metabolic alterations indicate that in Parkinson's disease, the SN is in a state of oxidant stress that plays a direct role in cell death. This hypothesis would be more strongly supported if an animal model with similar disturbances could be identified.

Zitter mutant rat

The zitter rat is an autosomal recessive mutant derived from the Sprague-Dawley (SD) rat strain (Rehm et al., 1982). The zitter rat exhibits several neurological abnormalities such as body tremors and a flaccid paresis that progresses with aging (Gomi et al., 1990; Inui et al., 1990; Kondo et al., 1992, 1995). Abnormal metabolism of H_2O_2 has been reported in this mutant rat (Gomi et al., 1994). The Zitter brain exhibits a significant reduction in DA and dihydroxyphenylacetic acid (DOPAC) as well as a reduction in catalase activity and these biochemical abnormalities gradually progress with aging. In the zitter rats, the reduction of DA was more prominent in the caudate-putamen than in the nucleus accumbens and olfactory tubercle (Ueda et al., 2000). These changes are similar to those seen in Parkinson's disease (Table 1).

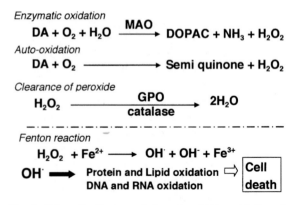

Fig. 2. Schematic diagram of dopamine (DA) metabolism in substantia nigra neurons. DOPAC: dihydroxyphenylacetic acid. GPO: gultathion peroxidase. MAO: monoamine oxidase.

Table 1. Metabolic alternations in Parkinson's disease

DA turnover	increased
MAO-B activity	increased
H_2O_2	increased
Glutathione peroxidase	decreased
Catalase	decreased
Superoxide dismutase	increased
Iron	increased

To examine the morphological changes in the dopaminergic neuron system, we carried out immuno-histochemical and *in situ* hybridization analyses using tyrosine hydroxylase (TH) antibodies and a dopamine receptor probe (Ueda et al., 2000; Joyce et al., 2000). In the control SD rat, TH-immunoreactive fibers are homogeneously distributed throughout the striatum. On the other hand, in the age-matched zitter rat, there is a characteristic reduction in TH-immunoreactive fibers in the striatum. Thus, in the dorso-lateral caudate-putamen, a reduction of TH-immunoreactive fibers was observed in the matrix-like areas, whereas in the ventro-medial striatum the reduction occurred in the patch-like areas (Fig. 3).

Figure 4 shows age-related changes in TH-immunore-active fibers in the striatum of a 12-month-old zitter rat. The arrows indicate abnormal TH-immunoreactive fibers that are characterized by swollen varicosities and irregular thickened intervaricose segments. These abnormal fibers are most likely degenerating dopaminergic fibers. The swollen varicosities indicate an accumulation of TH in the proximal stump of the dopaminergic fibers as a result of interrupted axonal flow. This morphology is very similar to that of the retraction balls in Cajal's drawings. Table 2 summarize the age-related changes of the density of abnormal TH-immunoreactive fibers in the caudate-putamen, nucleus accumbens and olfactory tubercle. Furthermore, degenerative TH-immunoreactive fibers were also observed in the spinal cord (Saitoh et al., 1996, Okuda et al., 1999) but not in the olfactory bulb (Egawa et al., 1999).

Dopaminergic cell death in the SN of the zitter rat

In order to determine the number of TH-immunoreactive neurons in the SN pars compacta (SNc), SN pars

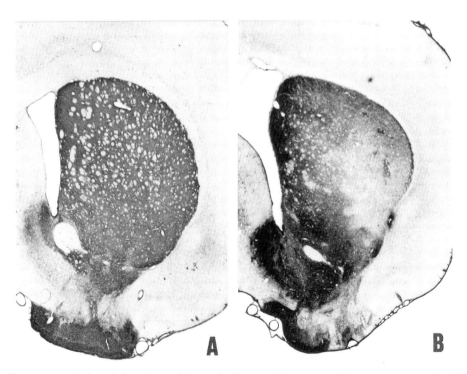

Fig. 3. Photomicrographs through the striatum of 12-month-old control (A) and zitter (B) rats immunostained for TH. × 12.

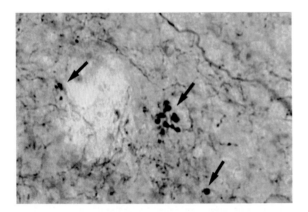

Fig. 4. A photomicrograph of TH-immunohistochemically stained sections through the striatum of 6-month-old zitter rat. Arrows indicate degenerating TH-immunoreactive fibers. × 400.

Table 2. Summary of age-related changes of the density of abnormal and normal TH-immunoreactive fibers.

	Age-related changes of the density of abnormal TH-immunoreactive fibers			
	2M	4M	6M	12M
CPU	+	++	+++	++
NA	+	+	++	++
OT	−	−	−	−

	Age-related changes of the density of normal TH-immunoreactive fibers			
	2M	4M	6M	12M
CPU	++++	+++	++	+
NA	++++	++++	+++	+++
OT	++++	+++	++	++

reticulata (SNr), ventral tegmental area (VTA) and retrorubural area (RRA), cell counts were performed. We analyzed 10 to 15 serial sections at 300-μm intervals throughout the mesencephalic DA neuron system. A total of 342 photographic montages were created from serial midbrain sections at the same magnification (× 150). To clarify the nucleus in the TH-immunostained cell body, we used a high magnification with a high voltage beam. Cells with a nucleus or a nuclear fragment greater than one-half the average nuclear diameters were marked on the photographic montages. From these, the number of marked TH-immunoreactive neurons were counted

unilaterally in the SNc, SNr, VTA and RRA of 2, 4, 6 and 12-month-old zitter rats and age-matched SD rats in a blind protocol (4 each; each group was represented in 13 to 15 photographic montages). Cell sizes were measured in each TH-immunoreactive cell group in each of three animals (Table 3). In order to determine the correction factor, the long and short axes of the cell were measured at high magnification (× 400). Fifty TH-immunoreactive cells with clearly visible nuclei were measured in each region in each age group (Table 4). The raw cell counts were corrected for split nuclei using the equation of Abercrombie (1946) as modified by Konigsmark (1970). The correction factor ranged from 0.5 to 0.8 in TH-immunohistochemical preparations. Data were analyzed by a single-factor analysis of variance (ANOVA) followed by Sheffe's multiple-comparisons-test. Figure 5 illustrates the distribution of TH-immunoreactive cells in 4 pairs of sections from the midbrain area of a 12-month-old zitter mutant rat and an age-matched SD rat. There was a significant loss of TH-immunoreactive cells in the midbrain of the zitter rat.

TH-immunoreactive neurons of SD and zitter rats (12-month-old) were mapped with a computer imaging analysis system with 3-dimensional (3-D) analysis software (OZ-95, Rise System Integrate Co., Ichikawa, Japan). The outline of midbrain sections and TH-immunoeactive neurons were traced using a computer assisted microscope system (PROVIS, Olympus, Tokyo, Japan) using a CCD camera (Fuji HC-2500, Fujifilm, Tokyo, Japan). Subsequently, contours of the sectional image were translated to 3-D coordinate values, with the vertical-coordinate (Z value) given by the number of serial sections and the inter-sectional intervals. Figure 6 displays 3-D reconstruction of DA neurons in the SN (blue), VTA (green) and RRA (red) of 12-month-old SD (A) and zitter (B) rats. Table 3 provides cell counts of TH-immunoreactive cells in the different areas of the midbrain. There was a significant difference in the total number of TH-immunoreactive cells between zitter and age-mached SD rats (Fig. 7).

Antioxidative treatment

Neuroprotective strategies for possible therapy in Parkinson's disease have been considered at several steps in the DA metabolism chain (Fig. 8). In the first step, the monoamine oxidase—type B (MAO-B) inhibitor

Table. 3. Size of TH-immunoreactive neurons in the mesencephalon

groups	SNc		SNr		VTA		RRA	
	long axis	short axis	long axis	short axis	long axis	short axis	long axis	short axis
2-month-old								
SD	20.0±3.6	12.6±2.7	19.9±3.6	12.6±1.9	17.8±2.7	11.5±1.2	22.2±3.2	12.3±1.9
Zitter	20.6±3.6	12.3±1.8	19.7±4.6	12.8±2.6	15.2±1.9	11.5±1.1	21.3±4.3	12.6±2.1
6-month-old								
SD	21.8±4.4	11.1±1.9	20.7±3.4	12.2±1.6	16.9±2.7	10.7±1.6	21.8±3.7	12.9±2.5
Zitter	20.7±4.4	10.9±1.6	21.1±4.1	11.7±1.4	17.0±3.4	11.9±2.7	21.4±4.6	12.3±2.2
12-month-old								
SD	20.4±2.6	10.8±1.7	20.1±4.0	11.3±2.0	18.4±2.9	10.9±1.4	20.3±3.1	12.4±1.5
Zitter	21.6±4.3	10.8±1.7	19.4±4.0	12.9±2.1	17.3±1.4	10.3±1.4	19.3±4.6	11.9±2.3

The mean ± S.D. length of the long and short axis (μm). Twenty five cells were measured in each group. SNc: substantia nigra pars compacta. SNr: substntia nigra pars reticulata. VTA: ventral tegmental area. RRA: retrorubular area.

Table 4. Corrected estimates of counts of TH-immunoreactive neurons in the mesencephalon of SD and zitter rats.

	Age	Area			
		SNc	SNr	VTA	RRA
SD	2M	12156.0±695.2	657.0±71.8	12612.0±2773.7	2340.0±349.9
	4M	11958.0±732.6	633.5±40.9	12353.0±1209.7	2395.5±583.4
	6M	11896.5±1945.1	721.5±163.8	12129.8±612.7	2129.5±582.1
	12M	10379.0±1863.5	659.5±127.5	11870.3±135.2	2207.0±316.5
Zitter	2M	9374.0±2030.2	462.0±154.6	7902.7±861.4	1342.0±253.5
	4M	7461.0±616.1	404.5±106.4	7486.5±1184.5	822.0±555.9
	6M	5467.5±591.8*	533.5±41.1	7528.5±882.7	739.5±316.4
	12M	4028.0±435.7* **	401.5±61.4	6223.0±662.2*	592.7±164.2*

Numbers in each group represent mean ± SD. All data from zitter rats significantly different from those of age-matched SD rats. *Value significantly different from 2-month-old zitter rat. **Value significantly different from 4-month-old zitter rats.

deprenyl was the first drug to merit serious consideration as a possible neuroprotective substance. Inhibition of MAO-B with selegiline prevents the degeneration of dopaminergic neurons induced by MPTP or 6-OHDA exposure in animal models of Parkinsonism (Kieburtz and Shoulson, 1996). In the second step, iron chelators have been demonstrated to effectively prevent the degeneration of dopaminergic neurons (Olanow and Youdim, 1996). Free radical scavengers have also been tested in Parkinson's disease. Vitamin E had no apparent effect in early Parkinson's disease in the DATATOP (deprenyl and tocophenol antioxidative therapy of parkinisonism) study (Shoulson, 1992). However, it is possible that the doses were insufficient, since vitamin E does not easily penetrate into the brain.

The endogenous hormone melatonin is known to be a strong hydroxyl radical scavenger. Due to its extreme lipophilicity, melatonin crosses every morphological barrier—that is, the blood-brain barrier—and gets into every bodily fluid and cell (Reiter et al., 1993; Reiter 1995). A marked reduction in the number of labeled neurons is seen in the group with no melatonin in the drinking water. However, the zitter rat—with drinking water containing melatonin had more labeled neurons in the substantia nigra pars compacta compared to the tap water group with no melatonin. Furthermore, the degenerating

298

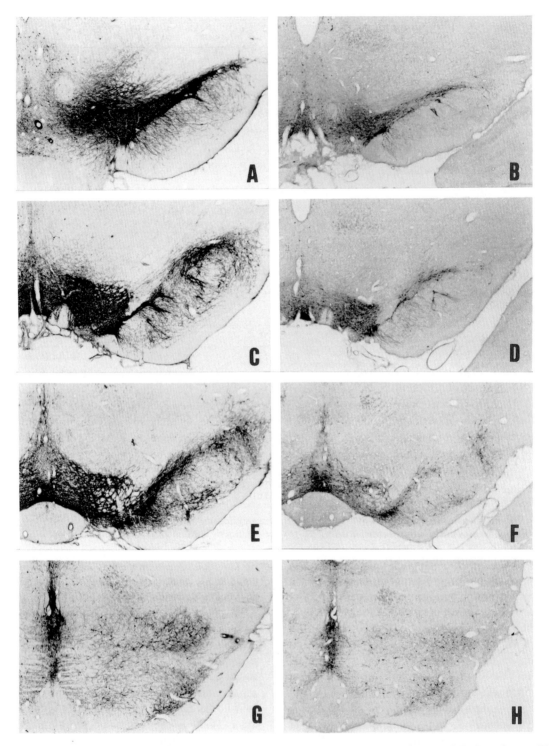

Fig. 5. TH-immunoreactivity in the midbrain from rostral to caudal levels. Photomicrographs in the left column (A, C, E, G) are from a wild-type rat, while photomicrographs in the right column (B, D, F, H) are from a homozygous zitter rat. The age of both groups is 6-months. × 20.

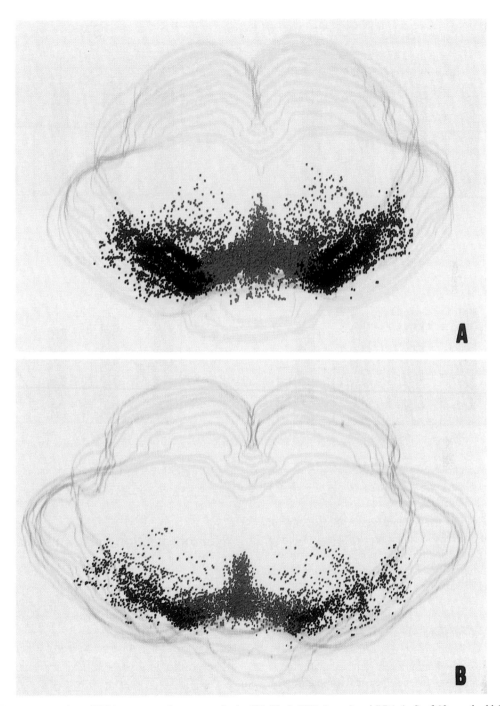

Fig. 6. A 3-D reconstruction of TH-immunoreactive neurons in the SN (blue), VTA (green) and RRA (red) of 12-month-old SD (A) and zitter (B) rats.

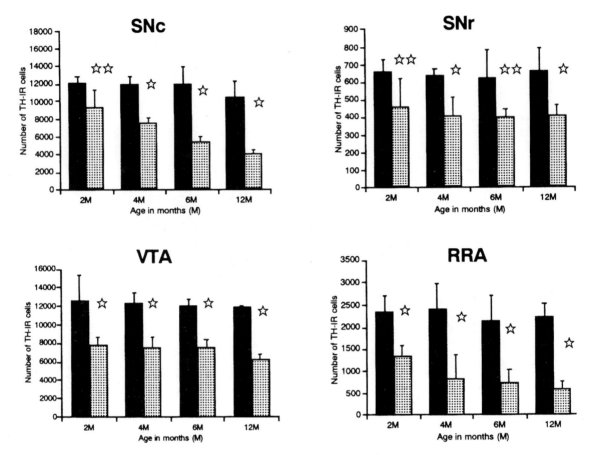

Fig. 7. Age related differences of TH-immunoreactive neurons in the SNc, SNr, VTA and RRA of SD (shaded bar) and zitter (dotted bar) rats.

TH-immunoreactive fibers decreased in the striatum of the zitter rat with melatonin (Fig. 9). These findings indicate that daily drinking of melatonin exerts a protective effect on nigrostriatal dopaminergic neurons in this animal model of Parkinson's disease.

Transplantation study

To determine whether grafted fetal dopaminergic neurons can survive in the host environment with progressive oxidative stress *in vivo*, grafts of fetal ventral mesencephalic tissue were taken from normal rats and transplanted into the striatum of adult zitter rats. Zitter rats with this graft in the left striatum showed an amphetamine-induced rotational bias to the contralateral side, which was not seen in the control zitter rat. Tyrosine

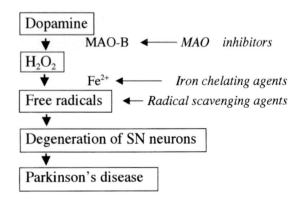

Fig. 8. Neuroprotection in Parkinson's disease.

301

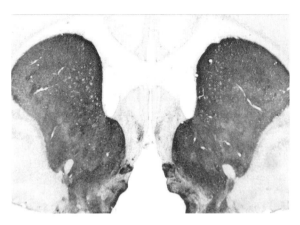

Fig. 9. A photomicrograph through the striatum of a 10-month-old zitter rat with melatonin treatment. × 20.

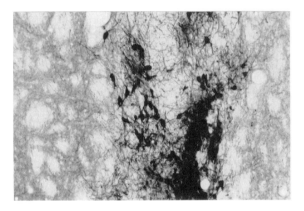

Fig. 10. A photomicrograph of a coronal section through the host striatum showing a fetal substantia nigra transplant. Two months after transplantation. TH-immunohistochemistry. × 80.

hydroxylase (TH)-positive neurons were packed in the graft and their processes densely innervated the graft (Fig. 10). The outgrowing TH-positive neurite could be traced to the adjacent host striatum, but the distal end of these fibers underwent degeneration.

To visualize and isolate live dopamine neurons in the embryonic ventral mesencephalon, we have transgenic mice expressing green fluorescent protein (GFP) under the control of the rat TH promoter (Sawamoto et al., 2001). Ventral mesencephalic neurons with GFP fluorescence from these fetal transgenic mice were sorted by fluorescence-activated cell sorting and then the collected dopamine neurons were transplanted into the striatum of zitter rats. A decreased number of surviving dopaminergic neurons as well as a degeneration of

neurites was demonstrated by TH- and GFP-immunohistochemical analyses. This information provides further evidence to support the hypothesis that host oxidant stress can influence the survival and growth of grafted dopaminergic neurons.

Conclusion

Today, the admirable drawings of Santiago Ramón y Cajal can be replaced by molecular-specific probes, such as antibodies, that can detect the specific neurons most vulnerable to the pathological process of Parkinson's disease. Morphological studies—combined with biochemistry and molecular biology—have yielded important discoveries about the molecular interactions in this disease. Furthermore, genetically tailor-made neurons will become powerful tools to examine not only the morphology and function of the brain, but also for therapies in neurological disease.

References

Abercrombie, M. (1946) Estimation of nuclear population from microtome Sections. *Anat. Rec.*, 94: 239–247.

Cajal, S.R. (1928) Degeneration and regeneration of the nervous system. Vol. I, II, (translated by May, R.M.) Hafner Pub. Co., New York.

Egawa, H., Kitajima, T. and Ueda, S. (1999) Tyrosine hydroxylase-, calbindine- and parvalbumine-immunoreactive neurons in the main olfactory bulb of the zitter rat. *J. Brain Sci.*, 25: 17–25.

Gomi, H., Inui, K., Taniguchi, H., Yoshikawa, Y. and Yamanouchi K. (1990) Edematous changes in the central nervous system of zitter rats with genetic spongiform encephalopathy. *J. Neuropathol. Exp. Neurol.*, 49: 250–259.

Gomi, H., Ueno, L. and Yamanouchi, K. (1994) Antioxidant enzymes in the brain of zitter rats: abnormal metabolism of oxigen species and its relevance to pathogenic changes in the brain of zitter rats with genetic spongiform encephalopathy. *Brain Res.*, 653: 66–72.

Inui, T., Yamamura, T., Yuasa H., Kawai, Y., Okaniwa, A., Serikawa, T. and Yamada, J. (1990) The spontaneous epileptic (SER), a zitter tremore Double mutant rat: histopathological findings in the central nervous system. *Brain Res.*, 517: 123–133.

Joyce, J.N., Yoshimoto, K. and Ueda, S. (2000) The zitter mutant rat exhibits loss of D3 Receptors with degeneration of the dopamine system. *NeuroReport*, 11: 2173–2175.

Kieburtz, K. and Shoulson, I. (1996) Treatment of Parkinson's disease with deprenyl (selegiline) and other monoamine oxidase inhibitors. In: C.W. Olanow, P. Jenner and M. Youdim (Eds.), *Neurodegeneration and neuroprotection in Parkinson's disease.* Academic Press, London, pp. 47–54.

Kondo, A., Sendoh, S., Akazawa, K., Sato, Y. and Nagara, H. (1992) Early myelination in zitter rat: morphological, immuno-cytochemical and morphometric studies. *Dev. Brain Res.*, 67: 217–228.

Kondo, A., Sendoh, S., Takamatsu, J. and Nagara, H. (1993) the zitter rat: membranous abnormality in the Schwann cells of myelinated nerve fibers. *Brain Res.*, 613: 173–179.

Kondo, A., Sendoh, S., Miyata, K. and Takamatsu, J. (1995) Spongy degeneration in the zitter rat: ultrastructural and immunohisto-chemical studies. *J. Neurocyto.*, 24: 533–544.

Konigsmark, B.W. (1977) Methods for counting of neurons. In: W.J.H. Nauta and S.O.E. Ebbesson (Eds.), *Contemporary Research Methods in Neuroanatomy.* Springer, Berlin, pp. 315–340.

Okuda, K., Saitoh, Y., Kitajima, T., Yamaoka, S. and Ueda, S. (1999) Evidence for degeneration of monoaminergic fibers in the spinal cord of zitter mutant rat. *Acta Histo. Cyto.*, 32: 341–344.

Olanow, C.W. (1993) A radical hypothesis for neurodegeneration. *Trends in Neuroscience*, 16: 439–444.

Olanow, C.W. and Youdim, M.B.H. (1996) Iron and neurodegenera-tion: prospects for neuroprotection. In: C.W. Olanow, P. Jenner and M. Youdim (Eds.), *Neurodegeneration and Neuroprotection in Parkinson's Disease.* Academic Press, London, pp. 55–67.

Reiter, R.J., Poeggeler, B., Tan, D.-X., Chen, L.-D., Manchester, L.C. and Guerrero, J.M. (1993) Antioxidant capacity of meta-tonin: a novel action not requiring a receptor. *Neuroendocrinol. Lett.*, 15: 103–116.

Reiter, R.J. (1995) Oxidative processes and antioxidative defense mechanisms in the aging brain. *FASEB J.*, 9: 526–533.

Rohm, S., Mehraein, P., Anzil, A.P. and Deerberg, F. (1982) A new rat mutant with defective overhaires and spongy degeneration of the central nervous system: clinical and pathological studies. *Lab. Anim. Sci.*, 32: 70–73.

Saitoh, Y., Kitajima, T., Yamaoka, S. and Ueda, S. (1996) Degenerative changes in the serotonergic fibers in the spinal cord of zitter mutant rat. *Acta Histo. Cyto.*, 29: 265–268.

Sawamoto, K., Nakao, N., Kobayashi, K., Matsusita, N., Takahashi H., Kishita, K., Yamamoto, A., Yoshizaki, T., Terashima T., Murakami, F., Itakura T. and Okano H. (2001) Visualization, direct isolation, and transplantation of midbrain dopaminergic neurons. *Pro. Natl. Acad. Sci. U.S.A.*, 98: 6423–6428.

Shoulson, I. (1992) Neuroprotective clinical strategies for Parkinson's disease. *Ann. Neurol.*, 32: s143–145.

Ueda, S., Aikawa, M., Ishizuya-Oka, A., Koibuchi H., Yamaoka, S. and Yoshimoto, K. (1998) Age-related degeneration of sero-toniergic fibers in the zitter rat brain. *Synapse*, 30: 62–70.

Ueda, S., Aikawa, M., Ishizuya-Oka, A., Yamaoka, S., Koibuchi H. and Yoshimoto, K. (2000) Age-related dopamine defficiency in the mesostriatal dopamine system of zitter mutant rats: regional fiber vulnerability in the striatum and the olfactory tubercle. *Neuroscience*, 95: 389–398.

E.C. Azmitia, J. DeFelipe, E.G. Jones, P. Rakic and C.E. Ribak (Eds.)
Progress in Brain Research, Vol. 136
© 2002 Elsevier Science B.V. All rights reserved

CHAPTER 24

CNS Schwann-like glia and functional restoration of damaged spinal cord

M. Nieto-Sampedro*

*Department of Neural Plasticity, Instituto Cajal de Neurobiología, CSIC, Av. Doctor Arce 37, 28002 Madrid, Spain and
Unit of Experimental Neurology, Hospital Nacional de Parapléjicos, 45071 Toledo, Spain*

Introduction

Cajal concluded in 1914 that spontaneous regeneration of the injured CNS was not possible. The major obstacles observed at the time were lack of neuronal replacement and abortive growth of regenerating axons, caused primarily by the growth-hostile environment created by reactive astrocytes. This situation contrasted with the response in the PNS, where Schwann cells promoted robust axonal regrowth after nerve damage. Research during the last two decades, pioneered by our group first at the University of California at Irvine and then at the Cajal Institute in Madrid, has permitted a more realistic (and optimistic) view of repair of CNS damage. Our work has covered four complementary aspects of the CNS lesion repair problem, to show: (i) that neurotrophic and neuritogenic activities expressed in brain and spinal cord under normal circumstances are up-regulated after injury; (ii) that the concentration of neurite inhibitors in normal brain also increases after injury; (iii) that glioblast division inhibitors exist in normal CNS and that their concentration decreases after injury; (iv) that Schwann-like macroglia, capable of promoting axon regeneration in injured spinal cord, exist in normal CNS.

Our second line of work confirmed Cajal's view of gliotic tissue as a major obstacle to axonal regeneration.

After injury, a 200,000 kDa heparansulfate/chondroitin sulfate proteoglycan is greatly up-regulated first in neurons, then in fibrous reactive astrocytes. When added in solution to cultured neurons, the proteoglycan prevented differentiation of new growth cones and caused the collapse of existing ones. When bound to the culture substrate, the proteoglycan repelled growing neurites. *In vivo* it was located in the plasma membranes of enlarged fibrous reactive astrocytes.

Astrocyte number during CNS development or after an open injury is regulated by the coordinated action of mitogens and antimitotics, to reach a steady-state. Whereas mitogens are well-known and abundant in the CNS, the existence of natural astroblast antimitotics has only been known during the last decade. We purified one of these molecules and identified it as an O-acetylated ganglioside of the series *b*. Its physiological role in 'glial scar' formation and fibrous reactive astrocyte differentiation is not clear yet.

Finally, we found Schwann-like macroglial cells in the brain. These cells, that we have called aldynoglia or growth-promoting glia, have the appearance and properties of early radial glia, but are found in the adult. They occur in CNS loci where axon regeneration is observed throughout life, like the olfactory system, hypothalamus-hypophysis and pineal gland. Contrary to Schwann cells, they mingle with astrocytes. Olfactory bulb ensheathing cells (OBEC) have been cultured, purified and transplanted to promote sensory and central axon growth in the spinal cord. We will briefly report anatomical,

*Corresponding author: Tel.: (34) 915854720; Fax: (34) 915854754;
E-mail: mns@cajal.csic.es

electrophysiological and behavioural recovery from multiple rhizotomy, promoted by OBEC transplants. Although OBECs are not a panacea for every lesion, the latest findings from our laboratory indicate that transplanted OBECs suppress astrocyte reactivity, thus generally favouring axonal growth.

Injury-induced growth factors: secondary neuronal death arrest and neural transplant survival and integration

Minimizing or preventing secondary neuronal death after injury may greatly contribute to a favorable prognosis for recovery after CNS injury, without further interventions to replace the lost cells. NGF plays a key role in the survival of brain cholinergic neurons (Nieto-Sampedro et al., 1983; Korschig et al., 1985; Shelton and Reichardt, 1986; Whittemore et al., 1986) and exogenous supply of crude of injured brain tissue extract made possible the survival of fetal striatal tissue implanted immediately after an open injury (Nieto-Sampedro et al., 1984). Septal neuron loss following fimbria transection (Wictorin et al., 1985) could be prevented almost completely by intraventricular infusion of NGF (Gage et al., 1988) or combined NGF and FGF (Otto et al., 1989). Purified neurotrophic factors have been used to promote regeneration in the spinal cord of sensory (Ramer et al., 2000) and corticospinal axons (Schnell, et al., 1994). These results and others (Silver and Whittemore, 1997) clearly indicate that neurotrophic factors (NTFs) may be used as pharmacological agents in the treatment of CNS injury.

Regardless of the success in preventing secondary neuronal death, a variable number of cells will be lost during the acute phase of injury. Furthermore, preventing neuronal loss is of little help to chronic CNS injury patients. In these cases, transplantation of fetal tissue into the injured CNS has been proposed as a means of replacing lost neurons. In order to be useful as therapeutic tools, transplants must survive in the wound cavity and integrate with the host. Reliably successful survival and integration of masses of neurons, that is, survival of tissue grafts, is necessary. However, the survival of solid fragments of embryonic CNS tissue in a wound cavity made in the host parenchyma depends not only on the age of the donor tissue, but also on the type of neuron transplanted. Many cortical neurons survive well, septal or

monoamine neurons less well and striatal acetyl-cholinesterase-positive neurons survive poorly or not at all. The survival and growth of striatal neurons in a wound cavity was dramatically enhanced by placing the transplant in the host after neurotrophic factor production had began to rise (Nieto-Sampedro et al., 1982, 1983). There was a close correlation between NTF activity for striatal neurons in the tissue immediately adjacent to the cavity and survival of transplants of the same type of neurons (Nieto-Sampedro et al., 1982, 1983, 1984; Manthorpe et al., 1983; Whittemore et al., 1985). Optimal survival coincided with maximal production of NTFs and exogenous supply of injured-brain extracts at the time of transplantation made the delay unnecesary (Nieto-Sampedro et al., 1984). Any donor tissue tested so far survives successfully when grafted using the delayed transplantation paradigm.

The delayed transplantation technique was introduced before information on injury-induced NTFs was available (Stenevi et al., 1976; Lewis and Cotman, 1983). The delay was assumed to allow the formation of a vascular bed which facilitated transplant survival (Stenevi et al., 1976). In adult rats, vascularization of a cortical wound occurs at the same time as the rise in NTF activity. However, whereas the number of capillaries in the new CNS surface levels off after 10 days postlesion, both neuronotrophic activity and transplant survival reach a maximum at about 8–10 days postlesion and decay thereafter (Nieto-Sampedro et al., 1987). Neurite-promoting activity was enhanced also greatly after injury (Needels et al., 1986). The decreased availability of neurotrophic and neurite-promoting activities with increasing delay accounts for the diminished viability of transplants with delays longer than 10 days, inspite of the presence of a well established capillary bed in the host wound cavity.

The success or failure of axonal regeneration seems to depend on signals that the regenerating neurons exchange with their immediate environment. Transplantation of embryonic CNS tissue into adult hosts provides a way to test whether CNS extracellular territory permits axons to navigate over long distances once connections are established during development, and whether embryonic CNS tissue transplants homologous to that lost by injury, would function as a relay station, receiving the original input from the host and sending to the original target projections similar to those interrupted by the lesion. This arrangement permits one to examine long-distance navigation in the adult CNS by both developing and adult fibers.

Embryonic fibers are remarkably successful in growing over long distances within the adult CNS and forming appropriate synapses with their target. Implants of embryonic locus coeruleus (Bjorklund et al., 1979), septum (Bjorklund and Stenevi, 1977), raphe (Bjorklund et al., 1976; Azmitia et al., 1981) and entorhinal cortex (Gibbs et al., 1985) form their own distinctive pattern of connections in the rat dentate gyrus, identical to that of the original synapses. The positioning of the implants in very abnormal locations, i.e. occipital cortex, does not prevent the fibers from reaching their correct target (Lewis and Cotman, 1983; Nieto-Sampedro et al., 1983). Furthermore, it appears that the specificity of the connections formed by a given type of afferent is determined by the neurotransmitter used by that type of fiber. For example, after fimbria-fornix transection in the adult rat, transplants of cholinergic cells from embryonic corpus striatum (Nieto-Sampedro et al., 1983) or habenula (Gibbs et al., 1986) form similar termination fields as those of septal transplants or the original septal fibers. Thus, the specificity of synapse formation resides in both the afferent originating in the transplant and the host target cells. The embryonic axons reach their target independently of whether they will eventually be myelinated (such as the perforant path) or unmyelinated (i.e. septal fibers). In summary, the adult CNS environment does not seem to offer obstacles to the progress of embryonic axons. However, adult axon sprouts seem to find greater difficulties.

The possible therapeutic value of transplants in neural circuit repair requires that projections from the transplant reach the correct host target, and that host axons innervate the appropriate cells in the transplant. Non-myelinated adult host septal or dorsal raphe fibers are capable of entering embryonic transplants and correctly innervating the hippocampal (Kromer et al., 1980; Sunde and Zimmer, 1983) or cortical (Gibbs et al., 1985) cells. This is quite remarkable, considering that the cellular organization of embryonic transplants tends to be more disarranged than that of the normal tissue (Oblinger and Das, 1982; Sunde and Zimmer, 1983; Kromer et al., 1984; Gibbs et al., 1985). However, damaged myelinated fiber systems are rarely able to penetrate into a transplant. Innervation from adult host thalamus, contralateral entorhinal cortex, presubiculum or subiculum never reach transplanted embryonic entorhinal neurons.

Typically, these myelinated fibers grow around the transplant but do not enter it. However, in one case, contralateral entorhinal and subicular fibers entered the implant (Gibbs et al., 1985). The zone of the implant where host fibers were seen entering was that where the layer of glial cells usually surrounding transplants (Lundberg and Møllgard, 1979; Azmitia and Whittaker, 1983; Lindsay and Raisman, 1983) was either very sparse or absent (Nieto-Sampedro et al., 1987). It appears that the layer of glia in the surface of implants, like the surface of injured tissue, cannot be crossed by myelinated axons. Thus, in general, CNS transplants are incomplete relay stations. They send acurate output, but receive only a minor proportion of input. In order to achieve effective transplant-host integration, the problem of the glial boundary has to be solved. At the time, it appeared essential to define the various roles that astroglia could play and search for the molecules that controlled the number and type of these cells.

Gliotic tissue neurite outgrowth inhibitors

The failure of injured axons to regenerate in the adult mammalian central nervous system (CNS) seems due to the neurite inhibitory properties of CNS glia, rather than to any intrinsic lack of growth capacity of the central fibers (Cajal, 1928; Richardson, et al., 1980; Nieto-Sampedro, 1999). Comparison of the CNS with the peripheral nervous system (PNS) where spontaneous regeneration is the rule, shows that the main difference is linked to their respective glial environments (Aguayo, 1985). Whereas Schwann cells in the peripheral nervous system favour axon regeneration by producing growth-promoting cell-surface and extracellular matrix molecules and soluble growth factors (Fawcett and Keynes, 1990), oligodendrocytes, reactive astrocytes and reactive microglia appear responsible for the unfavorable axon regenerating environment of the CNS. Oligodendrocyte components NI 35 and NI 250, of apparent molecular weight 35 kD and 250 kD, respectively, as well as extracellular matrix glycoproteins of the tenascin family, J1/160 and J1/180 (apparent mol. wt. 160 kD and 180 kD), inhibit *in vitro* cell spreading and neurite outgrowth (Schwab and Caroni, 1988; Caroni and Schwab, 1988a,b; Fawcett et al., 1989; Bandtlow et al., 1990; Pesheva et al., 1989; Schachner, 1991). The regeneration of damaged cortico-spinal axons in the rat was favoured by blocking

306

antibodies against NI 35/250 alone or together with growth factors (Schnell and Schwab, 1990, 1993; Schnell et al., 1994; Thallmair et al., 1998).

Unfortunately, oligodendrocytes alone do not entirely explain lack of CNS regeneration as damaged CNS axons also fail to regenerate in grey matter. The boundary between PNS and CNS in the spinal cord, the dorsal root entry zone (DREZ) contains astrocytes and Schwann cells. The astrocytes invade the PNS and act as a stop signal for Schwann cells, thus preventing the ingrowth in the spinal cord of both Schwann cells and regenerating axons (Liuzzi and Lasek, 1987). Because spinal cord sensory afferents show high intrinsic growth capacity and their morphological and physiological properties are well characterized (Fraher, 2000), dorsal rhizotomy has been used extensively to investigate CNS regeneration. The gliotic tissue formed at the DREZ /dorsal horn after sensory axon injury (Liuzzi and Lasek, 1987) or in other CNS loci (Bovolenta et al., 1993), has neurite inhibitory properties that prevent spinal cord penetration of the abundant sprouts formed after damage of the sensory axon central branch (Cajal, 1928). Axon regeneration seems inhibited by the disorganized mass of cells formed at lesion sites, the so-called "*glial scar*" (Cajal, 1928; Reier and Houle, 1988). Both, oligodendrocytes and astrocytes, appear involved.

CNS lesions are classified as isomorphic and anisomorphic, depending on their effect on gross tissue morphology (Greenfield, 1958). Anisomorphic lesions, like stab wounds, laceration, or hemorrhagic necrosis, disrupt gross tissue morphology. In contrast, tissue architecture is preserved inspite of cellular loss in isomorphic lesions like wallerian degeneration, anoxic, neurotoxic or degenerative damage. Isomorphic and anisomorphic lesions evoke the change of normal or "*resting*" glia into *reactive* glia, i.e. glia that reacts to a perturbation such as a lesion. The most common morphological image of a *reactive* astrocyte is that of a cell bigger than a resting astrocyte and with more numerous fibrous processes. Reactive and fibrous are synonyms for cells with numerous, associated GFAP filaments, although white matter astrocytes present a fibrous appearance in the absence of any lesion. The misnomer "glial scar" describes the accumulation of reactive astrocytes overlayed by fibroblasts and collagen. It is generally found at anisomorphic lesion sites, probably the attempt of the organism to reconstitute a new *glia limitans* (Nieto-Sampedro, 1988). Glia respond differently to different types of injury and

the use of the same name, i.e. "reactive astrocyte", for cells with different or even opposite properties generates unnecessary confusion. In any case, regenerating axons fail to grow past the "glial scar" (Cajal, 1928) and no axon growth occurred into transplanted gliotic tissue (Reier et al., 1983).

"Reactive" astrocytes and "activated" microglial cells are the major cellular components of the glial scar. These cells, conveniently recognized by specific markers such as glial fibrillary acidic protein (GFAP), expressed in high levels by reactive astrocytes, or complement receptor protein CD11b, differentially expressed in activated microglial cells (Graeber et al., 1988), have other unique characteristics not shared by normal adult glia. Cajal (1928) proposed that reactive astroglia prevented axonal outgrowth by acting as either a passive mechanical barrier or as an active source of inhibitory molecules. Since growth cones release proteases that degrade extracellular matrix components, the glial scar is unlikely to act as a physical barrier (Günther et al., 1985; Pittman, 1985; McGuire and Seeds, 1990). Putative inhibitory molecules were detected immunohistochemically in the damaged mammalian CNS (McKeon et al., 1991; Laywell et al., 1992; Levine and Levine, 1992), but direct evidence of involvement of gliotic tissue in CNS regeneration failure could not be presented. A major difficulty was that reactive glia could not be maintained in culture as such, either dying during the isolation process or reverting to a "blast-like" form. Neonatal astroblasts in monolayer culture are an excellent substrate for axonal growth (Noble et al., 1984; Fallon, 1985; Pixley et al., 1987), regardless of whether they grew as flat polygonal cells or whether they were differentiated to stellate cells with the help of dibutiryl-cAMP (Wandosell et al., 1993). Although stellate cells were considered an *in vitro* model of reactive glia (Federoff et al., 1984), their neuritogenic properties differed drastically from those of injured tissue glia (Streit et al., 1988; Bovolenta et al., 1991a; Wandosell et al., 1990, 1993). Geometry seemed to play a role, because astroblasts grown in culture as a three-dimensional network could not be penetrated by growing axons (Fawcett et al., 1989).

Astrocytes undergo two concomitant (but not necessarily related) phenomena in both anisomorphic and isomorphic lesions: (i) proliferation and (ii) differentiation into fibrous astrocytes. At least part of the astrocytes in the 'glial scar' arise as the result of injury-induced proliferation and proliferating astroglia have been called also reactive astrocytes. However, the astrocytes that proliferate are not necessarily those that become reactive and the properties and appearance of proliferating astrocytes are very different from those of fibrous reactive astrocytes. Whereas hypertrophic fibrous astrocytes appear after any CNS insult, astroglia proliferation seems influenced by the lesion type (Hatten et al., 1991; Norenberg, 1994). Astrocytes proliferating in the adult mammalian CNS may be either mature astrocytes that have undergone de-differentiation, remaining astrocyte precursors, new astroblasts arising from stem cells, or all these possibilities. Although the question is clearly asked now, its definite answer needs further research.

Astrocytes cannot be cultured from adult mammalian CNS, except from tissue adjacent to an injury site (Lindsay et al., 1982; Lindsay, 1986; Nieto-Sampedro, unpublished) in which case they proliferate as cells with the same morphology and immunological properties than type 1 neonatal brain astroblasts (Lindsay et al., 1982; Lindsay, 1986). A portion of the dividing astrocytes after brain and spinal cord anisomorphic injury definitely arose from stem cells (Holmin et al., 1997; Johansson et al., 1999), attracted to damaged tissue (Johansson et al., 1999; Helmuth, 2000). Astroblasts promote neuritogenesis, are a preferred substrate for neurite extension (Noble et al., 1984; Fallon, 1985; Pixley et al., 1987; Tommaselli et al., 1988) and during development often they are seen associated to growth cones *in vivo* (Silver, 1984; Bovolenta and Mason, 1987). In contrast, the membranes of fibrous reactive astrocytes induced by Wallerian degeneration or toxin injection, contain proteoglycans that cause growth cone collapse, inhibit neurite outgrowth and repel growing neurites (Bovolenta et al., 1991, 1992, 1993, 1997, Table 1). In summary, although central neurons are capable of long distance growth over the appropriate glial substrate (Tello, 1911; Aguayo et al., 1987), gliotic tissue constitutes the most general obstacle to re-establishment of lost connections, preventing the growth of regenerating sprouts, or supplying them with misguidance cues and preventing them from reaching their target (Nieto-Sampedro, 1999).

Molecular bases of gliotic tissue inhibitory properties

A direct approach was developped in our laboratory to study the cellular and molecular bases of inhibition of axon regeneration by gliotic tissue. Plasma membranes purified from gliotic tissue were used as an *in vitro* 'glial scar' model that permitted to examine directly the effect of gliotic tissue on neurite initiation and outgrowth. We found that gliotic tissue plasma membranes prevented axonal regeneration *in vitro* by two contrasting mechanisms, neurite inhibition and neurite "misguidance", both of which involved reactive astrocytes (Bovolenta et al., 1991a,b, 1992) and their expression of growth-promoting or inhibitory membrane proteoglycans (Table 1; Bovolenta et al., 1993, 1997). Our conclusion was that the ratio of fibrous reactive astrocytes to astroblasts determined the overall neurite promoting or neurite inhibiting properties of gliotic tissue. This ratio changed with post-lesion time, determining the proteoglycans expressed in gliotic tissue and, as a consequence, its growth properties (Nieto-Sampedro, 1999).

Astrocytes form molecular boundaries that limit axonal territories after CNS lesions. The growth inhibitory molecules expressed by hypertrophic reactive astrocytes belong to different families, but the most general after injury are proteoglycans (Snow et al., 1990; Bovolenta et al., 1991, 1997, Laywell and Steindler, 1991; McKeon et al., 1991; Haas et al., 1999; Table 1). A number of CNS proteoglycans contribute to regulate synaptogenesis by promoting or inhibiting neurite outgrowth both, during development and after lesions. The initial belief that certain proteoglycan types were associated to either neurite outgrowth promotion (heparan sulphate; Lander et al., 1983; Sandrock and Matthew, 1987) or its inhibition (chondroitin sulphate; Cole and McCabe, 1991; Fichard et al., 1991; Snow et al., 1991) has proven too simplistic. General rules do not seem to apply (Dou and Levine, 1995; Bandtlow and Zimmermann, 2000) and chondroitin sulfate proteoglycans (CSPGs) sometimes co-localize with axonal growth barriers and other times are neurite outgrowth promoters (Faissner et al., 1994) in recognized axon growth pathways (Rauch, 1997). Plasma membranes purified from normal or gliotic hippocampus (deafferented or neurotoxin injured; Fernaud-Espinosa et al., 1993), contained molecule/s capable of preventing neurite initiation, repelling and causing the collapse of growth cones initiated by laminin (Bovolenta et al., 1991, 1992). The injured tissue inhibitory molecule was a heparan-sulfate/chondroitin-sulfate proteoglycan (Bovolenta et al., 1993), abbreviated as IMPg. The glycosaminoglycan chains of IMPg are responsible for its neurite

Table 1. Proteoglycans in normal and damaged CNS

Name	Type	Molecular Weight × 10		Neurites*	Cell source	Ref.
		PG	Core			
UMPG	CS/HS	200–220	48	±	Neurons	1
IMPG	CS/HS	200–220	48	–	Astrocytes	1, 2
PMPG	CS/HS	200–220	48	–	Neurons	1, 2, 3
NG2	CS	500	300	–	O2A, oligo progen.	4, 5, 6
Neurocan	CS		136	–	Neurons/Astroc.	7, 8
Brevican	CS		145	–	Astroc.	9, 10, 11
Perlecan	HS/CS/DS		467	±	Blood vessels	12
Appican	CS	200	90	–	Glia	13
Glypican-5	HS	220	58	±	Neurons	14, 15
Phosphacan	CS/KS	400–500	173	±	Glia	16, 17
DSD-1-PG	Mouse phosphacan homologue			±	Glia/neurons	17
Syndecans 2-3	HS	40–200	20-120	?	Neurons	23, 24
Syndecan-4	HS/CS	200	25, 30, 50	±	Glia	18, 19, 24
Agrin	HS	500	25	–	Neurons/glia	20
Ryudocan	HS	160	30, 50	syndecan-4	Endothelium	18, 21
Neuroglycan C	CS	150	56–120	?	Neuroblasts	22

CS, chondritin sulphate; HS, heparan sulphate; KS, keratan sulphate; DS, dermatan sulphate. References: **1**, Bovolenta et al., 1993; **2**, Bovolenta et al., 1997; **3**, Fernaud-Espinosa et al., 1998; **4**, Dawson et al., 2000; **5**, Dou and Levine, 1994, 1995; **6**, Fidler et al., 1999; **7**, Rauch et al., 1992; **8**, Friedlander et al., 1994; **9**, Thon et al., 2000; **10**, Yamada et al., 1994, 1997; **11**, Thon et al., 2000; **12**, Noonan et al., 1991; **13**, Shioi et al., 1995; **14**, Karthikeyan et al., 1994; **15**, Saunders et al., 1997; **16**, Maurel et al., 1994; **17**, Garwood et al., 1999; **18**, Kojima et al., 1992; **19**, David et al., 1992; **20**, Chang et al., 1997; **21**, Tsuzuki et al., 1997; **22**, Watanabe et al., 1995; **23**, Carey, 1997; **24**, Hsueh and Sheng, 1999.

*, +, neurite promotion; –, neurite inhibition; ±, promoting or inhibitory activity, depending on the presence of other growth modifiers; ?, data not available.

inhibitory activity (Bovolenta et al., 1993; Bovolenta et al., 1997). Immunostaining of sections of normal and injured brain with specific monoclonal antibodies to IMPg, permitted us to identify its cellular location. Whereas IMPg-immunoreactivity in normal brain was found on the surface of neurons, after kainic acid injection intense IMPg staining was found on the plasma membranes of fibrous reactive astrocytes (Bovolenta et al., 1997). Proteoglycans with molecular and biological properties similar to IMPg but located in neurons were isolated from perinatal brain (PNPg; Fernaud-Espinosa et al., 1998). IMPg immunoreactivity has been found in reactive astrocytes in all injured tissue examined so far, including injured spinal cord (Verdu et al., 2001). Several proteoglycans purified from CNS tissue in the last decade have been characterized and their properties are compared to IMPg and PNPg in Table 1. The possible identity (or lack of it) of IMPg and PNPg with any of the other proteoglycans in Table 1 will be established after these proteoglycans are sequenced. Meanwhile, its combined properties resemble most those of glypican-5 or syndecan-4 (Table 1).

Neurostatin, an inhibitor of astroblast division

CNS injury induces astrocyte proliferation and at least part of the astroglia in the 'glial scar' arises from glia division. Proliferating astrocytes have been called also reactive astrocytes. After injury to the adult mammalian CNS, such cells may originate from either mature astrocytes that have undergone de-differentiation, from remaining astrocyte precursors, from new astroblasts arising from stem cells, or from all these sources. Although mitogens are abundant in brain, astrocyte number remains stationary throughout adulthood (Sturrock, 1974; Korr, 1986). We hypothesized that the number of glial cells was controlled by the concomitant presence of mitogen inhibitors. Circumstantial support for this hypothesis was provided by the higher than 100% recovery of mitogenic activity from brain extracts after molecular filtration (Nieto-Sampedro et al., 1985). Furthermore, brain extracts showed mitogenic activity the dose-response curves of which were bell-shaped, suggesting the concomitant presence of both, mitogens and mitogen inhibitors (Nieto-Sampedro, 1987). Definite evidence for the existence in brain of specific mitogen inhibitors, was obtained more recently, using specific antibodies (Nieto-Sampedro, 1988b). The inhibitor, which had epitopes in common with both, the carbohydrate moiety of the epidermal growth factor receptor (EGFR) and human blood groups (Nieto-Sampedro and Broderick, 1989), was designated EGFR related inhibitor (ERI). Because of its source and biological activity, the glial inhibitor is now called *neurostatin*. Neurostatin is cytostatic for neonatal astrocytes with ID_{50} values of 200 to 300 nM (Abad-Rodríguez et al., 1998). At these concentrations, the inhibitor shows no activity on fibroblasts, 3T3 cells or A431 epidermoid carcinoma cells. Inhibition of cell division did not imply cell death, until concentrations 3 or 4-fold higher than the ID_{50} were reached. Concentrations of 800 nM or higher, caused non-specific cytotoxicity. Neurostatin and its synthetic oligosaccharide analogs inhibited the division of astrocytes, glioma and neuroblastoma cells in culture (Nieto-Sampedro, 1988; Abad-Rodríguez et al., 1998) and one structural analogue promoted the destruction *in vivo* of an experimental rat brain glioma (Nieto-Sampedro et al., 1996).

Determination of the precise structure of neurostatin required the purification of comparatively large amounts of the molecule, which was facilitated by preparation of brain ganglioside extracts (Tettamanti et al., 1973). Neurostatin was purified to homogeneity from these extracts, using a combination of conventional and high performance ion-exchange chromatographies. The structure of the purified inhibitor was determined by combining bidimensional nuclear magnetic resonance (NMR), MALDI-TOF mass spectrometry and biochemical studies. The conclusion was that neurostatin is the 9-O-acetylated form of ganglioside GD1b. It inhibited the proliferation in culture of both primary astroblasts and glioma cells (both rat and human) at nanomolar concentrations, either in defined medium or in the presence of 10% foetal calf serum (Abad-Rodríguez et al., 2000). The possible activity of neurostatin on stem cell or glial precursor division and differentiation are being investigated.

CNS Schwann-like macroglia and spinal cord lesion repair

Oligodendrocytes, reactive astrocytes and reactive microglia are responsible for the unfavorable environment for regenerating axons found in injured CNS. By contrast, Schwann cells in the peripheral nervous system favour axon regeneration by producing growth-promoting cell-surface and extracellular matrix molecules and soluble growth factors (Fawcett and Keynes, 1990). Because spinal cord sensory afferents show high intrinsic growth capacity and their morphological and physiological properties are well characterized (Fraher, 2000), dorsal rhizotomy has been used extensively to investigate CNS regeneration. The neurite inhibitory properties of gliotic tissue formed after injury at the dorsal horn/dorsal root entry zone (DREZ; Liuzzi and Lasek, 1987) or in other CNS loci (Bovolenta et al., 1993), prevent spinal cord penetration of the abundant sprouts formed after damage to the central branch of the sensory axons (Cajal, 1928).

Cajal's laboratory initiated peripheral nerve transplantation in the CNS (Tello, 1911), although these promising studies were only taken up successfully much later by Aguayo's group (Aguayo et al., 1985, 1987). Schwann cells in the peripheral nervous system favour axon regeneration by producing growth-promoting cell-surface and extracellular matrix molecules and soluble growth factors (Fawcett and Keynes, 1990). However, a more general and promising alternative was recently developed at the Cajal Institute (Nieto-Sampedro and Ramón-Cueto, 1994; Ramón-Cueto and Nieto-Sampedro, 1994), using transplants of olfactory bulb ensheathing cells (OBEC). OBECs are a macroglia type with phenotypic properties intermediate between those of astrocytes and Schwann cells (Doucette, 1990, 1995). Several characteristics make OBECs similar to Schwann cells but different from mature astrocytes and oligodendrocytes. One is that OBECs can be cultured from adult tissue (Ramón-Cueto and Nieto-Sampedro, 1992). A second distinctive feature is that they express low affinity neurotrophin receptor (p. 75 NTR) immunoreactivity (Gómez-Pinilla et al., 1987), like Schwann cells (Fields and Dammermann, 1985; Bunge et al., 1986; Johnson et al., 1988; Assouline and Pantazis, 1989). Again like non-myelinating Schwann cells, OBECs show potent neurite-promoting properties (Kafitz and Greer, 1999; Sonigra et al., 1999) and are capable of rapid ensheathment of axons (Doucette, 1986, 1990; Ramón-Cueto et al., 1993). However, unlike Schwann cells

310

and like regular CNS glia, OBECs mingle with astrocytes and are capable of long distance migration in adult brain (Gudiño-Cabrera and Nieto-Sampedro, 1996).

Transplantation of OBECs near the DREZ (Nieto-Sampedro and Ramón-Cueto, 1994; Ramón-Cueto and Nieto-Sampedro, 1994) modifies the spinal environment, causing astrocyte reactivity to diminish or disappear (Verdú et al., 2001) and promoting regeneration and spinal ingrowth of damaged dorsal root fibers. However, damage to a single dorsal root does not cause a clear functional deficit that may permit to assess the recovery achieved with the help of OBEC transplants, due to innervation overlap by adjacent dorsal roots. Accordingly, we performed multiple rhizotomy at the lumbar (Navarro et al., 1999), lumbosacral (Pascual et al. 1997, 2002) and cervical (Taylor et al. 1999, 2000) levels, determining the extent of sensory function recovery and its anatomical and electrophysiological correlates. Variations of the OBEC transplantation technique has

now been used to repair multiple dorsal rhizotomies at these cord levels, achieving significant recovery of functions. These studies show that OBEC transplantation induces recovery of cutaneous, proprioceptive and autonomic sensory function by promoting axonal regrowth leading to: (1) reinnervation of the dorsal horn; (2) activation of postsynaptic dorsal horn neurons; (3) restitution of polysynaptic reflex activity. Furthermore anatomical and electrophysiological recovery was translated at the behavioral level in the restoration of withdrawal reflexes and organized supraspinal nocifensive responses to forepaw stimulation.

Multiple cervical rhizotomy: recovery of sensory function

Unilateral C4 to T2 dorsal rhizotomy in the rat (Fig. 1) leads to severe sensory deficits in the forepaw.

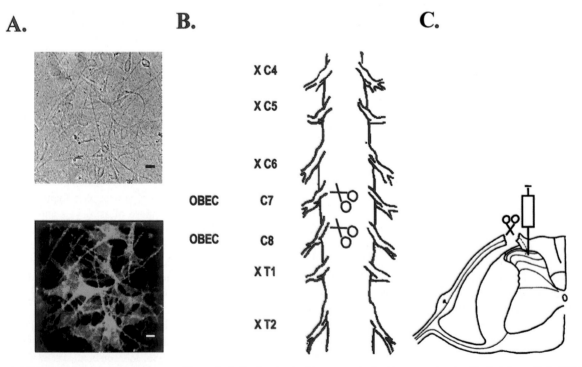

Fig. 1. (A) Purified ensheathing glia from rat olfactory bulb (10 days *in vitro*) immunostained with a monoclonal antibody to low affinity NGF receptor. Scale bar 40 μm. (B) The central branch of dorsal roots C4 to T2 was transected and (C) Dorsal roots C7/C8 were reapposed to their respective dorsal root entry zone using fibrin glue and a suspension of OBECs (75,000 cells/root in 2.5 μl of Dulbecco's modified Eagle's medium) was transplanted into the ipsilateral dorsal horn at the entry zone level (transplanted group); the same volume of DMEM alone was injected in the control untreated group. The remaining brachial plexus dorsal roots (C4, C5, C6, T1 and T2) were resected proximally towards the ganglion.

Transplantation of OBECs medial to the DREZ of cut dorsal roots C7/C8 promoted significant recovery of sensory function (Taylor et al., 1999) and response to noxious stimuli as judged by C-fos protein expression (Hunt et al., 1987). The expression of c-fos protein in intrinsic dorsal horn neurons of the superficial dorsal horn laminae, increased after thermal stimulation (immersion of the ipsilateral forepaw in water at 52°C) in nonoperated animals or in sham-operated controls. It was lost in rhizotomized animals and partially restored in the ipsilateral dorsal horn of OBEC-transplanted animals. Therefore, OBEC transplants help to re-establish functional contacts between injured sensory axons and intrinsic dorsal horn neurones.

Direct evidence of functional restitution of cutaneous reflex circuits was obtained by recording biceps reflex activity in response to stimulation of the median nerve ipsilateral to the C4-T2 rhizotomy and C7/C8 transplantation (Fig. 2). Stimulus–response curves were obtained for non-operated animals (Norm), rhizotomized rats transplanted with cell culture medium (Rhiz. + DMEM) and rats transplanted with ensheathing cells (Rhiz + OBEC; Fig. 2A and B). Median nerve activation with short (0.1 ms; Fig. 2A) or long (0.5 ms; Fig. 2B) pulse duration stimuli, indicated that only small diameter afferents had regenerated in transplanted animals (Fig. 2B). Biceps reflexes recovered after OBEC transplantation and showed a higher "gain" than either normal

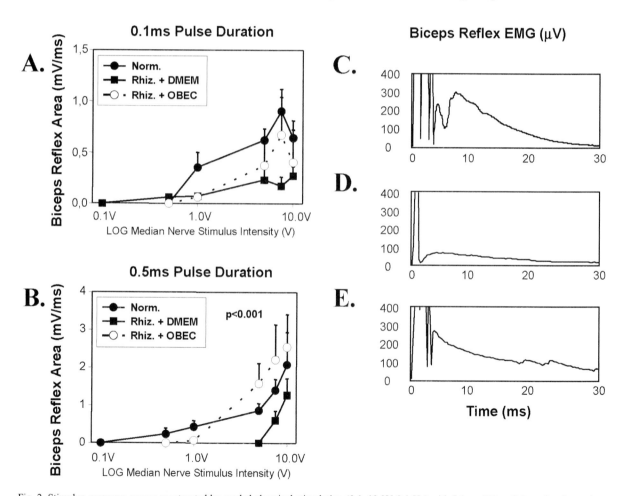

Fig. 2. Stimulus–response curves constructed by graded electrical stimulation (0.1–10.0V, 0.1 Hz) with 0.1 ms (**A**) or 0.5 ms duration pulses (**B**) of the ipsilateral median nerve and the integration of averaged, rectified biceps EMG reflex responses in normal and in rhizotomized animals transplanted with DMEM or OBECs. (**C–E**) Biceps reflex responses evoked by stimulation of the ipsilateral median nerve at 7.5 V in a normal rat (**C**), up to two months (D) and 6 months after complete dorsal rhizotomy in an OBEC-transplanted rat (**E**).

or non-transplanted rhizotomized rats. The synchronized electromyographic discharge evoked in the biceps muscle by median nerve stimulation in normal adult rats (Fig. 2C) was lost after rhizotomy or transplant of DMEM alone (Fig. 2D). In contrast, similar stimulation in OBEC transplanted animals six months after injury evoked unsynchronized biceps discharge (Fig. 2E).

Recovery of sensory input observed electrophysiologically, occurred in parallel to the restoration of sensory reflexes in the awake animal. Withdrawal reflex and supraspinal nocifensive responses to both radiant heat stimuli and mechanical stimuli, applied to the ipsilateral forepaw plantar pad, were assessed behaviourally before and up to 2 months after cervical dorsal rhizotomy. No reflex activity was evoked by mechanical stimuli applied to the forepaw after brachial rhizotomy in either the non-transplanted group or in the OBEC-transplanted group (data not shown). In contrast, reflex responses of the ipsilateral forepaw to thermal stimuli showed significant

recovery in OBEC-treated animals. During the first month following rhizotomy, ipsilateral withdrawal reflex responses were abolished in both experimental groups. In contrast, the withdrawal reflex recorded in the transplanted group during the second month after injury (latency 10–15 s; Fig. 3A) was significantly better than the response evoked in the non-transplanted control group (20–22 s). The same behavioural test was also used to measure the recovery of organized and unlearned supraspinal responses in transplanted animals. A defined non-parametric scale was developed to grade orientation of the head and paw-licking behaviour in response to thermal stimulation of the forepaw. The score of this supraspinal nocifensive scale (SNS) fell from a maximal value of '3' in normal animals to '0' after rhizotomy. The score remained at '0' in non-transplanted animals, indicating lack of orientation and contact of the ipsilateral forepaw in response to thermal stimulation (Fig. 3B and C). In contrast, the group of OBEC-transplanted rats

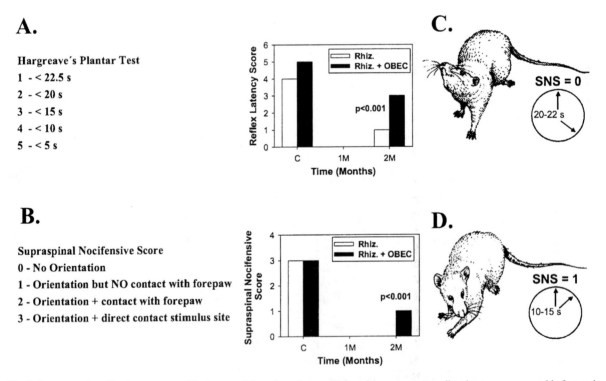

Fig. 3. Recovery of nocifensive responses. The latency of the reflex of paw withdrawal in response to radiant heat, was measured before and up to 2 months after complete ipsilateral brachial plexus (C4-T2) dorsal rhizotomy. (**A**) Rhizotomized rats received dorsal horn injections of DMEM alone (open bars) or a suspension of OBECs in DMEM (filled bars). (**B**) Supraspinal nocifensive response to radiant heat as in A, before and up to 2 month after rhizotomy (format as in **A**). (**C** and **D**). Schematic of the rats' behaviour observed during the second month after rhizotomy indicating the reflex latency and supraspinal nocifensive score in non-transplanted (**C**) and OBEC-transplanted (**D**).

recovered an SNS score of '1' during the second month following rhizotomy indicating orientation towards the stimulated forepaw (Fig. 3B and D). Furthermore, the development of these supraspinal nocifensive responses following OBEC implantation correlated significantly with the recovery of flexor withdrawal activity, indicating that both reflexive and supraspinal behavioural responses measured activity evoked by regenerating afferents.

OBEC transplantation could be a general strategy for CNS injury repair (Ramón-Cueto and Nieto-Sampedro, 1994; Gudiño-Cabrera and Nieto-Sampedro, 1996), except that is limited by the well-defined migration preferences of OBECs in adult CNS (Gudiño-Cabrera and Nieto-Sampedro, 1996). It appears that regeneration may be promoted by OBECs only when the preferred direction of OBEC migration coincides with the growth direction of regenerating sprouts (Gudiño-Cabrera et al., 2000).

Schwann-like immunoreactive glia in adult brain

Because OBEC-like glia with varying migration preferences may occur elsewhere in brain, we screened adult rat brain for glial cells that like OBECs would be GFAP, Vimentin and p75-positive and could grow in culture from adult tissue dissociates. OBEC-like macroglial cells fulfilling these criteria were found in several brain loci.

Two of these macroglial types, tanycytes and pituicytes, have a function that involves rapid and reversible ensheathment of axons (Theodosis and MacVicar, 1996; García-Segura et al., 1996). Furthermore, tanycytes and pituicytes have regeneration promoting properties similar to both OBECs and Schwann cells (Chauvet et al., 1995, 1996, 1998). Tanycytes, pituicytes, OBECs and a type of pineal glia, in common with non-myelinating Schwann cells, survive well when cultured from adult rodent brain tissue, exhibit morphologies similar to OBECs, and express a common distinctive set of immunological markers (Table 2), namely p75 neurotrophin receptor, O4 antigen, estrogen receptor-α type (Gudiño-Cabrera and Nieto-Sampedro, 1999), and insulin-like growth factor 1 (IGF-1). In co-culture with neurons, they associate with neurites in a manner suggestive of enveloping and express a peripheral myelinating phenotype (Gudiño-Cabrera and Nieto-Sampedro, 2000).

The Schwann-like properties shown by these macroglial cells, define a CNS macroglial class that would not fit in any of the conventional central glia types. We have called this distinct group of growth-promoting CNS macroglia, "aldynoglia" (greek αλδαινο, make grow). The proliferative and growth-promotin properties of aldynoglia seem to be retained during the lifetime of the organism in those CNS loci where normal function depends on continuous axon renewal. Aldynoglia

Table 2. Comparative immunological markers of conventional central macroglia, aldynoglia and Schwann cells

Cell Type	O4	p75	S100	ER	Vim	GFAP
Ast.[†]	−	−	+	−	−	++
Olig[†]	++	-	±	-	-	-
SC*	+	++	++	++	++	++
Tan[†]	+	+	++	++	++	++
Tan*	+	++	++	+	++	+
Pit[†]	+	+	++	++	++	++
Pit*	+	++	++	+	++	+
OBECs[†]	+	+	++	+	++	++
OBECs*	+	++	++	+	++	+

Cell immunoreactivity was: (++), very intense; (+), clearly positive; (−) negative. Reaction with the immunological markers indicated was examined: (†), in adult tissue *in situ*; (*), in cultures prepared from adult tissue. Astrocytes (**Ast.**), oligodendrocytes (**Olig**) and cultured non-myelinating Schwann cells (**SC**), were used as standards of immunostaining intensity, under the same experimental conditions as the rest of the cell types. **Tan**, tanycytes; **Pit**, pituicytes; **OBECs**, olfactory ensheathing cells. O4, seminolipid, sulfatide antigen; **p75**, low affinity NGF receptor; **S100**, Ca^{2+}-binding protein S100; **ER**, estrogen receptor-α; **Vim**, vimentin; **GFAP**, glial fibrillary acidic protein (polyclonal IgG). Immunostaining of tissue sections with polyclonal anti-S100 was not selective, i.e. weak staining of every type of glial cell was superimposed over intense **OBEC** or tanycyte staining.

plasticity seems totally or partially lost with age where and when it is no longer essential, as in the case of adult retinal Müller cells and Bergmann glia and cortical and spinal cord radial glia. The concomitant expression of estrogen receptor and low affinity neurotrophin receptor may confer Schwann-like plasticity to these glial cells.

Conclusions

The work of our group in the last two decades has confirmed and extended Cajal's observations on the regeneration inhibiting role of reactive glia, while recognizing its positive side, as source of injury-induced neurotrophic and neuritogenic activities. We have added some complementary ways of overcoming inhibition with blocking antibodies to the inhibitors. The recognition of the existence in the CNS of macroglia with Schwann-like properties and its value in promoting central axon regeneration when transplanted in spinal cord injuries, would have made Cajal very happy.

References

Abad-Rodríguez, J., Vallejo-Cremades, M. and Nieto-Sampedro, M. (1998) Control of glial number: purification from mammalian brain extracts of an inhibitor of astrocyte division. *Glia.*, 22: 160–171.

Abad-Rodríguez, J., Bernabe, M., Romero-Ramírez, L. and Vallejo-Cremades, M.T., Fernández-Mayoralas, A. and Nieto-Sampedro, M. (2000) Purification and structure of neurostatin, an inhibitor of astrocyte division from mammalian brain. *J. Neurochem.*, 74: 2547–2556.

Aguayo, A.J. (1985) Axonal regeneration from injured neurons in the adult mammalian central nervous system. In: C.W. Cotman (Ed.), *Synaptic Plasticity.* Guildford, New York, pp. 457–484.

Aguayo, A.J., Vidal-Sanz, M., Villegas-Pérez, M.P. and y Bray, G.M. (1987) Growth and connectivity of axotomized retinal neurons in adult rat with optic nerves substituted by PNS grafts linking the eyes and midbrain. *Ann. NY Acad. Sci.*, 495: 1–9.

Assouline, J.G. and Pantazis, N.J. (1989) Detection of a nerve growth factor receptor on fetal human Schwann cells in culture: absence of the receptor on fetal human astrocytes. *Dev. Brain Res.*, 45, 1–14.

Azmitia, E.C., Perlow, M.J., Brennan, M.J. and Lauder, J.M. (1981) Fetal raphe and hippocampal transplants into adult and aged C57 BL/6N mice: a preliminary immunocytochemical study. *Brain Res. Bull.*, 7: 703–710.

Azmitia, E.C. and Whittaker, P.M. (1983) Formation of a glial scar following microinjection of fetal neurons into the hippocampus or midbrain of adult rat: an immunocytochemical study. *Neurosci. Lett.*, 38: 145–150.

Bandtlow, C., Zachleder, T. and Schwab, M.E. (1990) Oligodendrocytes arrest neurite growth by contact inhibition. *J. Neurosci.*, 10: 3837–3848.

Bandtlow, C.E. and Zimmermann, D.R. (2000) Proteoglycans in the developing brain: new conceptual insights for old proteins. *Physiol. Rev.*, 80: 1267–1290.

Bjorklund, A., Stenevi, U. and Svengaard, N.-A. (1976) Growth of transplanted monoaminergic neurons into the adult hippocampus along the perforant path. *Nature*, 262: 787–790.

Bjorklund, A. and Stenevi, U. (1977) Reformation of the severed septohippocampal cholinergic pathway in the adult rat by transplanted septal neurons. *Cell Tis. Res.*, 185: 289–302.

Bjorklund, A., Segal, M. and Stenevi, U. (1979) Functional reinnervation of rat hippocampus by locus coeruleus implants. *Brain Res.*, 170: 409–426.

Bovolenta, P. and Mason, C.A. (1987) Growth cone morphology varies with position in the developing mouse visual pathway from the retina to first targets. *J. Neurosci*, 7: 1447–1460.

Bovolenta, P., Wandosell, F. and Nieto-Sampedro, M. (1991a) Neurite outgrowth over resting and reactive astrocytes. *Res. Neurol. Neurosci.*, 2: 221–228.

Bovolenta, P., Wandosell, F. and Nieto-Sampedro, M. (1991b). Central Neurite outgrowth over glial scar tissue *in vitro*. In: S.B. Kater, P.C. Letourneau and E.R. Macagno (Eds.), *The Nerve Growth Con.* Raven Press, pp. 477–488.

Bovolenta, P., Wandosell, F. and Nieto-Sampedro, M. (1992) CNS glial scar tissue: a source of molecules which inhibit central neurite outgrowth. *Progress Brain Res.*, 94: 367–379.

Bovolenta, P., Wandosell, F. and Nieto-Sampedro, M. (1993) Characterization of a neurite outgrowth inhibitor expressed after CNS injury. *Eur. J. Neurosci.*, 5: 454–465.

Bovolenta, P., Fernaud-Espinosa, I., Rosalía Méndez-Otero and Nieto-Sampedro, M. (1997) Neurite outgrowth inhibitor of gliotic brain tissue. Mode of action and cellular localization, studied with specific monoclonal antibodies. *Eur. J. Neurosci.*, 9: 977–989.

Bunge, R.P., Bunge, M.B. and Eldridge, C.F. (1986) Linkage between axonal ensheathment and basal lamina production by Schwann cells. *Ann. Rev. Neurosci.*, 9: 305–328.

Cajal, S.R. (1928) *Degeneration and Regeneration in the Nervous System*, Hafner, New York.

Carey, D.J. (1997) Syndecans: multifunctional cell-surface co-receptors. *Biochem. J.*, 327: 1–16.

Caroni, P. and Schwab, M.E. (1988a) Two membrane protein fraction from rat central myelin with inhibitory properties for neurite growth and fibroblast spreading. *J. Cell Biol.*, 106: 1281–1288.

Caroni, P. and Schwab, M.E. (1988b) Antibodies against myelin associated inhibitor of neurite growth neutralizes non-permissive substrate properties of CNS white matter. *Neuron.*, 1: 85–96.

Chang, D., Woo, J.S., Campanelli, J., Scheller, R.H. and Ignatius, M.J. (1997) Agrin inhibits neurite outgrowth but promotes attachment of embryonic motor and sensory neurons. *Dev. Biol.*, 181: 21–35.

Chauvet, N., Parmentier, M.L. and Alonso, G. (1995) Transected axons of adult hypothalamic-neurohypophysial neurons regenerate along tanicytic processes. *J. Neurosci. Res.*, 41: 129–144.

Chauvet, N., Privat, A. and Alonso, G. (1996) Aged median eminence glial cell cultures promote survival and neurite outgrowth of cocultured neurons. *Glia*, 18: 211–223.

Chauvet, N., Prieto, M. and Alonso, G. (1998) Tanycytes present in the adult rat mediobasal hypothalamus support the regeneration of monoaminergic axons. *Exp. Neurol.*, 151: 1–13.

Cole, C.G. and McCabe, C.F. (1991) Identification of a developmentally regulated keratan sulphate proteoglycan that inhibits cell adhesion and neurite outgrowth. *Neuron*, 7: 1007–1018.

David, G., van der Schueren, B., Marynen, P., Cassiman, J.J. and van der Berghe, H. (1992) Molecular cloning of amphiglycan, a novel integral membrane heparan sulfate proteoglycan expressed by epithelial and fibroblastic cells. *J. Cell Biol.*, 118: 961–969.

Dawson, M.R.L., Levine, J.L., and Reynolds, R. (2000) NG2-expressing cells in the central nervous system: are they oligodendroglial progenitors? *J. Neurosci. Res.*, 61: 471–479

Dou, C.L. and Levine, J.M. (1994) Inhibition of neurite growth by the NG2 chondroitin sulfate proteoglycan. *J. Neurosci.*, 14: 7616–7628.

Dou, C.L. and Levine, J.M. (1995) Differential effects of glycosaminoglycans on neurite outgrowth on laminin and L1 substrates. *J. Neurosci.*, 15: 8053–8066.

Doucette, J.R. (1986) Astrocytes in the Olfactory Bulb. In: S. Fedoroff, and Vernardakis, A. (Eds.), *Astrocytes*, Vol. 1, Academic Press, Orlando, pp. 293–310.

Doucette, R. (1990) Glial influences on axonal growth in the primary olfactory system. *Glia*, 3: 433–449.

Doucette, R. (1995) Olfactory ensheathing cells: potential for glial cell transplantation into areas of CNS injury. *Histol. Histopathol.* 10: 503–507.

Faissner, A., Clement, A., Lochter, A., Streit, A., Mandl, C. and Schachner, M. (1994) Isolation of a neural chondroitin sulfate proteoglycan with neurite outgrowth promoting properties. *J. Cell Biol.*, 126: 783–799.

Fallon, J. (1985) Preferential outgrowth of central nervous system neurites on astrocytes and Schwann cells as compared with nonglial cells *in vitro*. *J. Cell Biol.*, 100: 198–207.

Fawcett, J.W., Housden, E., Smith-Thomas, L. and Meyer, R.L. (1989) The growth of axons in three-dimensional astrocyte cultures. *Dev. Biol.*, 135: 449–458.

Fawcett, J.W. and Keynes, R.J. (1990) Peripheral nerve regeneration. *Annu. Rev. Neurosci,*. 13: 43–60.

Fedoroff, S., McAuley, W.A.J., Houle, J.D. and Devon, R.M. (1984) Astrocyte cell lineage. V Similarity of astrocytes that form in the presence of dBcAMP in culture to reactive astrocytes *in vivo*. *J. Neurosci. Res.*, 12: 15–27.

Fernaud-Espinosa, I., Nieto-Sampedro, M. and Bovolenta, P. (1993) Differential activation of microglia and astrocytes in aniso- and iso-morphic gliotic tissue. *Glia*, 8: 277–291.

Fernaud-Espinosa, I., Nieto-Sampedro, M. and Bovolenta, P. (1998) A neurite outgrowth-inhibitory proteoglycan expressed during development is similar to that isolated from adult brain after isomorphic injury. *J. Neurobiol.*, 36: 16–29.

Fichard, A., Verna, J.M. and Saxod, R. (1991). Involvement of a chondroitin sulfate proteoglycan in the avoidance of chick epidermis by dorsal root ganglia fibers: a study using β-D-xyloxide. *Dev. Biol.*, 148: 1–9.

Fidler, P.S., Schuette, K., Asher, R.A., Dobbertin, A., Thornton, S.R., Calle-Patiño, Y., Muir, E., Levine, J.M., Geller, H.M., Rogers, J.H., Faissner, A. and Fawcett, J.W. (1999) Comparing astrocytic cell lines that are inhibitory or permissive for axon growth: the major axon-inhibitory proteoglycan is NG2. *J. Neurosci.*, 19: 8778–8789.

Fields, K.R. and Dammerman, M. (1985) A monoclonal antibody equivalent to anti-rat neural antigen-1 as a marker for Schwann cells. *Neurosci.*, 15, 877–886.

Fraher, J.P. (2000) The transitional zone and CNS regeneration. *J. Anat.*, 196: 137–158.

Friedlander, D., Milev, P., Karthikeyan, L., Margolis, R.K., Margolis, R.U. and Grumet, M. (1994). The neuronal chondroitin sulfate proteoglycan neurocan binds to the neural cell adhesion molecules Ng-CAM/L1/NILE and N-CAM, and inhibits neuronal adhesion and neurite outgrowth. *J. Cell Biol.*, 125: 669–680.

Gage, F.H., Armstrong, D.M., Williams, L.R. and Varon, S. (1988) Morphological response of axotomized septal neurons to nerve growth factor. *J. Comp. Neurol.*, 269: 147–155.

García-Segura, L.M., Chowen, J.A. and Naftolin, F. (1996) Endocrine glia: roles of glial cells in the brain actions of steroid and thyroid hormones and in the regulation of hormone secretion. *Front Neuroendocrin.*, 17: 180–211.

Garwood, J., Schnädelbach, O., Clement, A., Schütte, K., Bach, A. and Faissner, A. (1999). DSD-1-proteoglycan is the mouse homolog of phosphacan and displays opposing effects on neurite outgrowth dependent on neuronal lineage. *J. Neurosci.*, 19: 3888–3899.

Gibbs, R.B., Harris, E.W. and Cotman, C.W. (1985) Replacement of damaged cortical projections by homotypic transplants of entorhinal cortex. *J. Comp. Neurol.*, 237: 47–64.

Gibbs, R.B., Anderson, K. and Cotman, C.W. (1986) Factors affecting innervation in the CNS: Comparison of three cholinergic cell types transplanted to the hippocampus of adult rats. *Brain Res.*, 383: 362–366.

Gómez-Pinilla, F., Cotman, C.W. and Nieto-Sampedro, M. (1987) NGF Receptor immunoreactivity in rat brain: topographic distribution and response to entorhinal ablation. *Neurosci. Lett.*, 82, 260–266.

Graeber, M.B., Streit, W.J. and Kreutzberg, G.W. (1988) Axotomy of the rat facial nerve leads to increased expression of CR3 complement receptor expression by activated microglial cells. *J. Neurosci. Res.*, 21, 18–24.

Greenfield, J.G. (1958) General pathology of nerve cell and neuroglia. In: J.G. Greenfield, W. Blackwood, A. Meyer, W.H. McMenemey, and R.M. Norman, (Eds.), *Neuropathology* London: Ed. Arnold, Ltd., pp. 1–66.

Gudiño-Cabrera, G. and Nieto-Sampedro, M. (1996) Ensheathing cells: large scale purification from adult olfactory bulb, freeze-preservation and migration of transplanted cells in adult brain. *Restor. Neurol. Neurosci.*, 10, 25–34.

Gudiño-Cabrera, G. and Nieto-Sampedro, M. (1999) Estrogen receptor immunoreactivity in Schwann-like brain macroglia. *J. Neurobiol.*, 40: 458–470.

Gudiño-Cabrera, G., Pastor, A.M., de la Cruz, R.R., Delgado-García, J.M. and Nieto-Sampedro, M. (2000) Limits to the capacity of olfactory ensheathing glia to promote axonal regrowth in the CNS. *NeuroReport*, 11(3): 467–471.

Gudiño-Cabrera, G. and Nieto-Sampedro, M. (2000) Schwann-like macroglia in adult rat brain. *Glia*, 30: 49–63.

Guenther, J., Nick, H. and Monard, D. (1985) A glial derived neurite promoting factor with protease inhibitory activity. *EMBO J.*, 4: 1963–1966.

318

Schnell, L. and Schwab, M.E. (1990) Axonal regeneration in the rat spinal cord produced by an antibody against myelin associated neurite growth inhibitors. *Nature*, 343: 269–272.

Schnell, L. and Schwab, M.E. (1993) Sprouting and regeneration of lesioned corticospinal tract fibers in the adult rat spinal cord. *Eur. J. Neurosci.*, 5: 1156–1171

Schnell, L., Schneider, R., Kolbeck, R., Barde, Y.-A. and Schwab, M.E (1994) Neurotophin-3 enhances sprouting of corticospinal tract during development and after adult spinal cord lesion. *Nature*, 367: 170–173.

Schwab, M.E. and Caroni, P. (1988) Oligodendrocytes and fibroblast spreading *in vitro. J. Neurosci.*, 8: 2381–2393.

Shelton, D.L. and Reichardt, L.F. (1986) Studies on the expression of the β nerve growth factor (*NGF*) gene in the central nervous system: level and regional distribution of NGF mRNA suggest that NGF functions as a trophic factor for several distinct populations of neurons. *Proc. Natl. Acad. Sci. USA*, 83: 2714–2718.

Shioi, J., Pangalos, M.N., Ripellino, J.A., Vassilacopoulou, D., Mytilineou, C., Margolis, R.U. and Robakis, N.K. (1995) The Alzheimer amyloid precursor proteoglycan (Appican) is present in brain and is produced by astrocytes but not by neurons in primary neural cultures. *J. Biol. Chem.* 270: 11839–11844.

Silver, J. (1984) Studies on the factors that govern directionality of axonal growth in the embryonic optic nerve and at the chiasm of mice. *J. Comp. Neurol.*, 223: 238–251.

Silver, J. and Whittemore, S.R. (1997) *Exp. Neurol.*, 148, Number 2. R.P. Bunge memorial issue.

Snow, D., Lemmon, V., Carrino, D., Caplan, A. and Silver, J. (1990) Sulfated proteoglycans in astroglial barriers inhibit neurite outgrowth *in vitro. Exp. Neurol.*, 109: 111–130.

Snow, D., Watanabe, M., Letourneau, P. and Silver, J. (1991) A chondroitin sulfate proteoglycan may influence the direction of retinal ganglion cell outgrowth. *Development*, 113: 1473–1485.

Sonigra, R.J., Brighton, P.C., Jacoby, J., Hall, S. and Wigley, C.B. (1999) Adult rat olfactory nerve ensheathing cells are effective promoters of adult central nervous system neurite outgrowth in coculture. *Glia*, 25: 256–259.

Stenevi, U., Bjorklund, A. and Svendgaard, N.-A. (1976) Transplantation of central and peripheral monoamine neurons to the adult rat brain: techniques and conditions for survival. *Brain Res.*, 114: 1–20.

Streit, W.J., Graeber, M.B. and Kreutzberg, G.W. (1988) Functional plasticity of microglia: a review. *Glia*, 1: 301–307.

Sturrock, R.R. (1974) Histogenesis of the anterior limb of the anterior commissure of the mouse brain. A quantitative study of changes in the glial population with age. *J. Anat.*, 117: 17–25.

Sunde, N. and Zimmer, J. (1983) Cellular, histochemical and connective organization of the hippocampus and fascia dentata transplanted to different regions of immature and adult rat brain. *Dev. Brain Res.*, 8: 165–191.

Taylor, J.S., Muñetón, V.C., Bui, C., Gudiño-Cabrera, G. and Nieto-Sampedro, M. (1999) Reparación funcional del sistema sensorial tras rizotomía del plexo braquial mediada por trasplantes de glia envolvente. *Revista de Neurología*, 30: 256.

Taylor, J.S., Muñetón-Gómez, V.C., Eguía-Recuero, R. and Nieto-Sampedro, M. (2001) Transplants of olfactory bulb ensheathing cells promote functional repair of multiple dorsal rhizotomy. *Prog. Brain Res.*, 132: 651–664.

Tello, J.F. (1911) La influencia del neurotropismo en la regeneración de los centros nerviosos. *Trab. Lab. Invest. Biol.* 9: 123–159.

Tettamanti, G., Bonali, F., Marchesini, S. and Zambotti, V. (1973). A new procedure for the extraction, purification and fractionation of brain gangliosides. *Biochim. Biophys. Acta.*, 296: 160–170.

Thallmair, M., Metz, G.A.S., Graggen, W.J.Z., Raineteau, O., Kartje, G.L. and Schwab, M.E. (1998) Neurite growth inhibitors restrict plasticity and functional recovery following corticospinal tract lesions. *Nature Neurosci.*, 1: 124–131.

Theodosis, D.T. and MacVicar, B. (1996) Neurone–glia interactions in the hypothalamus and pituitary. *TINS*, 19: 363–367.

Thon, N., Haas, C.A., Rauch, U., Merten, T., Fässler, R., Frotscher, M. and Deller, T. (2000) The chondroitin sulphate proteoglycan brevican is upregulated by astrocytes after entorhinal cortex lesions in adult rats. *Eur. J. Neurosci.*, 12: 2547–2558.

Tommaselli, K.J., Neugebauer, K.M., Bixbey, J.L., Lilien, J. and Reichardt, L.F. (1988). N-Cadherin and integrins: two receptor system that mediate neuronal process outgrowth on astrocyte surface. *Neuron*, 1: 33–43.

Verdú, E., García-Alías, G., Forés, J., Gudiño-Cabrera, G., Nieto-Sampedro, M. and Navarro, X. (2001) Effects of ensheathing cells transplanted into photochemically damaged spinal cord. *NeuroReport*, 12: 2303–2309.

Wandosell, F., Bovolenta, P. and Nieto-Sampedro, M. (1990) Reactive astrocytes and dBcAMP-treated astrocytes have different surface markers. *Soc. Neurosci. Abst.*, 16: 351.

Wandosell, F., Bovolenta, P. and Nieto-Sampedro, M. (1993) Differences between reactive astrocytes and cultured astrocytes treated with Dibutiryl-cyclic AMP. *J. Neuropathol. Exper. Neurol.*, 52: 205–215.

Whittemore, S.R., Nieto-Sampedro, M., Needels, D. and Cotman, C.W. (1985) Neuronotrophic factors for mammalian brain neurons: injury induction in neonatal, adult and aged rat brain. *Develop. Brain Res.*, 20: 169–178.

Whittemore, S.R., Ebendal, T., Lärkfors, L., Olson, L., Seiger, A., Strömberg, I. and Persson, H. (1986) Developmental and regional expression of ß nerve growth factor mRNA and protein in the rat central nervous system. *Proc. Natl. Acad. Sci. USA*, 83: 817–821.

Wictorin, K., Fischer, W., Williams, L.R., Varon, S., Bjorklund, A. and Gage, F.H. (1985) Loss of acetylcholine esterase positive cells and choline acetyl transferase activity in the septal area and diagonal band of Broca following fimbria-fornix transection. *Soc. Neurosci. Abstr.* 11: 257.

Yamada, H., Watanabe, K., Shimonaka, M. and Yamaguchi, Y. (1994) Molecular cloning of brevican, a novel brain proteoglycan of the aggrecan/versican family. *J. Biol. Chem.*, 269: 10119–10126.

Yamada, H., Fredette, B., Shitara, K., Hagihara, K., Miura, R., Ranscht, B., Stallcup, W.B. and Yamaguchi, Y. (1997) The brain chondroitin sulfate proteoglycan brevican associates with astrocytes ensheathing cerebellar glomeruli and inhibits neurite outgrowth from granule neurons. *J. Neurosci.*, 17: 7784–7795.

E.C. Azmitia, J. DeFelipe, E.G. Jones, P. Rakic and C.E. Ribak (Eds.)
Progress in Brain Research, Vol. 136

CHAPTER 25

Neuroplasticity in the damaged dentate gyrus of the epileptic brain

Charles E. Ribak* and Khashayar Dashtipour[1]

Department of Anatomy and Neurobiology, University of California at Irvine, College of Medicine, Irvine, CA 92697-1275, USA

Abstract: Using Golgi preparations, Cajal described many cell types and connections of the dentate gyrus. He described granule cells as having a round or elliptical cell body with their long axis perpendicular to the granule cell layer, dendrites arising from one pole and an axon arising from the other. Cajal apparently never studied the brains from epileptic animals or humans, and thus did not report on changes in granule cell morphology after epilepsy. Several neuroplastic changes have been described in the dentate gyrus of epileptic mammals in the past decade or so using modern methods. Two changes involving their processes include mossy fiber sprouting of granule cell axons into the inner molecular layer of the dentate gyrus and the formation of hilar basal dendrites. Two changes associated with increased neurogenesis of granule cells in the epileptic brain include hilar ectopic granule cells and the dispersion of the granule cell layer. The significance of the first two changes is that granule cell axon collaterals establish additional synapses with apical and basal dendrites of granule cells, and these connections contribute to new recurrent excitatory circuitry. The significance of increased neurogenesis is that granule cells are migrating into inappropriate areas (deep hilus) or excessive numbers of granule cells accumulate in the layer (dispersion). These data on the epileptic dentate gyrus show that granule cells may change their axonal and dendritic arbors as well as their numbers and position to respond to altered activity possibly caused by decreased inhibition. These findings indicate that the dentate gyrus shows several neuroplastic changes following temporal lobe epilepsy.

Introduction

Santiago Ramón y Cajal described the morphology of the dentate gyrus in rodents and other mammals in his textbook, *the Histology of the Nervous System* (see Fig. 479 in Cajal, 1911). His scheme of this structure shows that granule cells, the main neuron type of the dentate gyrus, have a bipolar shape with apical dendrites arising from one pole and a single process emerging from the opposite pole. The axons of granule cells are characterized as having large mossy fibers in the hilus and stratum lucidum of

CA3 but also show smaller axon collaterals in the hilus. Cajal's addition of arrows to his drawings correctly demonstrated the direction in which messages from granule cells are forwarded to hilar neurons and the pyramidal cells of CA3.

These features of granule cells were used in the past decade to base a number of neuroplastic changes observed in the epileptic brain that were probably never envisioned by Cajal. However, it needs to be noted that Cajal was aware of chromatolytic (degenerative) changes of neurons, the loss of dendritic spines and the atrophy of dendrites in the brains of epileptic humans (Cajal, 1897). In the present chapter, we will show data that demonstrate four major neuroplastic changes in the epileptic brain. These include modification of the axonal projections of granule cells in that mossy fibers sprout into the inner molecular layer. Also, the formation of hilar basal

_____
*Corresponding author: Tel.: (949) 824-5494; Fax: (949) 824-8549;
E-mail: ceribak@uci.edu
[1]Department of Neurology, Southern Illinois University, School of Medicine, Springfield, IL 62794-9637, USA.

dendrites will be discussed as another neuroplastic change for the granule cell's processes. Two other changes involving granule cells in the epileptic brain are associated with an increased neurogenesis of granule cells. One is the abnormal migration of large numbers of granule cells into the hilus and the other is the thickening of the granule cell layer, often referred to as the dispersion of the granule cell layer. These changes represent important findings because they impact on the neural circuitry of the dentate gyrus. In fact, it will be shown that three of these changes contribute to additional recurrent excitatory circuitry in the brains of epileptic animals.

Mossy fiber sprouting

The sprouting of mossy fibers into the inner molecular layer is a well-known neuroplastic change that occurs in the dentate gyrus following seizures (Fig. 1). Previous studies of the hippocampus have demonstrated that axons in the developing and adult brain have the capacity for growth and synaptogenesis in response to a loss of neighboring axons (Cotman and Lynch, 1976). Studies by Sutula et al. (1989) and Represa et al. (1989) were the first to describe this phenomenon whereby mossy fibers sprouted axons into the inner molecular layer of the dentate gyrus from epileptic humans. Subsequent studies of human temporal lobes from epileptic patients confirmed this observation (Houser et al., 1990; Babb et al., 1991). In addition, several experimental models of epilepsy showed a similar morphological change (Nadler et al., 1980; Tauck and Nadler, 1985; Sutula et al., 1988; Cronin et al., 1992; Ribak et al., 1998). The significance of these findings is that the sprouted mossy fibers are in a position to form synapses with the apical dendrites of granule cells.

Several electron microscopic studies attempted to resolve this issue (Sutula et al., 1988; Babb et al., 1991; Represa et al., 1993; Franck et al., 1995; Okazaki et al., 1995; Ribak et al., 1998; Zhang and Houser, 1999). First, the sprouted axons needed to be identified as mossy fibers. Second, these axons needed to be shown to form asymmetric synapses with granule cell dendrites in the inner molecular layer. These studies demonstrated both points in rats, monkeys and humans. Thus, the targets of many sprouted mossy fibers are the proximal apical dendrites and dendritic spines of granule cells. These new

connections may provide a basis for spontaneous seizures in that the sprouted mossy fibers establish a novel recurrent excitatory circuit among granule cells.

Hilar basal dendrites

The formation of basal dendrites on granule cells is the most recently described neuroplastic change that was found in rats with status epilepticus using several anatomical methods, including the one used by Cajal, the Golgi method (Fig. 2). Hilar basal dendrites (HBDs) were shown in three different models of temporal lobe epilepsy, perforant path stimulation, kainic acid-induced and pilocarpine-induced (Spigelman et al., 1998; Buckmaster et al., 1999; Ribak et al., 2000). HBDs originate from the hilar pole of granule cell somata and then extend into the hilus for varying distances (Figs. 2 and 3). Less commonly they originate from the lateral sides of granule cell somata or from the base of the apical dendrites (Spigelman et al., 1998). HBDs could be a single basal dendrite or branched. Basically they are restricted to the subgranular region of the hilus, that part which is the first 50–100 μm subjacent to the granule cell layer. It was hypothesized that the loss of hilar neurons and their dendrites in the subgranular zone of epileptic rats acts as a catalyst for granule cells to sprout their dendrites into this region to replace a major postsynaptic target of mossy fibers (Spigelman et al., 1998). Although the exact cause of the formation of HBDs remains unclear, the presence of these dendrites in the hilus may be to produce additional recurrent excitatory circuits in the dentate gyrus of the epileptic brain.

Once again, this question was addressed using electron microscopy. Ribak et al. (2000) examined preparations from both pilocarpine and kainate models of temporal lobe epilepsy to determine whether HBDs provide an additional postsynaptic target for the large concentration of mossy fibers in the hilus. They observed labeled granule cell axon terminals forming asymmetric synapses with labeled HBDs (Fig. 4). Also, large mossy fiber boutons were presynaptic to HBDs of granule cells. These results indicated that new mossy fiber synapses with HBDs are formed following epilepsy and that these new synapses contribute to additional recurrent excitatory circuitry for granule cells (Fig. 5). If many granule cells are involved in this increased recurrent excitatory circuit, it could provide a basis for the increased excitability of granule cells and subsequent spontaneous seizures.

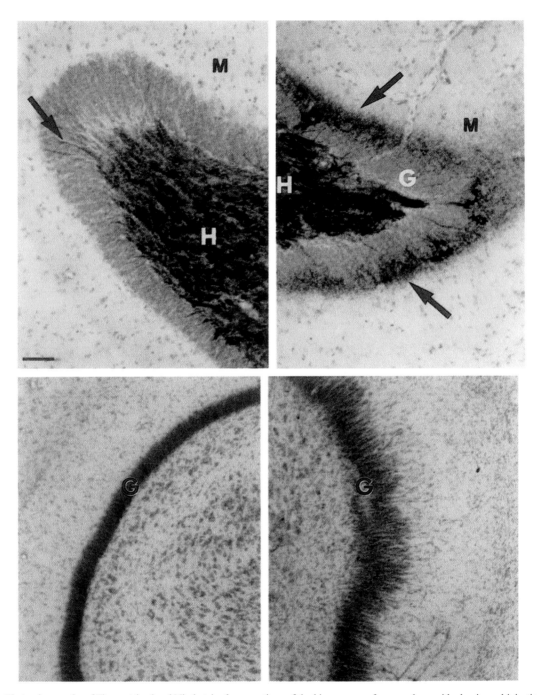

Fig. 1. Photomicrographs of Timm-stained and Nissl-stained preparations of the hippocampus from monkeys with alumina gel injections into the amygdala. **Top panels**—Timm stained sections from the control (left) and ipsilateral (right) sides of the dentate gyrus. The control side shows the normal distribution pattern of mossy fibers in the hilus (H) and a few fibers (arrow) in the granule cell layer (G) that are associated with interneurons. In contrast, the ipsilateral dentate gyrus shows massive sprouting of mossy fibers (arrows) into the inner molecular layer (M) of the dentate gyrus. **Bottom panels**—Nissl stained sections of the dentate gyrus to show a normal granule cell layer (G) on the **left** and granule cell dispersion on the **right**. Note the radially oriented rows of granule cells that extend into the molecular layer. Scale bar in top left panel = 100 μm for top panels and 200 μm for the bottom panels. Printed with permission from Ribak et al. (1998).

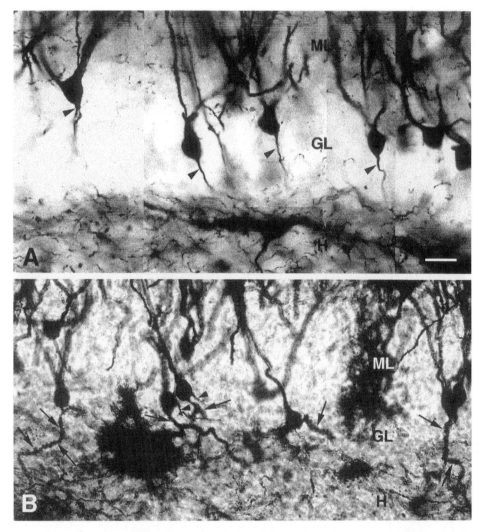

Fig. 2. Golgi-impregnated granule cells from control (**A**) and perforant path-stimulated (**B**) rats. Note the thin axons (arrowheads) emerging from the base of granule cells in the control preparation as described by Ramón y Cajal (1911). In contrast, the granule cells from the dentate gyrus from stimulated rats show basal dendrites (arrows) at the base of the granule cells. In these cases, the axons (arrowheads) are shifted to the side of the cell body. ML, molecular layer; GL, granule layer; H, Hilus. Scale bar = 10 μm. Reprinted with permission from Spigelman et al. (1998).

Neurogenesis of granule cells in the normal and epileptic dentate gyrus

Another neuroplastic change in the dentate gyrus involves the recent discovery that neurogenesis of granule cells occurs throughout adulthood. Altman and Das (1965) provided the first piece of evidence for postnatal hippocampal neurogenesis in rats using thymidine autoradiography. Later, other studies in the guinea-pig, rabbit and rhesus monkey also showed postnatal neurogenesis of granule cells but indicated that it was limited to a brief postnatal period (Altman and Das, 1967; Gueneau et al., 1982; Eckenhoff and Rakic, 1988). It appears that Kaplan and Hinds (1979) were the first to show adult neurogenesis of granule cells when they analyzed newly generated neurons in the electron microscope to show that they were postsynaptic to axon terminals. Subsequently, other studies have confirmed

323

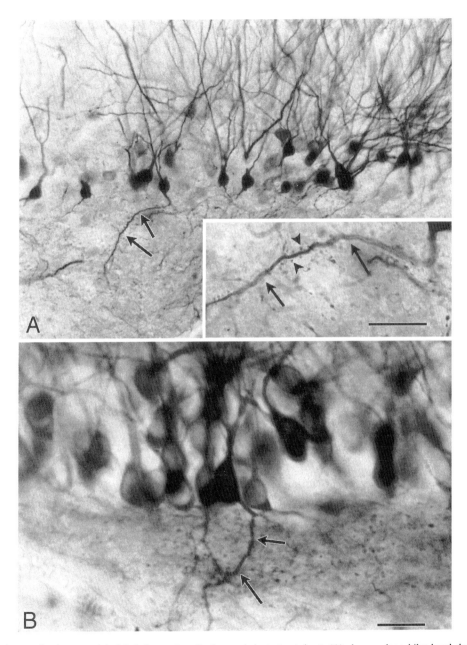

Fig. 3. Photomicrograph of retrogradely labeled granule cells from a kainate treated rat. (**A**) shows a long hilar basal dendrite (arrows) that arises from a labeled granule cell. The inset shows an enlargement of the same dendrite (arrows) and its dendritic spines (arrowheads). (**B**) Enlargement of another granule cell with a branched hilar basal dendrite (arrows). Scale bars = 50 μm in **A** and 10 microns in **B** and inset. Reprinted with permission from Ribak et al. (2000).

this observation in rats and humans (see Kempermann and Gage, 1999). It needs to be noted that newly generated granule cells are produced below the granule cell layer and migrate mainly into this layer.

The brains of epileptic rats were analyzed to determine whether the rate of neurogenesis in the granule cell layer of the dentate gyrus was affected. Parent et al. (1997) showed increased neurogenesis of granule cells following SE.

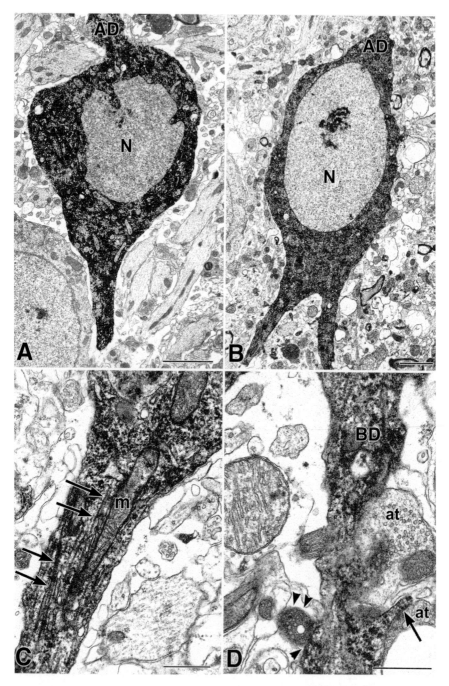

Fig. 4. Electron micrographs of retrogradely labeled granule cells with biocytin from control (**A**) and kainic acid treated (**B**) rats. (**A**) shows a normal granule cell with an unlabeled nucleus (N) showing a small dendrite (AD) arising from its apical pole and an axon from its opposite pole. (**B**) This labeled granule cell shows an axon and basal dendrite arising from its hilar pole and an apical dendrite (AD) from its opposite pole. Note the unlabeled nucleus. (**C**) Enlargement of the axon initial segment with a long thin mitochondrion (m) from the granule cell in **B**. (**D**) Enlargement of the basal dendrite (BD) of the granule cell in **B**. Note the two unlabeled axon terminals (at) apposed to this dendrite. One of them forms a synapse (arrow) with a spine. A labeled axon terminal (double arrowheads) forms a synapse (arrowhead) with the shaft of this basal dendrite. Scale bars = 2.5 microns in **A** and **B**; 0.5 microns in **C** and **D**. Reprinted with permission from Ribak et al. (2000).

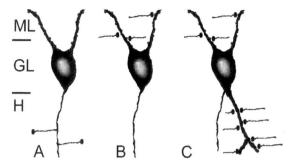

Fig. 5. Schematic diagram of granule cells from the normal and epileptic dentate gyrus. **A** shows a normal granule cell with its dendrites in the molecular layer (ML), cell body in the granule cell layer (GL) and axon and axon terminals (filled circles) in the hilus (H). **B** is a granule cell from a rat that had seizures and subsequent mossy fiber sprouting (3 axon terminals in the ML). Synapses made by these axon terminals provide the basis for a recurrent excitatory circuit. **C** shows a granule cell with a basal dendrite in the hilus that is postsynaptic to mossy fiber collaterals (7 axon terminals in H) and sprouted mossy fibers in the ML (3 axon terminals). The basal dendrite also contributes to new recurrent excitatory circuits in the epileptic brain. Reprinted with permission from Ribak et al. (2000).

Thus, status epilepticus stimulates neurogenesis of dentate granule cells, and hippocampal network plasticity associated with epileptogenesis may arise from aberrant connections formed by these newly born cells. Subsequent studies confirmed this finding in other models of temporal lobe epilepsy (Parent et al., 1998; Scott et al., 1998; Covolan et al., 2000; Nakagawa et al., 2000).

Increased neurogenesis might not only be involved in the aberrant connections formed by mossy fibers and HBDs of newly born granule cells but also might play a major role in inducing other morphological changes such as ectopic hilar granule cells and granule cell dispersion. The following sections will explore these two other phenomena of granule cells in the dentate gyrus of epileptic animals and humans. One of these, the appearance of many hilar ectopic granule cells after epilepsy, is most likely caused by increased neurogenesis and abnormal migration of granule cells (see Scharfman et al., 2000). The other section involves the dispersion of the granule cell layer that is most likely a result of increased neurogenesis of granule cells but the proof for this link is still elusive.

Hilar ectopic granule cells

Several investigators indicated that granule cell bodies may normally exist in the hilus of the dentate gyrus where they are referred to as ectopic granule cells (Amaral, 1978; Seress and Pokorny, 1981; Gaarskjaer and Laurberg, 1983; Marti-Subirana et al., 1986). Two studies have recently shown that such hilar ectopic granule cells are increased in number in the dentate gyrus of epileptic rats (Parent et al., 1997; Scharfman et al., 2000). Scharfman et al. (2000) observed a large increase in the number of calbindin immunoreactive neurons in the hilus after pilocarpine-induced status epilepticus. Such cells were identified using morphological and physiological parameters and were shown to be similar to granule cells. They suggested that the location of these granule cells in the deep hilus would contribute to the hyperexcitability found in this model of epilepsy. The electrophysiology of these hilar ectopic granule cells from epileptic rats indicated normal electrophysiological characteristics but they also discharged synchronously with spontaneous epileptiform bursts of CA3 pyramidal cells (Scharfman et al., 2000). This abnormal bursting property of hilar ectopic granule cells suggested that they receive mossy fiber input as do the CA3 pyramidal cells.

More recently, Dashtipour et al. (2001) analyzed hilar ectopic granule cells at the ultrastructural level using retrogradely transported biocytin that was injected into stratum lucidum of CA3 where mossy fibers send their axons. In this way, granule cells were labeled because they are the main cell type of the dentate gyrus with projections to this region (Fig. 6). They showed that for the most part hilar ectopic granule cells have similar ultrastructural features to those of granule cells in the granule cell layer (Dashtipour et al., 2001). However, a striking difference was shown in that hilar ectopic granule cells exclusively had asymmetric synapses on their somata and proximal dendrites. In fact, some of these synapses were made by labeled mossy fibers (Dashtipour et al., 2001). These results indicated that hilar ectopic granule cells are postsynaptic to mossy fibers contributing to additional recurrent excitatory circuitry. These latter results together with those of Scharfman et al. (2000) suggest that bursting of the relatively few hilar ectopic granule cells may recruit the normal granule cell population into epileptiform activity via their reciprocal synaptic connections. In this way, hilar ectopic granule cells could be critical for the synaptically driven reverberating excitation characteristic of the dentate gyrus in the epileptic, but not in the normal, brain.

326

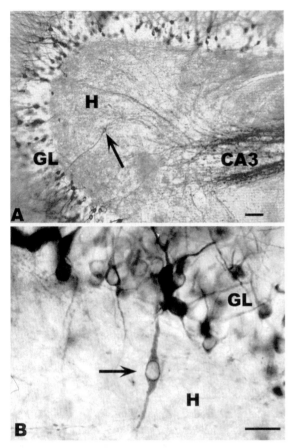

Fig. 6. Photomicrographs of biocytin-labeled granule cells from an epileptic rat. (**A**) shows a low magnification of the granule cell layer (GL) containing biocytin-labeled cells and the labeled bundle of mossy fibers in CA3. An ectopic biocytin-labeled granule cell (arrow) is shown in the hilus (H) with a long dendrite extending into the granule cell layer. (**B**) shows an enlargement of another biocytin-labeled ectopic granule cell in the hilus (H). Note the thick dendrite extending toward the GL and its long axis that is perpendicular to the hilar border with the GL. Scale bars = 50 μm in **A** and 25 μm in **B**. Reprinted with permission from Dashtipour et al. (2001).

Granule cell dispersion

Another feature that is observed in the dentate gyrus following epilepsy is the dispersion of the granule cell layer. Normally, the granule cell layer is densely packed and the cells are staggered and organized randomly (Seress, 1992). The dispersed granule cells were frequently aligned in columns (Fig. 1), and many of these neurons

displayed elongated bipolar forms. Also, the granule cell layer typically has a regular border with the molecular layer, but this border is irregular in the dentate gyrus from epileptic brains (Fig. 1). Houser (1990) provided a detailed qualitative description of granule cell dispersion in the brains of young patients with temporal lobe epilepsy (TLE). She suggested that the dispersion of granule cells is caused by a problem in neuronal migration. More recently, Ribak et al. (1998) induced complex partial seizures by alumina gel injections into the temporal lobe of rhesus monkeys. In addition to several behavioral, electrographic and pathological changes, they observed granule cell dispersion in adult monkeys ipsilateral to the injections while the contralateral hippocampus appeared normal (Fig. 1). The dispersed granule cells were analyzed with electron microscopy where they were shown to be organized in orthogonal rows with intervening radially oriented processes of reactive astrocytes (Fig. 7). It was suggested that the astrocytic processes caused the granule cells to form these linear arrays (Ribak et al., 1998). Thus, they proposed that granule cell dispersion is related to seizure activity and is not due to a developmental disorder as argued by Houser (1990).

The epileptic dentate gyrus characterized by dispersion of the granule cell layer appears to have greater numbers of granule cells than in the normal dentate gyrus. How are these extra granule cells generated? Experiments have not yet addressed this question, but it seems plausible that increased neurogenesis of granule cells, typically found in epileptic brains, may be playing a crucial role. Future studies will be needed to prove this suggestion.

Acknowledgments

The authors gratefully acknowledge our collaborators on these studies Drs. Igor Spigelman, Xiao-Xin Yan, Andy Obenaus, Claude Wasterlain, J. Victor Nadler, Maxine Okazaki, Roy Bakay, Peter Weber, Laszlo Seress, Charles Epstein, Thomas Henry and Peter Tran. We also acknowledge Dr. Bao Xue, Angela X. Torres and Alan M. Wong for comments on the manuscript. This book chapter is dedicated to the victims of the New York City World Trade Center attack on September 11, 2001. This work was supported by NIH grant NS 38331 to C.E. Ribak.

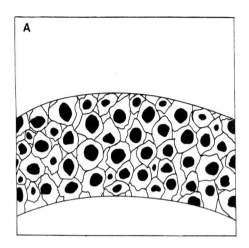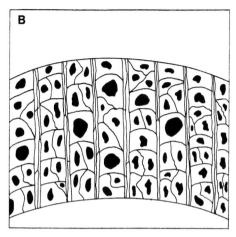

Fig. 7. Schematic diagram of granule cell dispersion. (**A**) shows the normal random distribution of granule cells in the granule cell layer from a control animal. (**B**) represents the changes from the ultrastructural findings from Ribak et al., (1998) where processes of reactive astrocytes radiate at regular intervals through the granule cell layer and cause granule cells to form linear arrangements. As a result the granule cell layer appears to thicken. It remains to be determined whether granule cell dispersion is caused by increased neurogenesis of granule cells that occurs in the epileptic brain.

References

Altman, J. and Das, G.D. (1965) Autoradiographic and histological evidence of postnatal hippocampal neurogenesis in rats. *J. Comp. Neurol.*, 124: 319–335.

Altman, J. and Das, G.D. (1967) Postnatal neurogenesis in the guinea-pig. *Nature*, 214: 1098–1101.

Amaral, D.G. (1978) A Golgi study of cell types in the hilar region of the hippocampus in the rat. *J. Comp. Neurol.*, 195: 851–914.

Babb, T.L., Kupfer, W.R., Pretorius, J.K., Crandall, P.H. and Levesque, M.F. (1991) Synaptic reorganization by mossy fibers in human epileptic fascia dentata. *Neurosci.*, 42: 351–363.

Buckmaster, P.S. and Dudek, F.E. (1999) In vivo intracellular analysis of granule cell axon reorganization in epileptic rats. *J. Neurophysiol.*, 81: 712–721.

Cajal, S.R. (1897) *Texture of the Nervous System of Man and the Vertebrates*, Springer, Vienna (translated by Pasik, P. and Pasik, T.).

Cajal, S.R. (1911) *Histologie du Systeme Nerveux de l'Homme et des Vertebres*, Vol. 2. Maloine, Paris.

Cotman, C.W. and Lynch, G.S. (1976) Reactive synaptogenesis in the adult nervous system: the effects of partial deafferentation on new synapse formation. In: S. Barondes (Ed.), *Neuronal Recognition*, Plenum Press, New York, pp. 109–130.

Covolan, L., Ribeiro, L.T., Longo, B.M. and Mello, L.E. (2000) Cell damage and neurogenesis in the dentate granule cell layer of adult rats after pilocarpine- or kainate-induced status epilepticus. *Hippocampus*, 10: 169–180.

Cronin, J., Obenaus, A., Houser, C.R. and Dudek, F.E. (1992) Electrophysiology of dentate granule cells after kainate-induced synaptic reorganization of the mossy fibers. *Brain Res.*, 573: 305–310.

Dashtipour, K., Tran, P.H., Okazaki, M.M., Nadler, J.V. and Ribak, C.E. (2001) Ultrastructural features and synaptic connections of hilar ectopic granule cells in the rat dentate gyrus are different from those of granule cells in the granule cell layer. *Brain Res.*, 890: 261–271.

Eckenhoff, M.F. and Rakic, P. (1988) Nature and fate of proliferative cells in the hippocampal dentate gyrus during the life span of the rhesus monkey. *J. Neurosci.*, 8: 2729–2747.

Franck, J.E., Pokorny, J., Kunkel, D.D. and Schwartzkroin, P.A. (1995) Phyisologic and morphologic characteristics of granule cell circuitry in human epileptic hippocampus. *Epilepsia*, 36: 543–558.

Gaarskjaer, F.B. and Laurberg, S. (1983) Ectopic granule cells of hilus fasciae dentatae projecting to the ipsilateral regio inferior of the rat hippocampus. *Brain Res.*, 274: 11–16.

Gueneau, G., Privat, A., Drouet, J. and Court, L. (1982) Subgranular zone of the dentate gyrus of young rabbits as a secondary matrix. A high-resolution autoradiographic study. *Dev. Neurosci.*, 5: 345–358.

Houser, C.R. (1990) Granule cell dispersion in the dentate gyrus of humans with temporal lobe epilepsy. *Brain Res.*, 535: 195–204.

Houser, C.R., Myashiro, J.E., Swartz, B.E., Walsh, G.O., Rich, J.R. and Delgado-Escueta, A.V. (1990) Altered patterns of dynorphin immunoreactivity suggest mossy fiber reorganization in human hippocampal epilepsy. *J. Neurosci.*, 10: 267–282.

Kaplan, M.S. and Hinds, J.W. (1979) Neurogenesis in the adult rat: electron microscopic analysis of light radioautographs. *Science*, 197: 1092–1094.

Kempermann, G. and Gage, F.H. (1999) New nerve cells for the adult brain. *Sci. Amer.*, 280: 48–53.

328

Marti-Subirana, A., Soriano, E. and Garcia-Verdugo, J.M. (1986) Morphological aspects of the ectopic granule-like cellular populations in the albino rat hippocampal formation: a Golgi study. *J. Anat.*, 144: 31–47.

Nadler, J.V., Perry, B.W. and Cotman, C.W. (1980) Selective reinnervation of hippocampal area CA1 and the fascia dentata after destruction of CA3–CA4 afferents with kainic acid. *Brain Res.*, 182: 1–9.

Nakagawa, E., Aimi, Y., Yasuhara, O., Tooyama, I., Shimada, M., McGeer, P.L. and Kimura, H. (2000) Enhancement of progenitor cell division in the dentate gyrus triggered by initial limbic seizures in rat models of epilepsy. *Epilepsia*, 41: 10–18.

Okazaki, M.M., Evenson, D.A. and Nadler, J.V. (1995) Hippocampal mossy fiber sprouting and synapse formation after status epilepticus in rats: visualization after retrograde transport of biocytin. *J. Comp. Neurol.*, 352: 515–534.

Parent, J.M., Yu, T.W., Leibowitz, R.T., Geschwind, D.H., Sloviter, R.S. and Lowenstein, D.H. (1997) Dentate granule cell neurogenesis is increased by seizures and contributes to aberrant network reorganization in the adult rat hippocampus. *J. Neurosci.*, 17: 3727–3738.

Parent, J.M., Janumpalli, S., McNamara, J.O. and Lowenstein, D.H. (1998) Increased dentate granule cell neurogenesis following amygdala kindling in the adult rat. *Neurosci. Lett.*, 247: 9–12.

Represa, A., Robain, O., Tremblay, E. and Ben-Ari, Y. (1989) Hippocampal plasticity in childhood epilepsy. *Neurosci. Lett.*, 99: 351–355.

Represa, A., Jorquera, I., Le Gal La Salle, G. and Ben-Ari, Y. (1993) Epilepsy-induced collateral sprouting of hippocampal mossy fibers: does it induce the development of ectopic synapses with granule cell dendrites? *Hippocampus*, 3: 257–268.

Ribak, C.E., Seress, L., Weber, P., Epstein, C.M., Henry, T.R. and Bakay, R.A.E. (1998) Alumina gel injections into the temporal lobe of rhesus monkeys cause complex partial seizures and morphological changes found in human temporal lobe epilepsy. *J. Comp. Neurol.*, 401: 266–290.

Ribak, C.E., Tran, P.H., Spigelman, I., Okazaki, M.M. and Nadler, J.V. (2000) Status epilepticus-induced hilar basal dendrites on rodent granule cells contribute to recurrent excitatory circuitry. *J. Comp. Neurol.*, 428: 240–253.

Scharfman, H.E., Goodman, J.H. and Sollas, A.L. (2000) Granule-like neurons at the hilar/CA3 border after status epilepticus and their synchrony with area CA3 pyramidal cells: functional implications of seizure-induced neurogenesis. *J. Neurosci.*, 20: 6144–6158.

Scott, B.W., Wang, S., Burnham, W.M., De Boni, U. and Wojtowicz, J.M. (1998) Kindling-induced neurogenesis in the dentate gyrus of the rat. *Neurosci. Lett.*, 248: 73–76.

Seress, L. (1992) Morphological variability and developmental aspects of monkey and human granule cells: differences between the rodent an d primate dentate gyrus. In: C.E. Ribak, C.M. Gall and I. Mody (Eds.), *The Dentate Gyrus and Its Role in Seizures*, Amsterdam, Elsevier, pp. 3–28.

Seress, L. and Pokorny, J. (1981) Structure of the granular layer of the rat dentate gyrus. *J. Anat.*, 133: 181–195.

Spigelman, I., Yan, X.-X., Obenaus, A., Lee, E.Y.-S., Wasterlain, C.G. and Ribak, C.E. (1998) Dentate granule cells form novel basal dendrites in a rat model of temporal lobe epilepsy. *Neurosci.*, 86: 109–120.

Sutula, T., Xiao-Xian, H. Cavazos, J. and Scott, G. (1988) Synaptic reorganization in the hippocampus induced by abnormal functional activity. *Science*, 239: 1147–1150.

Sutula, T., Cascino, G., Cavazos, J., Parada, I. and Ramirez, L. (1989) Mossy fiber synaptic reorganization in the epileptic human temporal lobe. *Ann. Neurol.*, 26: 321–330.

Tauck, D.L. and Nadler, J.V. (1985) Evidence of functional mossy fiber sprouting in hippocampal formation of kainic acid treated rats. *J. Neurosci.*, 5: 1016–1022.

Zhang, N, and Houser, C.R. (1999) Ultrastructural localization of dynorphin in the dentate gyrus in human temporal lobe epilepsy: a study of reorganized mossy fiber synapses. *J. Comp. Neurol.*, 405: 472–490.

Complex connections and organization

E.C. Azmitia, J. DeFelipe, E.G. Jones, P. Rakic and C.E. Ribak (Eds.)
Progress in Brain Research, Vol. 136
© 2002 Elsevier Science B.V. All rights reserved

CHAPTER 26

Complex connections and organization (an overview)

Ricardo Martínez Murillo*

Instituto Cajal (CSIC), Avenida del Doctor Arce 37, 28002 Madrid, Spain

As the Director of the Cajal Institute (CSIC) in Madrid, it gave me a great deal of pleasure to participate in the first meeting of the Cajal Club to be held outside of the United States. It was also a great honor to be able to welcome such a host of distinguished neuroscientists to Madrid, each a leader in their field. As well as the special tribute paid to Cajal by holding this meeting in Spain, the wide variety of areas within the field of the neurosciences that were covered and the diversity of the individual contributions served to emphasize the influence that his original studies have had on the field. As such, it is easy to see why many consider Santiago Ramón y Cajal as the founding father of modern neuroscience.

The Cajal Club/Cajal Institute International Conference provided an opportunity for the participants to get together and discuss questions of general interest to neuroscientists. Particular attention was paid during the meeting to Cajal's original concepts, reported about 100 years ago, and how they have shaped our current thinking as well as how they have evolved. The way in which we conceive the neuron was addressed from many different viewpoints, relative to those first formulated by Cajal at the end of the 19th and beginning of the 20th centuries.

This section contains chapters that include review data and original results on: (i) the understanding of the functional organization of the spinal cord (by P. Rudomin), (ii) modern methods for identifying classes of thalamic neurons and the intrinsic circuitry of the thalamus (by Edward G. Jones), (iii) the basal forebrain organization (by L. Zaborszky), (iv) anatomical substrates for the visual receptive fields of single neurons and for their surrounding (by A. Angelucci, J. B. Levitt and J. S. Lund), (v) and the structural and functional organization of the visual cortex (by V. A. Casagrande, X. Xu, and G. Sáry).

The present review by Rudomin examines the experimental evidence supporting the existence of central mechanisms able to modulate the synaptic effectiveness of sensory fibers ending in the spinal cord of vertebrates. Rudomin emphasizes that *"we are just at the beginning of the road"* for the understanding of the rather complex structure of the spinal cord and that particular attention should be paid on the functional role of the mechanisms of presynaptic control. Cajal's discoveries strengthened the view that the spinal cord is a rather complex structure contributing to the concept that the spinal cord is composed of many different classes of neurons that receive specific connections from other neuronal elements. Frank and Fuortes described in 1957 a new mechanism for the regulation of the synaptic effectiveness of sensory fibers in the vertebrate spinal cord, namely presynaptic inhibition. It was not until the early sixties that Eccles and his collaborators related this inhibition to primary afferent depolarization (PAD; for review see Rudomin and Schmidt, *Exp. Brain Res.*, 129: 1–37, 1999). Today, it is well known that the synaptic effectiveness of sensory fibers ending in the spinal cord of vertebrates can be centrally controlled by means of specific sets of GABAergic interneurons that establish axo-axonic synapses with the terminal arborizations of the afferent fibers. It seems that the intraspinal branches of the sensory fibers are not hard wired routes that diverge excitation to spinal neurons,

*Corresponding author: Tel.: 91 5854 752; Fax: 91 5854 754;
E-mail: director.inrc@csic.es

in the 20–50 Hz ("40 Hz") range are embedded in the so-called desynchronized wave form of the awake electroencephalogram (Steriade and Amzica, 1996; Timofeev and Steriade, 1997; Steriade, 2001).

An effect of corticothalamic stimulation on relay cells is inhibition, leading to spindle oscillations

Despite the obvious glutamatergic nature of corticothalamic synapses, which is evidenced by the ability to record

NMDA-, AMPA- and metabotropic glutamate receptor-based EPSCs in relay cells under appropriate conditions (Figs. 9, 10) (McCormick and von Krosigk, 1992; Kao and Coulter, 1997; Golshani et al., 1998; Turner and Salt, 1998), another effect of corticothalamic stimulation on relay cells is the disynaptic, feed-forward inhibition resulting from coactivation of the reticular nucleus. A single weak electrical pulse applied to the corticothalamic fibers leads to a small, short latency EPSP in a relay cell, but this is quickly obliterated by a deep and prolonged IPSP lasting up to 100 ms and representing the input from the reticular nucleus

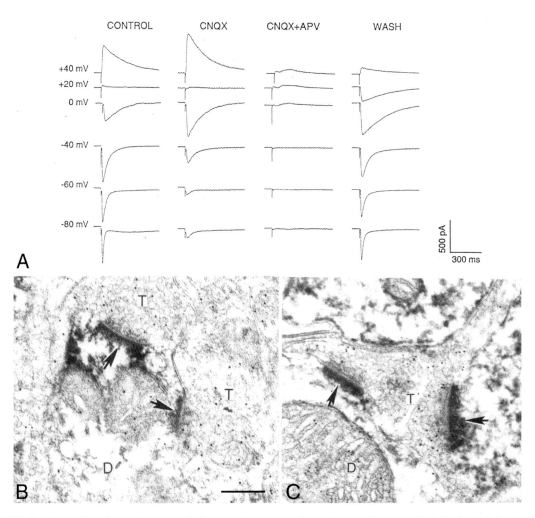

Fig. 9. **A.** Whole cell recordings from a relay neuron in the ventral posterior nucleus of a mouse thalamocortical slice *in vitro*, showing EPSCs recorded in response to stimulation of corticothalamic fibers, in the presence of AMPA (CNQX) and NMDA (APV) receptor antagonists. From Golshani et al. (1998). **B,C.** Electron micrographs of glutamate immunoreactive corticothalamic axon terminals (T) ending on dendrites at synapses in which the postsynaptic densities (arrows) are strongly immunoreactive for NMDA (A) and AMPA (B) receptors. Bar 0.5 μm.

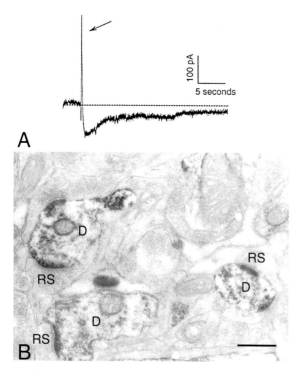

A

B

Fig. 10. **A.** Long lasting EPSC representing metabotropic glutamate receptor-based response of a relay cell to stimulation of cortico-thalamic fibers in the presence of NMDA, AMPA- and GABA$_A$-receptor antagonists. Arrow indicates preceding GABA$_B$-mediated IPSC. From Golshani et al. (1998). **B.** Corticothalamic terminals (RS) in the ventral posterior nucleus of a rat, ending on dendrites that are strongly immunoreactive for metabotropic glutamate receptor mGluR$_{1a}$. Bar 0.5 μm.

(Fig. 11A). This IPSP can be shown, as would be expected, to consist of both GABA$_A$ and GABA$_B$ receptor-mediated components. The importance of corticothal-amic-induced inhibition of the relay cells is that it drives them towards the burst firing mode. As they recover from this inhibition, the low threshold calcium conductance is deinactivated and the cells fire a burst of action potentials (Fig. 11B). This has the effect of re-exciting, via the collaterals of thalamocortical fibers, the reticular nucleus cells which then fire a new burst of action potentials. These re-inhibit the relay cells which burst again on recovering, and so the cycle continues at 7–14 Hz, the spindle frequency. Recordings made simultaneously from reticular nucleus and relay cells in the underlying ventral posterior nucleus clearly demonstrate synchrony of their discharges at spindle frequencies, as well as

the synaptic interplay between the two sets of cells (Fig. 11C). The initial effect of corticothalamic activation upon the reticular nucleus cell is a steeply-rising EPSP, leading to a short train of action potentials (Fig. 11B). That on the relay cells is predominantly the disynaptic inhibition described above, succeeded by a burst of action potentials. Re-excitation of the reticular nucleus cell is evident in the second and subsequent trains of discharges, all of which are preceded by a step-wise EPSP in which each step increment in amplitude can be correlated with one of the action potentials of the burst in a connected relay cell. Each successive event in the oscillation of the relay cell is a facsimile of its predecessor: inhibition succeeded by burst firing (von Krosigk et al., 1993; Warren et al., 1994; Bal et al., 1995).

Apart from causing repetitive burst firing in relay cells, a reticular nucleus cell, by reason of the widespread terminations of its axon alone, has the effect of distributing the disynaptic inhibitory effects of corticothalamic stimulation across many relay cells, thus helping to promote synchrony throughout the whole thalamo-cortico-thalamic network. Spread of corticothalamic effects across many reticular nucleus cells and recruitment of others by collateral inputs from the thalamo-cortical axons of bursting relay cells will also serve to spread spindle oscillations across most of the thalamus and cortex. Studies *in vivo* indicate that spindle oscillations start more or less simultaneously throughout the thalamus, rather than spreading slowly across it (early reports of slowly spreading synchrony *in vitro* are thought to have been due to absence of intact corticothalamic connections in the preparation) (Kim et al., 1995; Steriade and Amzica, 1996). The simultaneous onset of spindles throughout cortex and thalamus implies rapid diffusion of reticular nucleus effects on relay cells and equally rapid collateral excitation of widespread sectors of the reticular nucleus by bursting relay cells. Although the corticothalamic system is particularly powerful in inducing spindle oscillations, it is the reticular nucleus that is the prime mover in synchronizing the oscillations of virtually all cells in the network. Its capacity to do this is enhanced when the weak inhibitory effects of one reticular nucleus cell on another are removed (Sohal et al., 2000).

The power of the corticothalamic projection to induce low frequency oscillations in the spindle range clearly depends upon the capacity of the disynaptic inhibitory effect of the reticular nucleus to overcome the direct,

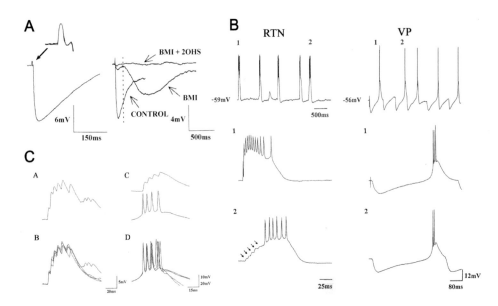

Fig. 11. **A.** Left panel: Whole cell recording from a relay neuron in the ventral posterior nucleus of a mouse thalamocortical slice *in vitro*, showing that a single weak electrical stimulus (arrow) applied to the corticothalamic fibers elicits a small monosynaptic EPSP that is quickly obliterated by the deep and long lasting disynaptic IPSP which reflects the collateral corticothalamic excitation of the reticular nucleus. Right panel shows that this IPSP consists of GABA$_A$ and GABA$_B$ components revealed by application of selective antagonists bicuculline (BMI) and 2-hydroxysaclofen (2OHS). **B.** Low frequency oscillations induced by a single, weak electrical stimulus to corticothalamic fibers in two neurons of the reticular (RTN) and ventral posterior (VP) nucleus of the mouse thalamocortical slice. First response on the part of the RTN cell is a steep EPSP surmounted by a burst of action potentials. First and all subsequent responses of the VP cell are characterized by the disynaptic inhibition from RTN cells, with burst firing as the cell recovers from the hyperpolarization. Second and subsequent responses of the RTN cell are characterized by step-wise pattern of increasing EPSP amplitude, reflecting collateral excitation from axons of the bursting VP cell, leading to renewed burst firing. **C.** Details of single (A, C) and superimposed repreated EPSCs in RTN cells and of bursts of action potentials (C, D) in a connected VP Cell. B,C from Warren et al. (1994).

monosynaptic excitatory effect of corticothalamic fibers upon the relay cells of the dorsal thalamus. To effect this, the strength of the corticothalamic input to the reticular nucleus should, of necessity, be stronger than that to the relay cells. Modeling studies in which the inputs to reticular nucleus relay cells are set at equal strengths result in a failure to elicit oscillatory activity in the network (Destexhe et al., 1998). How can synapses made by branches of the same axons on reticular nucleus cells and relay cells differ in strength or efficacy? Recent observations provide a resolution of this dilemma.

Using a minimal stimulation paradigm and low Ca^{2+} conditions in which the probability of vesicle release is reduced to close to zero, it is possible to record unitary EPSCs in relay cells and reticular nucleus cells in response to stimulation of a small number of corticothalamic fibers (Fig. 12). Under these conditions, and with GABA and NMDA receptor-based responses excluded, corticothalamic EPSCs in the reticular nucleus cells are nearly three times larger than in relay cells (Fig. 12B) (Golshani et al., 2001). A basis for this difference in AMPA-receptor based synaptic strength has been discovered in the presence of nearly three times as many GluR$_4$ receptor subunits at the corticothalamic synapses on the reticular nucleus cells than at corticothalamic synapses on relay cells (Fig. 12C, D). GluR$_3$ subunits are present in equal numbers and GluR$_1$ and GluR$_2$ subunits are not expressed in the thalamus (Liu et al., 2001). Hence, corticothalamic synapses on reticular nucleus cells are enriched with GluR$_4$ receptor subunits, and increases in channel opening time consequent upon this enrichment should account for the larger EPSCs in the reticular nucleus cells.

Collateral corticothalamic and thalamocortical inputs to reticular nucleus cells possess different properties

As mentioned above, in *in vitro* slices of rodent thalamus, it is possible to separate in reticular nucleus cells' EPSCs derived from orthodromic activation of corticothalamic fibers and EPSCs derived from collaterals of antidromically activated thalamocortical axons on the basis of latency (Fig. 13) (Liu et al., 2001). In the mouse thalamocortical slice, minimal EPSCs elicited in reticular nucleus cells by antidromic invasion of thalamocortical collaterals occur at latencies of less than 3 ms while those elicited by orthodromic activation of the thinner corticothalamic fibers occur with latencies longer than 6 ms. The amplitudes of minimal corticothalamic EPSCs are remarkably consistent, probably reflecting the presence of a single vesicle release site at the relatively small,

single synaptic contacts (Fig. 13). The rise times of these EPSCs are, however, quite variable, reflecting the scatter of corticothalamic terminals across the dendritic tree of the reticular nucleus cell. By contrast, minimal EPSCs resulting from activation of thalamocortical collateral synapses in reticular nucleus cells have variable amplitudes, reflecting the presence of multiple release sites at the large perforated synaptic contacts with their multiple synaptic segments (Fig. 13). Rise times are, however, very consistent, reflecting the localization of the thalamocortical synapses close to the cell soma. Unlike the corticothalamic synapses at which $GluR_4$ receptor subunits are enriched in comparison with $GluR_3$ subunits. $GluR_4$ and $GluR_3$ subunits appear in equal proportions at collateral thalamocortical synapses (Figs. 12, 13). At the larger collateral thalamocortical synapses, however, the overall number of AMPA receptor subunits is much higher than at the corticothalamic

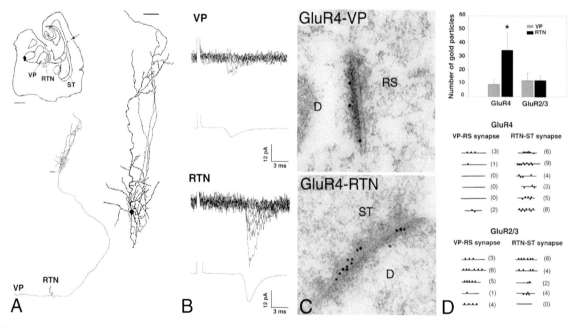

Fig. 12. **A.** Location and camera lucida drawings of a typical layer VI corticothalamic cell from a mouse thalamocortical slice preparation. The axon branches to innervate both the reticular nucleus (RTN) and the ventral posterior nucleus (VP). **B.** 10 superimposed consecutive traces and their mean, showing EPSCs recorded from a VP cell and an RTN cell in response to minimal stimulation of corticothalamic fibers. Minimnal EPSCs in RTN cells have approximately three times greater amplitudes than those in VP cells. **C.** Immunogold labeling for GluR4 receptor subunits at corticothalamic (RS) synapses in VP and RTN showing larger number of particles in the RTN. **D.** Quantification of immunogold particles representing GluR4 and GluR 2/3 receptor subunits at postsynaptic densities of four serially sectioned corticothalamic synapses in VP and RTN. Number of GluR4 particles at corticothalamic synapses on RTN cells are approximately three times greater than at corticothalamic synapses on VP cells. From Golshani et al. (2000).

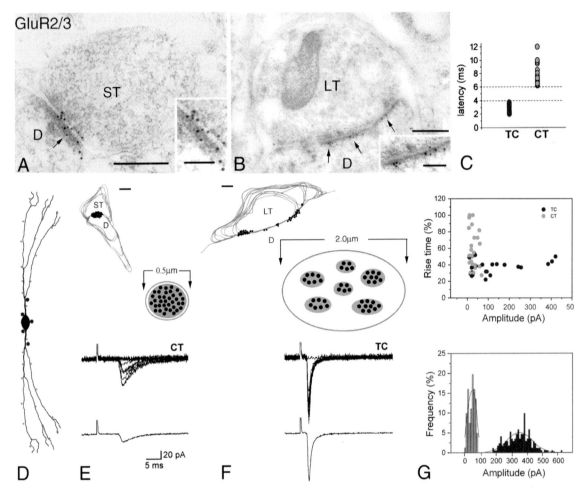

Fig. 13. **A,B**. Electron micrographs of terminals of corticothalamic (ST) and thalamocortical (LT) collaterals in the reticular nucleus of a mouse, showing immunogold labeling for GluR2 and 3 receptor subunits at their synapses. Corticothalamic terminals are characterized by a single vesicle release site, thalamocortical collateral terminals by multiple release sites (arrows). Bars 0.25 μm and 0.1 μm (insets). **C.** Bimodal latencies of EPSCs recorded from reticular nucleus cells in response to stimulation of subcortical white matter. Shorter latency responses reflect antidromic invasion of thalamocortical fibers (TC) and excitation of reticular cells via their collaterals. Longer latency EPSC's represent orthodromic activation of corticothalamic (CT) collaterals. **D.** Schematic view of a reticular nucleus cell showing proximal location of thalamocortical collateral synapses and more distributed distribution of corticothalamic collateral synapses. **E,F.** Upper: reconstructions from serial electron micrographs of corticothalamic (ST) and thalamocortical (LT) collateral synapses terminating on dendrites (D) of reticular nucleus cells, with the postsynaptic densities immunogold labeled for GluR 2/3 subunits. En face views of each synapse indicate single release sites at thalamocortical collateral synapse and multiple release sites at thalamocortical collateral synapse. Lower: overlay of 10 successive EPSCs and mean of these EPSCs recorded from reticular nucleus cells in response to minimal stimulation of corticothalamic or thalamocortical fibers. Minimal thalamocortical EPSCs have larger amplitudes and faster rise and decay times than minimal corticothalamic EPSCs. **G.** Upper: rise times of minimal thalamocortical EPSCs are relatively constant, reflecting proximal location of synapses, but amplitudes vary, probably reflecting wider variability in number of release sites. Minimal corticothalamic EPSCs have variable rise times reflecting more undespread distribution of the synapses, but constant amplitudes, reflecting the single release site. Based on Liu et al. (2001).

synapses. This may provide the capacity for the powerful re-entrant excitation of the reticular nucleus cells by bursts of action potentials in relay cells during the course of spindle oscillations. Some of the variance in the rise times of the EPSCs engendered in reticular nucleus cells by the thalamocortical collaterals may be attributable to the variable number of subunits located at each of the segments of the perforated synapse.

Interactions between cortex and thalamus during high frequency oscillatory activity

Although by no means universally accepted (Shadlen and Movshon, 1999), current thinking looks to coherent, higher frequency oscillations of large populations of cortical and thalamic neurons in the γ (20–50 Hz) range as concomitants of forebrain activities that underlie perception, cognition and directed attention (Llinás and Paré, 1991, 1997; Singer and Gray, 1995). In the sensory systems of the cerebral cortex, large scale synchrony of neurons in the areas that form links in the chain of corticocortical processing is thought necessary to ensure the binding of separate elements of sensory experience into a single cognitive event. It is inconceivable, however, that the thalamic nuclei with which these areas are reciprocally connected should not also oscillate in synchrony with these cortical areas. In seeking for thalamocortical connections that might serve to disperse thalamic activity across multiple cortical areas, attention in the past has tended to focus on the intralaminar nuclei which have traditionally been thought to possess axons that project diffusely to the cortex and to terminate there in layer I on the peripheral apical dendritic branches of pyramidal cells of all layers. Attractive as this hypothesis may seem, it rests upon evidence that is at best incomplete. It is now clear that the classical intralaminar nuclei project to relatively restricted regions of the cerebral cortex, that their axons are not excessively widely distributed and some appear to end in deeper layers rather than in layer I (reviewed in Steriade et al., 1997a). Moreover, a large number of intralaminar cells, perhaps the majority, project not to the cortex at all but to the striatum. This striatal projection of the intralaminar nuclei, unknown to Cajal, remains little investigated, even today. In circuit diagrams of the basal ganglia and thalamus used to "explain" the pathophysiology of movement disorders, it commonly goes unrepresented (Jones, 2001a).

Recent findings in monkeys reveal a hitherto unrecognized pattern of thalamic organization that provides a basis for the dispersion of thalamic activity across multiple cortical areas and for recruiting large constellations of thalamic and cortical neurons in synchronous activity that underlies discrete cognitive events (Jones, 1998a,b; 2001b). The data upon which this hypothesis rests are described in the following section.

The core and matrix of the primate thalamus

Immunocytochemical staining for the two major calcium binding proteins, parvalbumin and 28 kDa calbindin, reveals two distinct classes of relay neurons in the thalamus of monkeys and certain other primates (Jones and Hendry 1989; Diamond et al., 1993) (Fig. 14). Neurons immunoreactive for calbindin are distributed widely throughout the dorsal thalamus and can be found in every nucleus, however defined—relay, intralaminar, nonspecific, etc. Parvalbumin immunoreactive cells, by contrast, are found in certain nuclei only, typically in the principal sensory and motor relay nuclei, certain nuclei of the pulvinar and in some intralaminar nuclei. They are absent from all other dorsal thalamic nuclei. When present, they are typically found in large, dense clusters associated with densely terminating afferent fibers which are themselves parvalbumin immunoreactive. They appear as a core imposed on a diffuse background matrix of calbindin cells, hence the terminology used to describe the two cell classes. Calbindin cells tend to be slightly smaller than parvalbumin cells but are much larger than the intrinsic GABAergic neurons (Rausell et al., 1992). Unlike in some species such as cats, the intrinsic GABA cells do not express parvalbumin. The reticular nucleus cells do but these are not relay cells.

In some locations, there is a superficial impression of complementarity in the distributions of calbindin and parvalbumin cells and, where parvalbumin cells are absent, calbindin cells often appear in increased numbers. In the dorsal lateral geniculate nucleus, parvalbumin cells are found only in the magno- and parvocellular layers, while calbindin cells are concentrated in the S layers and interlaminar plexuses between these layers (Jones and Hendry, 1989; Hendry and Calkins, 1998) (Fig. 15). Closer inspection reveals, however, that the calbindin cells spread throughout the nucleus and are continuous with the larger population of calbindin cells in the adjoining inferior pulvinar nucleus (Jones, 1998a). In the ventral posterior nucleus zones of calbindin only cells are intercalated among the larger masses of parvalbumin cells and are especially concentrated in a parvalbumin absent zone along the posteromedial border of the ventral posterior medial (VPM) nucleus (Figs. 14, 15). Here, they are continuous with the larger population of calbindin cells in the posterior nucleus and anterior pulvinar nucleus. In the medial geniculate complex,

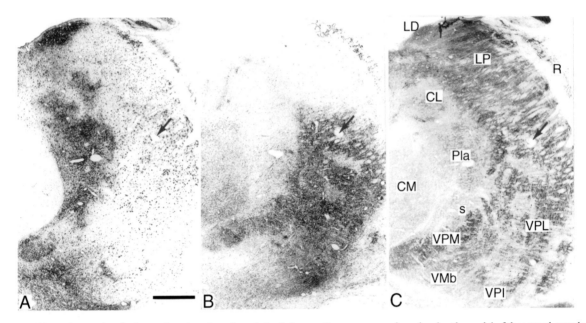

Fig. 14. Photomicrographs of adjacent frontal sections through the thalamus of a macaque monkey, showing the nuclei of the ventral complex stained immunocytochemically for calbindin (A), or parvalbumin (B), or histochemically for cytochrome oxidase (C). Note the restriction or concentration of parvalbumin core cells in certain nuclei, the widespread distribution of calbindin matrix cells, their increased concentration in nuclei from which core cells are absent, and the correlation of weak cytochrome oxidase activity with the concentration of matrix cells. Arrows indicate profiles of the same sectioned blood vessel. Bar 0.5 mm. From Jones (2001b).

the ventral nucleus is dominated by parvalbumin cells with only a few background calbindin cells of the matrix (Fig. 15). The more anterior of the dorsal nuclei has a mixed population of the two cell types, while the posterior dorsal nucleus possesses mainly calbindin cells, continuous with those of the inferior pulvinar nucleus. The magnocellular nucleus exhibits islands of calbindin cells alternating with islands of parvalbumin cells. In all nuclei where parvalbumin cells are concentrated, metabolic activity is high and histochemical staining for enzymes such as cytochrome oxidase (CO) is correspondingly high. Calbindin-rich zones, however, show weak CO staining (Fig. 14).

Parvalbumin cells and calbindin cells project differently upon the cerebral cortex. Parvalbumin cells show the well-known topographically organized projection in which adjacent groups of cells project to adjacent regions of one or at most two cytoarchitectonic areas of the cortex where they terminate in small (~600 μm), localized zones of terminals in the middle layers (deep III and IV) (Fig. 16). Calbindin cells, by contrast, project more diffusely. Adjacent cells can project to separated zones of cortex, including to different (though usually adjacent)

cortical areas (Rausell et al., 1991a, 1992). In these areas, their axons terminate in superficial layers (I, II and upper III). Every thalamic nucleus that contains both parvalbumin and calbindin cells, thus, has both focused, area-specific, middle-layer projections from parvalbumin cells of the core, and diffuse superficial-layer projections from calbindin cells of the matrix that are unconstrained by borders between functional areas in the cerebral cortex (Fig. 16). This dual projection can be found in both relay nuclei and the intralaminar nuclei. In nuclei in which only calbindin cells are found, diffuse superficial layer projections predominate. These may have a special significance, as outlined below.

The focused and diffuse characters of axonal projections to the cerebral cortex from core and matrix cells is reflected in their inputs from subcortical afferent pathways. Nuclei characterized by a high density of parvalbumin core cells, such as the ventral posterior nucleus, laminar dorsal lateral geniculate nucleus, and the ventral medial geniculate nucleus receive the terminations of ascending afferent pathways that are typically highly organized topographically and in which neurons at the various relay stations exhibit highly localized receptive fields and specific stimulus-response properties. The fibers of these pathways, e.g. the medial lemniscus, P and M components of the optic tract, and the brachium of the inferior colliculus are themselves parvalbumin immunoreactive and terminate in localized, topographically ordered domains within the borders of the parvalbumin core.

Nuclei and portions of nuclei characterized by a high density of calbindin matrix cells, on the other hand, typically receive the terminations of ascending pathways such as the spinothalamic tract and brainstem tegmental auditory pathways that are more diffusely organized, less directly connected with their peripheral receptors, and whose fiber terminations characteristically spread quite diffusely through large regions of the thalamus unrestricted by borders between nuclei (Fig. 15). Neurons

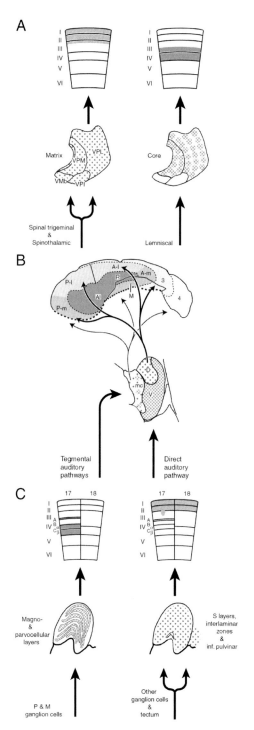

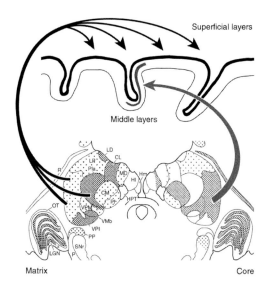

Fig. 16. Lower part of figure shows relative distributions and concentrations of calbindin matrix cells (left) and parvalbumin core cells (right) in a frontal section through the middle of a macaque monkey thalamus. Upper part of figure shows schematically the projection of the matrix to superficial layers of cortex over a relatively wide extent and unconstrained by borders between areas. Core cells restricted to individual nuclei, here exemplified by the ventral posterior nucleus, project in topographically ordered manner upon middle layers of single functional cortical fields. From Jones (2001b).

Fig. 15. Schematic views of diffuse and focused subcortical inputs to the matrix and core compartments of the ventral posterior (A), medial geniculate (B) and lateral geniculate (C) nuclei of the macaque monkey, their layer-specific and widespread and focused projections to the cerebral cortex. In A and C, cortical areas are indicated by schematic vertical sections with the layers indicated; in B the surface of the supratemporal plane with the auditory fields delineated by different intensities of parvalbumin immunoreactivity are indicated. Based on Jones (2001b).

receiving inputs from the less direct auditory pathways in the dorsal nuclei of the medial geniculate complex, for example, are not tonotopically organized, fatigue easily and tend to require novel stimuli to activate them. The spinothalamic tract, although containing a population of nociceptive-specific fibers is dominated by fibers with large receptive fields and multi-modal inputs. Patch-like terminations of these fibers are found wherever there are calbindin rich zones in and around the ventral posterior nucleus (Rausell et al., 1992). In the dorsal lateral geniculate nucleus, fibers ascending from the deeper layers of the superior colliculus and terminating in large numbers in the calbindin-rich inferior pulvinar nucleus, spill over into the dorsal lateral geniculate nucleus and terminate among the matrix cells of the S layers and interlaminar plexuses. These matrix regions are also innervated specifically by the least well characterized population of retinal ganglion cells which includes blue-on cells but apparently many other types as well (Martin et al., 1997).

Two kinds of corticothalamic fiber have different patterns of thalamic termination

Retrograde labeling studies have for many years shown that although the majority of cells projecting to a particular thalamic nucleus are found in layer VI of the cortical area related to that nucleus, a smaller but significant number is almost invariably found in layer V of the same area (Steriade et al., 1997a). Studies in rodents and carnivores have revealed not only that layer VI and layer V corticothalamic cells have very different morphologies but also that the terminations of their fibers adopt very different ramification and terminal patterns in the thalamus.

Corticothalamic neurons of layer VI typically are small, modified pyramidal cells with a narrow, ascending dendritic field centered on a short apical dendrite that ends in the middle layers of the cortex among the terminations of thalamocortical fibers (Fig. 4). Here, they receive monosynaptic inputs from the thalamocortical fibers. The axon of a layer VI corticothalamic cell, before leaving the cortex, gives off two or three recurrent collaterals which typically ascend within the confines of or closely adjacent to the vertical dendritic field of the cell (Ojima et al., 1992; Ojima, 1994). Each cell, therefore, influences a relatively narrow zone of the cortical area in

which it lies. The primary axon of the cell is directed only to the thalamus. As it enters the thalamus it gives off one or two short collaterals in the reticular nucleus and then terminates in a relatively narrow zone, in appropriate topographic order, only in the dorsal thalamic nucleus from which its parent cortical area receives input (Fig. 4). Some deep layer VI cells in rodents can have terminations extending across two related nuclei such as the ventral posterior and medial nucleus of the posterior group (Hoogland et al., 1987; Bourassa et al., 1995). Although ending in a relatively restricted zone of the related thalamic nucleus, the terminals of a single layer VI corticothalamic cell can apparently influence thalamic relay cells that project to regions of cortex outside the narrow cortical zone in which it resides. Corticothalamic axons terminating in the A laminae of the dorsal lateral geniculate nucleus of the cat, for example, concentrate their terminals in a 500 µm wide zone but some terminals extend for up to 1500 µm beyond that (Murphy and Sillito, 1996). In other words, the corticothalamic axon can influence an extent of the visual field representation in the lateral geniculate nucleus many times greater than that represented in the cortical column in which its parent cell resides. In rodents, too, fibers derived from a cell beneath a single cortical barrel in the somatosensory cortex may extend terminals into VP barreloids adjacent to the barreloid that provides input to that cortical barrel, and thus into thalamic regions representing other facial vibrissae (Hoogland et al., 1987; Bourassa et al., 1995).

Corticothalamic cells whose somata lie in layer V are quite different from those of layer VI. Where the layer VI cells are characterized by focused axonal ramifications in both cortex and thalamus, the layer V cells are characterized by diffuseness. The layer V cells are typically pyramidal in form with larger somata than the layer VI cells, and have a stout apical dendrite ending in a tuft of branches in layer I of the cortex. The axon is thick and as it descends towards the white matter it gives off a number of horizontal collaterals that extend for a considerable distance (Fig. 4). The primary axon descends towards the thalamus but this is only one of its targets for, depending on the area in which the parent cell lies, the axon will have branches to the tectum, other parts of the brainstem or spinal cord. Although the thalamic branch almost invariably traverses the reticular nucleus en route to the dorsal thalamus, it does not give off collaterals in the reticular nucleus. Within the dorsal thalamus, its terminations are not restricted to the nucleus from which its parent cortical area receives inputs. Instead, branches extend across one or more adjacent nuclei. In the case of cells with somata located in the motor and somatosensory areas of the cortex, these additional nuclei commonly include those of the intralaminar system. In the case of cells in the primary visual cortex, nuclei of the pulvinar-lateral posterior complex are the targets, and in the case of cells in the primary auditory area of the cortex, the dorsal and magnocellular nuclei of the medial geniculate complex are the targets (Fig. 4). It is not without significance that many of the additional nuclei to which the layer V corticothalamic cells project, tend to be dominated by cells of the thalamic matrix. In them, the axons of the layer V corticothalamic cells terminate in small numbers of large boutons, quite unlike the numerous small boutons of layer VI corticothalamic cells. These larger boutons may enter into synaptic relationships with relay cells that are more like those of ascending afferent fibers than those of the terminals of the layer VI cells.

Widespread synchrony of the thalamus and cerebral cortex in cognition

During the alert, waking state, stimuli generated naturally in the external world or experimentally by artificial stimulation of a major subcortical afferent pathway, commonly lead to synchronous high frequency discharges in the 20–50 Hz ("40 Hz") range in discrete populations of thalamic relay neurons and in the cortical area or areas to which these project (Gray et al., 1989; Usrey and Reid, 1999). In the cortex, discrete populations of neurons in connected cortical areas can show similar synchrony which may serve to unite them temporarily as part of the process that ensures binding of distributed components of a sensory percept into a single experiential event (Gray et al., 1989; Singer and Gray, 1995). In magnetoencephalographic traces, 40 Hz activity can be seen moving across the cortex as new areas are recruited as part of what can be construed as a discrete conscious event (Ribary et al., 1991). Similarly, long range recruitment of parieto-temporal and frontal cortical areas into synchronous activity of this kind, may promote interactions that unite perception with the planning of strategies for action (Tononi et al., 1992).

The cells of the thalamic matrix clearly form a basis for dispersion of activity across larger areas of cortex

than those of the core with their focused projections to an individual area. Within an area, the terminations of matrix cell axons on distal dendrites in superficial layers and of core cell axons on more proximal dendrites in middle layers should serve as a coincidence detetection circuit leading to a high degree of temporal integration (Llinás and Paré, 1997) (Fig. 17). This in turn should promote synchronous activity in the cells of individual cortical columns and in a group of columns activated by the same stimulus. Oscillatory activity in these cortical columns should be fed back by layer VI corticothalamic cells to the thalamic nucleus from which they receive input, serving to reinforce the synchrony. Synchronous activity would be spread across other cortical columns in the same cortical area and in adjacent cortical areas by the diffuse projections of matrix cells in the thalamic nucleus. However, other thalamic nuclei and, through their matrix cells, other cortical areas should also be recruited into large scale coherent activity by the diffuse intracortical and corticothalamic projections of layer V corticothalamic neurons (Fig. 17). As an oscillation fades, these temporary links between discrete populations of cortical and thalamic cells with different relationships to a cognitive event would be broken. They would be reformed in new patterns as part of the process underlying new cognitive experiences.

Summing up

What Cajal would have thought of all the new data that have appeared on the thalamus in recent times can only be a subject of conjecture. He would no doubt have been gratified that his briefly-described observations on the reticular nucleus and on the thick and thin corticothalamic fibers should have proven to be so prescient. He would have related well to the remarkable two-way traffic that occurs between cortex and thalamus, since it provides a functional correlate of what he called the centrifugal and centripetal pathways, and he responded with renewed excitement whenever he revealed new two way connections of this kind associated with a brain or spinal center. As one who continually sought to perfect and apply new techniques that could reveal aspects of nerve cells hidden to the Golgi technique, he would have relished the wide variety of new methods that are now available for delineating neurons morphologically and chemically. What he would have made of the

354

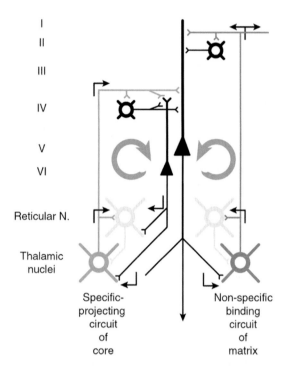

I
II
III
IV
V
VI

Reticular N.

Thalamic
nuclei

Specific-
projecting
circuit
of
core

Non-specific
binding
circuit
of
matrix

Fig. 17. Coincidence detection circuit formed by differential laminar terminations of matrix and core cells on cortical pyramidal cells. Inputs from core and matrix cells oscillating at high frequencies would be integrated over the dendritic tree and promote oscillatory activity in the cortical cells, activity that would be further promoted by feedback to the initiating thalamic nucleus by layer VI corticothalamic cells. Widespread extent of matrix cell terminations in cortex and of layer V corticothalamic axons in thalamus would promote synchrony of oscillations across wide regions of cortex and thalamic nuclei. From Jones (2001b). Based in part on Llinás and Paré (1997).

physiological discoveries on the dynamics of the system is open to question. For all his morphological insights and his remarkable capacity to derive fundamental biological principles from morphological observations, he was not, even by the standards of his time, particularly sophisticated physiologically. Early physiological observations pointing to the character of synaptic transmission, for example, did not enter into his thinking that led up to the formulation of the neuron doctrine. Where he did engage in physiological speculation, for example, about activity-dependent changes in the numbers and morphology of dendritic spines, he usually obtained it from others. While convinced of the active nature of connectivity between neurons, his contributions were primarily in mapping the static organization of connections

within and between neurons in the different nuclei and cortices of the central nervous system, based on the principle of dynamic polarization, and how these defined the routes for the transmission of information through the brain and spinal centers.

It was a remarkable feat that the internal, cell-to-cell circuitry of virtually every nucleus and cortex as we know it today was built by Cajal's hands in the brief period between commencing work with the Golgi method in 1888 and the publication of the first volume of the *Textura del Sistema Nervioso* in 1899. The thalamus, despite all the new data outlined in this review, is no exception.

Acknowledgments

Supported by grant numbers NS 21377 and NS 39094 from the National Institutes of Health, United States Public Health Service.

References

Agmon, A., Yang, L.T., Jones, E.G. and O'Dowd, D.K. (1995) Topological precision in the thalamic projection to neonatal mouse barrel cortex. *J. Neurosci.*, 15: 549–561.

Asanuma, C. (1992) Noradrenergic innervation of the thalamic reticular nucleus: a light and electron microscopic immunohistochemical study in rats. *J. Comp. Neurol.*, 319: 299–311.

Asanuma, C. (1994) GABAergic and pallidal terminals in the thalamic reticular nucleus of squirrel monkeys. *Exp. Brain Res.*, 101: 439–451.

Bal, T., von Krosigk, M. and McCormick, D.A. (1995) Role of the ferret perigeniculate nucleus in the generation of synchronized oscillations *in vitro*. *J. Physiol. (Lond.)*, 483: 665–685.

Bal, T., von Krosigk, M. and McCormick, D.A. (1995) Synaptic and membrane mechanisms underlying synchronized oscillations in the ferret lateral geniculate nucleus *in vitro*. *J. Physiol. (Lond.)*, 483: 641–663.

Benson, D.L., Isackson, P.J., Hendry, S.H.C. and Jones, E.G. (1991) Differential gene expression for glutamic acid decarboxylase and type II calcium-calmodulin-dependent protein kinase in basal ganglia, thalamus and hypothalamus of the monkey. *J. Neurosci.*, 11: 1540–1564.

Benson, D.L., Isackson, P.J., Gall, C.M. and Jones, E.G. (1992) Contrasting patterns in the localization of glutamic acid decarboxylase and Ca^{2+}/calmodulin protein kinase gene expression in the rat central nervous system. *Neurosci.*, 46: 825–850.

Bickford, M.E., Günlük, A.E., Van Horn, S.C. and Sherman, S.M. (1994) GABAergic projection from the basal forebrain to the visual sector of the thalamic reticular nucleus in the cat. *J. Comp. Neurol.*, 348: 481–510.

Bloomfield, S.A. and Sherman, S.M. (1989) Dendritic current flow in relay cells and interneurons of the cat's lateral geniculate nucleus. *Proc. Natl. Acad. Sci. USA*, 86: 3911–3914.

Bourassa, J., Pinault, D. and Deschênes, M. (1995) Corticothalamic projections from the cortical barrel field to the somatosensory thalamus in rats: A single-fibre study using biocytin as an anterograde tracer. *Europ. J. Neurosci.*, 7: 19–30.

Cajal, S.R. (1899) *Textura del Sistema Nervioso del Hombre y de los Vertebrados.* Vol. 1. Madrid, Moya.

Cajal, S.R. (1904) *Textura del Sistema Nervioso del Hombre y de los Vertebrados.* Vol.2, parts 1 and 2. Madrid, Moya.

Cajal, S.R. (1891) Sur la structure de l'écorce cérébrale de quelques mammifères. *La Cellule*, 7: 125–176.

Cajal, S.R. (1899a) Estudios sobre la corteza cerbral humana I: Corteza visual. *Rev. trim. Micrográf.*, 4: 1–63.

Cajal, S.R. (1899b) Estudios sobre la corteza cerebral humana II: Estructura de la corteza motriz del hombre y mamíferos superiores. *Rev. trim. Micrográf.*, 4: 117–200.

Cajal, S.R. (1900) Contribución al estudio de la vía sensitiva central y estructura del talamo óptico. *Rev. trim. micr.*, 5: 185–198.

Cajal, S.R. (1902) Estructura del tubérculo cuadrigémino posterior, cuerpo geniculado interno y vías acústicas centrales. *Trab. Lab. Invest. Biol. Madrid*, 1: 207–227.

Cajal, S.R. (1903) Estudios talámicos. *Trab. Lab. Invest. Biol. Univ. Madrid*, 2: 31–69.

Cajal, S.R. (1903) Las fibras nerviosas de origen cerebral del tubérculo cuadrigémina anterior y tálamo óptico. *Trab. Lab. invest. Biol. Madrid*, 2: 5–21.

Cox, C.L., Huguenard, J. and Prince, D.A. (1996) Heterogeneous axonal arborizations of rat thalamic reticular neurons in the ventrobasal nucleus. *J. Comp. Neurol.*, 366: 416–430.

Crabtree, J.W. (1992a) The somatotopic organization within the rabbit's thalamic reticular nucleus. *Europ. J. Neurosci.*, 4: 1343–1351.

Crabtree, J.W. (1992b) The somatotopic organization within the cat's thalamic reticular nucleus. *Europ. J. Neurosci.*, 4: 1352–1361.

Crabtree, J.W. (1996) Organization in the somatosensory sector of the cat's thalamic reticular nucleus. *J. Comp. Neurol.*, 366: 207–222.

Crabtree, J.W. (1998) Organization in the auditory sector of the cat's thalamic reticular nucleus. *J. Comp. Neurol.*, 390: 167–182.

Cucchiaro, J.B. and Uhlrich DJ, Sherman SM (1991) Electron-microscopic analysis of synaptic input from the perigeniculate nucleus to the A-Laminae of the lateral geniculate nucleus in cats. *J. Comp. Neurol.*, 310: 316–336.

Deschênes, M., Madariaga-Domich, A. and Steriade, M. (1985) Dendrodendritic synapses in the cat reticularis thalami nucleus: a structural basis for thalamic spindle synchronization. *Brain Res.*, 334: 165–168.

Destexhe, A., Contreras, D. and Steriade, M. (1998) Mechanisms underlying the synchronizing action of corticothalamic feedback through inhibition of thalamic relay cells. *J. Neurophysiol.*, 79: 999–1016.

Diamond, I.T., Fitzpatrick, D. and Schmechel, D. (1993) Calcium binding proteins distinguish large and small cells of the ventral posterior and lateral geniculate nuclei of the prosimian galago

and the tree shrew (*Tupaia belangeri*). *Proc. Natl. Acad. Sci. USA*, 90: 1425–1429.

Erisir, A., Van Horn, S.C. and Sherman, S.M. (1997) Relative numbers of cortical and brainstem inputs to the lateral geniculate nucleus. *Proc. Natl. Acad. Sci. USA*, 94: 1517–1520.

Friedlander, M.J., Lin, C.S. and Sherman, S.M. (1979) Structure of physiologically identified X and Y cells in the cat's lateral geniculate nucleus. *Science*, 204: 1114–1117.

Friedlander, M.J., Lin, C.-S., Stanford, L.R. and Sherman, S.M. (1981) Morphology of functionally identified neurons in lateral geniculate nucleus of cat. *J. Neurophysiol.*, 46: 80–129.

Golshani, P., Liu, X.B. and Jones, E.G. (2001) Differences in quantal amplitude reflect GluR4- subunit number at corticothalamic synapses on two populations of thalamic neurons. *Proc. Natl. Acad. Sci. USA*, 98: 4172–4177.

Golshani, P., Warren, R.A. and Jones, E.G. (1998) Progression of change in NMDA, nonNMDA, and metabotropic glutamate receptor function at the developing corticothalamic synapses. *J. Neurophysiol.*, 80: 143–154.

Gray, C.M., König, P., Engel, A.K. and Singer, W. (1989) Oscillatory responses in cat visual cortex exhibit inter-columnar synchronization which reflects global stimulus properties. *Nature*, 338: 334–337.

Hamos, J.E., Van Horn, S.C., Raczkowski, D., Uhlrich, D.J. and Sherman, S.M. (1985) Synaptic connectivity of a local circuit neuron in lateral geniculate nucleus of the cat. *Nature*, 317: 618–621.

Hendry, S.H.C. and Calkins, D.J. (1998) Neuronal chemistry and functional organization in the primate visual system. *Trends Neurosci.*, 21: 344–349.

Hoogland, P.V., Welker, E. and Van der Loos, H. (1987) Organization of the projections from barrel cortex to thalamus in mice studied with phaseolus vulgaris-leucoagglutinin and HRP. *Exp. Brain Res.*, 68: 73–87.

Hunt, C.A., Pang, D.Z. and Jones, E.G. (1991) Distribution and density of GABA cells in intralaminar and adjacent nuclei of monkey thalamus. *Neurosci.*, 43: 185–196.

Huntsman, M.M., Porcello, D.M., Homanics, G.E., DeLorey, T.M. and Huguenard, J.R. (1999) Reciprocal inhibitory connections and network synchrony in the mammalian thaalmus. *Science*, 283: 541–543.

Jahnsen, H. and Llinás, R. (1983a) Electrophysiological properties of guinea-pig thalamic neurons: an *in vitro* study. *J. Physiol. (Lond.)*, 349: 205–226.

Jahnsen, H. and Llinás, R. (1983b) Ionic basis for the electroresponsiveness and oscillatory properties of guinea-pig thalamic neurones *in vitro*. *J. Physiol. (Lond.)*, 349: 227–248.

Jones, E.G. (1998a) Viewpoint: The core and matrix of thalamic organization. *Neuroscience*, 85: 331–345.

Jones, E.G. (1998b) A new view of specific and nonspecific thalamocortical connections. In: H.H. Jasper, L. Descarries, V.F. Castellucci and S. Rossignol (Eds.), *Consciousness: At the Frontiers of Neuroscience.* Lippincott-Raven, Philadelphia, pp. 49–74.

Jones, E.G. (2001a) Morphology, nomenclature and connections of the thalamus and basal ganglia. In: K. Krauss, J. Jankovic and R.G. Grossman (Eds.), *Surgery for Parkinson's Disease and*

356

Movement Disorders. Lippincott, Williams and Wilkins, New York, pp. 24–47.

Jones, E.G. (2001b) The thalamic matrix and thalamocortical synchrony. *Trends Neurosci.*, 24: 593–599.

Kao, C.Q. and Coulter, D.A. (1997) Physiology and pharmacology of corticothalamic stimulation-evoked responses in rat somatosensory thalamic neurons *in vitro. J. Neurophysiol.*, 77: 2661–2676.

Jones, E.G. and Hendry, S.H.C. (1989) Differential calcium binding protein immunoreactivity distinguishes classes of relay neurons in monkey thalamic nuclei. *Europ. J. Neurosci.*, 1: 222–246.

Jones, E.G. and Powell, T.P.S. (1969) Electron microscopy of synaptic glomeruli in the thalamic relay nuclei of the cat. *Proc. R. Soc. Lond. B*, 121: 153–171.

Jones, E.G., Tighilet, B., Tran, B.-V. and Huntsman, M.M. (1998) Nucleus- and cell-specific expression of NMDA and nonNMDA receptor subunits in monkey thalamus. *J. Comp. Neurol.*, 397: 371–393.

Kim, U., Bal, T. and McCormick, D.A. (1995) Spindle waves are propagating synchronized oscillations in the ferret LGNd *in vitro. J. Neurophysiol.*, 74: 1301–1323.

Kim, U. and McCormick, D.A. (1998) The functional influence of burst and tonic firing mode on synaptic interactions in the thalamus. *J. Neurosci.*, 18: 9500–9516.

Kölliker A. von (1896) *Handbuch der Gewebelehre des Menschen*, Sixth edition, Vol. 2 Nervensystem des Menschen und der Thiere. Engelmann, Leipzig.

Liu, X.-B. (1997) Subcellular distribution of AMPA and NMDA receptor subunit immunoreactivity in ventral posterior and reticular nuclei of rat and cat thalamus. *J. Comp. Neurol.*, 388: 587–602.

Liu, X.-B. and Jones, E.G. (1991) The fine structure of serotonin and tyrosine hydroxylase immunoreactive terminals in the ventral posterior thalamic nucleus of cat and monkey. *Exptl. Brain Res.*, 85: 507–518.

Liu X.-B. and Jones, E.G. (1996) Localization of alpha type II calcium calmodulin-dependent protein kinase at glutamatergic but not gamma-aminobutyric acid (GABAergic) synapses in thalamus and cerebral cortex. *Proc. Natl. Acad. Sci. USA*, 93: 7332–7336.

Liu, X.-B. and Jones, E.G. (1999) Predominance of corticothalamic synaptic inputes to thalamic reticular nucleus neurons in the rat. *J. Comp. Neurol.*, 414: 67–79.

Liu, X.-B., Honda, C.N. and Jones, E.G. (1995a) Distribution of four types of synapse on physiologically identified relay neurons in the ventral posterior thalamic nucleus of the cat. *J. Comp. Neurol.*, 352: 69–91.

Liu, X.-B., Warren, R.A. and Jones, E.G. (1995b) Synaptic distribution of afferents from reticular nucleus in ventroposterior nucleus of cat thalamus. *J. Comp. Neurol.*, 352: 187–202.

Liu, X.-B., Bolea, S., Golshani, P. and Jones, E.G. (2001) Differentiation of corticothalamic and thalamocortical collateral synapses on mouse reticular nucleus neurons by EPSC amplitude and AMPA receptor subunit composition. *Thalamus and Related Systems*, 1: 15–29.

Llinás, R.R., Paré, D. (1991) Of dreaming and wakefulness. *Neuroscience*, 44: 521–536.

Llinás, R.R., Paré, D. (1997) Coherent oscillations in specific and nonspecific thalamocortical networks and their role in cognition.

In: M. Steriade, E.G. Jones and D.A. McCormick (Eds.), *Thalamus Volume II Experimental and Clinical Aspects*, : Elsevier, Amsterdam, pp. 501–516.

Martin, P.R., White, A.J.R., Goodchild, A.K., Wilder, H.D. and Sefton, A.E. (1997) Evidence that blue-on cells are part of the third geniculocortical pathway in primates. *Europ. J. Neurosci.*, 9: 1536–1541.

McCormick, D.A. and von Krosigk, M. (1992) Corticothalamic activation modulates thalamic firing through glutamate "metabotropic" receptors. *Proc. Natl. Acad. Sci. USA*, 89: 2774–2778.

McCormick, D.A., Bal, T. and von Krosigk, M. (1993) Cellular basis and neurotransmitter control of thalamic oscillation and sensory transmission. In: D. Minciacchi, M. Molinari, G. Macchi and E.G. Jones (Eds.), *Thalamic Networks for Relay and Modulation*, Pergamon, Oxford, pp. 357–374.

McCormick, D.A. and Bal, T. (1997) Sleep and arousal: thalamocortical mechanisms. *Annu. Rev. Neurosci.*, 20: 185–215.

McCormick, D.A., Huguenard, J., Bal, T. and Pape, H.-C. (1997) Electrophysiological and pharmacological properties of thalamic GABAergic interneurons. In: M. Steriade, E.G. Jones and D.A. McCormick (Eds.), *Thalamus, Volume 2. Experimental and Clinical Studies*, Elsevier, Amsterdam, pp. 155–212.

Montero, V.M. (1989) The GABA-immunoreactive neurons in the interlaminar regions of the cat lateral geniculate nucleus: light and electron microscopic observations. *Exp. Brain Res.*, 75(3): 497–512.

Montero, V.M. and Zempel, J. (1986) The proportion and size of GABA-immunoreactive neurons in the magnocellular and parvocellular layers of the lateral geniculate nucleus of the rhesus monkey. *Exp. Brain Res.*, 62: 215–223.

Mulle, C., Madariaga, A. and Deschênes, M. (1986) Morphology and electrophysiological properties of reticularis thalami neurons in cat: In vivo study of a thalamic pacemaker. *J. Neurosci.*, 6: 2134–2145.

Murphy, P.C. and Sillito, A.M. (1996) Functional morphology of the feedback pathway from area 17 of the cat visual cortex to the lateral geniculate nucleus. *J. Neurosci.*, 16: 1180–1192.

Nissl, F. (1913) Die Grosshirnanteile des Kaninchens. *Arch. Psychiat.*, 52: 867–953.

Ojima, H. (1994) Terminal morphology and distribution of corticothalamic fibers originating from layers 5 and 6 of cat primary auditory cortex. *Cereb.Cortex*, 4: 646–665.

Ojima, H., Honda, C.N. and Jones, E.G. (1992) Characteristics of intracellularly injected infragranular pyramidal neurons in cat primary auditory cortex. *Cereb.Cortex*, 2: 197–216.

Pape, H.C. and McCormick, D.A. (1995) Electrophysiological and pharmacological properties of interneurons in the cat dorsal lateral geniculate nucleus. *Neuroscience*, 68: 1105–1125.

Pinault, D., Bourassa, J. and Deschênes, M. (1995) Thalamic reticular input to the rat visual thalamus: a single fiber study using biocytin as an anterograde tracer. *Brain Res.*, 670: 147–152.

Rafols, J.A. and Valverde, F, (1973) The structure of the dorsal lateral geniculate nucleus in the mouse. A Golgi and electron microscopic study. *J. Comp. Neurol.*, 150: 303–332.

Rausell, E. and Avendaño, C. (1985) Thalamocortical neurons projecting to superficial and to deep layers in parietal, frontal and prefrontal regions in the cat. *Brain Res.*, 347: 159–165.

Rausell, E. and Jones, E.G. (1991a) Chemically distinct compartments of the thalamic VPM nucleus in monkeys relay principal and spinal trigeminal pathways to different layers of the somatosensory cortex. *J. Neurosci.*, 11: 226–237.

Rausell, E. and Jones, E.G. (1991b) Histochemical and immunocytochemical compartments of the thalamic VPM nucleus in monkeys and their relationship to the representational map. *J. Neurosci.*, 11: 210–225.

Rausell, E., Bae, C.S., Viñuela, A., Huntley, G.W. and Jones, E.G. (1992) Calbindin and parvalbumin cells in monkey VPL thalamic nucleus: distribution, laminar cortical projections, and relations to spinothalamic terminations. *J. Neurosci.*, 12: 4088–4111.

Ribary, U., Ioannides, A.A., Singh, K.D., Hasson, R., Bolton, J.P.R., Lado, F., Mogilner, A. and Llinás, R. (1991) Magnetic field tomography of coherent thalamocortical 40- Hz oscillations in humans. *Proc. Natl. Acad. Sci. USA*, 88: 11037–11041.

Sanchez-Vives, M.V., Bal, T., Kim, U., von Krosigk, M. and McCormick, D.A. (1996) Are the interlaminar zones of the ferret dorsal lateral geniculate nucleus actually part of the perigeniculate nucleus? *J. Neurosci.*, 16: 5923–5941.

Sawyer, S.F., Martone, M.E. and Groves, P.M. (1991) A GABA immunocytochemical study of rat motor thalamus: light and electron microscopic observations. *Neuroscience*, 42: 103–124.

Shadlen, M.N. and Movshon, J.A. (1999) Synchrony unbound: a critical evaluation of the temporal binding hypothesis. *Neuron*, 24: 67–77.

Sherman, S.M. and Friedlander, M.J. (1988) Identification of X versus Y properties for interneurons in the A-laminae of the cat's lateral geniculte nucleus. *Exp. Brain Res.*, 73: 384–392.

Singer, W. and Gray, C.M. (1995) Visual feature integration and the temporal correlation hypothesis. *Ann. Rev. Neurosci.*, 18: 555–586.

Sohal, V.S., Huntsman, M.M. and Huguenard, J.R. (2000) Reciprocal ihibitory connections regulate the spatiotemporal properties of intrathalamic oscillations. *J. Neurosci.*, 20: 1735–1745.

Spacêk, J. and Lieberman, A.R. (1974) Ultrastructure and three-dimensional organization of synaptic glomeruli in rat somatosensory thalamus. *J. Anat.*, 117: 487–516.

Spreafico, R., Frassoni, C., Arcelli, P. and de Biasi, S. (1994) GABAergic interneurons in the somatosensory thalamus of the guinea-pig: a light and ultrastructural immunocytochemical investigation. *Neuroscience*, 59: 961–974.

Stanford, L.R., Friedlander, M.J. and Sherman, S.M. (1981) Morphology of physiologically identified W cells in the C-laminae of the cat's lateral geniculate nucleus. *J. Neurosci.*, 1: 578–584.

Steriade, M. (2001) Corticothalamic resonance, states of vigilance and mentation. *Neuroscience*, 101: 243–276.

Steriade, M. and Amzica, F. (1996) Intracortical and corticothalamic coherency of fast spontaneous oscillations. *Proc. Natl. Acad. Sci. USA*, 93: 2533–2538.

Steriade, M., Jones, E.G. and McCormick, D.A. (1997a) Thalamic organization and chemical neuroanatomy. In: *Thalamus*. Vol. 1., Elsevier, Amsterdam, pp. 31–174.

Steriade, M., Jones, E.G. and McCormick, D.A. (1997b) Diffuse regulatory systems of the thalamus. In: *Thalamus*. Vol. 1., Elsevier, Amsterdam, pp. 269–338.

Steriade, M., Jones, E.G. and McCormick, D.A. (1997c) Electrophysiological properties of thalamic neurons. In: *Thalamus*. Vol. 1., Elsevier, Amsterdam, pp. 339–391.

Timofeev, I. and Steriade, M. (1997) Fast (mainly 30–100 Hz) oscillations in the cat cerebellothalamic pathway and their synchronization with cortical potentials. *J. Physiol. (Lond.)*, 496: 81–102.

Tononi, G., Sporns, O. and Edelman, G.M. (1992) Reentry and the problem of integrating multiple cortical areas: simulation of dynamic integration in the visual system. *Cereb.Cortex*, 2: 310–335.

Tsumoto, T. and Suda, K. (1981) Three groups of cortico-geniculate neurons and their distribution in binocular and monocular segments of cat striate cortex. *J. Comp. Neurol.*, 193: 223–236.

Turner, J.P. and Salt, T.E. (1998) Characterization of sensory and corticothalamic excitatory inputs to rat thalamocortical neurones *in vitro*. *J. Physiol. (Lond.)*, 510: 829–843.

Uhlrich, D.J., Cucchiaro, J.B., Humphrey, A.L. and Sherman, S.M. (1991) Morphology and axonal projection patterns of individual neurons in the cat perigeniculate nucleus. *J. Neurophysiol.*, 65: 1528–1541.

Usrey, W.M. and Reid, R.C. (1999) Synchronous activity in the visual system. *Ann. Rev. Physiol.*, 61: 435–456.

von Krosigk, M., Bal, T. and McCormick, D.A. (1993) Cellular mechanisms of a synchronized oscillation in the thalamus. *Science*, 261: 361–364.

von Krosigk, M., Monckton, J.E., Reiner, P.B. and McCormick, D.A. (1999) Dynamic properties of corticothalamic excitatory postsynaptic potentials and thalamic reticular inhibitory postsynaptic potentials in thalamocortical neurons of the guinea-pig dorsal lateral geniculate nucleus. *Neuroscience*, 91: 7–20.

Warren, R.A., Agmon, A. and Jones, E.G. (1994) Oscillatory synaptic interactions between ventroposterior and reticular neurons in mouse thalamus *in vitro*. *J. Neurophysiol.*, 72: 1993–2003.

Warren, R.A. and Jones, E.G. (1997) Maturation of neuronal form and function in a mouse thalamocortical circuit. *J. Neurosci.*, 17: 277–295.

Warren, R.A., Golshani, P. and Jones, E.G. (1997) $GABA_B$-receptor-mediated inhibition in developing mouse ventral posterior thalamic nucleus. *J. Neurophysiol.*, 78:.550–553.

Williams, S.R., Turner, J.P. andersen, C.M. and Crunelli, V. (2001) Electrophysiological and morphological properties of interneurones in the rat dorsal lateral geniculate nucleus *in vitro* *J. Physiol., (Lond.)*, 490: 129–147.

Williamson, A.M., Ohara, P.T., Ralston, D.D., Milroy, A.M. and Ralston, H.J., III (1994) Analysis of gamma-aminobutyric acidergic synaptic contacts in the thalamic reticular nucleus of the monkey. *J. Comp. Neurol.*, 349: 182–192.

Wilson, J.R. (1989) Synaptic organization of individual neurons in the macaque lateral geniculate nucleus. *J. Neurosci.*, 9: 2931–2953.

Wilson, J.R., Friedlander, M.J. and Sherman, S.M. (1984) Fine structural morphology of identified X- and Y-cells in the cat's lateral geniculate nucleus. *Proc. R. Soc. London B.*, 221: 411–436.

Yen, C.-T., Conley, M. and Jones, E.G. (1985a) Morphological and functional types of neurons in cat ventral posterior thalamic nucleus. *J. Neurosci.*, 5: 1316.

Yen, C.-T., Conley, M., Hendry, S.H.C. and Jones, E.G. (1985b) The morphology of physiologically identified GABAergic neurons in the somatic sensory part of the thalamic reticular nucleus in the cat. *J. Neurosci.*, 5: 2254.

E.C. Azmitia, J. DeFelipe, E.G. Jones, P. Rakic and C.E. Ribak (Eds.)
Progress in Brain Research, Vol. 136

CHAPTER 28

The modular organization of brain systems. Basal forebrain: the last frontier

Laszlo Zaborszky*

*Center for Molecular and Behavioral Neuroscience, Rutgers, The State University of New Jersey,
197 University Avenue, Newark, NJ 07102, USA*

Abstract: Computational anatomical studies suggest that specific clusters of projection neurons in the basal forebrain together with specific prefrontal and posterior cortical associational regions constitute distributed parts of functional parallel circuits. The predictable sequence of cell clusters consisting of various types of noncholinergic cell populations in the basal forebrain suggests further subdivisions within these circuits. It is possible that similar to the parallel basal ganglia circuits (Alexander and Crutcher, 1990), large number of specialized channels and sub-channels exist within this triangular circuitry that permit parallel, multilevel processing concurrently. The location and size of the active modules may temporarily vary according to the prevalence of state-related diffuse ascending brain stem and specific telencephalic inputs. From this latter group of afferents, the prefrontal input may function as an external threshold control which allocates attentional resources via the basal forebrain to distributed cortical processes in a selective, self-regulatory fashion.

Introduction

Santiago Ramón y Cajal is widely acclaimed as the major player in establishing the neuron doctrine, however, Cajal's studies also were fundamental to the subsequent development of the concept of the modular organizational design of the brain. Although the first explicit statement about the modular arrangement of the neuropil, including some discussion on its possible functional significance, was made by Scheibel and Scheibel in 1958 in their description of the brainstem reticular formation, it is not difficult to see in Cajal's superb illustrations the forerunners of modern concepts about integrative units. In his final summary (Cajal, 1935), he listed various types of systematic synaptic arrangements, like the glomeruli of the olfactory bulb and the cerebellum, which essentially correspond to modular substructures.

Ironically, Camillo Golgi's idea of a nerve network appears as a valid attempt to deal with some of the holistic aspects of brain function (Shepherd, 1991). However, he could not conceive how behavior could be the product of the individual actions of nerve cells acting independently. Rather he envisioned the nervous system as a diffuse network with extensive interaction of its elements (Golgi, Nobel Lecture, 1967). In contrast to the diffuse net of axon collaterals of Purkinje cells according to Golgi, Cajal demonstrated that terminals of recurrent collaterals of Purkinje cells end on the dendritic trunks of neighboring Purkinje cells: "*This fact showed therefore, as we had admitted formerly, that the recurrent collaterals serve to associate in a dynamic ensemble the neurons of the same kind from the same area of the gray matter*" (Cajal, Nobel Lecture, p. 229, 1967). He also states in the *Histology* (pp. 93–127, Vol. 1, 1995): "*Therefore, we should not concern ourselves with the disposition of a single neuron, but rather with chains of neurons, which may be quite long and act in concert as a functional whole. Thus, no reflex chain of neurons is entirely linear;*

---

*Corresponding author: Tel.: 973-353-1080/ext. 3181;
Fax: 973-353-1844; E-mail: zaborszky@axon.rutgers.edu

each chain shares at least some neurons in common with its neighbors, and even with more remote chains in the various neural centers."

Modular organization at various levels of the neuraxis

Numerous elements of the module principle were implicit in Cajal's work on the architecture of the *spinal cord* by showing the systemic orientation of terminal axon arborizations in the dorsal horn. He emphasized that collaterals from the ascending and descending main branches of the primary afferents, after their bifurcation in the dorsal funiculus, are issued to the gray matter not at random but at determined distances (see Figs. 209–211, Cajal, 1995).

Certain regularities in the architecture of the *thalamic sensory relay nuclei* are well known both in terms of axonal arborizations or cellular layering. Cajal observed and illustrated (Fig. 257, Cajal, 1995) the fact that the bushy

terminal arborizations of the specific sensory (lemniscal) afferents give rise to a quasi-concentric lamination in the VPL of the thalamus. Figure 1A is a reproduction of his drawing from the *Histology* (Fig. 548, Cajal, 1995). An explanation for the systematic discontinuity in the architectural organization of the ventrobasal complex is given some seventy years later in the findings of Woolsey and van der Loos (1970) by showing the faithful reproduction of the whisker pad in the thalamus (Fig. 1B and C).

In spite of the limited knowledge at the time about the function of the individual neurons and without knowing about the existence of specific inhibitory interneurons, Cajal intuitively developed *cortical models* with a predominantly vertical orientation of neuron chains (e.g. Fig. 37, Cajal, 1892, reproduced as Fig. 13 in "Cajal on the Cerebral Cortex", 1988). The concept of modular architectonics of the cerebral cortex arose originally from the early physiological observations of Mountcastle (1957) of the vertical columnar organization of the somatosensory cortex. This was soon followed by an analogous architectural principle in the visual cortex

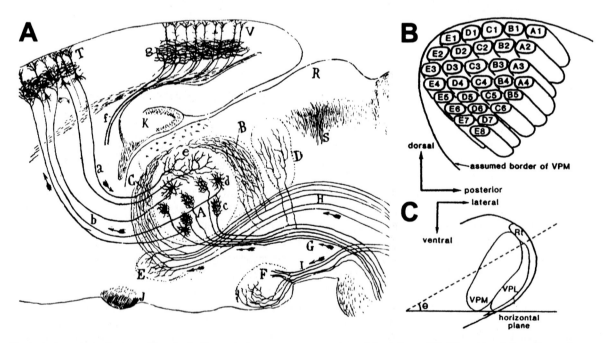

Fig. 1. **A:** Axonal arborizations of lemniscal afferents in the somatosensory nucleus of the thalamus (A). Other abbreviations: T, somatic sensory-motor area; V, visual area; a, corticothalamic fibers; b, thalamocortical fibers. Arrows indicate the direction of current flow. Reproduction of Cajal's original Fig. 548 (*Histology*, Vol. II, p. 718). **B:** Schematic drawing of columnar organization of vibrissal representation in VPM of the thalamus. The letters and numbers refer to the five rows of vibrissae on the face. **C:** Coronal section of the right thalamus. (B) is the medial view of the right VPM which was sectioned along the oblique horizontal plane shown by the broken line. The inclination (θ) is approximately 30°. Panels (B) and (C) are reproduced of Fig. 4 of Sugitani et al. (1990).

found by Hubel and Wiesel (1959). The modular architectonic principle of the cortex has received crucial support from studying the callosal and associational connections in primates by Goldman and Nauta (1977). Due to my tardiness in preparing material for publication, a photo of my original slide depicting degeneration in a callosal column in the rat appeared already in Szentagothai's Ferrier Lecture (Szentagothai, 1978; see legend to his Fig. 2), however as an independent source was published only as a book chapter in 1978 (Wolff and Zaborszky, 1978) and then as a full length paper much later in 1982 (Zaborszky and Wolff, 1982). The arborization spaces of callosal columns are one order of magnitude larger (300 to 30 μm) as compared to the orientation columns of Hubel and Wiesel (1972). Even after transections of large parts of the corpus callosum, the distribution of degenerated fibers show a discontinuous pattern: in coronal sections hourglass-shaped territories containing massive degeneration are alternating with areas containing little or no degenerated terminals (Fig. 2A) Cortico-cortical associational connections show an inhomogeneous distribution pattern similarly to callosal columns. With my student, Attila Csordas (Csordas and Zaborszky, 2001), we placed multiple retrograde tracer injections in various medio-lateral locations in the frontal/prefrontal cortex in rats and studied the distribution pattern of retrogradely labeled cells in posterior sensory-motor and associational cortical areas. Curiously enough, even after adding all cases with differently located frontal injections, the sharp borders are still apparent between territories containing massive projection neurons and others containing little if any (Fig. 2B–D). The systematic studies by Burkhalter, Malach, Killackey and more recently by Sakman and their colleagues (Koralek et al., 1990; Paperna and Malach, 1991; Coogan and Burkhalter, 1993; Malach, 1994; Johnson and Burkhalter, 1997; Lubke et al., 2000) in the rodent cortex and that in the prefrontal cortex in primates by Patricia Goldman-Rakic (e.g. 1984), Helen Barbas (Barbas and Rempel-Clover, 1997) and David Lewis (Pucak et al., 1996) amply confirmed the columnar nature of associational connections that can be utilized to predict the hierarchical organization of cortico-cortical connections as shown in the often cited diagram of Van Essen (Felleman and Van Essen, 1991). The size of Goldman-Rakic's associational columns compared with the size of the associational columns in rats show a remarkable congruence.

The idea of columnar organization of the neocortex[1] is part of the more general hypothesis of the modular organization of the nervous system, a widely documented principle of design for both vertebrate and invertebrate brains. Some of the main characteristics of the modular principle are summarized in a recent review by Liese (1990) and in the superb book on the anatomy and functions of cerebral cortex by Mountcastle (1998). The following features can be enlisted: (1) modules are local networks of cells in any regions of the CNS containing one or more electrically compact circuits active in a particular behavioral function; (2) modules are dynamic entities: modules, repeated iteratively within each larger structure, function independently, or they may act together when combined in groups whose composition may vary from time to time; (3) modules may differ in cell type and number in internal and external connectivity and in the mode of neuronal processing between different large entities; but within any single entity, like the neocortex, they have a basic similarity of internal design and operation, ranging in diameter from about 150–1000 μm; (4) the neighborhood relations between connected subsets of modules in different entities result in nested systems that serve distributed functions. A cortical area defined in classical cytoarchitectural terms may belong to more than one and sometimes to several such systems; (5) modules may develop through ontogenesis and phylogenesis by duplication of homeobox genes (Allman, 1998); (6) modules can be anatomically differentiable from the surrounding tissue. For example, in the striatum the striosome-matrix compartments can be defined using an AChE histochemical reaction (Graybiel and Ragsdale, 1978) or application of immunocytochemical and autoradiographic methods for the presence of various transmitters and receptors (Gerfen, 1985). AChE-staining also delineates patches in the superior colliculus that represent special sites where information from various sensory modalities can be integrated (Chevalier and Mana, 2000). In certain brain stem regions, computational anatomical methods helped to reveal a clustered, putatively modular organization, defined by patterns of connectivity (Malmierca et al., 1998; Leergaard et al., 2000).

---

[1]A more detailed discussion of the columnar-modular organization of the cortex is beyond the scope of this manuscript and the reader is referred to a recent review by Rockland (1998).

362

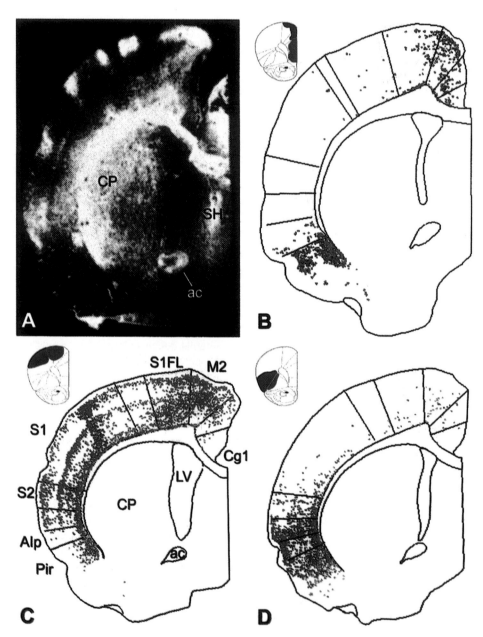

Fig. 2. **A:** Degenerating callosal columns following complete transection of the corpus callosum. Coronal section approximately at the level of the bregma, impregnated according to the method of Gallyas et al (1980). Modified from Fig. 4 of Zaborszky and Wolff (1982). **B–D:** Coronal sections from three cases showing discontinuous distribution of retrogradely labeled cells in posterior cortical areas following delivery of Fluoro-Gold (red) and Fast Blue (blue) in frontal cortical areas as indicated by the insets. Green dots represent double-labeled cells. Cortical area borders were superimposed from the Paxinos-Watson atlas. Abbreviations: ac, anterior commissure; cc, corpus callosum; CP, caudate putamen; LV, lateral ventricle; SH, degenerated hippocampo-septal fibers. Cg1, cingulate cortex; S1FL, forelimb area of the primary somatosensory cortex; S1, primary somatosensory cortex; S2 secondary somatosensory cortex; AIp, agranular insular cortex, posterior part; Pir, piriform cortex; M2, motor association cortex.

When multiple cell types are considered, the spatial variation of the relative density of different cell types is suggestive of the sites of integrative operations in the brain because these are areas where neurons would most likely share input and interact via local axonal connections. Utilizing novel computational methods (Nadasdy and Zaborszky, 2001), we investigated whether or not the imposition of numerical and spatial constraints may help to define hidden organizational patterns in the basal forebrain. Clustered structures can be revealed in a distributed population of a single cell type or can represent the topological association pattern of different chemically or hodologically defined cell populations. Careful reading of the structure of cellular segregation and association could contribute to a better understanding of how architectural features determine information processing.

In summary, based upon neuronal connectivity, dendritic and axonal arborization pattern, or cellular density distributions, networks can be disassembled into distinct pieces (units) of characteristic internal connectivity that are arranged into larger structures by repetition of similar architectural units. Modules are building blocks of the neural tissue that contain the necessary minimal pool of neurons to perform serial and parallel operations in the brain.

Basal forebrain

In a brief account, Cajal (1995) compared the large neurons, deep to the anterior perforate substance, to motor cells, based upon their size, abundant Nissl substance as well as rather large amounts of yellowish pigment (p. 598, Vol. II, *Histology*, 1995). Cajal, however, did not include these scattered large cells into a single system and did not realize their continuity with dispersed large neurons within the diagonal band of Broca as depicted in his Golgi specimens (Fig. 505, Cajal, 1995). Cajal thought that the large neurons underneath the globus pallidus are a special part of the corpus striatum. Interestingly, he understood that the scattered cells in the septum are associated with the hippocampus and cingulate cortex. Cajal also noted the overwhelming dorso-ventral orientation of the dendrites in the medial septum. However, the use of sophisticated computer reconstruction methods revealed one hundred years later that dendrites of basal forebrain neurons show a systematic, regionally selective orientation (Zaborszky et al., 2002).

It was Brockhaus in the early forties (1942), who rediscovered what Kölliker (1896) had already suggested half a century earlier that the aggregate, large neurons from the septal pole rostrally to the subthalamic nucleus caudally, embedded in the ill-defined regions of the substantia innominata, belonged to one system. This concept was confirmed later by histo-, immunocytochemical and connectional studies of the late seventies and early eighties by Butcher, Mesulam, Saper, Sofroniew and their colleagues (Sofroniew et al., 1982; Armstrong et al., 1983; Mesulam et al., 1983; Saper, 1984; Butcher, 1995). Recent interest in basal forebrain research was prompted by discoveries showing that a specific population of neurons in this region, namely those that use acetylcholine (ACh) as their transmitter and project to the cerebral cortex, are seriously compromised in Alzheimer's disease (Price et al., 1986). However, cholinergic corticopetal neurons represent only a fraction of the total cell population in these forebrain areas, which also contain various non-cholinergic neurons, including GABAergic and possibly glutamatergic corticopetal cells (Jones and Muhlethaler, 1999; Zaborszky et al., 1999).

Cortically projecting neurons in the basal forebrain are arranged along longitudinally oriented, segregated bands

Although there is considerable species variation in the precise locations of cholinergic projection neurons in the basal forebrain, the efferent projections of these cells follow basic organizational principles in all vertebrate species studied (Amaral and Kurz, 1985; Luiten et al., 1987; Mesulam et al., 1983; Rye et al., 1984, Saper, 1984). It is unclear, however, what is the functional equivalent of this topography, especially in light of a recent study in rat, showing that neighborhood relationships in the basal forebrain projection neurons do not correspond to near neighbors in the representational areas of sensorimotor cortices, thus arguing against a simple functional organization (Baskerville et al., 1993). In studies conducted with A. Csordas, we asked the question whether the organization of the basalo-cortical system can, in any sense, be related to the distributed and hierarchical organization of cortico-cortical connections, as proposed by Van Essen and his associates (Felleman and Van Essen, 1991). Figure 3A–H depicts a series of

364

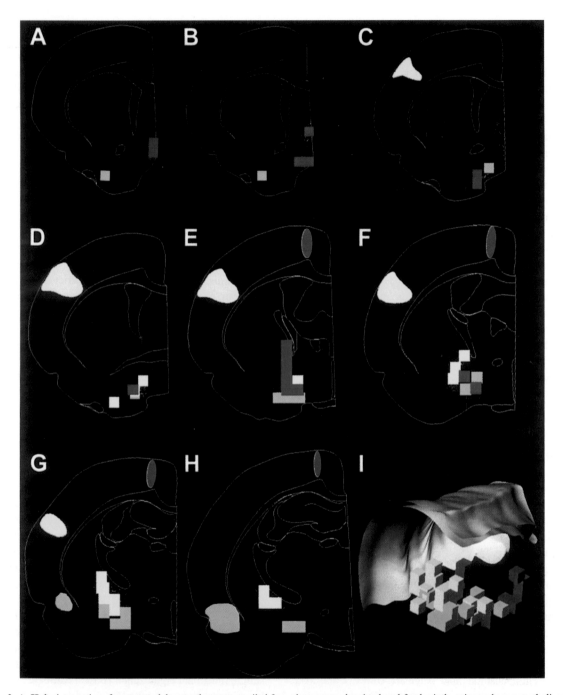

Fig. 3. **A–H** depict a series of rostro-caudal coronal maps compiled from three cases showing basal forebrain locations where non-cholinergic neurons projecting to different medio-laterally located frontal/prefrontal and posterior association areas occupy overlapping zones. Injection sites are marked with red, yellow and green colors and basal forebrain locations that contain projection neurons are marked with appropriately colored boxes. The different colored voxels (500 × 500 × 50 μm) in this figure represent spaces where non-cholinergic neurons in each individual animal, project to both a posterior association area and a corresponding frontal region are represented by at least 3 neurons from both cell populations. **I** shows the 3D distribution of these different voxels using the Micro3D program on a Silicon Graphics Octane computer. As can be seen only one voxel (panel D) is shared among the three animals.

rostro-caudal coronal maps compiled from three cases showing basal forebrain locations where noncholinergic neurons projecting to different medio-laterally located frontal/prefrontal and posterior association areas occupy overlapping zones. In order to extract important spatial and numerical features, we used a program that calculated local density values of neuronal populations by scanning equally subdivided units called voxels in each sections from each of the three brains (see Alloway et al., 1999; Leergard et al., 1999). The different colored voxels ($500 \times 500 \times 50$ µm) in this figure represent spaces where in each individual animal, noncholinergic neurons projecting to two specific cortical areas are represented by at least 3 neurons from both cell populations. Red voxels are from the animal that received a Fast Blue (FB) injection along the border of the M1/M2 associational cortex and a Fluoro Gold (FG) injection in the prelimbic cortex, approximately in a region as the 'red' injection site in the inset to Fig. 2B. Yellow voxels are from an animal where FB was deposited along a strip within the S1 sensory area and FG in the primary motor cortex similarly to the 'blue' injection site in the inset to Fig. 2C. Finally, green voxels are from a third animal that contain cell populations projecting to the perirhinal/posterior insular area and the sulcal prefrontal cortex. The selection of these brains from a larger pool of cases is based upon the fact that in each case the location of the injection sites in posterior associational areas maximally fit with the location of cortico-cortical columns containing a dense collection of neurons projecting to corresponding medio-laterally located frontal/prefrontal areas as documented in Fig. 2B–D. Figure 3I shows the 3D distribution of these different voxels. As can be seen only one voxel was shared among the three animals, indicating that these 3 longitudinally oriented noncholinergic bands in the basal forebrain are largely segregated from each other and thus can influence separately specific cortico-cortical associational fields. A similar arrangement can be obtained displaying cholinergic projecting neurons. Because brain size differences were corrected for, it is unlikely that the degree of overlap depends on misalignment. Figure 3I also suggests that the three projection bands are arranged in a twisted pattern where the location of the three markers shows a systematic association along the entire axis of the basal forebrain.

A detailed analysis of 9 cases with paired injections and some 30 'virtual' experiments constructed by using computer-generated combinations of the 9 cases indeed suggests that corresponding medio-laterally located frontal and posterior associational cortical areas receive their input from a partially overlapping area in the basal forebrain (Zaborszky and Csordas, in preparation). On the other hand, topographically noncorresponding frontal and parieto-insular areas receive their projections from nonoverlapping areas of the basal forebrain. In addition to the overlapping, band or band-like pattern of neurons projecting to associated cortical areas, these preliminary studies revealed another interesting feature that points to a precise interplay between associational cortical columns and specific basal forebrain bands. Namely, our studies revealed that the ratio of cholinergic and noncholinergic projection neurons systematically varies according to the cortical target area: this value is lower in frontal (on the average 0.3) than in posterior cortical areas (0.6), however in the cortical areas labeled by red or yellow colors in Fig. 3, this ratio is even higher (0.8–1.4). As mentioned above, these areas contain a heavy accumulation of cortico-cortical projection neurons. In contrast to these areas, in their immediate vicinity, cortical areas that only sparsely project to the frontal cortex, have their cholinergic/noncholinergic ratio significantly lower (0.4).

Spatial association of cholinergic and various types of noncholinergic neurons in the basal forebrain

Calbindin (CB), calretinin (CR) and parvalbumin (PV) are different calcium-binding proteins that are colocalized in different, nonoverlapping populations of noncholinergic neurons in the basal forebrain of rodents. When cholinergic and these three chemically identified neuronal populations are studied separately, each cell population shows a characteristic distribution pattern. Due to the lack of adequate multiple labeling techniques and the fact that differences between cases and different cell types are difficult to grasp in individual 2D histological sections, previous studies dealt only with the organization of basal forebrain subregions and failed to recognize that a systematic spatial relationship might exist among these cell populations along the entire extent of the basal forebrain (Zaborszky et al., 1986; Jakab and Leranth, 1995; Kiss et al., 1997).

We have shown in a recent publication (Zaborszky et al., 1999, Fig. 5 and Zaborszky et al., in preparation) that cholinergic (CH) and the three calcium-binding containing neuronal populations construct large-scale cell sheets or bands that seem to be twisted and attached to each other in a complicated fashion. However, a closer observation suggests that the four cell sheets display a pattern of association in the entire basal forebrain. By constructing volumetric databases of local cell counts for the four major cell populations in the basal forebrain, it is apparent that the density of cells in each cell population shows regional variation. One can delineate sub-spaces where cell densities are significantly higher from an average cell density. Figure 4A shows a scatter-plot distribution of CH and PV cells (red and green dots) including high density locations of either cell populations (large red and green symbols). Although using a relatively low threshold of high pass filtering on the density data (≥ 5 cells per $250 \times 250 \times 50$ μm voxel size) these clusters seem to be diffusely distributed. When using a relatively high threshold level ($d \geq 15$ cells/unit space) as in Fig. 4A, the clustering of CH and PV cell populations deviate from randomness. As can be seen, high density CH and PV clusters often share a narrow space. For a further analysis of the spatial relationships

among the four cell populations, we first determined locations where pairs of the four cell populations overlap and then combined these separate renderings into one scheme. The model in Fig. 4B displays a combined rendering of voxels where CH/PV (green) CH/CR (yellow) and CH/CB (dark blue) cell populations show overlapping distributions at a given threshold density. Because often more than two cell populations occupy the same space, to avoid misinterpreting topological relationships among multiple cell populations, several independent methods had to be used. Disregarding local details, Fig. 4B suggests that the large-scale relationships among the four cell populations arise from a twisted banded pattern along the entire basal forebrain. The similarity of the large-scale arrangement of the three noncholinergic projection bands of Fig. 3I and the systematic twisted banded pattern of the three calcium-binding neuronal populations relative to cholinergic neurons shown in Fig. 4B is striking. The model in Fig. 4C applies another algorithm on the same database. This so-called iso-relational surface rendering technique imposes a combination of density and spatial relational constraints

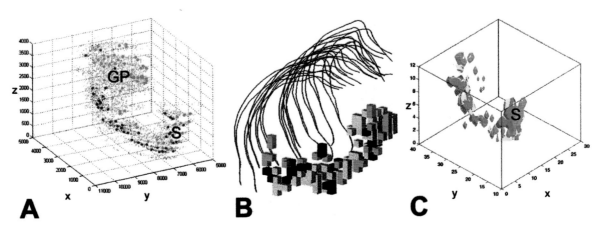

Fig. 4. **A:** Differential density scatter plot to show the spatial distribution of cholinergic (red dots) and parvalbumin (green dots) containing neurons in the basal forebrain. Filled circles mark the high-density locations where the density of cholinergic or parvalbumin cells is higher than 15 in the unit space ($250 \times 250 \times 50$ μm). Data from this and subsequent panels are derived from a brain alternately stained for choline acetyltransferase, parvalbumin, calretinin and calbindin. Cells were plotted using a computerized microscope and the Neurolucida® software. Axis scaling is in μm corresponding to the x, y and z coordinates according to the Neurolucida database. **B:** Combined rendering to show locations where cholinergic/parvalbumin (green), cholinergic /calretinin (yellow) and cholinergic /calbindin (dark blue) cells overlap in the basal forebrain from the same dataset as (A). Voxel size is the same as in (A), density ≥ 5 per voxels. Medial view, rostral is right, caudal is left. The wire frames are the outlines of the corpus callosum. **C:** Iso-relational maps. The spatial relationship of cholinergic neurons to the other three cell types was determined by mapping the change in their density ratios. The ratios between the cholinergic and other markers were calculated considering only those unit spaces where both cell types have a density ≥ 5 cells. These surfaces cover the space where the relationship of cholinergic cells to parvalbumin (green), calretinin (yellow) and calbindin (blue) neurons is at least $0.5\!:\!1$. The numbers along the x and y-axis indicate the voxel indices. Numbers along the z-axis indicate layers (sections). Note that the orientation of both models in panel (A) and (C) is the same. GP, globus pallidus; S, septum. Figure C is from Zaborszky et al. (2002).

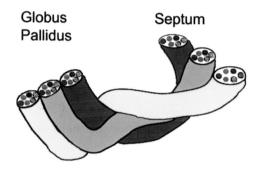

Fig. 5. Schematic illustration to show the relationship of the three projection bands from Fig. 3I and the notion that each of these bands contains several transmitter-specific sub-channels.

(Nadasdy and Zaborszky, 2001). In Fig. 4C each differently colored surface rendered around regions where the density of both the cholinergic and one from the other three cell populations met two criteria: (1) density is at least five for each cell type within the voxel dimension (250 × 250 × 50 μm) and (2) the ratio of cholinergic to the other cell type counts is 0.5 or higher. For example, the voxels covered by green surfaces contain at least twice as many parvalbumin as cholinergic neurons. Similarly, yellow surfaces cover voxels where the density of both calretinin and cholinergic cells are > 5 in each voxel and the ratio of calretinin/cholinergic cells is at least 0.5. Finally, blue surfaces highlight the iso-relational distributions of cholinergic and calbindin cells. Merging the three pairwise iso-relational surfaces into one scheme suggests that the gross cholinergic cell band can be parcelled into several smaller clusters or larger amalgamations, where cholinergic cells are mixed with the other three cell types in a specific fashion. Because CR, CB and PV have been found in at least a subpopulation of corticopetal neurons (Zaborszky et al., 1999; Gritti et al., 2001), it is likely that each noncholinergic projection band from Fig. 3I may consist of several transmitter-specific 'sub-bands'. A similar global pattern emerges when comparing similar types of renderings from different brains, suggesting that the configuration of the iso-relational surfaces is not by chance and that the high density clusters in the individual cell populations may correspond to the zones where the different cell bands overlap with each other resulting in mixed clusters (Zaborszky et al., in preparation). The location of these mixed clusters can be predicted based upon the twisted

pattern of 'macro' (topographically organized projection neurons) and 'micro' bands (the various chemically specified cell groups within a projection channel). Figure 5 shows the possible arrangement of the three projection bands from Fig. 3I. It is also indicated in this scheme that each projection band may contain several transmitter-specific sub-bands.

Differential tuning of various cortical areas from the basal forebrain

A systematic analysis of all voxels from a volumetric database that contains all four cell markers suggests that cholinergic neurons are admixed with the three other noncholinergic cell populations in a large number of combinations. However, the composition of these mixed clusters is predictable and characteristic of the location (Zaborszky et al., 2002; in preparation). In spite of the high percentage of mixed high-density voxels, a substantial proportion (23–45%) of the high-density voxels for each cell type remains 'lonely'; i.e., contains only one marker above the set threshold density level. The consequence of this arrangement is that for each cell type and structure a characteristic 'signature' combination of overlapping and lonely voxels exists. Unfortunately, at present, it is unknown how signaling factors along the longitudinal and transverse domains of the forebrain proliferative 'protomap' regulate gene expression and migration pattern (Rakic, 1995; and this volume; Rubinstein et al., 1998) as to establish the observed sequence of mixed clusters. It is also unknown how these specific clusters may establish connections during ontogenesis with specified cortical locations as proposed below.

It is interesting to note in this context that stimulations in spatially different locations in the basal forebrain result in different modulations of ongoing cortical activity (Jimenez-Capdeville et al., 1997). For example, activation of some basal forebrain sites provoked an intense discharge of many neurons in the vicinity of the cortical recording electrode and the same stimulus site provoked release of large amounts of ACh in the cortex. Stimulation of other sites produced strong inhibition and no increase in cortical ACh release. Jimenez-Capdeville et al. (1997) suggested that the immediate excitatory response was due to a disinhibition of the pyramidal cells by activation of the basalo-cortical GABAergic projection terminating on cortical interneurons as suggested earlier by Freund and his colleagues (Freund and Meskenaite, 1992). The excitation was then maintained by the slower onset excitatory ACh action. On the other hand, according to this study, the silencing of the cortical activity at the end of the basal forebrain stimulation is due to the activation of putative glutamatergic basalo-cortical neurons that may preferentially contact certain classes of cortical neurons, leading to intracortical inhibition. The authors also suggested without any experimental proof that basal forebrain sites generating inhibition of cortical neuronal activity are surrounded by basal forebrain regions that activated the cortex and provoked release of ACh. We hypothesize that these different responses could relate to the differential composition of clusters in the basal forebrain. For example, one can expect that stimulation electrodes located in predominantly PV/CH mixed regions would result in different cortical responses from that caused by stimulating locations in regions populated primarily with CB and CR cells that may contain glutamate (Gritti et al., 2001). This postulated organization could ensure that a combination of relatively few types of basal forebrain neurons may generate a large spectra of differential tuning in various cortical areas.

Input–output relations of cholinergic clusters

Using a double strategy of recording the location of putative contact sites between identified axons and cholinergic profiles as well as identifying the presence of synapses in representative cases under the electron microscope, one can get a fairly good idea about the extent of potential transmitter interactions in the basal forebrain. Although ascending brainstem noradrenergic and dopaminergic axons contact cholinergic neurons in extensive portions of the basal forebrain, the majority of telencephalic afferents (cortical, amygdaloid, striatal) appear to have a preferential distribution in subregions of the basal forebrain (Zaborszky et al., 1991; Zaborszky and Duque, 2000). The prefrontal cortex innervates exclusively noncholinergic neurons in the basal forebrain, including parvalbumin-containing cell populations (Zaborszky et al., 1997), suggesting some selectivity in the innervation pattern of various neurons. A partial 3D reconstruction of the dendrites of several hundred cholinergic neurons suggests a tendency of iso-orientation of

dendrites within a given cholinergic cell cluster (Zaborszky et al., 2002). Because many of the afferent axons also show regionally specific orientation, it is likely that cholinergic cell clusters in each major subdivision of the basal forebrain can sample a unique combination of afferents.

Prefrontal-basalo-cortical modular loops in allocation of the attentional spotlight

Cortical release of ACh from the basal forebrain appears to be essential for the enhancement of sensory evoked responses and cortical reorganization of the body surface representations (Juliano et al., 1991; Metherate and Ashe, 1991; Killgard and Mersenich, 1998; Rasmusson, 2000). Experiments with basal forebrain stimulation and measuring in vivo cortical release of ACh are somewhat equivocal in determining whether the basal forebrain contributes selectively to sensory processing or if the released ACh in the cortex is only part of a general cortical arousal mechanism as suggested by Sarter and Bruno (1997). Our anatomical and preliminary electrophysiological studies (Golmayo et al., 1999), however, raise the possibility that the basal forebrain may participate in selective sensory processing via its input from the prefrontal cortex and its output to distributed, functionally related cortical areas. This notion is diagrammatically visualized in Fig. 6 by showing several specific cortico-prefrontal-basal forebrain-cortical circuits. This hypothesis is based upon (a) the strict topography in cortico-prefrontal projections (Zaborszky and Csordas, in preparation), (b) prefrontal-basal forebrain projections (Sesack et al., 1989; Zaborszky et al., 1997), (c) basal forebrain-sensory projections (Zaborszky and Raza, in preparation), and (d) the close spatial relationship among basal forebrain cells that project to both prefrontal and posterior association cortex (Csordas and Zaborszky, 2001).

Many neurobehavioral studies have indicated the involvement of the prefrontal cortex in higher cognitive functions such as working memory and attention (Goldman-Rakic, 1987; Fuster, 1989; Miller and Cohen, 2001). PET imaging studies in humans (Paus et al., 1997) and orientation deficits in rats and monkeys after lesions of the basal forebrain (Whisaw et al., 1985; Voytko et al., 1994), together with our preliminary electrophysiological results (Golmayo et al., 1999), suggest that the role played by the prefrontal cortex in these cognitive

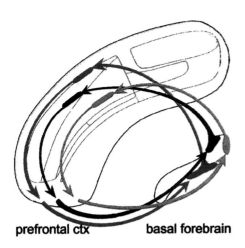

prefrontal ctx   **basal forebrain**

Fig. 6. Schematic model to show that specific cell groups in the basal forebrain together with specific prefrontal and associational cell groups constitute parts of distributed functional modules. The different colors represent three segregated parallel circuits. The background template is based upon Swanson: Brain Maps. Structure of the Rat Brain. (1992).

operations could be due in part to its close relation with the basal forebrain in modulating specific sensory responses.

Imaging studies revealed that combinations of multiple activated cortical fields in prefrontal and associational cortical areas are reproducible associated with specific cognitive components of mental operations (Roland, 1994; Raichle and Posner, 1997; Cabeza and Nyberg, 1997; Duncan and Owen, 2000). It seems to be that for each type of brain operation there is a working memory in the dorsolateral prefrontal-anterior cingulate regions that is responsible for the recruitment and maintenace of specific cortical fields via controlling selective attention (Roland, 1994; Desimone and Duncan, 1995; de Fockert et al., 2001). While the cortical network of attention is partially known (Posner and Dehaene, 1994; Raichle and Posner, 1997), the subcortical structures responsible for the necessary cortical coactivation and tuning are less well understood. From various physiological and limited imaging studies, it is likely that the pulvinar (LaBerge, 1995), the intralaminar nuclei, the mesopontine tegmentum (Kinomura et al., 1996) and the basal forebrain (Voytko, 1994) participate in this function. The proposed re-entrant circuitry of Fig. 6 could explain the timeline of attention-related evoked potentials in prefrontal and sensory cortical areas after

sensory stimulations (see discussion of this issue on p. 360 in Zaborszky et al., 1999) and fits with the idea that selective attention, recruitment of processors, tuning, working memory, vigilance, strategy selection and planning represent an interrelated multicomponent system (Baddeley, 1995).

In light of the possible significance of fast cortical oscillations in attention, perception and consciousness (Crick and Koch, 1990; Singer and Gray, 1995; Lumer et al., 1997; Singer, 1999; Gray, 2000; Steinmetz et al., 2000; Fries et al., 2001), the 20–40 Hz membrane potential fluctuations elicited by basal forebrain stimulation in cortical pyramidal neurons (Metherate et al., 1992) are of particular interest. We hypothesize that pyramidal cells in selected cortical regions could start to oscillate at high frequency when specifically located basal forebrain cell clusters receive signals from the prefrontal cortex about the significance of the sensory stimulus within 100 ms after sensory stimulation. Due to the possibility that the basal forebrain receives topographically organized input from the prefrontal cortex and its output preferentially targets associational cortical routes, the basal forebrain is well positioned anatomically to coordinate cortical oscillations among widely separated cortical regions and capable of binding these regions into larger functional networks. This proposed triangular circuitry for synchronized oscillations in large-scale networks may work concurrently with other proposed mechanisms, including cortico- thalamo-cortical (Ribari et al., 1991; Lumer et al., 1997; Steriade, 1999; Jones, 2001) or brain stem-thalamic oscillators (Munk et al., 1996; Steriade, 1996, 1999).

Acknowledgments

The original research summarized in this review was supported by PHS grant #23945. Special thanks are due to Dr. Z. Nadasdy for fruitful collaboration in recent years and reading an earlier version of this manuscript.

References

Alexander, G. E. and Crutcher, M. D. (1990) Functional architecture of basal ganglia circuits: neural substrates of parallel processing. *Trends Neurosci.*, 13: 266–271.

370

Allmann, J.M. (1998) *Evolving Brains*. Scientific American Library, W.H. Freeman and Co. New York, NY.

Alloway, D., Crist, J., Mutic, J.J. and Roy, S.A. (1999) Corticostriatal projections from rat barrel cortex have an anisotropic organization that correlates with vibrissal whisking behavior. *J. Neurosci.*, 19: 10908–10922.

Amaral, D.G. and Kurz, J. (1985) An analysis of the origins of the cholinergic and non-cholinergic septal projections to the hippocampal formation in the rat. *J. Comp. Neurol.*, 240: 37–59.

Armstrong, D.M., Saper, C.B., Levey, A.I., Wainer, B.H. and Terry, R.D. (1983) Distribution of cholinergic neurons in the rat brain demonstrated by immunohistochemical localization of choline acetyltransferase. *J. Comp. Neurol.*, 216: 53–68.

Baddeley, A. (1995) Working memory. In: M.S. Gazzaniga (Ed.), *The Cognitive Neurosciences.*, MIT Press, Cambridge, MA, pp. 755–764.

Barbas, H. and Rempel-Clower, N. (1997) Cortical structure predicts the pattern of cortico-cortical connections. *Cerebral Cortex*, 7: 635–646.

Baskerville, K.A., Chang, H.T. and Herron, P. (1993) Topography of cholinergic afferents from the nucleus basalis of Meynert to representational areas of sensorimotor cortices in the rat. *J. Comp. Neurol.*, 335: 552–562.

Brockhaus, H. (1942) Vergleichend-anatomische Untersuchungen uber den Basalkern Komplex. *J. Psychol. Neurol.*, Leipzig, 51: 57–95.

Butcher, L.L. (1995) The cholinergic system. In: G. Paxinos (Ed.), *The Rat Nervous System*, Academic Press, San Diego, pp. 1003–1015.

Cabezza, R. and Nyberg, L. (1997) Imaging cognition: an empirical review of PET studies with normal subjects. *J. Cogn. Neurosci.*, 9: 1–26.

Cajal, S.R. (1995) *Histology of the Nervous System*. Vol I-II. Translated by N. Sawnson and L. Swanson, Oxford University Press, New York.

Cajal, S.R. (1935) *Die Neuronlehre*. In: O. Bumke and O. Foester (Eds.), *Handbuch der Neurologie I*, Anatomie. Springer, Berlin, pp. 887–994

Cajal, S.R. (1967) The structure and connexions of neurons. Nobel Lecture, December 12, 1906. In: *Nobel Lectures. Physiology or Medicine*, 1901–1921. Elsevier, Amsterdam, pp. 220–253.

Cajal, S.R. (1892) El nuevo concepto de la histologia de los centros nerviosos. *Rev. Ciencias Med.*, 18: 457–476.

Chevalier, G. and Mana, S. (2000) Honeycomb-like structure of the intermediate layers of the rat superior colliculus, with additional observations in several other mammals: AChE patterning. *J. Comp. Neurol.*, 419: 137–153.

Coogan, T.A. and Burkhalter, A. (1990) Conserved patterns of cortico-cortical connections define areal hierarchy in rat visual cortex. *Exp. Brain Res.*, 80: 49–53.

Coogan, T.A. and Burkhalter, A. (1993) Hierarchical organization of areas in rat visual cortex. *J. Neurosci.*, 13: 3749–3772.

Crick, F. and Koch, C. (1990) Some reflections on visual awareness. Cold Spring Harbor Symposia on Quantitative Biology. 55: 953–962.

Csordas, A. and Zaborszky, L. (2001) Organization of the basal forebrain corticopetal system: a computational anatomical study.

Cajal Club/Cajal Institute Int. Conference May 2001, Madrid, Spain. Abstracts.

DeFelipe, J. and Jones, E.G. (1988) Cajal on the Cerebral Cortex. An Annotated Translation of the Complete Writings. Oxford University Press, New York.

DeFockert, J.W., Rees, G., Frith, C.D. and Lavie, N. (2001) The role of working memory in visual selective attention. *Science*, 291: 1803–1806.

Desimone, R. and Duncan, J. (1995) Neural mechanisms of selective attention. *Annu. Rev. Neurosci.*, 18: 193–222.

Duncan, J. and Owen, A.M. (2000) Common regions of the human frontal lobe recruited by diverse cognitive demands. *Trends Neurosci.*, 23: 475–483.

Felleman, D.J. and Van Essen, D.C. (1991) Distributed hierarchical processing in the primate cerebral cortex. *Cerebral Cortex*, 1: 1–47.

Freund, T.F. and Meskenaite, V. (1992) Gamma-aminobutyric acid-containing basal forebrain neurons innervate inhibitory interneurons in the neocortex. *Proc. Nat. Acad. Sci. USA*, 89: 738–742.

Fries, P., Reynolds, J.H., Rorie, A.E. and Desimone, R., (2001) Modulation of oscillatory neuronal synchronization by selective visual attention. *Science*, 291: 1561–1563

Fuster, J.M. (1989) *The Prefrontal Cortex: Anatomy, Physiology and Neuropsychology of the Frontal Lobe*, 2nd edition, Raven Press, New York.

Gallyas, F., Wolff, J.R., Bottcher, H. and Zaborszky, L. (1980) A reliable and sensitive method to localize terminal degeneration and lysosomes in the central nervous system. *Stain Technol.*, 55: 299–305.

Goldman, P.S. and Nauta, W.J.H. (1977) Columnar distribution of cortico-cortical fibres in the frontal association, limbic and motor cortex of the developing rhesus monkey. *Brain Res.*, 122: 393–413.

Goldman-Rakic, P.S. (1987) Circuitry of primate prefrontal cortex and regulation of behavior by representational memory. In: F. Plum (Ed.), *Handbook of Physiology, The Nervous System, Higher Functions of the Brain*, Am. Physiol. Soc. Bethesda, pp. 373–417.

Goldman-Rakic, P.S. (1984) Modular organization of prefrontal cortex. *Trends Neurosci.*, 7: 419–429.

Golgi, C. (1967) The neuron doctrine—theory and facts. Nobel Lecture December 11, 1906. In: *Nobel Lectures. Physiology or Medicine*, 1901–1921. Elsevier, Amsterdam, pp. 189–217

Gray, C.M. (1999) The temporal correlation hypothesis of visual feature integration: still alive and well. *Neuron*, 24: 31–47.

Graybiel, A.M. and Ragsdale, C.W. Jr. (1978) Histochemically distinct compartments in the striatum of human, moneky, and cat demonstrated by acetylthiocholinesterase staining. *Proc. Natl. Acad. Sci. USA*, 75: 5723–5726.

Gerfen, C.R., Baimbridge, K.G. and Miller, J.J. (1985) The neostriatal mosaic: compartmental distribution of calcium-binding protein and parvalbumin in the basal ganglia of rat and monkey. *Proc. Natl. Acad. Sci. USA*, 82: 8780–8784.

Golmayo, L., Zaborszky, L. and Nunez, A. (1999) Somatosensory cortical inputs to the basal forebrain contribute to somatosensory cortical processing. *Soc. Neurosci. Abst.*, 25: 1167.

Gritti, I., Manns, I.D., Mainville, L. and Jones, B.E. (2001) Calcium binding proteins reveal a distinct subgroup of cortically projecting basal forebrain neurons that may synthesize glutamate as a neurotransmitter. *Soc. Neurosci. Abstr.*, 27: 675.

Hubel, D.H. and Wiesel, T.N. (1959) Receptive fields of single neurons in the cat's striate cortex. *J. Physiol. (Lond).*, 148: 574–591.

Hubel, D.H. and Wiesel, T.N. (1972) Laminar and columnar distribution of geniculo-cortical fibers in the macaque monkey. *J. Comp. Neurol.*, 146: 421–450.

Jakab, R.L and Lernath, C. (1995) Septum. In: Paxinos, G. (Ed.), *The Rat Nervous System, 2nd ed.*, Academic Press, San Diego, pp. 405–422.

Jimenez-Capdeville, M.E., Dykes, R.W. and Myasnikov, A.A. (1997) Differential control of cortical activity by the basal forebrain in rats: a role for both cholinergic and inhibitory influences. *J. Comp. Neurol.*, 381: 53–67.

Johnson, R.R. and Burkhalter, A. (1997) A polysynaptic feedback circuit in rat visual cortex. *J. Neurosci.*, 17: 7129–7140.

Jones, E.G. (2001) The thalamic matrix and thalamocortical synchrony. *Trends Neurosci.*, 24: 595–601.

Jones, B.E. and Muhlethaler, M. (1999) Cholinergic and GABAergic neurons of the basal forebrain: role in cortical activation. In: Lydic, R. and Baghdoyan, H.A. (Eds.), *Handbook of Behavioral State Control—Cellular and Molecular Mechanisms*, CRC Press, New York, pp. 213–234.

Kilgard, M.P. and Merzenich, M.M. 1998. Cortical map reorganization enabled by nucleus basalis activity. *Science*, 279: 1714–1718.

Kinomura, S., Larsson, J., Gulyas, B. and Roland, P.E. (1996) Activation by attention of the human reticular formation and thalamic intralaminar nuclei. *Science*, 271: 512–514.

Kiss, J., Magloczky, Z., Somogyi, J. and Freund, T.F. (1997) Distribution of calretinin-containing neurons relative to other neurochemically identified cell types in the medial septum of the rat. *Neuroscience*, 78: 399–410.

Koelliker, A. (1896) Handbuch der Gewebelehre des Menschen. Vol 2. Nervensystem des Menschen und der Thiere. Verlag von Wilhelm Engelman, Leipzig.

Koralek, K.A., Olavarria, J. and Killackey, H. (1990) Areal and laminar organization of corticocortical projections in the rat somatosensory cortex. *J. Comp Neurol.*, 299: 133–150.

Juliano, S. L., Ma, W. Bear, M.F. and Eslin, D. 1990. Cholinergic manipulation alters stimulus-evoked metabolic activity in cat somatosensory cortex. *J. Comp. Neurol.*, 297: 106–120.

LaBerge, D. (1995) Computational and anatomical models of selective attention in object identification. In: MS Gazzaniga (Ed.), *The Cognitive Neurosciences*, MIT Press, Cambridge, MA, pp. 649–663.

Leergaard, B.T., Alloway, K.D., Mutic, J.J. and Bjaalie, J.G. (2000) Three-dimensional topography of corticopontine projections from rat barrel cortex: correlations with corticostriatal organization. *J. Neurosci.*, 20: 8474–8484.

Leise, E.M. (1990) Modular construction of nervous system: a basic principle of design for invertebrates and vertebrates. *Brain Res. Rev.*, 15: 1–23.

Lubke, J., Egger, V., Sakmann, B. and Feldmeyer, D. (2000) Columnar organization of dendrites and axons of single and synaptically coupled excitatory spiny neurons in layer 4 of the rat barrel cortex, *J. Neurosci.*, 20: 5300–5311.

Luiten, P.G., Gaykema, R.P., Traber, J. and Spencer, D.G., Jr. (1987) Cortical projection patterns of magnocellular basal nucleus subdivisions as revealed by anterogradely transported *Phaseolus vulgaris leucoagglutinin. Brain Res.*, 413: 229–250.

Lumer, E.D., Edelman, G.M. and Tononi, G. (1997) Neural dynamics in a model of thalamocortical systems. 1: Layers, loops, and the emergence of fast synchronous rhythms. *Cerebral Cortex*, 7: 207–227.

Malach, R. (1994) Cortical columns as devices for maximizing neuronal diversity. *Trends Neurosci.*, 17: 101–104.

Malmierca, M.S., Leergard, T.B., Bajo, V.M., Bjaalie, J.G., and Merchan, M.A. (1998) Anatomic evidence of a three-dimensional mosaic pattern of tonotopic organization in the ventral complex of the lateral lemniscus in cat. *J. Neurosci.*, 18: 10603–10618.

Mesulam, M.M., Mufson, E.J., Wainer, B.H., and Levey, A.I. (1983) Central cholinergic pathways in the rat: an overview based on an alternative nomenclature (Ch1–Ch6). *Neurosci.*, 10: 1185–1201.

Metherate, R. and Ashe, J.H. (1991) Basal forebrain stimulation modifies auditory cortex responsiveness by an action at muscarinic receptors. *Brain Res.*, 559: 163–167.

Metherate, R., Cox, C.L. and Ashe, J.H. (1992) Cellular bases of neocortical activation—modulation of neural oscillations by the nucleus basalis and endogenous acetylcholine. *J. Neurosci.*, 12: 4701–4711.

Miller, E.K. and Cohen, J.D. (2001) An integrative theory of prefrontal cortex function. *Annu. Rev. Neurosci.*, 24: 167–202.

Mountcastle, V.B. (1957) Modalities and topographic properties of single neurons of cat's sensory cortex. *J. Neurophysiol.*, 20: 408–434.

Mountcastle, V.B. (1998) *Perceptual Neuroscience. The Cerebral Cortex.* Harvard University Press, Cambridge, MA.

Munk, M.H.J., Roelfsema, P.R., Konig, P., Engel, A.K. and Singer, W. (1996) Role of reticular activation in the modulation of intracortical synchronization. *Science*, 272: 271–274.

Nadasdy, Z. and Zaborszky, L. (2001) Visualization of density relations in large scale neural networks. *Anatomy and Embryology*, 204: 303–318.

Paperna, T. and Malach R. (1991) Patterns of sensory intermodality relationships in the cerebral cortex of the rat. *J. Comp. Neurol.*, 308: 432–456.

Paus, T., Zatorre, R.J. Hofle, N., Caramanos, Z., Gotman, J., Petrides, M. and Evans, A.C. (1997) Time-related changes in neural systems underlying attention and arousal during the performance of an auditory vigilance task. *J. Cogn. Neurosci.*, 9: 392–408.

Paxinos, G. and Watson, C. (1998) *The Rat Brain in Stereotaxic Coordinates.* Academic Press, San Diego, CA.

Posner, M.I. and Dehaene, S. (1994) Attentional networks. *Trends Neurosci.*, 17: 75–79.

Posner, M.I., and Raichle, M.E. (1997) Images of Mind. *Scientific American Library*, WH Freeman and Co., New York.

Price, D.L., Whitehouse, P.J. and Struble, R.G. (1986) Cellular pathology in Alzheimer's and Parkinson's diseases. *Trends Neurosci.*, 9: 29–33.

Pucak, M.L., Levitt, J.B., Lund, J.S. and Lewis, D.A. (1996) Patterns of intrinsic and associational circuitry in monkey prefrontal cortex. *J. Comp Neurol.*, 376: 614–630.

Rakic, P. (1995) A small step for the cell, a giant leap for mankind: a hypothesis of neocortical expansion during development. *Trends Neurosci.*, 18: 383–388.

Rasmusson, D.D. (2000) The role of acetylcholine in cortical synaptic plasticity. *Behav. Brain Res.*, 115: 205–218.

Ribari, U., Ioannides, A.A., Singh, K.D., Hasson, R., Bolton, J.P.R., Lado, F., Mogilner, A. and Llinas, R. (1991) Magnetic field tomography of coherent thalamocortical 40-Hz oscillations in humans. *Proc. Natl. Acad. Sci. USA*, 88: 11037–11041.

Rockland, K.S. (1998) Complex microstructures of sensory cortical connections. *Curr. Opin. Neurobiol.*, 8: 545–551.

Roland, P.E. (1994) *Brain Activation*. Wiley-Liss, New York, 589 pp.

Rubenstein, J.L., Shimamura, K., Martinez, S. and Puelles, L. (1998) Regionalization of the prosencephalic neural plate. *Annu. Rev. Neurosci.*, 21: 445–77.

Rye, D.B., Wainer, B.H., Mesulam, M.M., Mufson, E.J. and Saper, C.B. (1984) Cortical projections arising from the basal forebrain: a study of cholinergic and noncholinergic components combining retrograde tracing and immunohistochemical localization of choline acetyltransferase, *Neuroscience*, 13: 627–643.

Saper, C.B. (1984) Organization of cerebral cortical afferent systems in the rat, I. Magnocellular basal nucleus. *J. Comp. Neurol.*, 222: 313–342.

Sarter, M. and Bruno, J.P. (1997) Cognitive functions of cortical acetylcholine: toward a unifying hypothesis. *Brain Res. Rev.*, 23: 28–46.

Scheibel, M.E. and Scheibel, A.B. (1958) Structural substrates for integrative patterns in the barin stem reticular core. In: H.H. Jasper, L.D. Proctor, R.S. Knighton, W.C. Noshay and R.T. Costello (Eds.), *Reticular Formation of the Brain*, Little Brown, Boston, MA.

Sesack, S.R., Deutch, Y., Roth, R.H. and Bunney, B.S. (1989) Topographical organization of the efferent projections of the medial prefrontal cortex in the rat: an anterograde tract-tracing study with *Phaseolus vulgaris* leucoagglutinin. *J. Comp. Neurol.*, 290: 213–242.

Shepherd, G.M. (1991) *Foundations of the Neuron Doctrine*. Oxford University Press, New York.

Singer, W. (1999) Neuronal synchrony: a versatile code for the definition of relations. *Neuron*, 24: 49–65.

Singer, W. and Gray, C.M. (1995) Visual feature integration and the temporal correlation hypothesis. *Annu. Rev. Neurosci.*, 18: 555–586.

Sofroniew, M.V., Eckenstein, F., Thoenen, H. and Cuello, A.C. (1982) Topography of choline acetyltransferase-containing neurons in the forebrain of the rat. *Neurosci. Lett.*, 33: 7–12.

Steinmetz P.N., Roy, A., Fitzgerald, P.J., Hsiao, S.S., Johnson, K.O. and Niebur, E. (2000) Attention modulates synchronized neuronal firing in primate somatosensory cortex. *Nature*, 404: 187–190.

Steriade, M. (1996) Arousal: revisiting the reticular activating system. *Science*, 272: 225–226.

Steriade, M. (1999) Coherent oscillations and short-term plasticity in corticothalamic networks. *Trends in Neurosci.*, 22: 337–345.

Sugitani, M, Yano, J., Sugai, T. and H Ooyama (1990) Somatotopic organization and columnar structure of vibrissae representation in the rat ventrobasal complex. *Exp. Brain Res.*, 81: 346–352.

Swanson, L.W. (1992) *Brain Maps: Structure of the Rat Brain*. Elsevier, Amsterdam.

Szentagothai, J, (1978) The Ferrier Lecture 1997. The neuron network of the cerebral cortex: a functional interpretation. *Proc. R. Soc. (Lond).*, 201: 219–248.

Voytko, M.L., Olton, D.S., Richardson, RT., Gorman, L.K., Tobin, J.R. and Price, D.L. (1994) Basal forebrain lesions in monkeys disrupt attention but not learning and memory. *J. Neurosci.*, 14: 167–186.

Whisaw, I.Q., O'Connor, W.T. and Dunnett, S.B. (1985) Disruption of central cholinergic systems in the rat by basal forebrain lesions or atropine: Effects on feeding, sensorimotor behavior, locomotor activity and spatial navigation. *Behav. Brain Res.*, 17: 103–115.

Wolff, J.R. and Zaborszky, L. (1979) On the normal arrangement of fibres and terminals and limits of plasticity in the callosal system of the rat. In: I.S. Russel, M.W. van Hof and V.G. Berlucchi (Eds.), *Structure and Function of the Cerebral Commissures*, MacMillan Press, London, pp. 147–154.

Woolsey, T.A. and Van der Loos, H. (1970) The structural organization of layer IV in the somatosensory region (SI) of mouse cerebral cortex. *Brain Res.*, 17: 205–242.

Zaborszky, L., Buhl, D.L., Pobalashingham, S., Somogyi, J. Bjaalie, J.G. and Nadasdy, Z. (in preparation) Three-dimensional chemoarchitecture of the basal forebrain: spatially specific clusters of cholinergic and calcium binding protein-containing neurons.

Zaborszky, L., Carlsen, J., Brashear, H.R. and Heimer, L. (1986) Cholinergic and GABAergic afferents to the olfactory bulb in the rat with special emphasis on the projection neurons in the nucleus of the horizontal limb of the diagonal band. *J. Comp. Neurol.*, 243: 488-509.

Zaborszky, L., Csordas, A., Buhl, D., Duque, A., Somogyi, J. and Nadasdy, Z. (2002) Computational anatomical analysis of the basal forebrain corticopetal system. In: A. Ascoli (Ed.), *Computational Neuroanatomy: Principles and Methods*, Humana Press (in press).

Zaborszky, L., Cullinan, W.E. and Braun, A. (1991) Afferents to basal forebrain cholinergic projection neurons: An update. In: T.C. Napier, P.W. Kaliwas and I. Hanin (Eds.), *Basal Forebrain: Anatomy to Function*. Plenum Press, New York, pp. 43–100.

Zaborszky, L. and Duque, A. (2000) Local synaptic connections of basal forebrain neurons. *Behav. Brain Res.*, 15: 143–158.

Zaborszky, L., Gaykema, R.P., Swanson, D.J. and Cullinan, W.E. (1997) Cortical input to the basal forebrain. *Neuroscience*, 79: 1051–1078.

Zaborszky, L., Pang, K., Somogyi, J., Nadasdy, Z. and Kallo, I. (1999) The basal forebrain corticopetal system revisited. In: *Advancing from the Ventral Striatum to the Extended Amygdala: Implications for Neuropsychiatry and Drug Abuse. Ann. NY. Acad. Sci.*, 877: 339–367.

Zaborszky, L. and Wolff, J.R. (1982) Distribution patterns and individual variations of callosal connections in albino rat. *Anat. Embryol.*, 165: 213-232.

E.C. Azmitia, J. DeFelipe, E.G. Jones, P. Rakic and C.E. Ribak (Eds.)
Progress in Brain Research, Vol. 136

CHAPTER 29

Anatomical origins of the classical receptive field and modulatory surround field of single neurons in macaque visual cortical area V1

Alessandra Angelucci[1], Jonathan B. Levitt[2] and Jennifer S. Lund[1,*]

[1]*Department of Ophthalmology and Visual Science, Moran Eye Center, University of Utah,*
50 North Medical Drive, Salt Lake City, UT 84132, USA
[2]*Department of Biology, City College of the City University of New York,*
138th Street and Convent Avenue, New York, NY 10031, USA

Abstract: From the analyses of our own and others' anatomical and physiological data for the macaque visual system, we arrive at a conclusion that three pathways can provide the V1 neuron with access to information from the visual field and affect its response. First, direct thalamic input can determine the size of the initial activating RF at high contrast. Second, lateral connections can enlarge the RF at low contrast by pooling information from larger regions of cortex that are otherwise ineffective when high contrast thalamic input is driving the cortical neuron. Thirdly, feedback from extrastriate cortex (possibly together with overlap or interdigitation of coactive lateral connectional fields within V1) can provide a large and stimulus specific surround modulatory field. The stimulus specificity of the interactions between the center and surround fields, may be due to the orderly, matching structure and different scales of intra-areal and feedback projection excitatory pathways. The observed activity changes of single recorded excitatory neurons could be a result of the relative weight of excitation on the excitatory neurons themselves and on local inhibitory interneurons that synapse on them. Inhibitory basket neurons, driven by the local excitatory neurons, could govern local interactions between cortical patches of different tuning properties, resulting in more distant changes in excitatory input in the laterally connected intra-areal neuronal pools.

Introduction

Santiago Ramón y Cajal's discoveries on the connectional architecture of the cortex were remarkable. However, in tracing axonal connections between neurons, he was hindered by the absence of the exquisitely sensitive neuronal labels that we have today, such as cholera toxin subunit B (CTB), biotinylated dextran amine (BDA) or biocytin. These labeling compounds are taken up mainly by the somata or dendrites of neurons within small injection

*Corresponding author: Tel.: +1 801 585 5554;
Fax: +1 801 585 1295; E-mail: jennifer.lund@hsc.utah.edu

sites and then transported anterogradely (to the axon terminals), and/or taken up by the axon terminals and transported retrogradely (back to the neurons' somata). We have used such labels to explore the anatomical pathways that provide neurons of macaque monkey primary visual cortex with access to information from the visual field (Angelucci et al., 1998, 2000, 2002). The cortical neuron's visual receptive field (RF) has classically been defined as that region of the outside visual world within which presentation of appropriate stimuli elicits action potentials from the neuron (Hartline, 1940; Barlow et al., 1967). The response of many cortical neurons to stimuli falling in their RF is modulated by parts of the visual image falling in the region surrounding the RF, even though neurons do not respond directly with action potentials to stimulation of the surround region alone (Blakemore and Tobin, 1972; Maffei and Fiorentini, 1976; Nelson and Frost, 1978; Allman et al., 1985; Gilbert and Wiesel, 1990; DeAngelis et al., 1994; Li and Li, 1994; Sillito et al., 1995; Levitt and Lund, 1997a; Walker et al., 1999; but see Rossi et al., 1998 and Li et al., 2001 for reports of late onset responses directly from regions beyond the classical RF). Most recently, this surround modulation has been modeled as overlapping excitatory and inhibitory mechanisms, where the inhibitory mechanism extends beyond the limits of the excitatory field (Sceniak et al., 2001). Here we review our and others' data from macaque monkey on the anatomical pathways by which the cortical neuron gains access to information from images falling on its RF and its RF surround, and discuss what might determine the size and interrelations of these two regions of the individual neuron's response field. We focus this discussion on parafoveal retinal eccentricities between 2° and 8°, as this region has been best explored in both anatomical and electrophysiological studies.

Thalamic inputs

Information from the visual field is first processed by the retinae of the two eyes and then relayed, via the lateral geniculate nucleus (LGN) of the thalamus, to the primary visual cortex (area V1). The retino-geniculo-cortical pathway consists of at least three channels derived from different ganglion cell populations. LGN relays of these three channels (magnocellular-M, parvocellular-P, and koniocellular or interlaminar-I) distribute to different depths in the cortical sheet, with the relays from right and left eyes segregated to interleaved stripe-like territories (see Levitt et al., 1996 for a review). Single unit recording within the principal termination zone of M and P thalamic inputs, layer 4C, shows the RFs of postsynaptic cells to be organized in a highly ordered retinotopic fashion reflecting the precision of their LGN inputs. This retinotopy is most precise for neurons that retain the clearest resemblance to LGN units, in having more or less circular RFs and lacking orientation specificity (Blasdel and Fitzpatrick, 1984). Single thalamic axons have very different arbor sizes depending on the channel to which they belong (Blasdel and Lund, 1983; Freund et al., 1989). For instance, the largest axons in the

magnocellular LGN channel (M1 axons) can have individual arbors that spread terminals up to 1.2 mm in extent, crossing 2 to 3 ocular dominance bands for the same eye, while the arbor of a single parvocellular channel axon spreads across only half an ocular dominance band- about 200 μm (Fig. 1).

The physical size of thalamic axon arbors relative to the size of the dendritic arbor of the thalamic recipient neurons in the cortex, and the overlap between them, determines the absolute limits of the cortical neuron's RF size due to direct thalamic inputs. The size of the RFs conveyed by the population of thalamic axons contacting a particular cortical neuron must be pooled in some fashion to form the basis for the cortical neuron's response field. Interestingly, RFs in layer 4C change in size and contrast sensitivity as a gradient in depth, being largest and most sensitive at the top of the layer (the M dominated zone), and smallest and least sensitive toward the bottom (the P dominated zone; Blasdel and Fitzpatrick, 1984; Hawken and Parker, 1984). This suggests that the neurons in the middle of the layer, with dendrites lapping to various degrees into the terminal zones of both M and P axons, sample from both types of thalamic inputs (see Bauer et al., 1999). Thus, the RF size and contrast

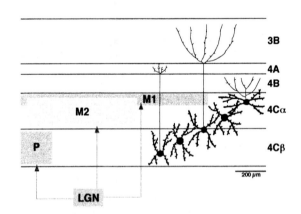

Fig. 1. Schematic diagram showing segregation of terminal territories of thalamic parvocellular (P) and magnocellular (M) afferents in layer 4C of macaque area V1. Note the different sizes of lateral geniculate (LGN) terminal axon arbors in this layer. The two populations of M axons (M1, M2) are thought to arise from different populations of M lateral geniculate neurons (see Lund et al., 1995). The distribution of postsynaptic layer 4C spiny stellate neurons is also schematically depicted; *thick processes* indicate dendritic trees of spiny stellate cells, *thin processes* depict their axons. Cells at different depths in layer 4C project to different output layers in V1. (Modified from Lund et al., 1995)

sensitivity of the postsynaptic cell is apparently a weighted average of the M and P inputs it receives.

V1 intra-areal lateral projections

Lateral projections between the cortical neurons of layer 4C could enlarge the size of the response field of individual neurons beyond that provided directly by thalamic axons. Within layer 4C, lateral projections are widest at the top of the layer (extending tangentially 2–3 mm from the cell of origin) and narrower toward the bottom of the layer, where they are quite local (within 300 μm) to the neurons of origin (Fitzpatrick et al., 1985; Yoshioka et al., 1994). Interlaminar projections into layer 4C from layer 6 neurons could also affect the response fields of layer 4C neurons, since in addition to thalamic inputs, layer 6 receives feedback inputs from extrastriate cortical neurons with RF sizes much larger than those in area V1.

Information is relayed in a columnar fashion from each point in layer 4C mainly to more superficial layers (Fig. 1; Fitzpatrick et al., 1985; Lachica et al., 1992; Yoshioka et al., 1994). Neurons in the most superficial tier of layer 4C project to layer 4B, where additional intralaminar lateral projections are made and received by the excitatory pyramidal and spiny stellate neurons in the layer (Blasdel et al., 1985; Asi et al., 1996). Mid-layer 4C cells project to layer 3B, and extensive intra-laminar lateral projections are made both at that level and in layers 2/3A, to which neurons of layer 3B project. Lowest layer 4C projects primarily to layer 4A, joining direct projections from the LGN P layers to the same 4A region. The lateral projections from excitatory neurons at any point in layers 4B and 2/3 are extensive (Fig. 2), covering elongated territories whose longer axis extends orthogonally to the ocular dominance domains (Yoshioka et al., 1996). Their spread along the long axis of the field can range between 3 and 10 mm in total length (on average 6–7 mm), depending on the size of the tracer injected column, and can reach up to 3–3.5 mm from the edge of the CTB (or BDA) injection sites to the furthest labeled point (Angelucci et al., 2002). The territory within the fields of the lateral projections is not uniformly innervated, but the terminals form bar-shaped fields around the injection sites in layer 4B (Fig. 2b; Asi et al., 1996), and columnar clusters with more circular cross section in layers 2–3 (Fig. 2a; Rockland and Lund, 1983; Lund et al., 1993). The bars and columns of

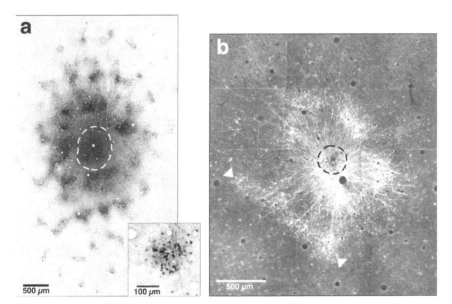

Fig. 2. Long-range intra-areal lateral connections in area V1. **a.** Top view of patchy lateral connections in layers 2/3 labeled by a CTB injection in these layers. Note the anisotropic distribution of the overall labeled region. *Inset*: higher magnification of a labeled patch showing cell body (retrograde) and terminal (anterograde) label, indicating the reciprocal nature of these projections. Modified from Angelucci et al. (2002). **b.** Top view of bar-like terminal territories of lateral connections in layer 4B labeled by a small injection of the anterograde tracer biocytin. *Arrowheads in b* point at a bar-shaped terminal region. *Dashed circles in a and b*: tracer uptake zones.

terminals have a similar regular center-to-center repeat distance of about 450–500 μm within the larger field of label. Using CTB, which yields both anterograde and retrograde labeling, each terminal region also contains retrogradely labeled cell bodies, an indication of the reciprocal nature of these connections (Fig. 2a, inset).

Feedback connections to V1

In addition to the thalamic afferents and the intra-areal lateral connections, there is another source of visual field information to individual V1 neurons. Several extrastriate visual cortical areas, some of which receive direct projections from area V1, send feedback projections to V1. Since neurons within these association areas have much larger RFs than V1 neurons, they feed back to V1 information concerning much larger areas of the visual field than the V1 neuron can access directly by other means (Angelucci et al., 1998, 2000, 2002; Lund et al., 1999). The size of these feedback fields can be measured after making small injections of the tracers CTB or BDA in V1 or in single extrastriate cortical areas. Small tracer injections in V1 produce extensive and elongated labeled fields in extrastriate cortical areas, whose longer axis in V2 extends orthogonal to the cytochrome oxidase (CO) stripes, and in all extrastriate areas appears to extend approximately parallel to the longer axis of the cortical area itself, following the overall anisotropy of visual field representation. The large size of these retrogradely labeled fields of cells in layers 5/6 of extrastriate cortex (long axis range = 4–10 mm, mean = 6.4 mm in V2; range = 4.5–10 mm, mean = 8 mm in V3; range = 7–11 mm, mean = 9 mm in MT), even after a small (400–500 μm diameter) V1 injection, gives an indication of the large aggregate RF that must reach single small regions of V1 via feedback pathways. Because of differences in cortical magnification factor, RF sizes and scatter among cortical visual areas, these labeled fields in extrastriate cortex span a much larger visuotopic extent than the V1 intra-areal connectional fields. Following single, small columnar injections involving all layers in areas V2, V3 or MT, large fields of both anterograde terminal and retrograde cell label are found mainly in layers 2/3, 4B and 5/6 of area V1. Some sparser anterograde (feedback) label is also seen in layer 1 following these injections. Interestingly, the V1 label in each of these layers is patterned in discontinuous patches that repeat at much the same scale as the intra-areal V1 connections (Fig. 3a).

Anterogradely labeled feedback connections and retrogradely labeled cells (i.e. the cells of origin of feedforward projections from V1 to extrastriate cortex) are superimposed in these patches (Fig. 3a inset). This observation suggests that the feedback pathways from any extrastriate region target the V1 efferent cells, or their immediate neighbors that project to that particular extrastriate area. These interareal connections are seen mainly in layers 4B and 5/6 after injections in areas MT, V3 and in the V2 thick CO-stripe compartments, and mainly in layers 2/3 and 5/6 after V2 injections in the thin CO-rich and CO-poor compartments. These feedback fields, much like the V1 intra-areal lateral connectional fields, appear anisotropic in V1 (Fig. 3b), with their longer axis extending roughly parallel to the V1–V2 border when near that border. This suggests that they follow visual field map anisotropies in V1. Feedback connections to V1 labeled by tracer injections in extrastriate cortex always exceed in size the intra-areal V1 connectional fields labeled by similarly sized V1 injection foci (long axis range = 6–14 mm, mean = 7–13 mm, depending on the extrastriate cortical area injected with the tracer).

Spatial anatomical scales, retinotopy and receptive field sizes

The three anatomical sources of visual field information–thalamic, lateral intra-areal, and feedback inter-areal inputs—could all contribute to determining the size of the receptive field and modulatory surround field for the V1 neuron. To identify the relative roles of these connections we have determined their spatial scale, in terms of cortical extent and corresponding visual field representation, and compared it to the sizes of RFs and surround modulatory fields measured physiologically for V1 neurons, and to RF sizes of extrastriate neurons (Angelucci et al., 2002). We have used small tracer (CTB or BDA) injections into electrophysiologically characterized cortical loci in areas V1, V2, V3 or MT, mapped and measured the resulting labeled connectional fields, and converted measurements in cortex into visual field extent. The latter was achieved either by overlaying anatomical maps of label on physiologically recorded maps of retinotopy from the same animal, or by estimating retinotopic extent using published equations relating magnification factor and RF scatter to retinal eccentricity, and our own measures of RF sizes (see Angelucci et al., 2002).

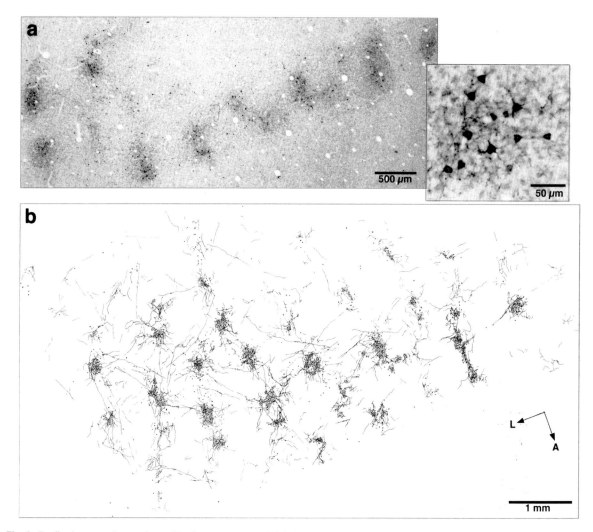

Fig. 3. Feedback connections to layer 4B of macaque area V1 labeled by a CTB injection involving the upper layers of cortical area V3. **a.** Micrograph of a low power view of a tangential section through V1 layer 4B, showing CTB labeled patches of corticocortical connections. *Inset*: higher magnification of a patch showing overlap of terminal label (terminals of feedback projections from V3 to V1) and cell body label (cells of origin of feedforward projections from V1 to V3). **b.** Two-dimensional composite reconstruction of anterograde and retrograde CTB label in V1 layer 4B, obtained by overlaying camera lucida drawings of several adjacent tangential sections through the layer. Same injection case as in a. Note the anisotropic distribution of the overall labeled region; this anisotropy follows that of the retinotopic field map in V1. *A*: anterior; *L*: lateral.

Thalamic input

In regard to the contribution of direct thalamic inputs to the RF of V1 layer 4C neurons, it is clear that receptive field size and contrast sensitivity are also dependent on the postsynaptic neuron threshold properties. RF size and sensitivity are measured by determining the minimum contrast, spatial location and extent of visual stimuli that

evoke suprathreshold responses (i.e. action potentials). Obviously, if its threshold is lower, a neuron may appear to be more sensitive or to have a larger RF, since less synaptic input will be needed to drive it. Intracellular recording and optical imaging studies (Grinvald et al., 1994; Das and Gilbert, 1995; Toth et al., 1996; Bringuier et al., 1999) have shown that subthreshold synaptic inputs to V1 neurons can arise from a much wider region of the visual field than can be identified on the basis of recording spikes. We confine our discussion here to suprathreshold measurements of RF size and properties, with the caveat that it is not yet known how the different types of inputs to a cortical neuron are integrated to produce suprathreshold responses.

In layer 4C of area V1, single unit recordings of nonoriented neurons, measured at retinal eccentricities between 5° and 8°, and hand mapped with small flashed high contrast black or white bars (Blasdel and Fitzpatrick, 1984), show them to have minimum response field diameters ranging between 0.4° and 0.1° from the top to the bottom of layer 4C. Using computer generated small grating patches of 75% contrast, we (Levitt and Lund, 2002) find RF diameters of 0.8°–1.5° for cells in layer 4C at the same eccentricity (these values are similar to those reported by Dow et al., 1981, for computer-mapped minimum response field sizes of V1 neurons at similar eccentricity). As has been appreciated for some time, and as we have seen from our own data compared to those of Blasdel and Fitzpatrick (1984), measurements of cortical RF size give very different dimensions when carried out using different test conditions (Schiller et al., 1976; Hubel and Wiesel, 1977; Dow et al., 1981; DeAngelis et al., 1994; Li and Li, 1994; Snodderly and Gur, 1995; Sceniak et al., 1999, 2001). These conditions include different stimulus contrasts, hand- versus computer mapping, single small flashed bars or grating stimuli presented at different locations or expanded in size (Fig. 4). One reason for these differences is that certain techniques do not reveal the full spatial extent of visual sensitivity. For example, isolated hand-held spot or slit stimuli and hand mapping of RF size may underestimate the extent of excitatory regions of the RF if the stimulus is too far from the RF center. In our experiments we have measured how neuronal responses vary with stimulus diameter, and have found that between 2° and 8° of retinal eccentricity, layer 4C neurons reach peak response using high contrast stimulus patches 0.8°–1.6° in diameter (Fig. 4, center). Furthermore, Sceniak et al. (1999) reported that by lowering the stimulus contrast, the RF summation area increases 2–3 fold; thus, our measures of RF peak summation area at high contrast given above for V1 neurons could instead be up to 2.4°–4.8° if measured at low contrast (Fig. 4, right).

One can try to estimate the potential receptive field diameter offered to each layer 4C cell by overlapped, retinotopically organized, thalamic axons. The cortical

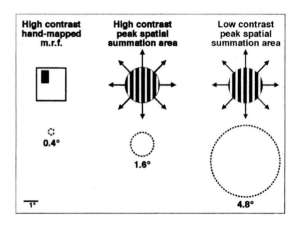

Fig. 4. Different methods used to map the receptive field (RF) size of cortical cells. *Left*: largest hand-mapped minimum response field (m.r.f.) size (bottom) of layer 4C neurons measured at 8° retinal eccentricity using a high contrast bar swiped over the cell's RF (top; based on results from Blasdel and Fitzpatrick, 1984). *Center*: largest computer-mapped peak summation area (bottom) of layer 4C neurons measured at 8° eccentricity using a high contrast grating stimulus expanding over the cell's RF (top; based on results from Levitt and Lund, 2002). *Right*: largest peak low contrast summation area of layer 4C neurons (bottom) estimated at 8° eccentricity on the basis of results from Sceniak et al. (1999).

neuron dendritic field (about 200 μm in diameter) could receive direct input from a total overlap of thalamic axon arbors equivalent to approximately two adjacent, non overlapped, thalamic axon terminal fields (Fig. 5a). Using published values of magnification factor (MF) across ocular dominance columns in V1 at 5°–8° retinal eccentricity (MF = 2.3–3.03 mm/degree at 5° eccentricity, and 1.43–2.06 mm/degree at 8° eccentricity; Van Essen et al., 1984; Tootell et al., 1988; Blasdel and Campbell, 2001), one can estimate that the arbor size of single M1 thalamic axons on the cortex (1.2 mm; Blasdel and Lund, 1983) covers a retinotopic area of 0.4°–0.8°. This retinotopic extent of M axon arbors is compatible with the measured size of large M LGN RFs (including center plus antagonistic surround; Derrington and Lennie, 1984; Spear et al., 1994; Levitt et al., 2001). Thus, the layer 4Cα neurons postsynaptic to the largest M axons could receive direct thalamic input from 0.8° to 1.6° of visual field (i.e. twice the retinotopic area covered in V1 by a single M1 axon terminal arbor; see Fig. 5a). These field estimates are larger than the minimum response field sizes (0.1°–0.4°) reported by Blasdel and Fitzpatrick (1984), but predict well the size of our computer-mapped

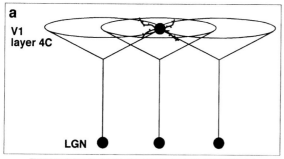

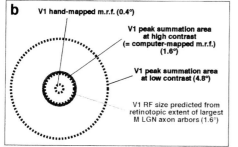

Fig. 5. Schematic diagram illustrating the potential contribution of thalamic inputs to the receptive field diameter of a V1 layer 4C spiny stellate neuron. **a.** Given the small size of a layer 4C neuron dendritic arbor (about 200 μm in diameter), and assuming orderly retinotopic organization of thalamic afferents in layer 4C, then each layer 4C neuron can receive information from a number of overlapped axons providing visual field information equivalent to approximately two adjacent nonoverlapped thalamic axon terminal arbors. **b.** *Dashed circles* indicate largest receptive field (RF) sizes of layer 4C neurons at 8° retinal eccentricity measured using different methods to map the size of cortical neurons' RFs (see Fig. 4). *Gray circle*: largest V1 RF size of layer 4C neuron predicted from the retinotopic extent of two adjacent, nonoverlapped, largest M thalamic axon arbors. Thalamic inputs can predict the largest high stimulus contrast summation area of V1 layer 4C neurons, but are too small to cover the size of the spatial summation area measured at low contrast. m.r.f.: minimum response field.

minimum response fields (0.8°–1.5°) and peak summation area (0.8°–1.6°) of V1 neurons measured at high contrast at similar retinal eccentricities (Fig. 5b). Our conclusions therefore differ from those of Sceniak et al. (2001), in that our estimates predict that LGN input to single neurons in layer 4C *could* underlie their high contrast spatial summation field (and high contrast minimum response field). Nonetheless, even the largest size of direct thalamic input field by this computation is still not likely to underlie the large sizes of layer 4Cα cell summation fields (2.4°–4.8°) measured at low contrast (Fig. 5b).

There is a further complication in that we now recognize that LGN neurons can also have an extended

modulatory field surrounding the classical (center-antagonistic surround) RF (Felisberti and Derrington, 1999, 2001). We must therefore acknowledge that LGN neurons providing the input to V1 may in fact have access to a much wider region of the visual field than previously appreciated, and that at least some of the surround modulatory region of cortical neuron RFs could be due to subcortical sources. However, since the subcortical surround effects seem not to be orientation-selective, as they are in cortex, intracortical processing clearly plays a major role in the generation of modulatory surrounds. In addition, it is highly unlikely that the dimensions of the surround field of LGN cells are reflected in the spatial scale of thalamocortical connections, since these surround fields are modulatory, and do not themselves evoke responses. Hebbian rules of connectivity imply that only the size of the LGN fields that can directly drive cortical neuronal responses should be of significance, and should be reflected in the spatial scale of thalamocortical connections.

Lateral connections in V1

We have compared physiological measures (between 2° and 8° eccentricity) of RF size with measures of the retinotopic extent of anatomical CTB (or BDA) labeled intra-areal lateral connections to an injected point in layers 4B or 2/3 of macaque area V1 (Angelucci et al., 2002). Figure 6 shows the retinotopic extent of lateral connections from a representative case in which a CTB injection was made in layers 2/3 of V1 at a retinal eccentricity of 6.5° close to the vertical meridian. The visual field extent of labeled V1 lateral connections is shown relative to the aggregate receptive field (ARF) size of neurons at the injected site that give rise to these connections. The concept of aggregate receptive field as used here reflects the cumulative RF of all neurons in a given cortical column (i.e. an injection site or a labeled connectional field), and it is computed by adding to the retinotopic extent of the labeled zone's diameter, the mean RF size of neurons at the edge of the labeled field, and the scatter in RF center position (see Angelucci et al., 2002). As noted above and shown in figure 6, for the same injection case, the size of the ARF of the injected neurons can vary depending on the method used to measure RF size. Accordingly, for the case in Fig. 6, when the ARF is computed using the neurons' minimum

384

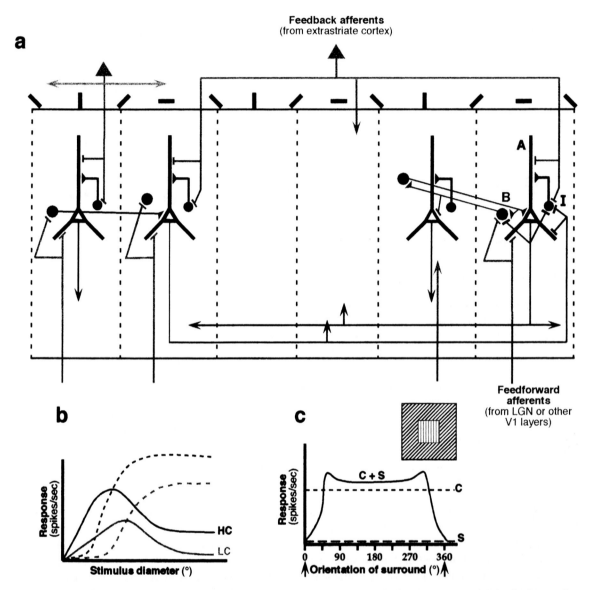

Fig. 9. **a.** Anatomical wiring used to explain center-surround interactions in area V1. Three main neuron types and their circuitry are shown. Pyramidal excitatory neuron A is the center recorded neuron. Neuron I is a local inhibitory interneuron reciprocally connected to pyramid A. Excitatory synapses (*flat endings*) onto pyramid A arise from: (1) feedforward afferents from the thalamus and other V1 layers; (2) long-range lateral connections from distant pyramidal neurons (shown to the left) located in the same V1 layer and in columns of similar orientation preference as pyramid A (*dashed lines* delimit cortical columns, and their orientation preference is indicated by the *black bars at the top*); (3) feedback connections from extrastriate cortex arising from neurons of similar orientation preference as pyramid A. Inhibitory synapses (*triangular endings*) onto pyramid A arise from: (1) local inhibitory neuron I; (2) basket neurons, another type of inhibitory interneuron, located in the same cortical hypercolumn as pyramid A, but in a column of orientation preference different from that of pyramid A (see two rightmost columns). Local interneuron I receives excitatory afferents from: 1) long-range lateral connections from distant pyramidal neurons with similar orientation preference as neuron I; 2) extrastriate feedback neurons of similar orientation preference as I; 3) its local pyramidal neuron A. Interneuron I controls the output of pyramid A. Basket neuron B inhibits pyramidal neurons and other basket neurons in adjacent columns of orientation preference different from that of B (Lund and Yoshioka, 1991). The same circuitry is repeated (but simplified for sake of clarity) in the two leftmost columns of the diagram. The pyramidal and basket neurons in these two left columns are driven by the "surround" stimulus and modulate the response of neuron A to the center stimulus. **b.** Graph showing the response dynamic of inhibitory neuron I (*dashed lines*)

and deep (5/6) layers. While extrastriate superficial layer cells feedback to the superficial layers of area V1, layers 5/6 of extrastriate cortex target both layers 5/6 and the superficial layers of V1 (Angelucci, Levitt and Lund, unpublished observations). The spread in area V1 of feedback connections arising from extrastriate cortical layers 5/6 is wider than that arising from the superficial layers, suggesting that the neurons of deeper layers of extrastriate cortex have larger RFs than those in superficial layers (Walton et al., 1999).

Neural substrates for receptive field and modulatory field

We have earlier suggested a pattern of connections that could underlie the surround modulation and inhibition observed in V1 neurons (Lund et al., 1995). At that time we had not explored the patterns of lateral connectivity using the most sensitive method of CTB now available, and we were unaware of the scaling of feedback pathways to V1 from extrastriate cortex. However, the basic premise of that model—i.e. that V1 excitatory neurons (e.g. pyramid A, Fig. 9a) would have local "symbiotic" inhibitory neurons (interneuron I, Fig. 9a) synapsing on them—may still be useful. Based on our recent data, we now propose a modified version of our earlier model. In this new model, shown in Fig. 9a, the local interneuron I receives the same intracortical excitatory relays (i.e. intra-areal lateral connections and inter-areal feedback connections) as the excitatory pyramidal neuron A, but does not receive direct thalamic or V1 interlaminar drive, which pyramid A does. Furthermore, interneuron I receives the output of pyramidal cell A via its collateral axon projections, and the response dynamic of interneuron I to excitatory input differs from that of pyramid A. The pyramidal neuron's firing rate simply depends linearly on the excitation afferent to it. In contrast, the local inhibitory interneuron has a higher response threshold, and is thus initially slow to start firing in response to excitatory input. However, with increasing excitatory input, the inhibitory neuron's response rapidly increases and thus begins to exert an effective brake on the excitatory neuron's firing, bringing it to asymptote or to actually decrease its rate of activity. Direct excitatory high contrast input from the thalamus or other V1 layers to pyramid A causes the interneuron to respond to input from pyramid A. In turn, this input from the pyramidal neuron, together with interareal feedback and intra-areal lateral excitatory inputs, causes interneuron I to exert enough inhibition to bring the excitatory neuron to asymptotic response (Fig. 9b). On the other hand, when thalamic inputs are driven at low contrast, lateral input can be more effective in driving up the activity of the excitatory pyramidal neuron; pyramid A can thus sum inputs coming from a larger area before the inhibitory neuron is driven sufficiently to bring about the pyramidal neuron's asymptotic response (Fig. 9b). In our model, surround modulation, via extrastriate feedback activity or further lateral input, is always present whatever the stimulus diameter. However, as a visual stimulus is expanded over the pyramidal neurons' RF and beyond, more weight of excitation from lateral and feedback connections reach pyramid A and its inhibitory interneuron partner, both directly and via laterally connected patches, eventually generating suppression of the excitatory neuron response. If, however, the stimulus in the surround is not matched to the stimulus in the neuron's receptive field, the offset patches that connect to the excitatory neuron via lateral connections are not contacted by the feedback excitatory activity (or by further lateral connectional fields), and thus the excitatory and local inhibitory neurons remain unaffected.

There is, however, experimental evidence of interaction between adjacent points of different response tuning—e.g. different orientations. When cross orientations are presented simultaneously to the classical RF,

and of its associated pyramidal neuron A (*continuous lines*) to a high contrast (*black*) and low contrast (*gray*) grating stimulus expanded over the receptive field of pyramid A. **c.** Graph showing the response of a V1 cell to concurrent stimulation of its central receptive field and surround (*C+S*). The center grating is at the cell's preferred orientation and direction of motion and at a lower contrast than the grating in the surround; the surround stimulus' orientation is systematically rotated around the clock (*inset*). There is no response to the surround stimulus alone (*S*). C: response to the central stimulus alone. There is marked inhibition of the response to center stimulation, when the surround stimulus matches the orientation of the central stimulus (*arrows*), but there is enhancement of the response to center stimulation, when the surround stimulus is at the oblique or orthogonal orientation to that of the center. We suggest this facilitation of the center pyramid A response by nonmatched surround stimulus orientation to be due to basket neuron inhibition between offset patches (see leftmost columns of a) reducing lateral excitation to pyramid A and interneuron I.

responses to either orientation are reduced. One anatomical substrate for this phenomenon could be mutual inhibition via inhibitory basket neurons (B in Fig. 9a), whose axons reach far enough laterally from any point to contact neurons (both excitatory and other basket neurons) tuned to the opposite orientation within the same hypercolumn (Fig. 9a, two rightmost columns). Thus, mutual suppression between interdigitated active zones in the lateral connectional fields of area V1 could lead to the observed cross orientation inhibition. An alternative mechanism, based on synaptic depression of feedforward (LGN) afferents, has recently been proposed to underlie cross orientation inhibition in V1 neurons (Carandini et al., 2001).

When the surround and center stimuli are nonoverlapping and of differing orientation, most commonly little modulatory effect of the surround is observed. However, by manipulating the relative contrast of center and surround stimuli; the activity of basket neuron inhibition may become evident. For some V1 cells, if the center contrast is low, surround stimuli of opposite orientation and high contrast may actually cause a slight increase in the firing of the cell to the low contrast center (Fig. 9c; Levitt and Lund, 1997a). We previously suggested (Lund et al., 1995) that this effect could be due to basket neurons (Lund and Yoshioka, 1991) driven by the surround located in columns of orthogonal orientation preference to that of the center neurons (Fig. 9a leftmost column); these basket neurons exert lateral inhibition on neurons located in adjacent patches of different orientation preference (Fig. 9a, second column from left) and connected to the center neurons. By this means, the basket neurons driven by a surround stimulus orthogonal to the center's could reduce lateral input to the center local inhibitor as well as to the excitatory pyramidal neuron, with further reduced excitation of the inhibitor. Such reduction of inhibition would be seen as a slight rise in the activity of the excitatory cell (Fig. 9c).

It is important to point out that for a subset of V1 neurons, when the center stimulus contrast is lower than that in the surround, center and surround stimuli of orthogonal orientation can instead have a suppressive, rather than a facilitatory, effect on the center cell's response (Levitt and Lund, 1997a). This can be expected if the contrast of the center stimulus is very low. At very low center stimulus contrast, the local inhibitory interneuron is virtually unresponsive. Thus, a high contrast surround stimulus of opposite orientation to the center would reduce lateral input predominantly to the center pyramid, with basically no effect on the local inhibitor. The net result would be lowering of the pyramid's activity. Futhermore, the specific type of center-surround interactions observed for V1 cells might depend on the neuron's position within the cortical orientation map (Das and Gilbert, 1999; Dragoi et al., 2001). Whereas the spatial relationship of the long-range intrinsic connectivity with the orientation map would not be significantly affected by the neuron's location within the map, its short-range connectivity (Lund and Yoshioka, 1991; Buzás et al., 2001) in relation to the orientation map would vary depending on the neuron being positioned near a singularity or a linear zone.

In some cells, local lateral inhibition may be stronger at closer angles than at the orthogonal—thus, two slight peaks in activity can be seen when the surround is oblique to the center orientation (see Fig. 9c; Levitt and Lund, 1997a). We are currently modeling the precise dynamics required of the two sorts of inhibitory interneurons and the local excitatory cell to see if these three neurons alone could provide a sound basis for the observed effects of basic center-surround interactions.

Acknowledgments

We thank Kesi Sainsbury for excellent technical assistance. This work was supported by MRC grants G9203679 and G9408137, EC grant Viprom Biomed 2, Wellcome Trust grant 050080/Z/97 and NIH grant EY12781.

References

Albright, T.D. and Desimone, R. (1987) Local precision of visuotopic organization in the middle temporal area (MT) of the macaque. *Exp. Brain Res.*, 65: 582–592.

Allman, J., Miezin, F. and McGuinness, E. (1985) Stimulus specific responses from beyond the classical receptive field: neurophysiological mechanisms for local-global comparisons in visual neurons. *Ann. Rev. Neurosci.*, 8: 407–430.

Angelucci, A., Lund, J.S., Walton, E. and Levitt, J.B. (1998) Retinotopy of connections within and between areas V1 to V5 of macaque visual cortex. *Soc. Neurosci. Abstr.*, 24: 897.

Angelucci, A., Levitt, J.B., Hupé, J.M., Walton, E.J.S., Bullier, J. and Lund, J.S. (2000) Anatomical circuits for local and global integration of visual information: intrinsic and feedback connections in macaque visual cortical area V1. *Eur. J. Neurosci.*, 12 (Suppl. 11): 285.

Angelucci, A., Levitt, J.B., Walton, E.J.S., Hupé, J.-M., Bullier, J. and Lund, J.S. (2002) Circuits for local and global signal integration in visual cortex. Submitted.

Asi, H., Levitt, J.B. and Lund, J.S. (1996) In macaque V1 lateral connections in layer 4B have a different topography than in layers 2/3. *Soc. Neurosci. Abstr.*, 22: 1608.

Barlow, H.B., Blakemore, C. and Pettigrew, J.D. (1967) The neural mechanisms of binocular depth discrimination. *J. Physiol.*, 193: 327–342.

Barone, P., Batardiere, A., Knoblauch, K. and Kennedy, H. (2000) Laminar distribution of neurons in extrastriate areas projecting to visual areas V1 and V4 correlates with the hierarchical rank and indicates the operation of a distance rule. *J. Neurosci.*, 20: 3263–3281.

Bauer, U., Scholz, M., Levitt, J.B., Obermayer, K. and Lund, J.S. (1999) A model for the depth-dependence of receptive field size and contrast sensitivity of cells in layer 4C of macaque striate cortex. *Vis. Res.*, 39: 613–629.

Bishop, P.O., Coombs, J.S. and Henry, G.H. (1973) Receptive fields of simple cells in the cat striate cortex. *J. Physiol. Lond.*, 231: 31–60.

Blakemore, C. and Tobin, E.A. (1972) Lateral inhibition between orientation detectors in the cat's visual cortex. *Exp. Brain Res.*, 15: 439–440.

Blasdel, G.G. and Lund, J.S. (1983) Termination of afferent axons in macaque striate cortex. *J. Neurosci.*, 3: 1389–1413.

Blasdel, G.G. and Fitzpatrick, D. (1984) Physiological organization of layer 4 in macaque striate cortex. *J. Neurosci.*, 4: 880–895.

Blasdel, G.G. and Campbell, D. (2001) Functional retinotopy of monkey visual cortex. *J. Neurosci.*, 21: 8286–8301.

Blasdel, G.G., Lund, J.S. and Fitzpatrick, D. (1985) Intrinsic connections of cells outside lamina 4C. *J. Neurosci.*, 5: 3350–3369.

Bringuier, V., Chavane, F., Glaeser, L. and Frégnac, Y. (1999) Horizontal propagation of visual activity in the synaptic integration field of area 17 neurons. *Science*, 283: 695–699.

Bullier, J., McCourt, M.E. and Henry, G.H. (1988) Physiological studies on the feedback connection to the striate cortex from cortical areas 18 and 19 of the cat. *Exp. Brain Res.*, 70: 90–98.

Bullier, J., Hupé, J.-M., James, A.J. and Girard, P. (2001) The role of feedback connections in shaping the responses of visual cortical neurons. *Progr. Brain Res.*, 134: 193–204.

Buzás, P., Eysel, U.T., Adorján, P. and Kisvárday, Z.F. (2001) Axonal topography of cortical basket cells in relation to orientation, direction, and ocular dominance maps. *J. Comp. Neurol.*, 437: 259–285.

Carandini, M., Heeger, D.J. and Senn, W. (2001) Cross orientation suppression in V1 explained by synaptic depression. *Soc. Neurosci. Abstr.*, 27: 12.12.

Das, A. and Gilbert, C.D. (1995) Long-range horizontal connections and their role in cortical reorganization revealed by optical recording of cat primary visual cortex. *Nature*, 375: 780–784.

Das, A. and Gilbert, C.D. (1999) Topography of contextual modulations mediated by short-range interactions in primary visual cortex. *Nature*, 399: 655–661.

DeAngelis, G., Freeman, R.D. and Ohzawa, I. (1994) Length and width tuning of neurons in the cat's primary visual cortex. *J. Neurophysiol.*, 71: 347–374.

Derrington, A.M. and Lennie, P. (1984) Spatial and temporal contrast sensitivities of neurones in lateral geniculate nucleus of macaque. *J. Physiol. Lond.*, 357: 219–240.

Domenici, L., Harding, G.W. and Burkhalter, A. (1995) Patterns of synaptic activity in forward and feedback pathways within rat visual cortex. *J. Neurophysiol.*, 74: 2649–2664.

Dow, B.M., Snyder, A.Z., Vautin, R.G. and Bauer, R. (1981) Magnification factor and receptive field size in foveal striate cortex of the monkey. *Exp. Brain Res.*, 44: 213–228.

Dragoi, V., Rivadulla, C. and Sur, M. (2001) Foci of orientation plasticity in visual cortex. *Nature*, 411: 80–86.

Felisberti, F. and Derrington, A.M. (1999) Long-range interactions modulate the contrast gain in the lateral geniculate nucleus of cats. *Vis. Neurosci.*, 16: 943–956.

Felisberti, F. and Derrington, A.M. (2001) Long-range interactions in the lateral geniculate nucleus of the New-World monkey, Callithrix jacchus. *Vis. Neurosci.*, 18: 209–218.

Fitzpatrick, D., Lund, J.S. and Blasdel, G.G. (1985) Intrinsic connections of macaque striate cortex: afferent and efferent connections of lamina 4C. *J. Neurosci.*, 5: 3329–3349.

Freund, T.F., Martin, K.A., Soltesz, I., Somogyi, P. and Whitteridge, D. (1989) Arborisation pattern and postsynaptic targets of physiologically identified thalamocortical afferents in striate cortex of the macaque monkey. *J. Comp. Neurol.*, 289: 315–336.

Gattass, R., Gross, C.G. and Sandell, J.H. (1981) Visual topography of V2 in the macaque. *J. Comp. Neurol.*, 201: 519–539.

Gattass, R., Sousa, A.P. and Gross, C.G. (1988) Visuotopic organization and extent of V3 and V4 of the macaque. *J. Neurosci.*, 8: 1831–1845.

Gilbert, C.D. and Wiesel, T.N. (1990) The influence of contextual stimuli on the orientation selectivity of cells in primary visual cortex of the cat. *Vision Res.*, 30: 1689–1701.

Girard, P., Hupé, J.-M. and Bullier, J. (2001) Feedforward and feedback connections between areas V1 and V2 of the monkey have similar rapid conduction velocities. *J. Neurophysiol.*, 85: 1328–1331.

Grinvald, A., Lieke, E.E., Frostig, R.D. and Hildesheim, R. (1994) Cortical point-spread function and long-range lateral interactions revealed by real-time optical imaging of macaque monkey primary visual cortex. *J. Neurosci.*, 14: 2545–2568.

Hartline, H.K. (1940) The receptive fields of optic nerve fibers. *Am. J. Physiol.*, 130: 690–699.

Hawken, M.J. and Parker, A.J. (1984) Contrast sensitivity and orientation selectivity in lamina IV of the striate cortex of the Old World monkeys. *Exp. Brain Res.*, 54: 367–372.

Hebb, D.O. (1949) *The Organization of Behavior.* J. Wiley & Sons, New York.

Hubel, D.H. and Wiesel, T.N. (1977) Ferrier lecture. Functional architecture of macaque monkey visual cortex. *Proc. R. Soc. Lond. B. Biol. Sci.*, 198: 1–59.

Hupé, J.-M., James, A.C., Payne, B.R., Lomber, S.G., Girard, P. and Bullier, J. (1998) Cortical feedback improves discrimination between figure and background by V1, V2 and V3 neurons. *Nature*, 394: 784–787.

Hupé, J.-M., James, A.C., Girard, P., Lomber, S.G., Payne, B.R. and Bullier, J. (2001) Feedback connections act on the early part of the responses in monkey visual cortex. *J. Neurophysiol.*, 85: 134–145.

Kennedy, H. and Bullier, J. (1985) A double-labeling investigation of the afferent connectivity to cortical areas V1 and V2 of the macaque monkey. *J. Neurosci.*, 5: 2815–2830.

388

Lachica, E.A., Beck, P.D. and Casagrande, V.A. (1992) Parallel pathways in macaque monkey striate cortex: anatomically defined columns in layer III. *Proc. Natl. Acad. Sci. USA.*, 89: 3566–3570.

Levitt, J.B. and Lund, J.S. (1997a) Contrast dependence of contextual effects in primate visual cortex. *Nature*, 387: 73–76.

Levitt, J.B. and Lund, J.S. (1997b) Spatial summation properties of macaque striate neurons. *Soc. Neurosci. Abstr.*, 23: 455.

Levitt, J.B. and Lund, J.S. (2002) The spatial extent over which neurons in macaque striate cortex pool visual signals. *Vis. Neurosci.*, in press.

Levitt, J.B., Lund, J.S. and Yoshioka, T. (1996) Anatomical substrates for early stages in cortical processing of visual information in the macaque monkey. *Behavioral Brain Res.*, 76: 5–19.

Levitt, J.B., Schumer, R.A., Sherman, S.M., Spear, P.D. and Movshon, J.A. (2001) Visual response properties of neurons in the lateral geniculate nucleus of normally-reared and visually-deprived macaque monkeys. *J. Neurophysiol.*, 85: 2111–2129.

Li, C.Y. and Li, W. (1994) Extensive integration field beyond the classical receptive field of cat's striate cortical neurons: classification and tuning properties. *Vision Res.*, 34: 2337–2355.

Li, W., Their, P. and Wehrhahn, C. (2001) Neuronal responses from beyond the classical receptive field in V1 of alert monkeys. *Exp. Brain Res.*, 139: 359–371.

Lund, J.S. and Yoshioka, T. (1991) Local circuit neurons of macaque monkey striate cortex: III. Neurons of laminae 4B, 4A and 3B. *J. Comp. Neurol.*, 311: 234–258.

Lund, J.S., Yoshioka, T. and Levitt, J.B. (1993) Comparison of intrinsic connectivity in different areas of macaque monkey cerebral cortex. *Cerebral Cortex*, 3: 148–162.

Lund, J.S., Wu, Q., Hadingham, P.T. and Levitt, J.B. (1995) Cells and circuits contributing to functional properties in area V1 of macaque monkey cerebral cortex: bases for neuroanatomically realistic models. *J. Anat.*, 187: 563–581.

Lund, J.S., Angelucci, A., Walton, E., Bullier, J., Hupé, J.-M., Girard, P. and Levitt, J.B. (1999) Topographic logic of connections within and between macaque monkey visual cortical areas V1, V2, and V5. *Investig. Opthalmol. Vis. Sci.*, S645: 3397.

Maffei, L. and Fiorentini, A. (1976) The unresponsive regions of visual cortical receptive fields. *Vision. Res.*, 16: 1131–1139.

Malach, R., Amir, Y., Harel, M. and Grinvald, A. (1993) Relationship between intrinsic connections and functional architecture revealed by optical imaging and in vivo targeted biocytin injections in primate striate cortex. *Proc. Natl. Acad. Sci. USA*, 90: 10469–10473.

Maunsell, J.H.R. and Van Essen, D.C. (1987) Topographic organization of the middle temporal visual area in the macaque monkey: representational biases and the relationship to callosal connections and myeloarchitectonic boundaries. *J. Comp. Neurol.*, 266: 535–555.

Morrone, M.C., Burr, D.C. and Maffei, L. (1982) Functional implications of cross-orientation inhibition of cortical visual cells. *Proc. R. Soc. Lond. B. Biol. Sci.*, 216: 335–354.

Nelson, J.I. and Frost, B. (1978) Orientation selective inhibition from beyond the classical receptive field. *Brain Res.*, 139: 359–365.

Rockland, K.S. and Lund, J.S. (1983) Intrinsic laminar lattice connections in primate visual cortex. *J. Comp. Neurol.*, 266: 303–318.

Roe, A.W. and Ts'o, D.Y. (1995) Visual topography in primate V2: multiple representation across functional stripes. *J. Neurosci.*, 15: 3689–3715.

Rossi, A.F., Desimone, R. and Ungerleider, L.G. (1998) Late onset response to extra-receptive field stimulation in V1. *Soc. Neurosci. Abstr.*, 24: 1978.

Sceniak, M.P., Ringach, D.L., Hawken, M.J. and Shapley, R.M. (1999) Contrast's effect on spatial summation by macaque V1 neurons. *Nat. Neurosci.*, 2: 733–739.

Sceniak, M.P., Hawken, M.J. and Shapley, R.M. (2001) Visual spatial characterization of macaque V1 neurons. *J. Neurophysiol.*, 85: 1873–1887.

Schiller, P.H., Finlay, B.L. and Volman, S.F. (1976) Quantitative studies of single-cell properties in monkey striate cortex. I. Spatiotemporal organization of receptive fields. *J. Neurophysiol.*, 39: 1288–1319.

Shmuel, A., Korman, M., Harel, M., Grinvald, A. and Malach, R. (1998) Relationship of feedback connections from area V2 to orientation domains in area V1 of the primate. *Soc. Neurosci. Abstr.*, 24: 767.

Sillito, A.M., Grieve, K.L., Jones, H.E., Cudeiro, J. and Davis, J. (1995) Visual cortical mechanisms detecting focal orientation discontinuities. *Nature*, 378: 492–496.

Snodderly, D.M. and Gur, M. (1995) Organization of striate cortex of alert, trained monkeys (*Macaca fascicularis*): ongoing activity, stimulus selectivity, and widths of receptive field activating regions. *J. Neurophysiol.*, 74: 2100–2125.

Spear, P.D., Moore, R.J., Kim, C.B.Y., Xue, J.-T. and Tumosa, N. (1994) Effect of aging on the primate visual system: spatial and temporal processing by lateral geniculate neurons in young adult and old rhesus monkeys. *J. Neurophysiol.*, 72: 402–420.

Tootell, R.B.H., Switkes, E., Silverman, M.S. and Hamilton, S.L. (1988) Functional anatomy of macaque striate cortex. II. Retinotopic organization. *J. Neurosci.*, 8: 1531–1568.

Toth, L.J., Rao, S.C., Kim, D.-S., Somers, D. and Sur, M. (1996) Subthreshold facilitation and suppression in primary visual cortex revealed by intrinsic signal imaging. *Proc. Natl. Acad. Sci. USA*, 93: 9869–9874.

Van Essen, D.C., Newsome, W.T. and Maunsell, J.H.R. (1984) The visual field representation in striate cortex of macaque monkey: asymmetries, anisotropies, and individual variability. *Vis. Res.*, 24: 429–448.

Walker, G.A., Ohzawa, I. and Freeman, R.D. (1999) Asymmetric suppression outside the classical receptive field of the visual cortex. *J. Neurosci.*, 19: 10536–10553.

Walton, E.J.S., Angelucci, A., Levitt, J.B. and Lund, J.S. (1999) Feedback connections from area V5/MT to areas V1 and V3 of macaque visual cortex. *Soc. Neurosci. Abstr.*, 25: 673.

Yoshioka, T., Levitt, J.B. and Lund, J.S. (1994) Independence and merger of thalamocortical channels within macaque monkey primary visual cortex: anatomy of interlaminar connections. *Vis. Neurosci.*, 11: 467–489.

Yoshioka, T., Blasdel, G.G., Levitt, J.B. and Lund, J.S. (1996) Relation between patterns of intrinsic lateral connectivity, ocular dominance and cytochrome oxidase reactive regions in macaque monkey striate cortex. *Cerebral Cortex*, 6: 297–310.

E.C. Azmitia, J. DeFelipe, E.G. Jones, P. Rakic and C.E. Ribak (Eds.)
Progress in Brain Research, Vol. 136
© 2002 Elsevier Science B.V. All rights reserved

CHAPTER 30

Static and dynamic views of visual cortical organization

Vivien A. Casagrande[1,2,3]*, Xiangmin Xu[2] and Gyula Sáry[1]

*Departments of [1]Cell Biology, [2]Psychology, and [3]Ophthalmology and Visual Sciences, Vanderbilt University,
Nashville, TN 37232-2175, USA*

Abstract: Without the aid of modern techniques Cajal speculated that cells in the visual cortex were connected in circuits. From Cajal's time until fairly recently, the flow of information within the cells and circuits of visual cortex has been described as progressing from input to output, from sensation to action. In this chapter we argue that a paradigm shift in our concept of the visual cortical neuron is under way. The most important change in our view concerns the neuron's functional role. Visual cortical neurons do not have static functional signatures but instead function dynamically depending on the ongoing activity of the networks to which they belong. These networks are not merely top-down or bottom-up unidirectional transmission lines, but rather represent machinery that uses recurrent information and is dynamic and highly adaptable. With the advancement of technology for analyzing the conversations of multiple neurons at many levels in the visual system and higher resolution imaging, we predict that the paradigm shift will progress to the point where neurons are no longer viewed as independent processing units but as members of subsets of networks where their role is mapped in space-time coordinates in relationship to the other neuronal members. This view moves us far from Cajal's original views of the neuron. Nevertheless, we believe that understanding the basic morphology and wiring of networks will continue to contribute to our overall understanding of the visual cortex.

Introduction

From the time of Cajal to the present day, the primary visual cortex of mammals has remained one of the most studied areas of the nervous system. Literally thousands of research papers have focused on this area starting well before Cajal began his classical studies. Cajal's elegant drawings of individual Golgi impregnated cells and of the arrangement of layers in the visual cortex describe the architecture of a structure that was already known during the peak of his career to be the recipient of visual signals from the retina. Cajal's genius was to go beyond the details of individual cells, beyond the limitations of the techniques of his day, beyond cytoarchitectural variations and to generalize about cortical structure in a

functional context. Without the aid of recording electrodes and modern imaging techniques Cajal speculated that cells in the visual cortex were connected in circuits involving cells with short axons and that vision involved successive steps of processing from the periphery through the thalamus to successive cortical areas. Cajal also was well ahead of his time in suggesting that connections in the adult cortex are not static but instead are dynamic and plastic.

Although it was known at the time of Cajal that the outside world was topographically mapped onto the visual cortex, no knowledge existed about the receptive fields of individual neurons, or how sensory quality might be represented by cortical neurons, or how neurons communicated with one another. The explosion of new technologies within the last 20–30 years has added an enormous wealth of detailed information about the cells, connections, pharmacology and physiology of the visual cortex. The big question is, however, to what degree has

---

*Corresponding author: Tel.: (615) 343-4538; Fax: (615) 343-4539;
Email: vivien.casagrande@mcmail.vanderbilt.edu

this knowledge changed our view of the structural and functional organization of this brain area or any other brain area. In other words, has current knowledge created a "paradigm shift" in the words of Kuhn (1970) in our thinking about the organization and operation of this area of the brain in the one hundred years since Cajal published his 1899 description of the human visual cortex (see pages 147–187 in DeFelipe and Jones, 1988 for translation)? In this chapter we will try to build a case in favor of the view that we are in the midst of a paradigm shift in the way science views the structure and function of the visual cortex and other brain areas, but with the following caveats. First, a paradigm shift is only recognized retrospectively; we are only proposing that one be in progress. Second, according to Kuhn's view paradigm shifts are abrupt changes in which new scientific theories replace old ones that are "proven wrong". In the strict sense arguing in favor of a paradigm shift would mean arguing that Cajal was wrong in his views. Instead, we would argue that the paradigm shift in progress is more similar to the main example given by Kuhn of the shift from classical mechanics to quantum mechanics. In quantum mechanics, the physicist calculates probabilities for particles following certain paths, rather than calculating the exact paths themselves as in classical mechanics. In other words, at one level quantum mechanics is dynamic while classical mechanics is more static. Although the approaches differ, classical mechanics is still applicable to most situations and is still considered a valid part of any curriculum in physics. In fact, natural science in today's world still rests on a foundation of Newtonian physics that has not changed much in hundreds of years. We will argue here that similarly to classical mechanics Cajal's contributions to brain structure remain and will in the future remain valid while a paradigm shift takes place in our view of functional organization. The rationale for focusing on the visual cortex is that it was studied in detail by Cajal and scientists of his time and remains one of the most studied areas of the brain today.

The remainder of this chapter is divided into four sections. In the first section we examine briefly Cajal's contributions to our knowledge of the anatomy of the visual cortex as well as relevant views of the day on the function of this region and its relation to sensation and perception. In the second section we focus on current views of the structure and function of the visual cortex showing how new technologies have not only added

details, but also provided a different framework for looking at function. In the third section we show how our current knowledge is leading us to view the behavior of neurons within visual cortex as a cooperative and dynamic network and how these views are forcing us to reexamine how information is coded by neurons. Finally, in the last section we return to our original question concerning paradigm shifts and summarize the evidence for and against the view that our perspective is different from Cajal's; we also address what shifting such a perspective predicts about future directions in the field. Throughout the chapter no effort is made to provide an exhaustive survey of the topic, but instead to provide the reader with specific examples to support relevant points.

Cajal's view of the visual cortex

When Cajal initiated his studies of the cerebral cortex he began at a time when there was already intense interest in the structure and function of this brain region. As reviewed in detail by Polyak (1957) and DeFelipe and Jones (1988) technological advances in the area of brain anatomy already had allowed for more detailed examination of the microscopic structure of cortex including advances in the fixation and hardening of tissue, microtome brain sectioning, and the use of carmine and other stains on tissue slices. Different cell types had already been identified in cortex by von Kölliker (1887), and Golgi (1884); and subsequently beginning with Meynert (see Jones, 1984) a significant effort was devoted to the cytoarchitecture of cortex with different laminar schemes proposed. On the functional side major debates concerning localization of mental activity within the brain had already appeared in the literature. Among the many contributions that preceded Cajal's work on visual cortex were discoveries based upon clinical observations of brain damaged patients and lesion and stimulation experiments in animals. By 1824 Wollaston had explained homonymous hemianopia in terms of partial decussation at the chiasm. Flourens (1824) had demonstrated the loss of vision following cortical lesions and provided the first proof that the cortex is involved in vision. Flourens, however, argued against functional localization within specific regions of cortex. Prior to Cajal's major works, Panizza (1861, see Polyak, 1957) had shown that the occipital lobe was essential for vision although Munk (1883, 1890) is generally credited with this discovery based upon his experimental observations of visual abnormalities after occipital lobe ablation studies in dogs. Munk later formulated the concept of a topographic projection of the retina onto occipital cortex. Contemporaneous with Cajal, major works on cortex such as those of Flechsig (1896 see Polyak, 1957) described the course of the visual radiation from the lateral geniculate nucleus (LGN) to primary visual cortex (striate cortex) providing the anatomical link between the eyes and the cortex. Cajal acknowledged the groundwork that went before him often summarizing the state of knowledge prior to presenting his own data. Cajal also made reference to past and on-going work in his defense of localization of function within the cortex and in his speculations concerning the roles of different regions of cortex in processing sensory information.

Cajal focused his efforts on details of the cellular architecture. His contributions to our understanding of cortical architecture including the visual cortex outlasted those of his contemporaries not only based upon the sheer volume of his scientific output (although this certainly didn't hurt), but also because he always constructed conceptual schemes in order to interpret his anatomical data in a functional context. Cajal classified cells, axons, connections and the laminar structure of cortex in an effort to define both what was fundamental about an area (its structural plan) and what differentiated functionally distinct areas. Although the unit of his investigation was the structure of the neuron and its processes, Cajal's goal was always to tie structure to function.

To examine how views have changed since Cajal investigated the visual cortex it is appropriate here to summarize his ideas and main contributions. Cajal believed that comparative anatomy was essential to providing an understanding of the fundamental principles of brain organization. Therefore, he began his cortical studies on small mammals including rats, mice and rabbits and used results in these species to compare with his findings in human cortex. Cajal provides his most extensive description of visual cortex at the peak of his studies of human cortex (1899–1902; see Chapter 14 DeFelipe and Jones, 1988). Cajal's basic tenets on visual cortical organization are presented in the latter chapter, although data are later provided on cat visual cortex and summarized in subsequent years in the context of newer physiological and anatomical data of others.

Cajal divided the human visual cortex into 7–9 cellular layers (see Fig. 1) based upon a combination of stains, comparisons with the schemes proposed by others and detailed Golgi studies of cell structure. Within this scheme Cajal argued that the cellular composition of the supragranular layers was similar to that found in other cortical regions. What he believed distinguished the striate cortex were: (1) the stria of Gennari made up of fibers of axons of intrinsic and extrinsic origin,

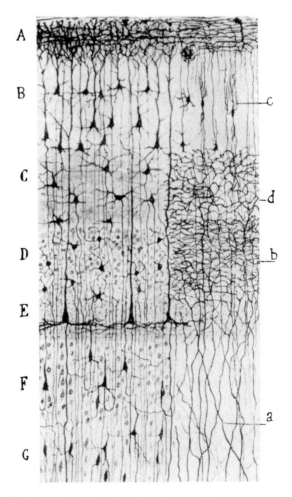

Fig. 1. Scheme of the main cells and layers of the visual cortex of man (calcarine fissure). A, molecular layer; B, layer of the small and medium pyramids ; C, layer of the large stellate cells; D, layer of the granule cells or of the minute star-shaped cells; E, layer of the giant cells; F, layer of the pyramids with arciform axon; G, layer of the polymorphic cells; a, b, d, terminal arborizations of the centripetal visual fibers. (From Cajal) Modified from DeFelipe and Jones (1988), figure 57, with permission of the publisher.

(2) a dense granular layer (his layer 5, layer IVC of Brodman, 1909) made up of small stellate cells that received input from the thalamus, and (3) the infragranular layers that contained both smaller pyramidal cells than seen in other regions of cortex, and cells with ascending axons not found in other areas.

Within the layers of visual cortex Cajal was able to describe most of the morphological cell types we recognize today even though he had no way to distinguish them except on the basis of morphology. In the area of morphology Cajal focused heavily on cell body shape and axonal morphology and less on the details of the dendrites themselves. Nevertheless, he believed that the intellectual power of human cortex over that of other species might be related to the elaboration of dendritic processes of pyramidal cells which Cajal referred to as "psychic" cells.

Cajal arranged his descriptions by layer because he believed that the laminar pattern of cortex, not just the cell structure itself, held functional significance. In Cajal's scheme the first layer or plexiform layer, layer I, contained special cells with long processes (today identified as the Cajal-Retzius cells), other cells with short axons, recurrent axons from cells in the lower layers and white matter, and the tufts of pyramidal cells lying in other layers. In Cajal's scheme layer I held special significance. Cajal believed signals from the association areas and from incoming sensations within striate cortex were combined in layer I to initiate action in the larger pyramidal cells of the infragranular layers. In visual cortex the "action" initiated within the pyramidal cells was seen by Cajal as driving special types of movements related to vision including movement of the head and eyes. Cajal's proposal concerning the motor functions of visual cortex made sense in light of the results of Munk (1889; see Polyak 1957) who had elicited head and eye movements following visual cortical stimulation in animals using high currents.

Layers II and III were described as containing mainly small and medium size pyramidal cells as well as several types of stellate and other nonpyramidal cells with short axons. Cajal showed that many of the pyramidal cells in layer III sent axons into the white matter as well as collaterals to other layers. As mentioned, Cajal believed that the cellular organization of the supragranular layers was common to all cortical regions reflecting some fundamental functional design. The short axon cells found in these and other layers, Cajal believed, played

two roles in visual cortex, namely, they were used to "increase the energy of the optic impulse to create sensation" and to propagate sensory signals to cells in other layers and different locations within a layer. This view has a decidedly modern ring.

Layers IV (the stria of Gennari, layer IVB of Brodmann) and V were identified by Cajal as the site of termination of optic fibers from the thalamus. We now know that such terminations are limited in human visual cortex to Cajal's layer V (layer IVC of Brodmann). Cajal characterized these layers as containing large (layer IV) and small (layer V) stellate cells. For Cajal these layers were the sites of initiation of sensation. He also believed that the axons of these cells transmitted sensory impulses directly to association cortex for memory formation. In addition to these stellate cells Cajal identified several other cell types within layers IV and V including both small pyramidal and nonpyramidal cells.

The infragranular layers VI–IX of visual cortex were described by Cajal as special because they contained some cells unique to visual cortex including pyramidal or ovoid cells that sent axons into the upper layers and giant pyramidal cells (Meynert cells) with descending axons. Cajal also described basket cell axons and other arrangements of axons and dendrites within these layers that he believed were unique elements. For Cajal the significance of the infragranular layers lay in their motor functions related to vision. The giant pyramidal cells (Meynert cells) he believed were part of optic reflex pathways concerned with movements of the eyes, lids, and pupils. In terms of function these ideas were not original with Cajal but reflected the prevailing view of other investigators of the time.

Generally when one thinks about Cajal's contributions to our understanding brain areas such as visual cortex, the emphasis is upon his description of the individual neuron. Yet Cajal's neurons are always placed within a scheme that emphasizes relation to function. Layers of visual cortex were considered functional units or modules, and, even though he fought throughout his career against the "reticularists" view of the nervous system defended by Golgi, Cajal certainly believed that groups of neurons must work together cooperatively as networks. This view is best exemplified in his diagrams not of visual cortex, but of the cerebellum and hippocampus where arrows are provided in his drawings of the proposed direction of flow of information within neural networks.

Advances in our knowledge of visual cortex

In the hundred years since Cajal published his major works describing the architecture and cell morphology of visual cortex there has been a technological revolution in neuroscience. Although the basic descriptions of cell morphology and anatomical architecture provided by Cajal remain valid today, great advances have been made in understanding the visual system and its functional architecture. The concepts of the visual receptive field and response properties of individual neurons did not exist during the peak period of Cajal's career. These concepts, initiated with the studies of Hartline working in the frog retina (1940), are now key to studies designed to understand the organization and function of the visual system at all levels. The visual system is currently viewed as a parallel distributed network designed to provide a description of the location and identification of objects that have survival value to the species. This is not done by transmission of a faithful camera-like representation of the sensory world as suggested at the time of Cajal. Instead, beginning with the construction of center-surround receptive fields in the retina the visual system selects what is needed to accomplish this goal. The retina contributes to this selection process by throwing away information about absolute light intensity, emphasizing local image contours, and compressing the wealth of information provided by receptors into manageable bits to be transmitted to the LGN via ganglion cells. The LGN regulates the flow of visual signals and informs the cortex about signal relevance while maintaining the basic sensory message transmitted from the retina. Primary visual cortex (hereafter referred to as V1) contributes by coding important aspects of local image features including their size, orientation, local direction of movement, and binocular disparity. All of these local descriptions of stimulus quality are critical for the more global and complex identification of objects ("what") and spatial relations ("where") that will take place in multiple extrastriate visual areas. We now know that in order for this to occur, V1 must solve the geometry puzzle of representing all stimulus qualities necessary for the subsequent steps of analyses within the different parts of the visual field map. V1 accomplishes this goal by a division of labor between different layers (as imagined by Cajal) and by different iterated modules within each layer. Below, we outline briefly specific advances in our understanding of V1.

V1 inputs

The revolution in anatomical techniques, particularly those that have allowed for tracing of connections using active transport mechanisms and a host of distinguishable labels, has allowed us to identify the majority (perhaps all) of the inputs to V1. Anatomical studies, often combined with physiological recording and immunocytochemical identification of transmitter/neuromodulator content, also have provided a detailed description of the structure and functional contribution of many of the V1 inputs. It was known at the time of Cajal that LGN cells sent axons to V1 but the system was viewed as serial in the sense that sensations arriving from the retina were processed in V1 and were sent to other cortical areas for "association" with other inputs and for memory storage; ultimately action was taken by motor cortex or projections to motor related subcortical structures. We now view information processing to and from V1 in terms of parallel inputs and outputs, complex feedback loops and interposed steps of integration. As shown in Fig. 2 on the input side at least 3 classes of LGN cells, the koniocellular (K), magnocellular (M) and parvocellular (P) cells send separate signals to V1 that terminate within different layers (see Casagrande, 1994; Hendry and Reid, 2000). Studies done in anaesthetized monkeys have shown that activation of V1 neurons depends completely on these inputs since chemical inactivation of the LGN blocks all visually evoked potentials (Malpeli et al., 1981). Additionally, we know based upon a variety of techniques including the down regulation of immediate early genes that input arriving from the left and right eye remains segregated in the form of ocular dominance columns in V1 of both humans and other primates, although the degree of segregation varies greatly between primate species (Florence and Casagrande, 1986; Florence and Kaas, 1992). Cajal was aware, from studies done by others, that binocular input reached V1. Only following the development of modern recording, labeling and optical imaging techniques, however, have the details of ocular dominance maps come to be appreciated. Figure 3 shows the complete pattern of ocular dominance columns on a flattened reconstruction through layer IV of V1 in a macaque monkey. In this case the pattern of eye input was revealed using a histochemical stain following loss of input from one eye. Such a loss results in local down regulation of cytochrome oxidase (CO) mitochondrial enzyme activity.

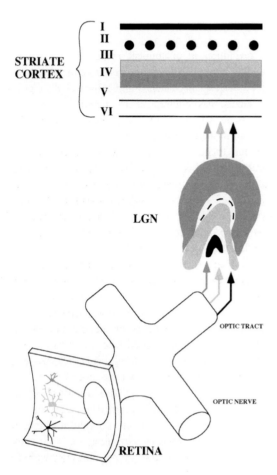

STRIATE CORTEX

LGN

OPTIC TRACT

OPTIC NERVE

RETINA

Fig. 2. In primates there are 3 parallel pathways from the retina through the lateral geniculate nucleus (LGN) to the striate cortex (V1): the parvocellular (P) pathway shown in medium grey, the magnocellular (M) pathway shown with light grey and the koniocellular (K) pathway shown with dark grey. Each pathway passes through separate LGN layers and terminates in different layers of cortex indicated by roman numerals. P and M LGN cells mainly terminate in lower and upper tiers of layer IV. These pathways also have other connections not shown. K LGN cells terminate within the cytochrome oxidase blobs in layer III and in layer I (see text for details).

CO staining is normally quite dark in all layers of V1 that receive input from the LGN; therefore loss of one eye results in lighter staining in zones connected to that eye. The result is shown in Fig. 3 in tangential sections through layer IV of V1 following flattening of the tissue. Black regions depict CO dense areas in cortex connected to the normal eye.

Besides the LGN, it is now known that V1 receives a variety of modulatory inputs both from subcortical and

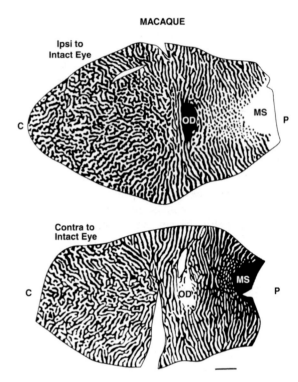

MACAQUE

Ipsi to Intact Eye

Contra to Intact Eye

Fig. 3. Distributions of ocular dominance columns in a macaque monkey ipsilateral and contralateral to the intact eye. These drawings were made from photographic montages. Black regions depict CO-dense reactivity related to the intact eye. The ocular dominance patterns in the two hemispheres are highly similar, although not identical. Splits that occurred during the flattening process are shown. The visual field is represented from central (C) to the peripheral (P) as indicated. The representation of the optic disc (OD) of the nasal retina is centered 17 deg from the fovea. The unbanded segments to the right correspond to the monocular temporal segment (MS) of the visual field. Scale bar = 5 μm. Reproduced from Florence and Kaas (1992), with permission of the publisher.

cortical areas. Although Cajal had speculated that the axons he identified in cortical layer I of V1 were from other cortical areas the technology did not exist that would allow him to directly identify the sources of incoming axons to V1. We now know that these extrageniculate inputs include serotonergic, noradrenergic, and cholinergic inputs from the brainstem and basal forebrain nuclei, respectively (Morrison et al., 1998), and that the latter inputs show differences in density within the V1 layers. Other input sources identified using modern tract tracing tools include the intralaminar nuclei of the thalamus and pulvinar, both of which send broad projections most heavily to layer I of V1. Additionally, there are retinotopically more specific sources of input to V1, many of which also receive projections from V1 including the claustrum, visual areas 2, 3, 4 (DL), and 5 (MT) (Casagrande and Kaas, 1994; Lyon and Kaas, 2001). Many higher order visual areas in the temporal and parietal lobes that do not receive direct projections from V1 nevertheless send axons to V1. These connectional details and the functional knowledge of various extrastriate visual areas are but a few of the many discoveries that have occurred since the time of Cajal.

The development of other technologies also has allowed us to ask questions concerning the functional significance of extrageniculate inputs to V1 in humans. An example of the impact that these nonLGN connections to V1 can have has been demonstrated using functional magnetic resonance imaging (fMRI) methods. Using these imaging methods it has been shown that topographic regions of V1 can be activated simply by asking normal subjects to imagine (with eyes closed) visual objects within particular areas of the visual field (i.e., in the *absence* of any direct stimulus to the retina, Chen et al., 1998). These findings argue that nonLGN inputs from extrastriate visual areas actually can have a strong impact on activity in V1. The noninvasive functional mapping methods of fMRI, positron emission tomography (PET) and other imaging methods have opened new doors for the investigation of brain function in humans. Prior to the development of these imaging technologies studies of brain function in humans were, as in Cajal's day, limited to clinical observations following brain damage or pathology.

V1 outputs

Cajal was aware that axons leaving V1 exited both from the superficial and deeper layers and that deep layer cells sent some axons subcortically. As with the inputs to V1, current knowledge of the outputs of V1 and their cellular origins and targets have allowed us to construct much more detailed anatomical wiring diagrams. These wiring diagrams combined with our knowledge of the cell properties and connections of output targets of V1 have fostered models of the flow of visual signals within the visual system. The important way that these details have changed our thinking concerns the function of the targets of V1 efferents. We now know that the lower layers, V and VI, send axons back to the thalamus and to the midbrain and pons. Layer VI is unique in that cells in this layer send both direct and indirect (via the thalamic reticular nucleus) feedback to the LGN and provide major pathways for V1 to regulate its own input. Cells in layer VI also send axons to the visual sectors of the claustrum, which appears also to modulate the responses of V1 neurons via feedback. Cells in layer V provide the major driving input to many cells in the pulvinar nucleus of the thalamus in monkeys; the pulvinar, in turn, provides input to a number of extrastriate areas that also feed signals back to V1. In addition, cells in layer V send a major projection to the superficial layers of the superior colliculus and other midbrain areas such as the pretectum, as well as nuclei in the pons that are concerned with eye movements. Thus, V1 is in a position to inform these structures of its activities and be informed by them indirectly through connections with the LGN or through feedback from extrastriate areas (see Casagrande and Kaas 1994 for overview).

As mentioned, Cajal was also aware that the superficial cortical layers of V1 provide output connections to some other cortical areas. Beginning with the seminal work of Ungerleider and Mishkin (1982) and Livingstone and Hubel (1988), working in macaque monkeys, we now know that V1 projects to a number of extrastriate cortical areas that are arranged within hierarchical-parallel systems designed to determine either object identification (the ventral stream) or location or visual action (the dorsal stream) (see Fig. 4). These connections emerge from different V1 layers or modules within layers suggesting that they carry different messages; a suggestion borne out by comparison of the response properties of cells within the different V1 layers in primates. In macaque monkeys the largest output connection is to visual area 2 (V2). Connections to V2 emerge from three populations of cells. Cells within the CO rich blobs of layer IIIA and IIIB send a major input to thin CO rich bands in V2, while the cells between the CO blobs (the interblobs) send projections to CO pale bands of cells (the interbands) in V2. Finally cells in layer IVB (also called the stria of Gennari) send axons to the thick CO bands in V2. In addition to these connections there are direct connections from layer IIIB to the dorsal medial visual area (DM, also called V3a) and patches of cells that lie below the CO blobs in layer IVB that project directly to extrastriate area MT (Boyd and Casagrande, 1999). Other output connections of layer III of V1 include projections to areas V3 and V4 (for review see Casagrande and Kaas, 1994).

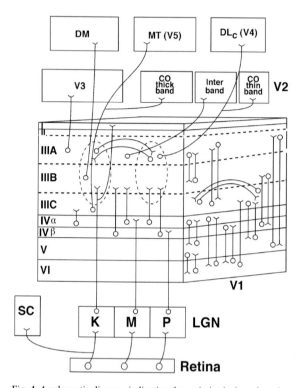

Fig. 4. A schematic diagram indicating the main intrinsic and extrinsic connections of V1 in primates as described in the text. No effort is made to define the strength of connections, or to indicate true axon collaterals or species-unique features. Feedback connections to V1 and the LGN as well as connections between extrastriate areas are not shown. The major input to V1 is from the lateral geniculate nucleus (LGN) which arrives via three pathways, the koniocellular (K), magnocellular (M) and parvocellular (P) pathways. The retina also projects to other targets, including the superior colliculus (SC) which also can in turn project to the LGN (connections not shown). Within V1, cell layers are heavily interconnected, not only by some of the axonal pathways shown but also via dendritic arbors (not shown). The main ipsilateral connections to extrastriate cortex exit from layer III. In layer IIIA, the cells within cytochrome oxidase (CO)-rich blobs, indicated by dotted ovals, and CO-poor interblobs send information to different target cells within bands in V2. In layer IIIB, cells within the CO blobs send projections to DM. Cells that lie under the CO blobs in layer IIIC send information to MT (V5). While the connection between V1 and V3 has been documented, it is not known from which layer or module this connection arises. Abbreviations of the visual areas are as follows: DL$_c$ (V4), dorsolateral caudal; DM, dorsomedial; MT (V5), middle temporal. Modified from Casagrande and Kaas (1994) with permission of the publisher.

In Cajal's day information processing was seen as serial from sensation through association to action. The notion of parallel inputs and outputs was restricted to the parallel processing of separate sensory modalities.

The prevailing views concern links between parallel input and output pathways *within* modalities. In vision it has been popular until recently to suggest that there is a direct link between the parallel input and output pathways of V1, namely that M LGN cells support motion perception (dorsal stream hierarchy) and P cells support color and form perception (ventral stream hierarchy). The best evidence for such a direct link comes from studies in which input from the macaque M and P pathways and associated K cells were briefly blocked with micro-injections of GABA (Nealey and Maunsell, 1994). This study clearly demonstrated that the majority of input to the middle temporal visual area (MT) comes from M cells or M and neighboring K cells since the two could not be inactivated separately in these studies. In spite of this, some MT cells could still be driven by the remaining P and/or K cells within the LGN. The importance of M input to area MT is not surprising given that cells in MT can detect rapid motion to which M cells are selectively sensitive. A fairly direct pathway for signals from M LGN cells to area MT has also been demonstrated anatomically; tract tracing studies have shown that cells in layer IVCα, the target layer for LGN M cells, send axons directly to cells in layer IVB which, in turn, can send signals to area MT. Nevertheless, cells in layer IVB that project to MT do not reflect the receptive field properties of M cells; instead most are complex direction selective cells whose receptive fields are constructed through circuits within the cortex (Movshon and Newsome, 1996). Even more opportunity for integration between pathways seems to exist before signals enter the ventral stream ("what" pathway). Blockade of the P layers and surrounding K layers does not silence cells within output layers IIIA and IIIB both of which respond well with either M or P layers blocked (Allison et al., 2000; see also below). Moreover, anatomically much of the output to the ventral stream leaves from layer IIIA which gets no direct input from layer IVC, but receives signals only after they have passed to other layers. Thus, both the wiring and physiology suggest that considerable integration of signals takes place in V1 before they are transmitted into the ventral stream for further analysis of object identity. Finally, the fact that lesions of either M or P layers in the LGN (together with associated K layers) do not eliminate either form or motion vision reinforces the view that it is inappropriate to equate complex visual behavior with the threshold properties of retinal and LGN cells (Schiller et al.1990; Merigan and Maunsell, 1990).

Cell types and receptive field properties

As mentioned earlier, one of the major advances in our knowledge of visual cortex since Cajal's day concerns the physiological characterization of properties of individual neurons. In the late 50s and early 60s Hubel and Wiesel (1962, 1968) began to characterize the properties of V1 receptive fields in cats and monkeys using a variety of patterns including line segments and spots of light displayed at discrete locations on a screen. In these seminal studies they showed that V1 cells could be subdivided based upon their responses to light. Hubel and Wiesel (1977) proposed that the cell types in V1 were arranged in serial order of complexity beginning with those that receive input directly from the LGN, which they termed simple cells. Hubel and Wiesel described these cells as orientation selective. Although there is still enormous debate over whether the property of orientation selectivity in V1 arises strictly from the arrangement of LGN cell inputs or is shaped by inhibitory connections within V1 (Bonds, 1989), there is no debate concerning the universal existence of this property in V1 of all primates. Hubel and Wiesel originally proposed that the receptive fields of each V1 cell class (namely simple, complex, and end-stopped cells) built upon the properties of their predecessors in serial order. We know now that the connections are more complex, that complex cells can receive input directly from the LGN and that end-stopped cells can either be simple or complex cells.

Hubel and Wiesel (1977) also introduced the idea that V1 must be made up of repeating columnar units. They described both the repeating cycles of orientation columns and ocular dominance columns. This concept of the vertical modular organization of individual cortical areas has had a tremendous impact on current thinking about the organization and function of cortex. Cajal never envisioned the visual cortex as modular. Hubel and Wiesel (1977) were cognizant of the problem that local stimulus attributes would need to be represented again and again at each locale. What they noticed early on in their studies was that orientation preference in cat and monkey V1 changes regularly as one moves an electrode tangentially within any layer (see Fig. 5). An advance of 1–2 mm was usually found to be sufficient to rotate twice through 180 degrees of orientation preference. This distance was also found to be sufficient to include at least one left and right eye ocular dominance column. From this information Hubel and Wiesel constructed a model in which they proposed that

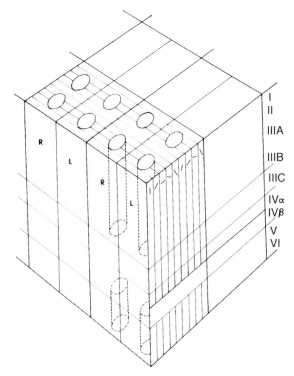

Fig. 5. Schematic diagram of the modular organization of V1. Each module (or hypercolumn; see text for details) consists of two ocular dominance columns (representing right and left eyes), a series of orientation columns (representing 180 degrees of rotation) and cytochrome oxidase blobs (representing color information). Reproduced from Livingstone and Hubel (1984) with permission of the publisher.

the cortex is composed of repeating modules called *hypercolumns*. They argued that each hypercolumn, whose exact boundaries were not fixed, should contain all of the machinery necessary to analyze one portion of visual space. More recently, Livingstone and Hubel (1984) argued that CO blobs should be added to this modular organization as zones uniquely equipped to transmit color signals to the next level. Although there is considerable debate as to whether CO blobs are actually uniquely designed for color processing since they appear to exist in all primates, even nocturnal species with only a single cone type (Casagrande, 1994), the fact that these modules are the targets of LGN input from a separate class of cells, the K cells, suggests that CO blobs do something special. Moreover, there appear to be enough CO blobs so that whatever is processed within these modules can clearly be represented across all topographic areas. Since CO blobs are positioned in the centers of ocular dominance columns in macaque monkeys they were added as another dimension to be included within a V1 hypercolumn (Fig. 5). The geometric problem is not so difficult for the cortex to solve when only three stimulus properties, orientation, ocular dominance, and color, must be constrained by topography, but when more properties known to be represented in V1 such as spatial frequency, direction selectivity, and binocular disparity are added, the task becomes more challenging.

Recently, optical imaging of intrinsic signals has been used in an attempt to determine the relationship between maps of different stimulus properties in single animals. Using this relatively high-resolution technique it has been found that changes in orientation selectivity are represented mainly in pinwheel formation with some regions also showing more gradual linear or abrupt fractures in the orientation map. The structure of orientation maps in different primates and in other species shows a great deal of similarity suggesting that orientation selective cells are organized the same way in humans. Maps of different stimulus qualities also suggest that, although not organized exactly as originally envisioned in the hypercolumn

model of Hubel and Wiesel (1977), maps of stimulus attributes are nevertheless iterated in such a manner that there are no "holes" in the map across space (see Fig. 6).

V1 cells and circuits

More than a hundred years ago Cajal described the morphology of most of the cells in V1 and postulated the direction of information flow. As mentioned earlier, Cajal's descriptions of V1 cells were always presented within a functional context. In spite of the fact that the functional roles of cells, layers and connections could only be guessed at, Cajal's guesses surprisingly often were correct (see above). Today, virtually all anatomical studies of cells and circuits in V1 are presented in a functional context. The numbers of cell classes and complexity of connections of V1 that have been identified and the controversies over the functional significance of the many circuits identified in V1 are beyond the scope of this short chapter (for recent review see Callaway, 1998).

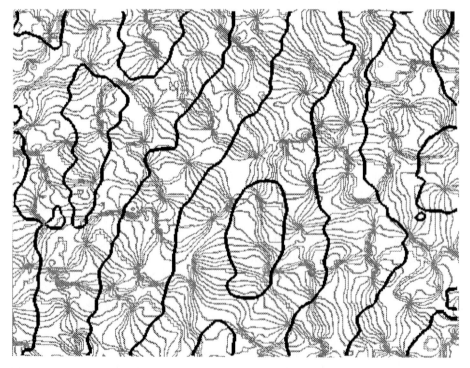

Fig. 6. Example of a contour plot of orientation preferences in overlay with the borders of ocular dominance bands imaged from macaque monkey V1. Iso-orientation lines (*gray*) are drawn in intervals of 11.25 degrees. *Black lines* indicate the border of ocular dominance bands. Reproduced from Obermayer and Blasdel (1993) with permission of the publisher.

Our aim here is to examine how the field has advanced over Cajal's contributions. The focus in current research at the level of cells and circuits in V1 is to compile sufficient detail on the morphology, neurochemistry and connections of individual cells in V1 that computer models of individual neurons and small and large groups of neurons can be generated.

Within these models V1 cells are divided into two main classes: pyramidal and nonpyramidal spiny cells containing glutamate (80% of V1 cells) and non-pyramidal, aspiny cells containing GABA (~20% of V1 cells). The former would fall into Cajal's long axon class while most of the latter would fall into varieties of Cajal's short axon class. Many subclasses of GABAergic interneurons have been identified based upon morphology, the presence of different calcium binding proteins such as calbindin and parvalbumin, or various peptides. The proportion of glutamate/GABA cells remains fairly constant across layers at least in macaque monkeys (Morrison et al., 1998).

We now know that connections between layers can be made by both excitatory and inhibitory neurons (for review see Lund, 1988; Callaway, 1998). Efforts to trace the general flow of information using pharmacological manipulations have suggested that layer IV becomes active first and after this the upper layers followed by the lower layers (Bolz et al, 1989). Circuits that connect layers III and V are especially robust as are circuits that connect layers IV and VI (at least from VI to IV, see Callaway, 1998). At the level of microcircuitry one concern to modellers has been the degree of precision in these circuits. If the local connectivity is based upon probability not on precision then efforts to document details of morphological differences between individual cells and their connections may not be meaningful. Recent studies, however, using dual recording, stimulation and calcium imaging techniques in slices of mouse visual cortex have suggested that cortical circuits of identified cells are surprisingly precise (Kozloski et al., 2001).

Most of the connections between V1 cells are local either within a layer or within a vertically defined column of cortex approximately 350–500 microns wide. There are, however, longer connections of up to 3 mm in macaque monkeys that occur typically between cells with similar properties (e.g., selectivity for the same orientation or ocular preference). These long tangential connections are found most commonly in layers I, III and V (Rockland and Lund, 1982). Cajal's drawings suggested that he had identified both types of connections although without the functional frame of reference we have today. The impact of these longer connections has been noted in the responses of V1 cells when areas beyond the classical receptive field are stimulated. Studies have shown that although V1 cells generally do not respond directly to stimuli presented outside of their receptive fields, if these cells are actively responding to a preferred stimulus within their classical receptive field this response can be modulated by stimuli presented simultaneously at other locations in the field (Levitt and Lund, 1997). Such interactions, which are considered in more detail below, suggest a means whereby responses to local features might begin to be put together to represent the global features of objects (Gilbert et al., 2000).

A dynamic view of visual cortex

The biggest change in our view of individual neurons within the visual system from Cajal's day until the present concerns their functional role. Although Cajal was well ahead of his time in suggesting that connections in adult cortex are not static but instead are dynamic and plastic, the tools were not available for him to eavesdrop on cells and sample their millisecond by millisecond conversations. We can now listen to the conversations of not one but many neurons while manipulating sensory inputs and pharmacology. We can sample neuronal activity at all levels from detailed neuronal interactions in slice preparations to fMRI imaging in awake humans. From all of these technological advances has emerged the idea that neurons do not have static functional signatures but instead change their messages depending upon the activity of the network at that instant in time. When speaking about neural networks one tends to think of a top-down or bottom-up flow of information. While these terms help us to dissect the network they fail to emphasize the recurrent nature of information flow in the nervous system. In other words the top-down or bottom-up view of information flow is, in fact, a bi-directional, continuous exchange of information between neurons and brain areas. In this section we consider the dynamic nature of V1 neurons beginning with "bottom-up" regulation of signals reaching V1 neurons and how these change the nature of their responses. Next, we examine how the concept of the receptive field of

V1 cells is changing based upon new information about network interactions. Finally, we review examples of "top-down" influences of V1 cell behavior and consider, in particular, the impact of arousal level, attention, and memory.

Bottom-up regulation

The concept of parallel input channels discussed earlier led to the idea that there might be labeled lines of communication between input and output pathways in V1. Evidence now shows that the majority of V1 cells integrate information from incoming pathways. Their response output appears to be dynamically regulated by the content of the stimulus. For example, it was shown recently that cells in all layers of V1 outside of layer IV show evidence of combined input from both the LGN M and P pathways (Allison et al., 2000). In other words these two pathways do not independently drive V1 cells. Evidence for this view was provided by selectively

blocking either the P or M pathways via GABA pressure injections into the appropriate LGN layers in the prosimian primate, bush baby (Allison et al., 2000). Prior to this blockade, the optimal orientation and spatial and temporal frequency of a drifting sine wave grating stimulus necessary to drive the cell was established. Contrast responses in V1 neurons were measured after blocking M or P layers in the LGN since M and P LGN cells are known to differ in contrast sensitivity. As can be seen in Fig. 7, V1 cells reflect different LGN inputs depending upon the contrast of the stimulus. At low contrast the V1 cells were entirely dependent upon the M pathway while at higher contrasts their responses reflected a combination of M and P inputs. Thus, whether a V1 cell is driven by one parallel input pathway or another is a reflection of stimulus content and its physical features.

Another example of dynamic "bottom-up" regulation of V1 inputs in relation to the LGN concerns the recent evidence that task relevance and other information can be

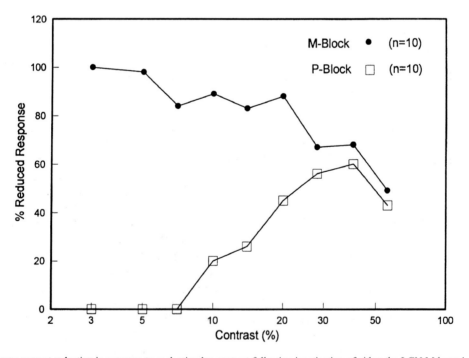

Fig. 7. The average percent reduction in response to each stimulus contrast following inactivation of either the LGN M layer 1 (filled circles) or P layer 6 (open squares) pathway. For the cells recorded during M layer 1 inactivation, the amount of response reduction decreased when stimulus contrast was increased, especially above 20% contrast. Conversely, the magnitude of response reduction during inactivation of P layer 6 increased when stimulus contrast was increased, especially above 10% contrast. The contributions of each pathway to the contrast-dependent response of V1 cells are clearly distinguishable. Reproduced from Allison et al. (2000) with permission of the publisher.

communicated directly to V1 cells along with sensory signals. In a recent study Sáry et al. (2001) were able to demonstrate in an awake monkey paradigm that LGN cell activity can either be enhanced or suppressed in relationship to a cue informing the monkey about task requirements. This enhancement or suppression of activity occurred while the monkey maintained fixation prior to any sensory stimulation of the receptive field of the LGN cell itself; the receptive fields of these cells were located an average of 10 degrees from the fixation point. An example of the enhancement in LGN activity under these conditions is shown in Fig. 8. This surprising result suggests that individual LGN cells carry multiple messages to their V1 targets. In addition, in the same study Sáry et al. (2001) were able to demonstrate that in a number of LGN cells response magnitude to the identical stimulus depends upon task requirements; some cells fire more vigorously to the stimulus if the monkey is required to make a saccade to the stimulus than when the monkey is required to keep its eyes

on the fixation point. Sáry et al (2001) have argued that modulation of LGN neurons (and thus V1 neurons as well) and increased response levels might achieve a better signal to noise ratio and ultimately lead to better localization of the target and better performance in a task where the target has behavioral relevance.

Dynamic regulation of V1 receptive field properties

The prevailing view since Hubel and Wiesel's (1962, 1965) seminal studies has been that each neuron in V1 is activated by stimuli over a limited range of visual space, which is called its receptive field. Recently, it has become clear that receptive fields of V1 cells are dynamically regulated. Classically, receptive fields were delimited based on the use of a single stimulus such as a light bar or an edge with a minimum discharge field defining the edges of the field (Hubel and Wiesel, 1962; Barlow et al., 1967). More recently, the size of each V1 cell's excitatory receptive field has been defined by use of patches of drifting sinusoidal gratings presented at the optimal orientation and spatial and temporal frequency (DeAngelis et al., 1992; 1994; Levitt and Lund, 1997). The length and width of these grating patches are varied independently; receptive-field length and width then are determined from the dimensions of the smallest grating patch required to elicit a maximal response (DeAngelis et al., 1992). This classical view of V1 receptive fields has been extended, because it was found that the responses of cells could be strongly modulated by stimuli or textural patterns placed far from the outer borders of their classically defined receptive fields (DeAngelis et al., 1992; Knierim and van Essen, 1992; Kapadia et al., 1995; Zipser et al., 1996; Levitt and Lund, 1997). The existence of facilitatory, inhibitory or disinhibitory surround effects has led to a broader definition of receptive field encompassing both the 'classical receptive field' and the 'nonclassical receptive field'. The key difference between the two definitions is that appropriate visual stimuli evoke responses from V1 cells within the 'classical receptive field '. In contrast, the impact of the nonclassical receptive field is only evident when both regions are stimulated simultaneously in which case the nonclassical receptive field can exert robust suppressive or facilitatory effects on the overall response of

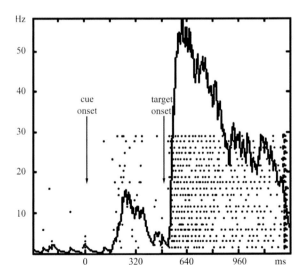

Fig. 8. Presentation of a behavioral cue influences LGN activity prior to target onset. Dots in the peristimulus time histogram represent individual neuronal spikes during the trials, the curve represents the average of 20 trials. Small triangles at the end of each raster line show reward for successful trials. The arrows point to the cue onset (time 0) and target onset, respectively. The first peak in the histogram shows the pretarget modulation with an onset latency of about 240 ms before presenting the visual stimulus. The second, larger peak shows the response of the LGN cell to the target presented in the receptive field. See also Sáry et al. (2001).

402

the cell (see Gilbert, 1992; 1998 and Fitzpatrick, 2000 for reviews). This distinction has important implications for the function of V1 neurons and suggests that these neurons may be performing more complex forms of analysis than previously thought. For instance, facilitatory surround effects may explain contour integration and illusory contours (Kapadia et al., 1995; Field et al., 1993), and suppressive effects could relate to perceptual 'pop-out' and curvature detection (Dobbins et al., 1987; Knierim and van Essen, 1992; Lamme, 1995).

Other evidence that the receptive fields of individual V1 cells are dynamic comes from work showing that the size of the classical receptive field in alert monkeys is not fixed but varies with stimulus contrast and the relationship between foreground and background (Kapadia et al., 1999). On average in these experiments, the length of the excitatory receptive field was 4-fold greater for a low-contrast stimulus than for a stimulus of high contrast (See Fig. 9). In addition, embedding a high-contrast stimulus in a textured background suppressed neuronal responses and produced an enlargement in receptive field

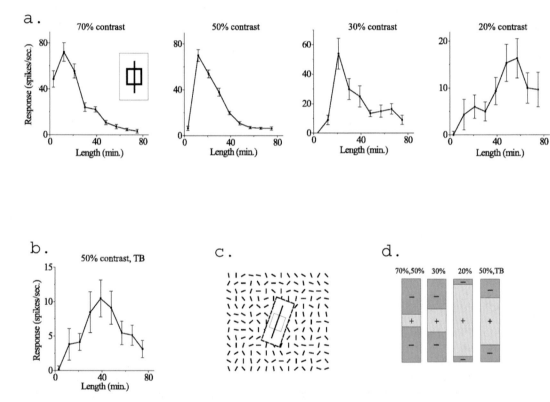

Fig. 9. The dimensions of V1 receptive fields are stimulus-dependent. (a) Length-tuning measurements in these four panels show the neuron's responses to optimally oriented bars of different lengths and 3' wide, presented at the central region of receptive field at four different contrasts. The extent of the excitatory receptive field is defined as the stimulus length that produces the maximal response at each contrast. The neuron shows spatial summation over a region 5-fold larger at low contrasts than at high contrasts. (b) Length-tuning measurements in a textured background. The stimulus is described in c. The background stimulus causes a suppression in the response to the bar stimulus and enhances spatial summation, even though the local contrast of the bar is still 50% (compare with 50% contrast condition in a). Response to background stimulus alone is 0.8 ± 1.2 spikes/sec. (c) Schematic of the textured background stimulus used in b and d. A 5° × 5° array of randomly oriented lines surrounds the receptive field (each bar measures 15' × 3' and the receptive field is depicted as an open square), whereas an optimally oriented bar is presented at different lengths at the central region of the receptive field. (d) Schematic summary of the changes in size of excitatory and inhibitory receptive field subregions under different stimulus conditions. Plus symbols (+) represent excitatory subregions and minus symbols (−) represent inhibitory subregions. As stimulus contrast is decreased, the excitatory region becomes larger and the inhibitory flanks become smaller. Embedding a high-contrast stimulus in a textured background produces changes similar to those produced by lowering its contrast. Modified with permission from Kapadia et al. (1999).

size similar to that produced by decreasing the contrast of an isolated stimulus. Kapadia and co-workers (1999) showed that receptive field dimensions are regulated in a dynamic manner that depends both on local stimulus characteristics, such as contrast, and on global relationships between the stimulus and its surroundings. The work of Sceniak et al. (1999) confirmed that the size of the receptive field (the extent of spatial summation) of macaque V1 cells depends on contrast, and was on average 2.3 fold greater at lower contrast. In the latter study, they measured cell response as a function of stimulus area to determine the spatial extent of the classical receptive field of V1 cells at various contrasts. The receptive field extent showed a strong stimulus dependence, and the extent of spatial summation shrank at high stimulus contrast. A similar dynamic dependence on stimulus contrast also has been reported in studies using multiple stimuli in the surround. The type of effect induced by presentation of a collinear stimulus outside the receptive field can often be switched from facilitation to suppression by increasing the contrast of the stimulus within the classical receptive field (e.g., Toth et al., 1996; Polat et al., 1998). If the size of the receptive field of V1 cells is not fixed but can vary with contrast and context, this means that the same region of visual space can exert no effect, a facilitatory effect, or a suppressive effect on a cell's response, depending on the stimulus characteristics.

In the above examples one could argue that the dynamic regulation of receptive field size does not actually alter other key properties such as direction selectivity or orientation selectivity. Recent studies show, however, that these key emergent properties also are not fixed but can be dynamically regulated (Bonds, 1989, 1991; Chapman et al., 1996; Ringach et al., 1997; Sharma et al., 2000; Dragoi et al., 2001). For example, Ringach et al. (1997) demonstrated that the development of orientation selectivity is time-dependent. Using the method of reverse correlation in the orientation domain over time they found that orientation tuning develops after a delay of 30–45 ms and persists for 40–85 ms. Neurons in layers $4C\alpha$ or $4C\beta$ of V1, which receive direct input from the LGN, show a single orientation preference which remains unchanged throughout the response period. In contrast, the preferred orientations of output layer neurons (in layers 2, 3 4B, 5 or 6) can change with time. In many cases the orientation tuning preferences can shift with time. These dynamic changes in response to different orientations is accompanied by a change in the sharpness of orientation tuning; cells in the input layers are more broadly tuned than cells in the output layers. The results of the latter study and others indicate that orientation selectivity is dynamically regulated within the V1 intracortical machinery, suggesting that V1 cells are more than a bank of static oriented filters (Ringach et al., 1997; See Vidyasagar et al., 1996; Ferster and Miller, 2000 for reviews).

Additional evidence that orientation selectivity of V1 cells can be dynamically regulated comes from a study in which input from the lower cortical layers was inactivated with GABA while responses of individual V1 cells were measured in the more superficial layers (Allison et al., 1995). Depending upon the location of the blocking electrode relative to the recording electrode, upper layer V1 cells exhibited a change in their orientation preference, a reduction in their orientation tuning, and/or an increase in their response amplitude. The effects on the orientation tuning of V1 cells were restricted in all cases to within ± 30 degrees of the preferred stimulus orientation. This means that layer blocking affects cells with preferred stimulus orientations similar to those of the recorded neurons. Only cells located within 500 microns tangential to the vertical axis of the injection site exhibited these effects. These results suggest that cells within layers 5 and 6 provide organized, orientation-tuned inhibition that regulates or dynamically sharpens the orientation tuning of cells in the upper cortical layers within the same, or closely neighboring, cell columns.

Adaptation effects on V1 cells

Other examples of the dynamic regulation of V1 responses are studies that show a reduction or shift in response depending upon the history of the cell. In an interesting recent demonstration of this effect on orientation, Dragoi et al. (2000) employed single-unit recording and intrinsic signal imaging (optical imaging) techniques to demonstrate systematic shifts in orientation preference away from the orientation used to adapt a V1 cell for 10 s to 10 min. In contrast to the common view of adaptation as a passive process that suppresses responses around the adapting orientation, this study showed that changes in orientation tuning occur due to response increases at orientations away from the adapting orientation. This suggests that adaptation-induced orientation plasticity is an active time-dependent process that involves network interactions and includes both response depression and enhancement (Dragoi et al., 2000).

More classical examples of such adaptation effects have been shown for both primate and cat V1 cells in contrast adaptation. Contrast sensitivity and gain of V1 cells are reduced after short exposure to high-contrast stimuli (Bonds, 1991; Allison et al., 1996). The temporal changes related to contrast adaptation were examined in detail by Bonds (1991). He explored these effects by stimulating cortical cells with drifting gratings in which contrast sequentially incremented and decremented in a stepwise fashion over time. All responses showed a clear hysteresis, in which contrast gain dropped on average 0.36 log units and then returned to baseline values within 60 s (Bonds, 1991).

Arousal level

V1 cells are also dynamically regulated based upon global changes in arousal. Recording from awake cats Livingstone and Hubel (1981) originally showed that visual signals are enhanced and spontaneous firing reduced on arousal compared to sleep. Many V1 cells also reduce the irregular burst-like firing and produce a more regular firing pattern when an animal awakes. These changes result in an increase in the signal-to-noise ratio and thus may lead to better transmission of visual signals during wakefulness. As discussed earlier these changes likely originate in the LGN. Neurons in the LGN appear to have two functional states: a bursting mode and a single spike mode. These modes determine the fidelity of response to sensory signals (McCormick and Feeser, 1990). During burst mode the LGN neurons are not capable of faithfully representing the incoming signal, while in the single spike mode, responses are tied more directly to the stimulus features themselves. In this way LGN cells can regulate the amount of sensory information that reaches V1 cells. Interestingly, Ramcharan and colleagues (2000) reported that the two modes of firing were also evident in the awake animal. Sherman (2001) has hypothesized that the two modes of activity of LGN neurons in awake animals serve two different purposes. V1 neurons receive a more linear representation of LGN input in the tonic mode. Tonic mode more faithfully describes stimulus features but with poorer detectability,

while in burst mode, V1 neurons receive more accurate information about stimulus change.

Attention

Other examples of dynamic regulation of responses of V1 cells concern the issue of attention. Although many studies suggest that V1 cells are not regulated by attentional shifts, a number of studies support such effects. Haenny and Schiller (1988) provided evidence that activity in V1 neurons can shift depending on attentional state. In the latter study the monkeys were required to perform a sequential matching task and had to detect the repetition of a particular pattern in a series of visual stimuli. This demanded that a decision be made which kept the attention level of the animal constant. Activity of V1 (and of V4) neurons was enhanced by as much as 20% during the presentation of a stimulus that the animal knew would be rewarded. It has been hypothesized that these attentional effects are produced by feedback to V1 cells from extrastriate areas.

To be effective, the feedback signals to V1 that relate to attention should be flexible and capable of rapidly "updating" the different regions of V1. What happens if the stimulus is not stationary, but moves relative to the receptive field while the animal performs a task? Or, the stimulus is stationary and the eyes perform a slow tracing movement along an elongated stimulus or contour line? In an experiment performed by Roelfsema and co-workers (1998) the monkey was involved in a curve-tracing task (using its eyes to trace the curve) while activity of V1 neurons was recorded. Whenever the receptive field of V1 neurons was located on the curve to be traced, neuronal activity was modulated by as much as 30%. Based on the latency differences between the modulation and the visual response proper (about 200 ms), the authors propose that the modulation observed in V1 is object-based. These results are particularly interesting since they suggest that V1 neurons are modified by higher order attentional shifts that can "lock" onto a target of interest.

There also is evidence that levels of attention can dramatically alter responses of V1 in humans. In an fMRI study, human subjects performed a speed discrimination task with sinusoidal gratings moving concentrically inward or outward, or had to view the grating stimuli passively. Performing the task actively resulted in a significant activation of V1 (Huk and Heeger, 2000). Performing the identical task passively resulted in no fMRI activation of V1. In a similar experiment Gandhi and colleagues (1999) presented a stimulus either in the right or left visual hemifield and measured changes in activity in V1 using fMRI. There was an increase in V1 activity, which shifted from hemisphere to hemisphere. The latter results raise two important points: V1 neurons can increase activity during a visual discrimination task on a population level, and this increase is spatially selective (follows the stimulus shift between the visual hemifields) and thus is likely to be the result of spatial attention.

In the examples given above, attention was shown to modify V1 neurons globally, but local effects have also been demonstrated (Ito and Gilbert, 1999). Earlier in this section we considered the impact of surround effects on the responses to V1 neurons to stimuli presented in the 'classical' receptive field. Ito and Gilbert (1999) also found that these surround effects were dependent upon attention. They found that if monkeys were trained in a brightness discrimination task containing flanking stimuli, and were required to focus their attention on a particular location of the stimulus screen or use it in a distributed way (not knowing where the change to be detected would show up), attention had a significant effect on the contextual facilitation seen in V1 neurons.

Working memory in V1

In the previous subsection we considered the impact of attention on the responses of V1 neurons. In this final subsection we provide evidence that V1 neuronal responses also are dynamically regulated based upon visual memory. Interestingly, Cajal would probably not have been surprised by such a finding because he proposed that centripetal fibers to V1 originated in association areas concerned with visual memory. Evidence for the impact of memory on V1 neuronal responses comes from a study by Super and colleagues (2001), who trained monkeys to perform a delayed-response figure-ground discrimination during which the animal had to remember the spatial location of a motion-defined target stimulus after it had been removed from the screen. After a variable period of time the monkeys had to make a saccade to the location of the remembered target. Neuronal responses in V1 were recorded during

the trials when either the target stimulus or the background fell on the receptive field. While initially V1 cells responded the same way to the target and the background, the authors observed a late modulation of the neuronal activity. This altered response persisted during the delay period even after removal of the stimulus. This modulation continued in trials when the stimulus was a target, whereas it decreased when the same stimulus was used as the background. The authors argue that the V1 cell memory related modulation is an active process and is related to the storage of information needed to successfully finish the task. The authors go on to propose that the altered activity they observe in V1 neurons may serve as a substrate for working memory.

Conclusions and future directions

We have now concluded our short tour highlighting the changes that have taken place in views of the visual cortical neuron since the time of Cajal. Most of the detailed descriptions of individual neurons and their relationships to each other and laminar cytoarchitecture made by Cajal still hold today. Cajal's concept of the neuron as the fundamental independent unit of the nervous system, of course, also still stands. Many of Cajal's speculations concerning the general flow of visual information and the circuits necessary to boost signals in V1 have been supported by modern experiments. There also have been enormous advances in our knowledge about V1 neurons and their connections and relationships to circuits, modules, layers and pathways. Although speculations by Cajal anticipated the simple to complex arrangement of neuronal receptive fields described by Hubel and Wiesel, this familiar concept of visual receptive fields did not exist at the time of Cajal. Moreover, Cajal diagramed circuits as excitatory; Cajal never anticipated that many of the circuits he drew involved inhibitory interneurons. Although Cajal speculated about chemical specificity in a developmental context, he never envisioned the complex intracellular signaling pathways that have been revealed by modern molecular neurobiology. Whether Cajal did or did not anticipate current views of neurons within V1 or any other region of the nervous system, however, does not address the main question we posed in the beginning of the chapter. The key question we posed earlier was whether the current approaches (as reviewed above,) constitute a "paradigm shift" in the words of

Kuhn (1970) in our thinking about the organization and operation of visual cortex over what was espoused by Cajal. What is the evidence for and against the occurrence of a paradigm shift?

The dynamic nature of processing in V1 neurons reviewed earlier provides the strongest evidence for a paradigm shift. Technology is now allowing the scientific community to address long standing conflicts between the psychology of perception and neurophysiology. Theories of perceptual processing have not attempted, until very recently, to bridge the divide between the views of neurophysiology and the subjective quality of a unified visual world. The reason for this is that these properties are inconsistent with classical neurophysiology. Classical neurophysiology is based upon Cajal's neuron doctrine where the input/output function of dendrites and axons, together with transmission across the synapse, suggests that neurons operate as quasi-independent processors in a sequential or hierarchical architecture that processes information in well defined pathways. Our subjective experience is, however, not like an assembly of abstract features but a stable unified whole. There is no accounting in the neuron doctrine for this constructive or generative aspect of perceptual processing. In fact, the apparent continuity of perception (known now as the "binding" problem) was one of the major arguments made against Cajal's neuron doctrine. Not only is perception unified but it is an active process where the acquisition of new sensory information is based upon the goal directed behavior of the organism. Because of these conflicts between classical neurophysiology and psychophysics, we would argue that there is currently an evolving paradigm shift in views of visual system processing. As reviewed under, "a dynamic view of visual cortex", models of V1 must take into account the continuous updating of information that takes place via both top-down and bottom-up signals. Individual V1 neurons are not static filters but instead clearly respond in a context dependent manner. Their responses depend both on their local connections and individual properties and on the global interactions of the networks to which they are connected—networks that carry information about sensory quality, behavioral relevance and context. These properties lead to the conclusion that the visual cortex is a node in an intricate distributed network, and that it can cooperatively extract high-order information from the visual scene. In this sense the contributions of the individual neuron are never independent of the network. As the technology for analyzing the conversations of multiple neurons at many levels in the visual system improves and is combined with higher resolution imaging, we predict that the paradigm shift will progress to the point where neurons are no longer viewed as independent processing units but as members of subsets of networks where their role is mapped in space–ime coordinates in relationship to the other neuronal members.

Does this mean that Cajal's contributions will disappear into obscurity? We hardly think so. Recent studies described earlier by Kozloski and co-workers (2001) clearly argue against the view that the morphology of neurons and their cortical circuits are random. Their studies provided evidence for very similar circuits for cells belonging to the same morphological class. Their message was that nature reproduces connections precisely. It is also the case that in tightly topographic systems such as the visual system, adequate coverage requires redundancy of circuits so that an understanding of the basic morphology and wiring of iterated modules will continue to contribute to our overall understanding of visual cortex.

Acknowledgements

We are grateful to Julia Mavity-Hudson for help with figures and Shirin S. Pulous for help with references. Aspects of the work reported in this chapter were supported by NIH grants EY01778 (VAC) and core grants HD 15052 and EY08126.

References

Allison, J.D., Casagrande, V.A. and Bonds, A.B. (1995) The influence of input from the lower cortical layers on the orientation tuning of upper layer V1 cells in a primate. *Visual Neurosci.*, 12: 309–320.

Allison, J.D., Kabara, J.F., Snider, R.K., Casagrande, V.A. and Bonds, A.B. (1996) GABAB-receptor-mediated inhibition reduces the orientation selectivity of the sustained response of striate cortical neurons in cats. *Visual Neurosci.*, 13: 559–566.

Allison, J.G., Melzer, P., Ding, Y., Bonds, A.B. and Casagrande, V.A. (2000) Differential contributions of magnocellular and parvocellular pathways to the contrast response of neurons in bush baby primary visual cortex (V1) *Visual Neurosci.*, 17: 71–76.

Barlow, H.B., Blakemore, C. and Pettigrew, J.D. (1967) The neural mechanism of binocular depth discrimination. *J. Physiol. (Lond.)*, 193: 327–342.

Bolz, J., Gilbert, C.D. and Wiesel, T.N. (1989) Pharamcological analysis of cortical circuitry. *TINS*, 12: 292–296.

Bonds, A.B. (1989) Role of inhibition in the specification of orientation selectivity of cells in the cat striate cortex. *Visual Neurosci.*, 2: 41–55.

Bonds, A.B. (1991) Temporal dynamics of contrast gain in single cells of the cat striate cortex. *Visual Neurosci.*, 6: 239-255

Boyd, J.D. and Casagrande, V.A. (1999) Relationships between cytochrome oxidase (CO) blobs in primate primary visual cortex (V1) and the distribution of neurons projecting to the middle temporal area (MT). *J. Comp. Neurol.*, 409: 573–91

Brodman, K. (1909) *Localization in the Cerebral Cortex*, translated and edited by L.J. Garey from *Vergleichen Lokalisationslehre der Grosshirnrinde in ihren Prinzipien dargestellt auf Grund des Zellenbaues* (Johann Ambrosius Barth, Leipzig), Smith-Gordon, London, pp. 37–59.

Cajal, S.R. (1899) Comparative study of the sensory areas of the human cortex. In W. E. Story and L.N. Wilson (Eds.), *Clark University 1889–1899 Decennial Celebration.* Clark Univ., Worcester, MA, pp. 311–382.

Cajal, S.R. (1954) Neuron Theory or Reticular Theory Objective Evidence of the Anatomical Unity of the Nerve Cells. Translated by M. Ubeda Purkiss and C.A. Fox, Cajal Institute, Madrid.

Callaway, E.M. (1998) Local circuits in primary visual cortex of the macaque monkey. *Ann. Rev. Neurosci.*, 21: 47–74.

Casagrande, V.A. (1994) A third parallel visual pathway to primate area V1. *TINS*, 17: 305–310.

Casagrande,V.A. and Kaas, J.H. (1994) The afferent, intrinsic and efferent connections of primary visual cortex in primates. In: A. Peters, K.S. Rockland, (Eds.), *Cerebral Cortex*, Vol. 10, Plenum Press, New York.

Chapman, B., Stryker, M.P. and Bonhoeffer, T. (1996) Development of orientation preference maps in ferret primary visual cortex. *J. Neurosci.*, 16: 6443–6453.

Chapman, B., Godecke, I. and Bonhoeffer, T. (1999) Development of orientation preference in the mammalian visual cortex. *J. Neurobiol.*, 41: 18–24.

Chen, W., Kato, T., Zhu, X.H., Ogawa, S., Tank, D.W. and Ugurbil, K. (1998) Human primary visual cortex and lateral geniculate nucleus activation during visual imagery. *Neuroreport*, 9: 3669–3774.

DeAngelis, G.C., Robson, J.G., Ohzawa, I. and Freeman, R.D. (1992) Organization of suppression in receptive fields of neurons in cat visual cortex. *J. Neurophysiol.*, 68: 144–163.

DeAngelis, G.C., Freeman, R.D. and Ohzawa, I. (1994) Length and width tuning of neurons in the cat's primary visual cortex. *J. Neurophysiol.*, 71: 347–374.

DeFelipe, J. and Jones, E.G. (1988) *Cajal on the Cerebral Cortex.* Oxford University Press, New York.

Dobbins, A., Zucker, S.W. and Cynader, M.S. (1987) Endstopped neurons in the visual cortex as a substrate for calculating curvature. *Nature*, 329: 438–441.

Dragoi V., Rivadulla C. and Sur, M. (2001) Foci of orientation plasticity in visual cortex. *Nature*, 411: 80–86.

Ferster, D. and Miller, K D. (2000) Neural mechanisms of orientation selectivity in the visual cortex. *Ann. Rev. Neurosci.*, 23: 441–471.

Field, D.J., Hayes, A. and Hess, R.F. (1993) Contour integration by the human visual system: evidence for a local 'association field'. *Vision Res.*, 33: 173–193.

Fitzpatrick, D.(2000) Seeing beyond the receptive field in primary visual cortex. *Curr. Opin. Neurobiol.*, 10: 438–443.

Flechsig, P. (1896) Die Localisation der geistigen Vorgänge. *Neurol. Centralbl.*, 15: 999–1003.

Florence, S.L. and Casagrande, V.A. (1986) Changes in the distribution of geniculocortical projections following monocular deprivation in tree shrews, *Brain Res.*, 374: 179–184.

Florence, S.L. and Kaas, J.H. (1992) Ocular dominance columns in area 17 of Old World macaque and talapoin monkeys: complete reconstructions and quantitative analyses. *Visual Neurosci.*, 8: 449–462.

Flourens, P.J.M. (1824) Recherches expérimentaes sur les propriétés et les fonctions du systéme nerveux dans les animaux vertébrés, par P.F.A Paris, chez Crevot, Libraire-éditeur. 2nd ed., J.-B. Bailliére, Paris.

Gandhi, S.P., Heeger, D.J. and Boyton, G.M. (1999) Spatial attention affects brain activity in human primary visual cortex. *Proc. Nat. Acad. Sci., USA*, 96: 3314–3319.

Gilbert, C.D. (1992) Horizontal integration and cortical dynamics. *Neuron*, 9: 1–13.

Gilbert, C.D.(1998) Adult cortical dynamics. *Physiol. Rev.*, 78: 467–485.

Gilbert, C., Ito, M., Kapadia, M. and Westheimer, G. (2000) Interactions between attention, context and learning in primary visual cortex. *Vision Res.*, 40: 1217–1226.

Golgi, C. (1884) Recherches sur l'histologie des centres nerveux. *Arch. Ital. Biol.*, 4: 92–123.

Haenny, P.E. and Schiller, P.H. (1988) State dependent activity in the monkey visual cortex I. Single cell activity in V1 and V4 on visual tasks. *Exp. Brain Res.*, 69: 225–244.

Hartline H.K. (1940) The receptive field of the optic nerve fibers. *Am. J. Physiol.*, 130: 690.

Hendry S.H. and Reid, R.C. (2000) The koniocellular pathway in primate vision. *Ann. Rev. Neurosci.*, 23: 127–153.

Hubel, D.H. and Wiesel, T.N. (1962) Receptive fields, binocular interaction and functional architecture in the cat's striate cortex, *J. Physiol. (Lond)*, 160: 106–154.

Hubel, D.H. and Wiesel, T.N. (1965) Binocular interaction in striate cortex of kittens reared with artificial squint. *J. Neurophysiol.*, 28: 1041–1059.

Hubel, D.H. and Wiesel, T.N. (1968) Receptive fields and functional architecture of monkey striate cortex, *J. Physiol. (Lond)*, 195: 215–243.

Hubel, D.H. and Wiesel, T.N. (1977) Ferrier lecture. Functional architecture of macaque monkey visual cortex. *Proc. R. Soc. Lond B.*, 198:1–59.

Huk, A.C. and Heeger, D.J. (2000) Task-related modulation of visual cortex, *J. Neurophysiol.*, 83: 3525–3536.

Ito, M. and Gilbert, C.D. (1999) Attention modulates contextual influences in the primary visual cortex of alert monkeys. *Neuron*, 22: 593–604.

Jones, E.G. (1984) History of cortical cytology. In: A. Peters and E.G. Jones (Eds.), *Cerebral Cortex*, Vol. 1: Cellular Components of the Cerebral Cortex. Plenum, New York, pp. 1–33.

Kapadia, M.K., Ito, M., Gilbert, C.D. and Westheimer, G. (1995) Improvement in visual sensitivity by changes in local context: parallel studies in human observers and in V1 of alert monkeys. *Neuron*, 15: 843–856.

408

Kapadia, M.K., Westheimer, G. and Gilbert, C.D. (1999) Dynamics of spatial summation in primary visual cortex of alert monkeys. *Proc. Natl. Acad. Sci. USA*, 96: 12073–12078.

Knierim, J.J. and van Essen, D.C. (1992) Neuronal responses to static texture patterns in area V1 of the alert macaque monkey. *J. Neurophysiol.*, 67: 961–980.

Kozloski, J., Hamzei-Sichani, F. and Yuste, R. (2001) Stereotyped position of local synaptic targets in neocortex. *Science*, 293: 868–872.

Kuhn, T.S. (1970) *The Structure of Scientific Revolutions*. Second Edition. The University of Chicago Press, Chicago, pp. 1–210.

Lamme, V.A. (1995) The neurophysiology of figure-ground segregation in primary visual cortex. *J. Neurosci.*, 15: 1605–1615.

Levitt, J.B. and Lund, J.S. (1997) Contrast dependence of contextual effects in primate visual cortex. *Nature*, 387: 73–76.

Livingstone, M. and Hubel, D.H. (1981) Effects of sleep and arousal on the processing of visual information in the cat. *Nature*, 291: 554–560.

Livingstone, M.S. and Hubel, D.H. (1984) Anatomy and physiology of a color system in the primate visual cortex. *J. Neurosci.*, 4: 309–356.

Livingstone, M.S. and Hubel, D.H. (1988). Segregation of form, color, movement, and depth: anatomy, physiology, and perception. *Science.*, 240: 740–749.

Lund, J.S. (1988) Anatomical organization of macaque monkey striate visual cortex. *Ann. Rev. Neurosci.*, 11: 253–288.

Lyon, D.C. and Kaas, J.H. (2001) Connectional and architectonic evidence for dorsal and ventral V3, and dorsomedial area in marmoset monkeys. *J. Neurosci.*, 21: 249–261.

Malpeli, J.G., Schiller, P.H. and Colby, C.L. (1981) Response properties of single cells in monkey striate cortex during reversible inactivation of individual lateral geniculate laminae, *J. Neurophysiol.*, 46: 1102–1119.

McCormick, D.A. and Feeser, H.R. (1990) Functional implications of burst firing and single spike activity in lateral geniculate neurons. *Neuroscience*, 39: 103–113.

Merigan, W.H., and Maunsell, J.H.R. (1990) Macaque vision after magnocellular lateral geniculate lesions. *Visual Neurosci.*, 5: 347–352.

Morrison, J.H., Hof, P.R. and Huntley, G.W. (1998) Neurochemical organization of the primate visual cortex. In: F. E. Bloom, A. Björklund and T. Hökfeld (Eds.), *The Handbook of Chemical Neuroanatomy*, Vol. 14, The primate nervous system, part II, Elsevier, Amsterdam, pp. 299–430.

Movshon, J.A. and Newsome, W.T. (1996) Visual response properties of striate cortical neurons projecting to area MT in macaque monkeys. *J. Neurosci.*, 16: 7733–7741.

Munk, H. (1883) Lecture on cerebral functions. *Nature,* 28: 431.

Munk, H. (1890) Of the visual area of the cerebral cortex, and its relation to eye movements. *Brain*, 13: 45.

Nealey T.A. and Maunsell J.H. (1994) Magnocellular and parvocellular contributions to the responses of neurons in macaque striate cortex. *J. Neurosci.*, 14, 2069–2079.

Obermayer K. and Blasdel G.G. (1993) Geometry of orientation and ocular dominance columns in monkey striate cortex. *J. Neurosci.*, 13: 4114–4129.

Polat, U., Mizobe, K., Pettet, M.W., Kasamatsu, T. and Norcia, A.M. (1998) Collinear stimuli regulate visual responses depending on cell's contrast threshold. *Nature*, 391: 580–584.

Polyak, S. (1957) H. Kluver (Ed.), *The Vertebrate Visual System*. The University of Chicago Press, Chicago, pp. 1–1390.

Ramcharan, E.J., Gnadt, J.W. and Sherman, M.S. (2000) Burst and tonic firing in thalamic cells of unasthetized, behaving monkey. *Visual Neurosci.*, 17: 55–62.

Ringach D.L., Hawken M. J. and Shapley R. (1997) Dynamics of orientation tuning in macaque primary visual cortex. *Nature*, 387: 281–284.

Rockland, K.S. and Lund, J.S. (1982) Widespread periodic intrinsic connections in the treeshrew visual cortex. *Science*, 215: 1532–1534.

Roelfsema, P.R., Lamme, V.A.F. and Spekreise, H. (1998) Object-based attention in the primary visual cortex of the macaque monkey. *Nature*, 395: 376–381.

Sáry Gy., Xu., X, Shostak, Y., Royal, D., Schall, J. and Casagrande V. (2001) Behavioral releveance influences LGN neurons of macaque monkey in the absence of receptive field stimulation. Abs., Vision Sciences Society Meeting, Sarasota, Florida B30.

Sceniak, M.P., Ringach, D.L., Hawken, M.J. and Shapley, R. (1999) Contrast's effect on spatial summation by macaque V1 neurons. *Nat. Neurosci.*, 2: 733–739.

Schiller P.H., Logothetis, N.K. and Charles, E.R. (1990) Role of the color-opponent and broad-band channels in vision. *Visual Neurosci.*, 5: 321–346.

Sharma, J., Angelucci, A. and Sur, M. (2000) Induction of visual orientation modules in auditory cortex. *Nature*, 404: 841–847.

Sherman, S.M. (2001) Tonic and burst firing: dual modes of thalamocortical relay. *TINS*, 24: 122–126.

Supèr, H., Spekreijse, H. and Lamme, V.A.F. (2001) Contextual modulation in primary visual cortex as a neuronal correlate for working memory. Abs., Vision Sciences Society Meeting, Sarasota, Florida, 344.

Toth, L.J., Rao, S.C., Kim, D.S., Somers, D. and Sur, M. (1996) Subthreshold facilitation and suppression in primary visual cortex revealed by intrinsic signal imaging. *Proc. Natl. Acad. Sci. USA*, 93: 9869–9874.

Ungerleider, L and Mishkin, M. (1982) Two cortical visual systems. In: D. Ingle, R. Mansfield, and M. Goodale (Eds.), *Analysis of Visual Behavior*, MIT Press, MA, pp. 549–586.

Vidyasagar, T.R., Pei, X. and Volgushev, M. (1996) Multiple mechanisms underlying the orientation selectivity of visual cortical neurones. *TINS*, 19: 272–277.

von Kölliker, A. (1887) Die Untersuchungen von Golgi über den feineren Bau des centralen Nerven-systems. *Anat. Anz.*, 2:480–483.

Wollaston, W.H. (1824) On semi-decussation of optic nerves. *Phil. Trans. R. Soc. Lond.*, 14: 222.

Zipser, K., Lamme, V.A. and Schiller, P.H. (1996) Contextual modulation in primary visual cortex. *J. Neurosci.*, 16: 7376–7389.

E.C. Azmitia, J. DeFelipe, E.G. Jones, P. Rakic and C.E. Ribak (Eds.)
Progress in Brain Research, Vol. 136

CHAPTER 31

Central control of information transmission through the intraspinal arborizations of sensory fibers examined 100 years after Ramón y Cajal

Pablo Rudomin*

Department of Physiology, Biophysics and Neurosciences, Centro de Investigación y Estudios Avanzados del Instituto Politécnico Nacional, 07000 Mexico D.F., Mexico

Abstract: About 100 years ago, Santiago Ramón y Cajal reported that sensory fibers entering the spinal cord have ascending and descending branches, and that each of them sends collaterals to the gray matter where they have profuse ramifications. To him this was a fundamental discovery and proposed that the intraspinal branches of the sensory fibers were "*centripetal conductors by which sensory excitation is propagated to the various neurons in the gray matter*". In addition, he assumed that "*conduction of excitation within the intraspinal arborizations of the afferent fibers would be proportional to the diameters of the conductors*", and that excitation would preferentially flow through the coarsest branches. The invariability of some elementary reflexes such as the knee jerk would be the result of a long history of plastic adaptations and natural selection of the safest neuronal organizations. There is now evidence suggesting that in the adult cat, the intraspinal branches of sensory fibers are not hard wired routes that diverge excitation to spinal neurons in an invariable manner, but rather dynamic pathways where excitation flow can be centrally addressed to reach specific neuronal targets. This central control of information flow is achieved by means of specific sets of GABAergic interneurons that produce primary afferent depolarization (PAD) via axo-axonic synapses and reduce transmitter release (presynaptic inhibition). The PAD produced by single, or by small groups of GABAergic interneurons in group I muscle afferents, can remain confined to some sets of intraspinal arborizations of the afferent fibers and not spread to nearby collaterals. In muscle spindle afferents this local character of PAD allows cutaneous and descending inputs to differentially inhibit the PAD in segmental and ascending collaterals of individual fibers, which may be an effective way to decouple the information flow arising from common sensory inputs. This feature appears to play an important role in the selection of information flow in muscle spindles that occurs at the onset of voluntary contractions in humans.

Descartes and the animal spirits

Three hundred years ago, René Descartes described the withdrawal behavior produced in humans in response to a nociceptive stimulus. He considered the nerves and the spinal cord as tubular structures that were able to conduct the impressions from the external world. The external

motions would affect the peripheral ends of the *nerve fibrils*, which would in turn displace their central ends. As the central ends were displaced, the pattern of *interfibrillar space* would be rearranged and the flow of *animal spirits* would be thereby directed into the appropriate nerves and muscles to produce the withdrawal movement (Fig. 1). The pineal gland in the brain would be the gateway between the body and soul. With sensory perception, information would be transferred to the pineal gland through animal spirits, blood and nerves. With motor commands, the gland would be moved by the soul, and

---

*Corresponding author: Tel.: 525 747 7099; Fax: 525 747 7099; E-mail: rudomin@fisio.cinvestav.mx

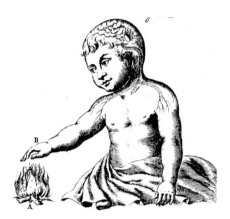

Fig. 1. Withdrawal reflexes to a nociceptive stimulus. Original drawing from Descartes. The fire (A), activates the animal spirits in the arm (B). Their vibrations are conducted up to the brain by means of tubular structures (peripheral nerves and spinal cord), where they are rearranged and directed back to the appropriate nerves to produce the withdrawal movement.

thrust the animal spirits towards the pores of the brain, and onto the nerves.

Clearly this view has been modified with time. Yet, the proposal of a causal relationship between stimulus and response had a remarkable impact in the development of Science. It provided a way to use measurable parameters to describe the behavior of living organisms. But it was not until the end of the nineteenth century, when electrical nature of the signals transmitted by nerve fibers was more firmly established. The anatomical studies of Lenhossek, Kölliker and Cajal, showed in addition that the spinal cord was a complicated network of interconnected fibers and neurons (see Cajal, 1904). This, together with the physiological observations of Sherrington (1906), were primary determinants of our actual understanding of the functional organization of the spinal cord.

The spinal cord of Cajal

The contributions of Cajal (1904) to spinal cord physiology have been enormous. Using the Golgi methods to stain myelinated fibers in longitudinal sections of the mouse spinal cord, Cajal found a series of transversal fibers merging into the gray matter. At that time the general belief was that these fibers were the continuation of individual sensory axons running in the dorsal columns. However, Cajal proposed that most of the transverse fibers were right angle collaterals of the longitudinal fibers in the white matter that ended in the gray matter at various segmental levels (Fig. 2).

This finding was received with some skepticism until Cajal attended the anatomical meeting in Berlin in 1889, and showed his histological preparations to Kölliker. The German anatomist was very impressed with Cajal's material and soon after he himself addressed the problem and described collaterals of sensory fibers in Clarke's column and in the substantia gelatinosa, as well as in the brainstem nuclei. In his book, Cajal commented that Kölliker considered the finding of the intraspinal collaterals of the sensory fibers as one of the "most important advances in the knowledge of the structure of the spinal cord".

To Cajal, the nerve impulses generated in the periphery would arrive to the dorsal columns where they would break down in one ascending and one descending current, of the same or different intensity. The nervous wave would then propagate through the intraspinal collaterals to be transmitted to motor and funicular neurons (Fig. 3). The excitatory current would be further propagated within the intraspinal arborizations of the axons like "*the blood current in the vascular tree, where the energy of the circulating waves would be proportional to the diameter of the conductors*". According to Cajal, the largest axon branches would "*absorb*" most of the nervous impulse that represented the ordinary pathway for spinal reflexes (Fig. 3).

The monolateral circumscribed spinal reflexes, such as the rotulian reflex, would be mediated by two neurons, one sensitive and one motor that were interconnected through the sensory motor collaterals. The circumscribed character of these reflexes would be a consequence of the reduced number of long collaterals emitted by each sensory fiber, which in turn activated a reduced number of motor neurons. Cajal considered that the neurons mediating the inborn reflexes such as the rotulian reflex had secure connections that were "fatally" established during the fetal stage or during the first months after birth. Their "invariability" and hereditary character would be the consequence of a long history of plastic adaptations of the nervous system to the most urgent defensive needs of the organism. Early in the phylogenetic development, these reflexes could have shown some variation, but with time and selection of the most secure arrangements, they would become invariable.

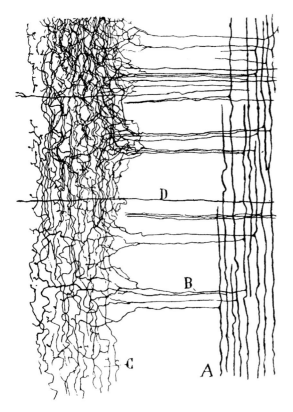
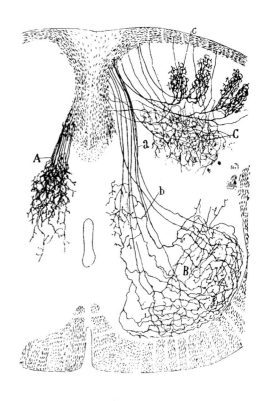

Fig. 2. Intraspinal collaterals of the sensory fibers. Two original drawings of Cajal. Left, longitudinal section of the dorsal column and Clarke's column of a 4 day-old-dog. A, white matter; B, collaterals to Clarke's column; C, longitudinal branches of the terminal arborizations. Right, main sensitive branches in a transversal section of the spinal cord of the newborn rat. A, collaterals in the intermediate nucleus of the gray matter; B, arborizations in motor pools. C, arborizations in the dorsal horn; a, sensitive-motor bundle; b, collaterals of fiber in the intermediate nucleus in the gray matter; c, deep collaterals in Rolando's substance.

Cajal also considered that after birth, before the definitive remodeling of the nervous arborizations, the collateral sensory-motor branches would have a relatively limited development. The excitatory currents would be conveyed preferentially through the coarsest ascending and descending branches in the dorsal columns, reaching the brainstem and the cerebral cortex with sufficient energy to cause a conscious reaction. Subsequently, and because of the continuous use, these collaterals would become hypertrophied at the expense of other terminals, whose diameter would remain more or less stationary, and the excitatory current would preferentially flow through them. This preference could be increased by means of the additional development (by branching and elongation) of the terminal arborizations of these collaterals, and by increasing the surface of contact and closeness with the neurons involved in the reflexes.

Cajal's views on synaptic transmission

The observations of Cajal in the spinal cord were essential to the formulation of the Neuron Theory that assessed the individuality of the neurons. Contiguity not continuity, as he used to state. This implied that excitation was transmitted from one neuron to the other following certain rules. He assumed that nerve impulses generated in the periphery were of electrical nature and were conducted until the terminals of the sensory fibers in the spinal cord and transmitted to other neurons by the same process. In this regard, he stated "there are reasons to believe that the cement that is interposed between the terminal arborizations of the collaterals and the body and dendrites of the nervous cells is not as perfect conductor as the nervous protoplasm, but offers some resistance, that is translated

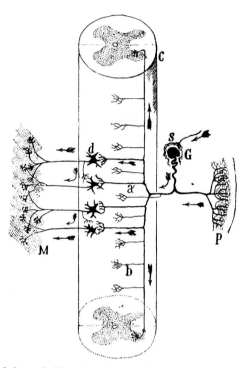

Fig. 3. Intraspinal branches of sensory fibers and their connections with motoneurons. Original drawing of Cajal that illustrates the intraspinal branches (b) of a sensory neuron (G) and their synaptic contacts with motoneurons (M) in several spinal segments. The arrows indicate the flow of excitation. Note that the peripheral branch of the sensory neuron innervates the skin (p), but we know now that muscle spindles, not cutaneous afferents, make mono-synaptic contacts with motoneurons.

by a delay in the traveling of the wave. This resistance is reduced when the tension of the current reaches a certain magnitude in the nervous arborization. This explains why the delay in conduction of the reflex current is larger the more neurons that are interposed in the pathway". He attributed inhibition of spinal reflexes, including the inhibition of the rotulian reflex by electrical excitation of a sensitive nerve, to depression resulting from intense excitation.

The view that impulse transmission between central neurons was of electrical nature prevailed in this, or in different forms, for about 50 years. Electrical transmission implied, to some extent, little variability in synaptic transmission. Yet, there were data suggesting that the conduction of impulses within the intraspinal arborizations of the afferent fibers could be curtailed either spontaneously (Barron and Matthews, 1938), or by a

conditioning stimulation of a neighboring dorsal root (Howland et al., 1955).

When the quantal nature of chemical transmission in peripheral synapses was more firmly established (Del Castillo and Katz, 1954), it became clear that variability of transmission in central synapses could also arise from variations in the amount of chemical transmitter released by the action potential in the presynaptic terminals (see Kuno, 1964). Later on, it was established that the synaptic effectiveness of the sensory fibers in the spinal cord could be modified by extrinsic mechanisms, among them, by specific sets of GABAergic interneurons that made synapses with the terminal arborizations of the afferent fibers (for review see Schmidt, 1971; Burke and Rudomin, 1977; Rudomin and Schmidt, 1999).

Central control of the synaptic effectiveness of sensory fibers

Present evidence indicates that the terminal arborizations of muscle and cutaneous afferents have GABAa as well as GABAb receptors. Activation of the GABAa receptors increases the permeability to chloride ions, which move according to their electrochemical gradient and produce primary afferent depolarization (PAD). Reduction of transmitter release (presynaptic inhibition) may occur either because of the depolarization of the terminal arborizations of the afferent fibers, or because the associated shunt that may prevent conduction of action potentials (see Rudomin and Schmidt, 1999). Activation of GABAb receptors appears to reduce the calcium currents associated with the action potential as well as transmitter release (Curtis et al., 1971; Levy, 1977; Peng and Frank, 1989; Quevedo et al., 1992; Zhang and Jackson, 1995).

It has been suggested that GABAa and GABAb receptors in muscle spindle afferents can be spatially separated (Stuart and Redman, 1992). However, it is not known if these two classes of receptors are activated by the same set or by independent sets of GABAergic interneurons. A separate activation of GABAa and GABAb receptors would allow for an independent control of impulse conduction in the intraspinal branch points (via GABAa receptors) and of the frequency behavior of synaptic transmission (via GABAb receptors; see Lev-Tov et al., 1988; Peshori et al., 1998).

Presynaptic control of the effectiveness of group I afferents

Work performed in functionally identified group I muscle afferents (Jiménez et al., 1988; Enríquez et al., 1996a,b) has indicated that intraspinal terminations of individual muscle spindle and tendon organ afferent fibers may have at least three different types of PAD patterns. Afferents with a type A PAD pattern are depolarized by stimulation of group I fibers (mainly from flexors) and by stimulation of the vestibular nuclei. In contrast, stimulation of cutaneous and of articular nerves, as well as

stimulation of the reticular formation, the nucleus raphe magnus, the cerebral cortex and the red nucleus, produces no PAD in these fibers, but is able to inhibit the PAD produced in them by activation of group I muscle fibers (see Fig. 4). Afferents with a type B PAD pattern are depolarized by stimulation of group I fibers, and also by stimulation of cutaneous afferents and by all of the above descending pathways. In contrast, afferents with a type C PAD pattern are depolarized by group I muscle and by descending, but not by cutaneous fibers, which instead inhibit the PAD.

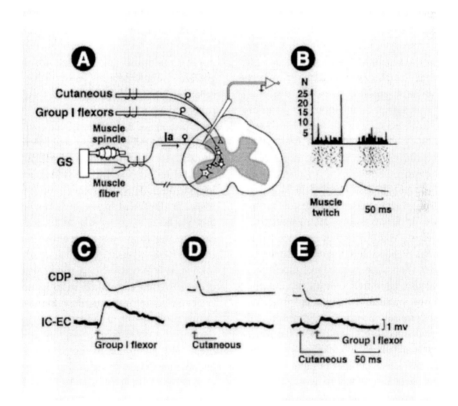

Fig. 4. PAD in a muscle spindle afferent. A, diagram of the method used to record intrafiber PAD from a functionally identified muscle spindle afferent. B–E, intrafiber recordings from a single afferent left in continuity with the gastrocnemius (GS) muscle. B, silencing of the background discharge of the afferent fiber during the contraction of the slightly stretched gastrocnemius muscle. Action potentials from the afferent fiber are shown as dots. Each row shows changes in background activity during a single muscle twitch. The histogram shows the sum of the action potentials in all trials. C, cord dorsum potentials (CDP) and transmembrane potential changes (IC–EC) in the same afferent fiber following stimulation of group I fibers from the flexor muscle posterior biceps and semitendinosus (PBSt) with a train of 3 pulses at 300 Hz, 2 xT (twice threshold) strength. These records were obtained while the gastrocnemius muscle was slackened to reduce background action potentials. D, same, but during stimulation of the cutaneous nerve superficial peroneus (SP) with single pulses 2 xT. Note that stimulation of the cutaneous nerve produced almost no membrane potential changes. E, SP inhibition of the PBSt-induced PAD. Traces C–E are averages of 64 responses elicited at 1 Hz. (Modified from Jiménez et al., 1988)

In the study of Enríquez et al., (1996a) fifty two percent of 131 functionally identified muscle spindles had a type A PAD pattern, 26% a type B and 13% a type C, while 11% of 41 fibers classified from tendon organs had a type A PAD pattern, 35% a type B and 54% a type C. These distributions changed significantly 2–12 weeks after crushing the axons of the afferent fibers in the peripheral nerve, and allowing them to regenerate and become reconnected with the muscle receptors. Under those conditions, 35% of 11 fibers that reconnected with muscle spindle afferents had a type A PAD pattern and 65% a type C PAD, while all 7 fibers that reconnected with tendon organs had a type B PAD pattern. The original distribution of type A, B and C PAD patterns in muscle spindles and tendon organs was partially recovered 6 months to 2.5 years after the nerve crush. (Enríquez et al., 1996b).

Although the functional implications of these changes in the profiles of PAD patterns have not been yet established, it is clear that the PAD patterns of muscle afferents are not an invariant feature of the neuronal pathways mediating presynaptic inhibition. They can be changed by peripheral nerve lesions, and, as shown below, by stimulation of sensory nerves and supraspinal structures (Lomelí et al., 1998).

There is another basic difference in the organization of PAD pathways and presynaptic inhibition of the Ia and Ib fiber systems. Repetitive activation of Ib fibers, either by electrical stimulation or during muscle contraction, generates a steady level of PAD (Lafleur et al., 1992) that leads to a transient disynaptic inhibition of motoneurons (Zytnicki et al., 1990). This appears to be due to a strong autogenetic presynaptic inhibition that filters out the input to the inhibitory interneurons generated from the tendon organs during muscle contraction (Zytnicki and L'Hôte, 1993; Zytnicki and Jami, 1998). On the other hand, as shown by Mendell and colleagues (Mendell, 1998; Peshori et al., 1998), single fiber Ia monosynaptic EPSPs of small amplitude do not decline with repetitive stimulation, but rather summate and produce a sustained depolarization, while large EPSPs grow initially and are subsequently depressed. However, after (-)-baclofen, a GABAb agonist, the large EPSPs are reduced in amplitude, but now summate during high frequency stimulation and lead to a sustained depolarization. Mendell (1998) and Peshori et al., (1998) suggested that, in addition to postsynaptic mechanisms, differences in the tonic levels of presynaptic inhibition in different terminals could play a relevant role in the frequency behavior of the synaptic actions mediated by the muscle afferents. It is possible that, unlike Ib afferents, Ia fibers display a low autogenetic PAD, but this remains to be investigated (however see Lev-Tov et al., 1983).

Local character of PAD

Studies made recently in our laboratory (Eguibar et al., 1997; Quevedo et al., 1997; Lomelí et al., 1998), together with ultrastructural observations (Lamotte et al., 1998) indicate that the distribution of GABAa synapses within the intraspinal arborizations of muscle spindle and tendon organ afferents *is not homogeneous*. Some collaterals appear to be the targets of one or more GABAergic interneurons, while others receive no axo-axonic connections from these interneurons. Studies on the PAD produced by *direct activation* (by means of intraspinal microstimulation) of single, or small groups of GABAergic interneurons, have further indicated that the monosynaptic PAD elicited in this way can remain *spatially confined* within a reduced set of intraspinal arborizations of the afferent fibers, without spreading to nearby collaterals (Quevedo et al., 1997).

Thus, the local character of PAD allows cutaneous, articular and descending inputs to inhibit the PAD elicited in specific collaterals of individual muscle spindle (Ia) fibers, as illustrated in Fig. 5. It has been suggested that this can be an effective way to decouple the information flow arising from common sensory inputs (see Lomelí et al., 1998). This differential control of presynaptic inhibition is subjected to a supraspinal control (Lomelí et al., 1998) and most likely plays an important role in the selection of information flow in muscle spindles that occurs at the onset of voluntary contractions in humans (Hultborn et al., 1987a, b) as well as in the resetting of presynaptic inhibition of muscle spindle afferents at the end of a step cycle, or when finding unexpected obstacles (Iles, 1996; Aimonetti et al., 1999).

Our more recent investigations have also indicated that different collaterals of individual afferents with a type B PAD pattern (mostly seen in tendon organ afferents) can exhibit different degrees of PAD in response to a common sensory or descending input. As shown in Fig. 6, stimulation of the PBSt and of the PAN nerves reduced the intraspinal threshold of the L3 and L6 collaterals of a single fiber (because of PAD), in contrast with stimulation of the motor cortex sites that produced PAD only in the L6 collateral.

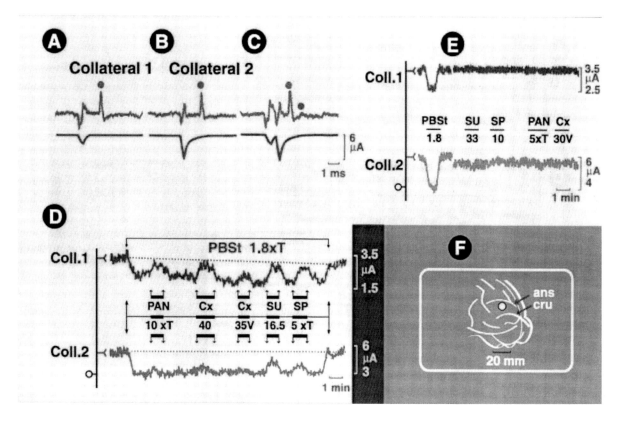

Fig. 5. Differential inhibition of PAD in two intraspinal collaterals of a single muscle afferent with a type A PAD pattern. A–C, antidromic action potentials produced in a single gastrocnemius afferent by stimulation through two separate micropipettes, both inserted within the intermediate nucleus at the L6 segmental level. At short time intervals, stimulation through one micropipette prevented generation of the action potential produced by stimulation through the other micropipette. This indicated that the antidromic action potentials recorded in the peripheral nerve were generated by activation of two collaterals of the same afferent fiber. E, threshold changes produced in these two collaterals following stimulation of the PBSt, sural (SU), SP, posterior articular (PAN) nerves and of the motor cortex (Cx, at the site indicated in F). Note that only stimulation of the PBSt nerve reduced the intraspinal threshold of both collaterals, because of PAD. D, differential inhibition of the PBSt-induced PAD following conditioning stimulation of the SU, SP, PAN nerves and of the motor cortex (location shown in F). Note that the conditioning stimuli to the PAN nerve and to the motor cortex inhibited almost completely the PAD elicited in collateral 1 (Coll. 1), practically without affecting the PAD produced in collateral 2 (Coll. 2). The PBSt nerve was stimulated with trains of 4 pulses at 300 Hz applied 25 ms before the intraspinal threshold testing pulses. Conditioning stimulation of the SU, SP and PAN nerves were single pulses preceding the PBSt train by 50 ms. The motor cortex was stimulated with a train of 8 anodal pulses at 700 Hz applied 75 ms before the PBSt train. Stimulus strengths are indicated in the figure. Afferent fiber with conduction velocity of 105 m/s and peripheral threshold 1.12 xT. (Modified from Eguibar et al., 1994)

These observations indicate rather strongly that the intraspinal arborizations of primary muscle spindle and tendon organ afferents are not hard-wired routes that diverge excitation to spinal neurons in an invariable manner, but rather dynamic pathways where information flow can be centrally addressed to reach specific neuronal targets (Lomelí et al., 1998). This central control of information flow is achieved, at least in part, by means of

GABAergic interneurons connected through axo-axonic synapses with the intraspinal terminals of the afferent fibers (see Rudomin and Schmidt, 1999).

Presynaptic control of group II afferents

The physiology and functional organization of the pathways leading to PAD and presynaptic inhibition of

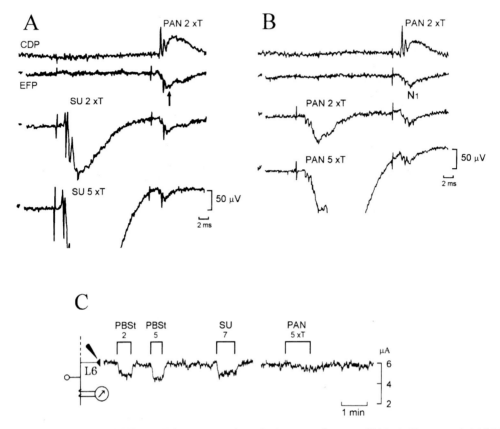

Fig. 7. Heterogenetic and autogenetic inhibition of the synaptic actions of joint nerve afferents and PAD. A, Heterogenetic inhibition of PAN actions. Effects of SU nerve stimulation on the PAN-evoked intraspinal field (EFP) potentials recorded at 2.12 mm depth in L6. Upper trace shows the cord dorsum potential (CDP) produced by the control PAN stimulus evoked at 2 xT strength. Note that SU pulses 5 xT strength depressed the slow component of the PAN-intraspinal field potential (N1 wave; Quevedo et al., 1993). B, Autogenetic inhibition of PAN actions. Effects of PAN conditioning on the PAN-evoked intraspinal field potentials. Note that conditioning stimulation with PAN pulses 5 xT also depressed the N1 component of the PAN-evoked field potential. C, intraspinal threshold changes of a single PAN afferent fiber measured at the same site where the field potentials shown in A and B were recorded. Note that stimulation of the PBSt and of the SU, but not of the PAN nerve, reduced the intraspinal threshold of the afferent fiber. This fiber had an antidromic latency of 3.8 ms (see arrow in A), a calculated conduction velocity of 53 m/s, and a peripheral threshold of 1.2 xT, and could well be involved in the generation of the N1 component of the PAN-evoked field potential. (From Lomelí and Rudomin, unpublished observations)

Concluding remarks

Cajal's finding, 100 years ago, that sensory fibers in the dorsal columns divided in ascending and descending branches, which in turn provided collaterals that entered the gray matter, and made synaptic contacts with a variety of spinal neurons, was a turning point for the understanding of the functional organization of the spinal cord. It contributed to the formulation of a series of useful concepts such as the principle of divergence and convergence of excitation flowing through sensory fibers and neuronal axons and the principle of polarization in the direction of excitation flow. But above all, it strengthened the view that the spinal cord is a rather complex structure, composed of many different classes of neurons, each of them giving and receiving specific connections from other neuronal elements. Many of these concepts are still valid. Pertaining the sensory fibers, it is now clear that their synaptic effectiveness can be modulated by extrinsic mechanisms, among them those mediated by GABAergic interneurons, and function as dynamic networks that allow addressing of information

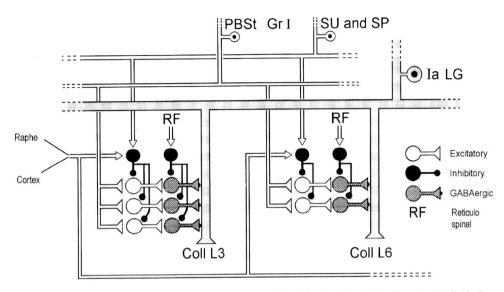

Fig. 8. Neuronal connections explaining the local character of inhibition of PAD in the L3 and L6 collaterals of individual muscle spindle afferents. PAD in a single Ia afferent from the lateral gastrocnemius (LG) produced by stimulation of group I PBSt afferents is mediated by at least two interposed interneurons. Separate groups of GABAergic interneurons produce PAD of L3 and L6 collaterals. Stimulation of cutaneous afferents and of cortico-spinal and raphe-spinal fibers inhibits PAD by acting on the first-order interneurons mediating PAD of muscle spindles, through separate sets of inhibitory interneurons. Reticulo-spinal (RF) fibers reduce PAD by inhibition of the last-order GABAergic interneurons. (Modified from Lomelí et al. 1998)

flow to specific neuronal targets. This is possible because (a) the local nature of PAD, in the sense that the PAD elicited in one intraspinal collateral does not necessarily spread to all the collaterals of the same afferent, and (b) because the intraspinal arborizations of individual afferents are the targets of more than one PAD-mediating GABAergic interneuron, as illustrated in Fig. 8.

It is clear that we are just at the beginning of the road and that a considerable amount of work is still needed to have a more complete understanding of the functional role of these mechanisms of presynaptic control. The synaptic effectiveness of each particular group of sensory fibers seems to be modulated by separate sets of spinal neurons, each responding with characteristic manners to supraspinal and sensory inputs. In this regard it is important to note that we know very little about the spatial distribution of GABAa and GABAb receptors within the terminal arborizations of individual afferent fibers and about the extent to which these receptors can be independently activated by the last-order GABAergic interneurons. A further step for the understanding of the functional role of central modulation of the synaptic effectiveness of sensory inputs will require studies in

behaving mammals during the execution of specific motor tasks, as well as during sensory discrimination.

Acknowledgments

I want to thank J. Lomelí for allowing reproduction of unpublished material. This work was partly supported by grants NIH NS 09196 and CONACyT 41739 and 3908N.

References

Aimonetti, J.M., Schmied, A., Vedel, J.P. and Pagni, S. (1999) Ia presynaptic inhibition in human wrist extensor muscles: effects of motor task and cutaneous afferent activity. *J. Physiol. (Lond.),* 93: 395–401.

Barron, D.H. and Matthews, B.H. (1938) The interpretation of potential changes in the spinal cord. *J. Physiol. (Lond.),* 92: 276–321.

Biella, G., Riva, L. and Sotgiu, M. L. (1997) Interaction between neurons in different laminae of the dorsal horn of the spinal cord. A correlation study in normal and neuropathic rats. *Eur. J. Neurosci.,* 9: 1017–1025.

Biella, G. and Sotgiu, M.L. (1995) Evidence that inhibitory mechanisms mask inappropriate somatotopic connections in the spinal cord of normal rat. *J. Neurophysiol.,* 74: 495–505.

420

Bras, H., Cavallari, P., Jankowska, E. and McCrea, D. (1989) Comparison of effects of monoamines on transmission in spinal pathways from group I and II muscle afferents in the cat. *Exp.Brain Res.*, 76: 27–37.

Bras, H., Jankowska, E., Noga, B. and Skoog, B. (1990) Comparison of effects of various types of NA and 5-HT agonists on transmission from group II muscle afferents in the cat. *Eur. J. Neurosci.*, 2: 1029–1039.

Burke, R.E. and Rudomin, P. (1977) Spinal neurons and synapses. In: J.M. Brookhart and V.B. Mountcastle (Eds.), *Handbook of Physiology. The Nervous System. Section 1*, Vol. 1, Part 2., American Physiological Society, Bethesda, Md., pp. 877–944.

Buss, R.R. and Shefchyk, S.J. (1999) Excitability changes in sacral afferents innervating the urethra, perineum and hindlimb skin of the cat during micturition. *J. Physiol. (Lond.)*, 514: 593–607.

Cajal, S.R. (1904) Textura del sistema nervioso del hombre y los vertebrados. *Madrid.*

Carpenter, D., Engberg, I., Funkenstein, H. and Lundberg, A. (1963) Decerebrate control of reflexes to primary afferents. *Acta Physiol. Scand.*, 59: 424–437.

Cervero, F. (1996) Spinal cord mechanisms of hyperalgesia and allodynia: role of peripheral input from nociceptors. *Prog. Brain Res.*, 113: 413–422.

Cervero, F. and Plenderleith, M.B. (1984) Dorsal root potentials are unchanged in adult rats treated at birth with capsaicin. *J. Physiol. (Lond.)*, 357: 357–368.

Curtis, D.R., Duggan, A.W., Felix, D. and Johnston, G.A.R. (1971) Bicuculline, an antagonist of GABA and synaptic inhibition in the spinal cord of the cat. *Brain Res.*, 32: 69–96.

Del Castillo, J. and Katz, B. (1954) Quantal components of the end-plate potential. *J. Physiol. (Lond.)*, 124: 566–573.

Eccles, J.C., Schmidt, R.F. and Willis, W.D. (1963) Depolarization of the central terminals of cutaneous afferent fibers. *J. Neurophysiol.*, 26: 646–661.

Eguibar, J.R., Quevedo, J. and Rudomin, P. (1997) Selective cortical and segmental control of primary afferent depolarization of single muscle afferents in the cat spinal cord. *Exp. Brain Res.*, 113: 411–430.

Enríquez, M., Jiménez, I. and Rudomin, P. (1996a). Changes in PAD patterns of group I muscle afferents after a peripheral nerve crush. *Exp. Brain Res.*, 107: 405–421.

Enríquez, M., Jiménez, I. and Rudomin, P. (1996b). Segmental and supraspinal control of synaptic effectiveness of functionally identified muscle afferents in the cat. *Exp. Brain Res.*, 107: 391–404.

Grubb, B.D., Stiller, R.U. and Schaible, H.-G. (1993) Dynamic changes in the receptive field properties of spinal cord neurons with ankle inputs in rats with chronic unilatteral inflammation in the ankle region. *Exp. Brain Res.*, 92: 441–452.

Harrison, P.J. and Jankowska, E. (1989) Primary afferent depolarization of central terminals of group II muscle afferents in the cat spinal cord. *J. Physiol. (Lond.)*, 411: 71–83.

Howland, B., Lettvin, J.Y., McCulloch, W.S., Pitts, W. and Wall, P.D. (1955) Reflex inhibitory by dorsal root interaction. *J. Neurophysiol.*, 18: 1–7.

Hultborn, H., Meunier, S., Morin, C. and Pierrot-Deseilligny, E. (1987a). Assessing changes in presynaptic inhibition of Ia fibres: a study in man and the cat. *J. Physiol. (Lond.)*, 389: 729–756.

Hultborn, H., Meunier, S., Pierrot-Deseilligny, E. and Shindo, M. (1987b). Changes in presynaptic inhibition of Ia fiber at the onset of voluntary contraction in man. *J. Physiol. (Lond.)*, 389: 757–772.

Iles, J.F. (1996) Evidence for cutaneous and corticospinal modulation of presynaptic inhibition of Ia afferents from the human lower limb. *J. Physiol. (Lond.)*, 491: 197–207.

Jankowska, E. and Riddell, J.S. (1998) Neuronal systems involved in modulating synaptic transmission from group II muscle afferents. In: P. Rudomin, R. Romo and L. Mendell, (Eds.), *Presynaptic Inhibition and Neural Control.* Oxford University Press, pp. 315–328.

Jankowska, E., Riddell, J.S. and McCrea, D.A. (1993) Primary afferent depolarization of myelinated fibres in the joint and interosseous nerves of the cat. *J. Physiol. (Lond.)*, 466: 115–131.

Jänig, W., Schmidt, R.F. and Zimmermann, M. (1967) Presynaptic depolarization during activation of tonic mechanoreceptors. *Brain Res.*, 5: 514–516.

Jänig, W., Schmidt, R.F. and Zimmermann, M. (1968a). Single unit responses and the total afferent outflow from the cat's food pad upon mechanical stimulation. *Exp. Brain Res.*, 6: 100–115.

Jänig, W., Schmidt, R.F. and Zimmermann, M. (1968b). Two specific feedback pathways to the central afferent terminal of phasic and tonic mechanoreceptors. *Exp. Brain Res.*, 6: 116–129.

Jiménez, I., Rudomin, P. and Solodkin, M. (1988) PAD patterns of physiologically identified afferent fibers from the medial gastrocnemius muscle. *Exp. Brain Res.*, 71: 643–657.

Kuno, M. (1964) Quantal components of excitatory synaptic potentials in spinal motoneurons. *J. Physiol. (Lond)*, 175: 81–89.

Lafleur, J., Zytnicki, D., Horcholle-Bossavit, G. and Jami, L. (1992) Depolarization of Ib afferent axons in the cat spinal cord during homonymous muscle contraction. *J. Physiol. (Lond.)*, 445, 345–354.

Lamotte, d.B., Destombes, J., Thiesson, D., Hellio, R., Lasserre, X., Kouchtir-Devanne, N., Jami, L. and Zytnicki, D. (1998) Indications for GABA-immunoreactive axo-axonic contacts on the intraspinal arborization of a Ib fiber in cat: a confocal microscope study. *J. Neurosci.*, 18: 10030–10036.

Lev-Tov, A., Fleshman, J.W. and Burke, R.E. (1983) Primary afferent depolarization and presynaptic inhibition of monosynaptic group Ia EPSPs during posttetanic potentiation. *J. Neurophysiol.*, 50: 413–427.

Lev-Tov, A., Meyers, D.E.R. and Burke, R.E. (1988) Modification of primary afferent depolarization in cat group Ia afferents following high frequency intra-axonal tetanization of individual afferents. *Brain Res.*, 438: 328–330.

Levy, R.A. (1977) The role of GABA in primary afferent depolarization. *Prog. Neurobiol.*, 9: 211–267.

Lomelí, J., Jankowska, E. and Rudomin, P. (2001) Indications that autogenetic inhibition of synaptic actions of articular afferents is not mediated by presynaptic GABAa receptors. *Proc. Soc. Neurosci.*, 26: 402–411.

Lomelí, J., Quevedo, J., Linares, P. and Rudomin, P. (1998) Local control of information flow in segmental and ascending collaterals of single afferents. *Nature*, 395: 600–604.

Mendell, L.M. (1998) Ia fiber architecture: implications for the functional role of presynaptic inhibition. In: P. Rudomin, R.

Romo and L. Mendell (Eds.), *Presynaptic Inhibition and Neural Control.* Oxford University Press, pp. 259–270.

Noga, R.R., Bras, H. and Jankowska, E. (1992) Transmission from group II muscle afferents is depressed by stimulation of locus coeruleus/subcoeruleus, Kolliker-fuse and raphe nuclei in the cat. *Exp. Brain Res.*, 88: 502–516.

Palecek, J., Paleckova, V., Dougherty, P.M., Carlton, S.M. and Willis, W.D. (1992) Responses of spinothalamic tract cells to mechanical and thermal stimulation of skin in rats with experimental peripheral neuropathy. *J. Neurophysiol.*, 67: 1562–1583.

Peng, Y. and Frank, E. (1989) Activation of GABAB receptors causes presynaptic inhibition at synapses between muscle spindle afferents and motoneurons in the spinal cord of bullfrogs. *J Neurosci.*, 9: 1502–1515.

Peshori, K.R., Collins, W.F. and Mendell, L.M. (1998) EPSP amplitude modulation at the rat Ia-alpha motoneuron synapse: effects of GABAB receptor agonists and antagonists. *J. Neurophysiol.*, 79: 181–189.

Quevedo, J., Eguibar, J.R., Jiménez, I. and Rudomin, P. (1992) Differential action of (-)-baclofen on the primary afferent depolarization produced by segmental and descending inputs. *Exp. Brain Res.*, 91: 29–45.

Quevedo, J., Eguibar, J.R., Jiménez, I., Schmidt, R.F. and Rudomin, P. (1993) Primary afferent depolarization of muscle afferents elicited by stimulation of joint afferents in cats with intact neuraxis and during reversible spinalization. *J. Neurophysiol.*, 70: 1899–1910.

Quevedo, J., Eguibar, J.R., Lomelí, J. and Rudomin, P. (1997) Patterns of connectivity of spinal interneurons with single muscle afferents. *Exp. Brain Res.*, 115: 387–402.

Riddell, J.S., Jankowska, E. and Eide, E. (1993) Depolarization of group II muscle afferents by stimuli applied in the locus coeruleus and raphe nuclei of the cat. *J. Physiol. (Lond.)*, 461: 723–741.

Riddell, J.S., Jankowska, E. and Huber, J. (1995) Organization of neuronal systems mediating presynaptic inhibition of group II muscle afferents in the cat. *J. Physiol. (Lond.)*, 483: 443–460.

Rudomin, P. and Schmidt, R.F. (1999) Presynaptic inhibition in the vertebrate spinal cord revisited. *Exp. Brain Res.*, 129: 1–37.

Schaible, H.G., Schmidt, R.F. and Willis, W.D. (1987a) Convergent inputs from articular, cutaneous and muscle receptors onto ascending tract cells in the cat spinal cord. *Exp. Brain Res.*, 66: 479–488.

Schaible, H.G., Schmidt, R.F. and Willis, W.D. (1987b) Enhacement of the responses of ascending tract cells in the cat spinal cord by acute inflammation of the knee joint. *Exp. Brain Res.*, 66: 489–499.

Schmidt, R.F. (1971) Presynaptic inhibition in the vertebrate central nervous system. *Ergeb. Physiol.*, 63: 20–101.

Sherrington, C.S. (1906) *The Integrative Action of the Nervous System.* Yale University Press, New Haven and London.

Stuart, G.J. and Redman, S.J. (1992) The role of GABAA and GABAB receptors in presynaptic inhibition of Ia EPSPs in cat spinal motoneurones. *J. Physiol. (Lond.)*, 447: 675–692.

Wall, P.D. (1994) Control of impulse conduction in long range branches of afferents by increases and decreases of primary afferent depolarization in the rat. *Eur. J. Neurosci.*, 6: 1136–1142.

Wall, P.D. (1995) Do nerve impulses penetrate terminal arborizations? A pre-presynaptic control mechanism. *Trends Neurosci.*, 18: 99–103.

Wall, P.D. and McMahon, S.B. (1994) Long range afferents in rat spinal cord. III. Failure of impulse transmission in axons and relief of the failure after rhizotomy of dorsal roots. *Philos. Trans. R. Soc. Lond B. Biol. Sci.*, 343: 211–223.

Weng, H.R., Laird, J.M., Cervero, F. and Schouenborg, J. (1998) GABAA receptor blockade inhibits A beta fibre evoked wind-up in the arthritic rat. *NeuroReport*, 9: 1065–1069.

Willis, W.D. (1999) Dorsal root potentials and dorsal root reflexes: a double-edged sword. *Exp. Brain Res.*, 124: 395–421.

Wilson, P. and Kitchener, P.D. (1996) Plasticity of cutaneous primary afferents projecting to the spinal dorsal horn. *Prog. Neurobiol.*, 48: 105–129.

Zhang, S.J. and Jackson, M.B. (1995) GABA$_A$ receptor activation and the excitability of nerve terminals in the rat posterior pituitary. *J. Physiol. (Lond.)*, 483: 583–595.

Zytnicki, D. and Jami, L. (1998) Presynaptic inhibition can act as a filter of input from tendon organs during muscle contraction. In: P. Rudomin, R. Romo and L. Mendell (Eds.), *Presynaptic Inhibition and Neural Control.* Oxford University Press, 303–314.

Zytnicki, D. and L'Hôte, G. (1993) Neuromimetic model of a neuronal filter. *Biol. Cybernetic.*, 70: 115–121.

Zytnicki, D., Lafleur, J., Horcholle-Bossavit, G., Lamy, F. and Jami, L. (1990) Reduction of Ib autogenetic inhibition in motoneurons during contractions of an ankle extensor muscle in the cat. *J. Neurophysiol.*, 64: 1380–1389.

Functional circuits, mental diseases and brain aging

E.C. Azmitia, J. DeFelipe, E.G. Jones, P. Rakic and C.E. Ribak (Eds.)
Progress in Brain Research, Vol. 136
© 2002 Elsevier Science B.V. All rights reserved

CHAPTER 32

Functional circuits, mental diseases and brain aging (an overview)

Luciano Angelucci*

Pharmacology 2, University La Sapienzia, 00185 Rome, Italy

The neuroscience presented in this section demonstrates that the post-Cajal era has substantially made progress in understanding the role of the neuron in integrative, cognitive and disease states. Indeed, the key to this progress in the post-Cajal era arose from the in-depth focusing on these problems using new methods, such as electronic microscopy, stereology, retrograde and anterograde axoplasmic labeling, blood flow analysis and metabolic brain imaging. Together, the results obtained with these methods have provided new morphological and architectural details that were out of sight, so to speak, for Cajal. Furthermore, these studies have provided new details about the neurochemical mechanisms involved with these functions. Thus, it is now possible to provide an understanding of brain functions that could only be located in Cajal's conceptual design of the nervous system and its connections.

This section starts with an excellent review of Cajal's Psychic Neuron by Patricia Goldman-Rakic. Her studies on prefrontal cortex have provided new insights into the role of neurons in this region to provide important information about mental representation. The analysis of "working memory" continues to be a central focus of her research and these studies show new functions for this brain region and how it can be affected by dopaminergic modulation. This section continues with an eloquent review of the reflexes associated with

respiratory control. Not only does Stephan Schwarzacher review the drawings of Cajal showing the innervation of the lungs and diaphragm, but he indicates that several new insights have been subsequently provided by researchers and have fine tuned Cajal's initial observations. Thus, new details on breathing centers in the brainstem are reviewed and compared with Cajal's ideas.

The next chapter in this section by Victoria Arango reports on her investigations in major depression in humans. She provides an excellent review on the malfunction of neurotransmitter transporters in the neuronal pathways subserved by serotoninergic activity. Although these pathways were only partially envisioned by Cajal, he suggested that the brain neuronal network may provide the basis for psychiatry. Thus, Cajal searched in architecturally differentiated neuronal circuits for the specific source of psychic alterations. At the same time, the great psychiatrist Sigmund Freud in "search" of the brain sites for repressed memories was certainly impressed by Cajal's work on the organization of the central nervous system (see Anderson and Green, 2001). These two great scientific figures were boldly engaged in the experimental demonstration that brain mechanisms are at the basis of memory suppression.

Investigations on normal and pathological brain aging were also presented at this Conference from the laboratories of Alan Peters and John Morrison. Although this type of study was not explicitly expressed in Cajal's work, his approach of showing age-dependent

*Corresponding author: Tel.: 39-06-49912596;
Fax: 39-06-494 0588; E-mail: luciano.angelucci@unirond1.it

426

morphological changes of the brain should be considered an important example of how to analyze the aging brain. Thus, these brain aging studies appear as a normal evolution of Cajal's interest in the connectivity of brain development.

References

Anderson, M.C. and Green, C. (2001) Suppressing unwanted memories by executive control. *Nature*, 410: 366–369.

E.C. Azmitia, J. DeFelipe, E.G. Jones, P. Rakic and C.E. Ribak (Eds.)
Progress in Brain Research, Vol. 136

CHAPTER 33

The "psychic cell" of Ramón y Cajal

Patricia S. Goldman-Rakic*

Department of Neurobiology, Yale University School of Medicine, 333 Cedar Street, New Haven, CT 06520-8001, USA

Abstract: Santiago Ramón y Cajal might have envisioned, but likely could not have anticipated, the scientific advances that have allowed the functional validation of the existence of a "psychic cell" in the prefrontal cortex and its extension to human cognition at the end of the 20th century. This achievement rests not only on the shoulders of giants but on many small steps in the development of primate cognition, single and multiple unit recording in behaving monkeys, light and electron microscopic analysis of cortical circuitry no less than on the evolution of concepts about memory systems and parallel processing networks, among other advances. We can only wonder what the next generation of neuroscientists will bring to our understanding of brain-behavior relationships and human information capacity.

The "psychic cell" of the cerebral cortex

Santiago Ramón y Cajal designated the pyramidal cell of the cerebral cortex the "psychic cell" of the brain (Cajal, 1892). When this designation was made in the late nineteenth century, knowledge of this neuron class was limited to its morphological characteristics, its pyramid-shaped cell body, its long axon that could only be followed for short distances in histological sections, its characteristic vertically extended, spine studded apical dendrite and its bushy basiliar dendritic arbor. Only with the introduction of the silver impregnation and axonal transport methods in the middle of the twentieth century did it become possible to define the destinations and synaptic targets of pyramidal cell axons and map their connections to neuronal targets in distant cortical areas and subcortical structures. By extrapolation from estimates made on hippocampal pyramidal neurons, the cortical pyramidal neuron integrates literally thousands of afferent inputs and through its efferent connections regulates skeletal and smooth muscles involved in movement and

affect. A significant feature of the cortical pyramidal cell, clarified only within the last two decades, is that it processes information and directs actions via glutamate transmission, differentiating it from the other major class of cortical neuron—the local circuit neuron which is nonpyramidal in shape, possesses smooth dendrites and for the most part utilizes the amino acid, gamma-amino-butyric acid (GABA) for neurotransmission. Unlike pyramidal neurons, the nonpyramidal cells do not innervate distant structures; rather their axonal terminations are confined to local targets, either near-by pyramidal neurons or other interneurons.

A major objective of systems neuroscience is to understand both the specific and generic functions of pyramidal neurons in different cortical areas and the cellular mechanisms by which they perform the operations which are essential to human cognition. A full understanding of the capacity of even a single pyramidal cell to integrate its myriad inputs and generate a decisive action requires knowledge not only of its biophysical properties but its circuitry, signaling mechanisms and contributions to information processing *in vivo*. In this chapter, I describe the efforts of my laboratory to understand the pyramidal cells of the prefrontal cortex, the area of the brain most closely and most often associated with the executive

---

*Corresponding author: Tel.: (203) 785-4808; Fax (203) 785-5263; E-mail: patricia.goldman-rakic@yale.edu

functions of the brain. We and others have been able to characterize prefrontal neurons functionally, i.e., "on-line", as they are actively engaged in a cognitive function for which the prefrontal cortex is specialized—working memory. We also address the circuit and receptor mechanisms which regulate pyramidal cell excitability *in vivo*.

Working memory: the "psychic" function of the prefrontal neuron

The appellation, "psychic" is particularly appropriate for the prefrontal neuron. The prefrontal cortex is in some sense uniquely positioned at the end of the "information highway", i.e., by virtue of extensive sensory monosynaptic connections with the higher order sensory cortices. Prefrontal neurons are privy to information of the outside world in the form of representations of on-going events in the current environment as well as to repositories of stored knowledge. This work may seem far afield from membrane biophysics, but I hope to demonstrate that a connection may exist between the disposition of neurotransmitter receptors and the localization of channels that could illuminate the biological basis of cognition. Neuroscientists are in position to integrate information from many levels of analysis in pursuit of the goal of understanding human cognition at a neurobiological level.

Studies in nonhuman primates dating back to the mid-fifties have established a role for the prefrontal cortex in higher cortical functions. Although the major primary sensory and primary motor domains of the cerebrum had been mapped, the functional map of the vast areas of the association cortex were provisional at best. However, a major discovery of this period was the critical role of the prefrontal cortex for performance on a particular kind of behavioral task—called the delayed-response task—which required animals to hold an item of information in mind for several seconds and to update a mental representation of that input on a moment by moment basis (Jacobsen, 1936). In the modern era, we have come to recognize that the function tapped by these laboratory tasks is essentially that which cognitive psychologists refer to as "working memory". Working memory is the inferred ability to hold information transiently 'on-line', essential for the temporal integration of ideas and action, for comprehension and thought (Baddeley, 1986; Just and Carpenter, 1992). A remarkable conjunction of physiology and behavior occurred when it was observed that

prefrontal neurons could exhibit sustained tonic activity triggered by the brief presentation of a stimulus (Fuster and Alexander, 1971; Kubota and Niki, 1971; Funahashi et al., 1989) as this distinguished neurons of the association cortex from sensory neurons that are time-locked to the stimulus. I have maintained that the prefrontal neuron's capacity for sustained activation in the absence of external stimulation is the cellular basis of mental representation and the essential building block for information processing systems in the human brain. This is the neural mechanism presumably disrupted in the condition: "out of sight—out of mind" that Sir John Ferrier used to describe monkeys with prefrontal lesions (Ferrier, 1886) and so often been used to describe patients with prefrontal lesions.

How is information represented in prefrontal neurons? We have shown that the sustained activity observed in many prefrontal neurons is, in fact, content specific. Prefrontal neurons have been shown to code specific items of information, such as the location of an object space mapped in egocentric coordinates (Fig. 1) (Funahashi et al., 1989; Fuster, 1973) and the direction of a prior response (Funahashi et al., 1993). This specificity is best illustrated by reference to the visuo-spatial memory system. While a monkey is being tested for its retention of the location of as many as 24 spatial locations with the visual field, a given well-tuned neuron that is recorded concurrently with the behavioral test, responds only on the memory trials of a given location, e.g., the 45° location, while its activity remains at baseline for almost every other location. Further, the activities of prefrontal neurons are often polarized, exhibiting excitatory responses to targets in preferred directions and inhibitory responses to targets in nonpreferred directions (Funahashi et al., 1989). In this way, the neuron is endowed with both a "memory field" and an opponent memory field (Fig. 1). Indeed, we now know that the neuron's memory field is in large part created by inhibitory inputs from nearby and distant interneurons, as described below.

Excitatory/inhibitory interactions in cortical circuits

Pyramidal and nonpyramidal cells constitute the major cellular constituents of the cerebral cortex and it is widely believed that understanding the interaction of

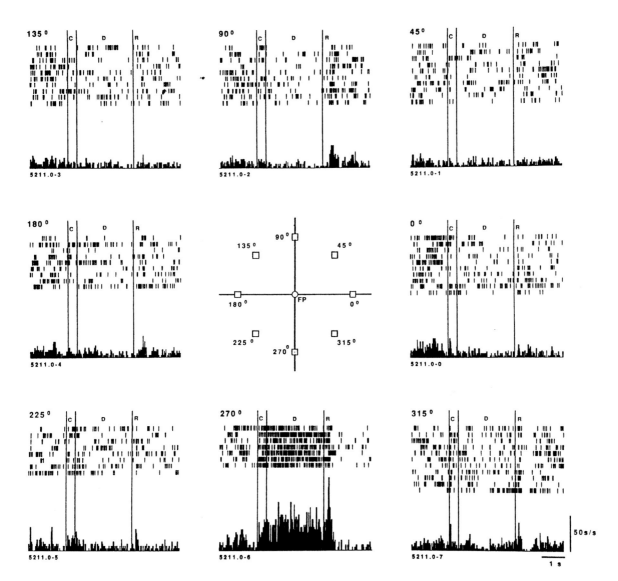

Fig. 1. The functional specificity of prefrontal neuronal activity recorded *in vivo* as a monkey performed a delayed-response task. The neuron's activity is precisely time-locked to the events in the task: the presentation of a spatial cue (500 ms); the delay period interposed between the cue and the response (3000 ms); and the response period after the delay (1000 ms). The raster display above each histogram reveals the neuron's firing rate on numerous trials during which the animal was required to remember targets located 13° from the fixation point. The neuron shown in this figure was tested during memory trials for each location but was activated only during the delay period when the target at the 270° location was recalled.; and not during trials when any other location was designated.. Furthermore, the neuron's firing rate, as shown in the rasters, was consistently enhanced during the delay period every trial the monkey recalled the 270° cue. The preferential activation of a prefrontal neuron during memory intervals (during which no stimulus is present and no response required) is termed the neuron's "memory field" in analogy with receptive field properties of neurons in sensory cortices. (From Funahashi et al., 1989.)

these two principal components of cortical architecture holds the key to a mechanistic understanding of cortical function. Based on an early observation, Mountcastle et al. (1969) were among the first to suggest that

"regular" and "thin" spikes observed in extracellular recording studies of primate cortical neurons corresponded to pyramidal and "stellate" nonpyramidal neuronal morphologies, respectively. Considerable progress has recently been made in deciphering the local circuits by which these major classes of neuron interact. *In vitro* intracellular work has confirmed that "regular spiking" (RS) and "fast spiking" (FS) neurons differ in their base widths and correspond to neurons with pyramidal and sparsely spiny stellate morphologies, respectively (McCormick et al., 1985). Furthermore, fast spiking neurons are parvalbumin positive, indicating that these GABAergic interneurons are likely the basket and chandelier cells (Kawaguchi, 1995) which provide a major source of inhibitory input to the soma, proximal dendritic regions and axon initial segments of pyramidal cells (e.g., Martin et al., 1983). As will be described below, the physiological distinction between fast-spiking (FS) and regular spiking (RS) neurons can be used to extrapolate the functional properties of putative interneurons and pyramidal neurons in extracellular recordings obtained from trained monkeys as they perform working memory tasks.

Until recently, all major progress on the excitatory-inhibitory interactions has come from the study of *in vitro* preparations with the one significant limitation that the activity of neurons examined in living slices cannot be time-locked to natural occurring events. On the other hand, while single unit studies in behaving animals have had the advantage of being able to time-lock neuronal activity to behaviorally relevant events, they have not generally been able to distinguish the neuronal type from which recordings were obtained or to perform intracellular recordings. Wilson et al. (1993) was the first to extend this line of investigation to the study of cognitive processes in the nonhuman primate. Based on findings in identified neurons in slice preparations, we used wave form analysis and firing rate to classify neurons as interneurons or pyramidal neurons *in vivo* as monkeys performed an oculomotor task which required them to make visually-guided or memory-guided eye movements to directional targets in space. In line with the studies mentioned above, cells were classified as putative interneurons if they exhibited thin spikes and high firing rates (FS, fast spiking cells) whereas the physiological signature used to define a pyramidal neuron was wide spike and lower firing rate (RS, regular spiking). A series of studies in the laboratory have now shown that (1) interneurons, like pyramidal neurons, express directional preferences, i.e., have memory fields (Wilson et al., 1993; Rao et al., 1999; Constantinidis et al., 2000, 2001); (2) that their pattern of activity relative to neighboring

pyramidal neurons is dependent on distance between the recorded neurons; and (3) at distances > 50 μm from each other, FS and RS neurons show complimentary firing patterns. Thus, using multiple electrodes *in vivo*, we have shown that neurons that lie in close proximity to each other not only are likely to have shared spatial tuning, i.e., to be iso-directionally related (Constantinidis et al., 2001), but also to be monosynaptically connected (Constantinidis et al., 2000). In contrast, neurons at wider distances, e.g., within 200–300 μm of each other, are more likely to have wide disparities in their spatial tuning and to be cross-directionally tuned, suggestive of a modular organization for visuo-spatial information processing. The striking local circuit and functional arrangements between adjacent and separated pyramidal and fast-spiking interneurons support a microcolumnar functional architecture in the dorsolateral prefrontal cortex for spatial memory fields and hence for psychic functions, similar to that found in other areas of cortex for sensory receptive fields.

A final observation relevant to the psychic neuron hypothesis comes from a recent combined physiological/anatomical analysis of prefrontal circuitry. To elucidate local circuit mechanisms subserving prefrontal cortical functions, we have characterized the responses of distinct subtypes of interneuron to their excitatory inputs in the prefrontal cortex of the ferret (Krimer and Goldman-Rakic, 2001). In dual somatic recordings from pyramidal-to-nonpyramidal pairs, we found that the unitary EPSPs, firing rates and action potential widths recorded in interneurons depended upon their size, correlated morphology and, importantly, the length of their axonal arbors. Small, fast-spiking interneurons with a restricted axonal arborization generally received only one excitatory synapse while larger interneurons with axons extending over 1 mm in either direction from the soma received up to five such connections and these multiple synapses exhibited linear summation (Fig. 2). The two types of pyramidal-to-interneuron circuits provide a foundation for the two physiological processes observed *in vivo*—iso-directional and cross-directional inhibition. An interneuron with short axonal extension may communicate mainly with its neighboring pyramidal neuron and other neurons within the same cortical microcircuit.

All together these findings on prefrontal cortex form the neural basis for the mental representation of visuo-spatial information. We are beginning to describe and elaborate the circuits in which "psychic cells" are

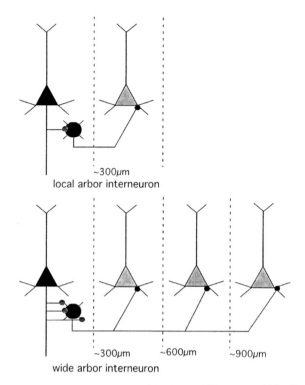

~300μm
local arbor interneuron

~300μm   ~600μm   ~900μm
wide arbor interneuron

Fig. 2. Diagram of two types of local pyramidal-nonpyramidal cell circuitry based on the membrane properties and morphological features of interneurons recorded in slices of ferret prefrontal cortex. The dendritic arbors and axonal plexus of both neurons were fully reconstructed using Neurolucida software. The axon of the interneuron ramified locally and did not extend beyond 300 μm and is considered a local arbor cell. Another type of pyramidal- nonpyramidal cell circuit is shown in the lower panel. In this type, the axon of the interneuron can be distributed as far as 1 mm from the pyramidal cell which innervates it and is referred to as a wide arbor cell. The membrane properties, response to excitatory input and morphological features of these two types of local circuits have been shown to be distinguishable in dual whole cell recording studies (Krimer and Goldman-Rakic, 2001). We have proposed that the upper and lower displayed circuits also differ with respect to the mediation of lateral inhibitory mechanisms—isodirectional and cross-directional inhibition, respectively. Figure based on data in Krimer and Goldman-Rakic, (2001).

embedded and the findings offer promise for a genuine neurobiology of cognition. They also provide a template for understanding other "psychic cells" and other prefrontal circuits, as described below.

Object/face responsive "psychic" neurons

The localization of neurons with visual-spatial tuning function in the dorsolateral prefrontal cortex, correlated

with the fact that these neurons receive preferential innervation from the posterior parietal cortex and constitute the central extension of the dorsal pathway, has suggested to us that category specific information may be mapped across the prefrontal promontory in a manner consistent with the terminal fields of cortical projections from other sensory association cortices. A logical place to search for such specificity would be the inferior convexity of the macaque prefrontal cortex where lesions commonly impair tasks which require the processing and memory of object features (Mishkin, 1964; Goldman et al., 1970; Passingham, 1975; Mishkin and Manning, 1978; Mishkin et al., 1982; Bachevalier and Mishkin, 1986). Accordingly, we have recorded from the inferior convexity while monkeys foveated a variety of visual stimuli presented at the center of the video monitor (Fig. 3) (O'Scalaidhe et al., 1997, 1999). The stimuli were photographs of animal and human faces in various orientations as well as of objects, familiar and abstract, and color swatches. We were able to identify neurons with strong specificities for particular stimuli. Indeed, we observed neurons that responded selectively to pictures of faces (Fig. 4). Remarkably, as shown in the figure, these cells are located in a circumscribed region of the inferior convexity which we have been shown to be connected with the inferotemporal region where "face" cells were first recorded (Gross, 1992). The same neurons were either far less responsive or unresponsive in the visuo-spatial delayed-response tasks that elicit strong and specialized responses from dorsolateral prefrontal cortex. Moreover, neurons with visuo-spatial sensory and memory fields recorded in the dorsolateral areas did not respond to the foveated stimuli used in the studies of inferior prefrontal convexity neurons. The dissociation of visuo-spatial and object coding features at both the areal and cellular levels strongly suggests that the neural systems subserving these two visual dimensions are organized as parallel and to a considerable extent segregated of information processing systems.

Auditory responsive "psychic" neurons

An important issue is whether the mapping of visually responsive neurons pertains only to the visual domain or extends more generally to informational processing in other systems. To examine the generality of the emerging "domain specific hypothesis", recent studies in this

432

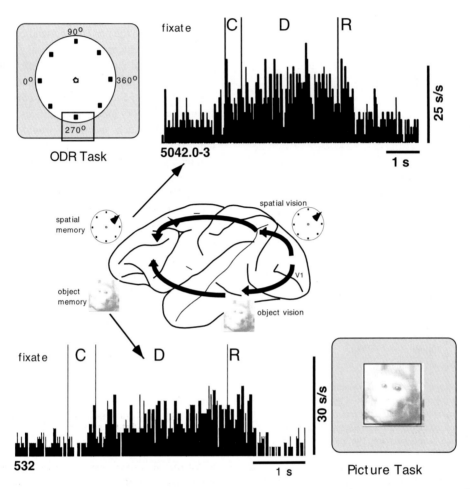

Fig. 3. Diagram representing the topographic architecture of prefrontal cortex. Neurons with specificities for representations of visuo-spatial stimuli are located in a dorsolateral or superior region of the prefrontal cortex which receives cortico-cortical afferents from the posterior parietal regions which process visual information originating in the magnocellular visual pathway. Neurons which respond to the identity of objects, e.g., faces, are located in the inferior convexity of the prefrontal cortex innervated by afferents from the inferotemporal cortex and parvocellular visual pathway. (From Goldman-Rakic, 1996.)

laboratory examined the prefrontal landscape for neurons that might be selectively responsive to auditory stimuli (Romanski and Goldman-Rakic, in press). Neuronal recordings were made as monkeys fixated a central point on a television monitor and either viewed visual stimuli or were presented with an auditory stimulus from a speaker located just below the monitor. Neurons were tested with one or more of ten lists of auditory stimuli consisting of monkey and human vocalizations, environmental sounds (bells, whistles, sirens, etc.), band-passed or white noise, FM sweeps, and tone bursts.

Vocalizations proved to be the most effective stimuli although most of the auditory responsive cells responded to both vocalization and nonvocalization stimuli) (Fig. 5). A small number of neurons, however, responded only to the category of vocalizations, indicating sparse representation of this class of stimulus. However, the selectivity of these prefrontal neurons for vocalization stimuli was demonstrated by the finding that both monkey or human vocalizations elicited a statistically stronger response in 71% (10/14) of these cells. In contrast to vocalizations, prefrontal neurons were much less responsive to pure tones. Thus, the macaque prefrontal cortex contains neurons that could mediate social and other nonspatial acoustic signaling. Supporting this conclusion, we found the auditory responsive neurons, not in the

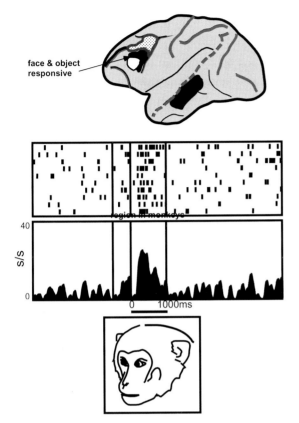

Fig. 4. Example of a prefrontal neuron which responded strongly to a picture of a monkey face and was unresponsive to pictures of other objects or to visuo-spatial stimuli, e.g. in oculomotor spatial delayed response tasks. The lateral view of the monkey brain shows that this and other face responsive neurons were found in an area on the inferior convexity of the prefrontal cortex (shown in black), ventral to the areas where visuo-spatially tuned neurons are observed. This area is interconnected with area TE in the temporal lobe where face cells have been recorded and where, in humans, lesions produced visual agnosias such as prosopagnoisa (also shown in black).

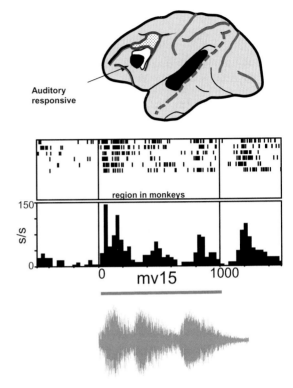

Fig. 5. Example of a prefrontal neuron which responded strongly to an auditory stimulus and was unresponsive to any visual stimulus presented. Notice that the neuron's response reflects the temporal and spectral characteristics of the sound, which in this case was a recording of a monkey vocalization (mv). The lateral view of the monkey brain shows that this and other auditory responsive neurons were found in an area on the inferior convexity of the prefrontal cortex (shown in black), anterior to the area where face and object responsive neurons have been recorded and ventral to the areas where visuo-spatially tuned neurons are observed. This area is interconnected with the auditory association regions in the temporal lobe that are associated with auditory perception (also shown in black).

dorsolateral prefrontal areas where the visual-spatial neurons reside, but rather in the inferior prefrontal convexity of macaque prefrontal cortex, presumably corresponding to Brodmann's areas 44, 45 and 47 (including Broca's area) where recent PET and fMRI studies of the human brain have shown activations in auditory working memory, phonological processing, comprehension and semantic judgement tasks (Fig. 5). Whereas our studies of visually responsive neurons found them located most commonly anterior to the inferior limb of the arcuate sulcus, the auditory responsive cells were tightly clustered anterolateral to visual neurons in the inferior limb as in the same

animals. No auditory responsive cells were found outside this ventrolateral quadrant of the recording cylinder.

References

Bachevalier, J. and Mishkin, M. (1986) Visual recognition impairment follows ventromedial but not dorsolateral prefrontal lesions in monkeys. *Behav. Brain Res.*, 20: 249–261.

Baddeley, A. (1986) *Working Memory*. Oxford University Press, London, pp. 1–289.

Cajal, S.R. (1892) A New Concept of the Histology of the Nerve Centers. In: *Cajal on the Cerebral Cortex. An Annotated Translation of the Complete Writings* by J. DeFelipe and

434

E.G. Jones. Chapter 7, Oxford University Press, New York 1988, pp. 69.

Constantinidis, C., Franowicz, M.N. and Goldman-Rakic, P.S. (2000) Psychophysical performance reflected in mnemonic activity of primate prefrontal cortex during a spatial working memory task. *Soc. Neurosci. Abstr.*, 26: 365.11.

Constantinidis, C., Franowicz, M.N. and Goldman-Rakic, P.S. (2001) Coding specificity in cortical microcircuits: a multiple-electrode analysis of primate prefrontal cortex. *J. Neurosci.*, 21: 3646–3655.

Ferrier, D. (1886) *The Functions of the Brain*. 2nd Edition, Putnam, New York.

Funahashi, S., Bruce, C.J. and Goldman-Rakic, P.S. (1989) Mnemonic coding of visual space in the monkey's dorsolateral prefrontal cortex. *J. Neurophysiol.*, 61: 331–349.

Funahashi, S., Chafee, M.V. and Goldman-Rakic, P.S. (1993) Prefrontal neuronal activity in rhesus monkeys performing a delayed anti-saccade task. *Nature*, 365: 753–756.

Fuster, J.M. (1973) Unit activity in prefrontal cortex during delayed-response performance: Neuronal correlates of transient memory. *J. Neurophysiol.*, 36: 61–78.

Fuster, J.M. and Alexander, G.E. (1971) Neuron activity related to short-term memory. *Science*, 173: 652–654.

Goldman, P.S., Rosvold, H.E. and Mishkin, M. (1970) Selective sparing of function following prefrontal lobectomy in infant monkeys. *Exp. Neurol.*, 29: 221–226.

Goldman-Rakic, P.S., Leranth, C., Williams, S.M., Mons, N. and Geffard, M. (1989) Dopamine synaptic complex with pyramidal neurons in primate cerebral cortex. *Proc. Natl. Acad. Sci. USA*, 86: 9015–9019.

Goldman-Rakic, P.S. (1996) The prefrontal landscape: implications of functional architecture for understanding human mentation and the central executive. *Phil. Trans. R. Soc. Lond. B.*, 351: 1445–1453.

Gross, C.G. (1992) Representation of visual stimuli in inferior temporal cortex. *Phil. Trans. R. Soc. Lond. B.*, 335: 3–10.

Jacobsen, C.F. (1936) Studies of cerebral function in primates. *Comp. Psychol. Monogr.*, 13: 1–68.

Just, M.A. and Carpenter, P.A. (1992) A capacity theory of comprehension: individual differences in working memory. *Psych. Rev.*, 99: 122–149.

Kawaguchi, Y. (1995) Physiological subgroups of nonpyramidal cells with specific morphological characteristics in layer II/III of rat frontal cortex. *J. Neurosci.*, 15: 2638–2655.

Krimer, L.S. and Goldman-Rakic, P.S. (2001) Prefrontal microcircuits: Membrane properties and excitatory input of local,

medium and wide arbor interneurons. *J. Neurosci.*, 21: 3788–3796.

Kubota, K. and Niki, H. (1971) Prefrontal cortical unit activity and delayed alternation performance in monkeys. *J. Neurophysiol.*, 34: 337–347.

Martin, K.A., Somogyi, P. and Whitteridge, D. (1983) Physiological and morphological properties of identified basket cells in the cat's visual cortex. *Exp. Brain Res.*, 50: 193–200.

McCormick, D.A., Connors, B.W., Lighthall, J.W. and Prince, D.A. (1985) Comparative electrophysiology of pyramidal and sparsely spiny stellate neurons of the neocortex. *J. Neurophysiol.*, 54: 782–806.

Mishkin, M. (1964) Perseveration of central sets after frontal lesions in monkeys. In: J.M. Warren and K. Akert (Eds.), *The Frontal Granular Cortex and Behavior*. McGraw-Hill, New York, pp. 219–241.

Mishkin, M. and Manning, F.J. (1978) Nonspatial memory after selective prefrontal lesions in monkeys. *Brain Res.*, 143: 313–323.

Mishkin, M., Ungerleider, L.G. and Macko, K.A. (1982) Object vision and spatial vision: two cortical pathways. *Trends Neurosci.*, 6: 414–417.

Mountcastle, V.B., Talbot, W.H., Sakata, H. and Hyvarinen, J. (1969) Cortical neuronal mechanisms in flutter-vibration studied in unanesthetized monkeys. Neuronal periodicity and frequency discrimination. *J. Neurophysiol.*, 32: 452–484.

O'Scalaidhe, S.P., Wilson, F.A.W. and Goldman-Rakic, P.S. (1997) Areal segregation of face-processing neurons in prefrontal cortex. *Science*, 278: 1135–1138.

O'Scalaidhe, S.P., Wilson, F.A.W. and Goldman-Rakic, P.S. (1999) Face-selective neurons during passive viewing and working memory performance of rhesus monkeys: evidence for intrinsic specialization of neuronal coding. *Cereb. Cortex.*, 9: 459–475.

Passingham, R.E. (1975) Delayed matching after selective prefrontal lesions in monkeys (*Macac mulatta*). *Brain Res.*, 92: 89–102.

Rao, S.G., Williams, G.V. and Goldman-Rakic, P.S. (1999) Isodirectional tuning of adjacent interneurons and pyramidal cells during working memory: evidence for microcolumnar organization in PFC. *J. Neurophysiol.*, 81: 1903–1916.

Romanski, L.M. and Goldman-Rakic, P.S. (2002) An auditory domain in primate prefrontal cortex. *Nat. Neurosci.*, 5: 15–16.

Wilson, F.A.W., Ó Scalaidhe, S.P. and Goldman-Rakic, P.S. (1993) Dissociation of object and spatial processing domains in primate prefrontal cortex. *Science*, 260: 1955–1958.

E.C. Azmitia, J. DeFelipe, E.G. Jones, P. Rakic and C.E. Ribak (Eds.)
Progress in Brain Research, Vol. 136
© 2002 Elsevier Science B.V. All rights reserved

CHAPTER 34

Cajal's prophetic functional considerations on respiratory reflexes: new questions about old answers

Stephan W. Schwarzacher*

Institute of Anatomy, University of Goettingen, Kreuzbergring 36, D-37075 Goettingen, Germany

Abstract: In the "Histology of the Nervous System" (*Histologie*, Spanish edition, 1899, 1904; French translation, 1909, 1911; all citations are from the American translation, 1995) Cajal did not only describe the origins and central pathways of cranial nerves but his detailed observations led him to numerous conclusions about the functional organization of brainstem reflexes. From studies of vagal and glossopharyngeal afferents he proposed a structural organization of the nucleus tractus solitarii (NTS). His view has been considerably changed by several authors on the basis of modern tracing studies. However, detailed histological examinations of functionally identified sensory fibers provided new understanding of a functional organization of the solitary nucleus that is very well in line with Cajal's original descriptions. The prophetic character of Cajal's concepts of structural–functional relations becomes even more evident by a reconsideration of his explanations of the reflexes underlying respiration, coughing and vomiting. Recent electrophysiological studies of spontaneously rhythmically active *in vitro* preparations have provided us with new insights in respiratory control. However, it appears that quite a number of Cajal's key questions concerning respiratory reflexes are still not solved. Therefore, a reconsideration of old and partly forgotten concepts might indeed provide a novel understanding of the structural and functional organization of brainstem reflexes.

Organization of the nucleus tractus solitarii (NTS)

In chapter 26 of the *Histologie* (Cajal, 1995) that describes the vagus and glossopharyngeal nerves or 9th and 10th cranial nerves, Cajal points out that "*the principal group of transverse or oblique fibers associated with the sensory roots of the 9th and 10th cranial nerves undergoes a simple bend to assume a descending course, such forming the solitary tract*". Accordingly, fibers and their collaterals descend and along their course send terminal fibers in the accompanying gray matter. Based on the distribution of these terminal fibers, Cajal determined a small "*interstitial or lateral nucleus*", and a larger "*medial nucleus*". This is accomplished by the "*comissural part of the nucleus of the solitary tract (NTS)*". This cell

group, which Cajal discovered, "*is formed by the fusion of the caudal ends of the two medial parts of the nucleus of the solitary tract*". "*Descending fibers interdigitate here with similar fibers from the other side.*" In addition, "*the vast majority of fibers in the solitary tract appear to end in the commissural part, where they produce an extremely dense plexus.*"

This principal description follows the idea of an organization of the NTS by the terminal regions of primary afferents, a logic that has the benefit of structural-functional consequences. Therefore, Cajal considers: "*It goes without saying that the crossing of these fibers is extremely important from the functional standpoint. Their existence suggests that all stimuli gathered by vagal nerve endings in the mucosae have the ability to evoke synergistic, bilateral responses in pulmonary smooth muscle, as well as in the striated inspiratory muscles.*" It was many decades later, that careful electrophysiological studies of functionally identified and

*Corresponding author: Tel.: 0049 551 397062;
Fax: 0049 551 397052; E-mail: sschwar@gwdg.de

intraaxonally recorded and labelled single vagal fibers have provided evidence for these prophetic statements (for refs. see Jordan, 2001).

Since the invention of axonal tracing techniques at the end of the seventies of the 20th century, a wide range of anatomical data has provided a more coherent picture of the central projections of the vagal and glossopharyngeal nerves and their branches in many different mammalian species (Spyer, 1990). Anterograde mapping mainly with horseradish peroxidase (HRP) or fluorescent tracers soon provided clear evidence for a principal somatotopic organization of the NTS. Whereas afferents of the supra-diaphragmatic, i.e. the cardiorespiratory vagal branches terminate in the lateral NTS, the subdiaphragmatic or gastrointestinal vagal parts end in the medial part of the NTS (for refs. see Spyer, 1990; Jordan, 2001). On the basis of HRP-labeling of different vagal branches Kalia and Mesulam (1980) proposed a new classification of different NTS subnuclei. However, this classification was inconsistent with other nomenclatures of the NTS sub-nuclei, that were based on cytoarchitectonic criteria (Loewy and Burton, 1978). The problem remained, however, that each of the labeled vagal and glossopharyngeal nerves and even small branches contains a heterogenous mixture of afferents, each with axons in myelinated and unmyeli-nated classes (Spyer, 1990). Moreover, afferents from one peripheral organ or target arise from a variety of different receptors. To overcome these problems, the laborious intraaxonal recording of individual afferent fibers with microelectrodes, their functional identi-fication and intraaxonal labeling has to be undertaken. In the following section the potential outcome and the limitations of such studies for a better understanding of the NTS organization will be exemplified by a descrip-tion of laryngeal afferents and their central projections.

Functional identification of primary afferent terminations in the NTS: projections of laryngeal mechano- and chemoreceptor afferents

The laryngeal mucosa is the localization of various receptors that are the origin of a number of important respiratory reflexes (for refs. see Widdicombe, 2001; Sant'Ambrogio and Widdicombe, 2001). In general, two major groups of reflexes can be distinguished: Those, that are involved in the maintanance of regular air movements during inhalation and exhalation, and those,

that register and defend irregular inhalation of toxic or vulnerable substances including aspiration. Despite the great importance for respiratory control, the laryngeal receptors and their central projections are still unsatis-factorily and inconsistently described and characterized in the current literature (Widdicombe, 2001). This is mainly due to the fact that the axons of laryngeal recep-tors are intermingled with pharyngeal fibers in the main afferent vagal branch of the laryngo-pharyngeal region, the superior laryngeal nerve. Therefore, stimulation of the superior laryngeal nerve alone does not identify laryngeal afferents. In addition, a local stimulation of the laryngeal mucosa has to be performed. This was achieved in *in vivo* cat experiments by insertion of a tra-cheal tube (Schwarzacher et al., 1991). Through a second tube in the superior esophagus, stimulation of the pha-ryngeal mucosa was done to clearly distinguish between laryngeal and pharyngeal receptors (Fig. 1A). This experimental setup opened the possibility for further discriminations of laryngeal receptors. Application of an irritant chemical such as cigarette smoke stimulated chemoreceptors, whereas application of negative or positive air pressure activated a completely different pop-ulation of mechanoreceptors (Fig. 1C,D). Intraaxonal recording and labeling of such identifed laryngeal receptor afferents within the solitary tract led to full reconstructions of single axons and their terminations (Fig. 1B). As already suggested by Cajal, these vagal axons entered the solitary tract (TS) rostrally and descended with 1–3 collaterals all the way through the TS. At more or less all rostrocaudal levels terminal fibers branched off the main collaterals and entered different subnuclei of the NTS where they ended with terminal boutons. This characteristic pattern of termination has been described for a couple of different vagal afferents, including lung strech receptor afferents and baroreceptor afferents (for refs. see Spyer, 1990; Jordan, 2001).

Both, laryngeal chemo- and mechanoreceptor afferents terminated in several different NTS subnuclei. As was expected from more general labeling studies (Kalia and Mesulam, 1980) the termination was restricted to the lat-eral parts of the NTS (see above). However, there was also a clear differentiation between the two types of tested laryngeal afferents. Chemoreceptor afferents terminated primarily in the ventrolateral NTS, a subnuculeus that is particularly involved in respiratory control (for refs. see Spyer, 1990; Jordan, 2001). Mechanoreceptor afferents exhibited a more widespread distribution in the NTS,

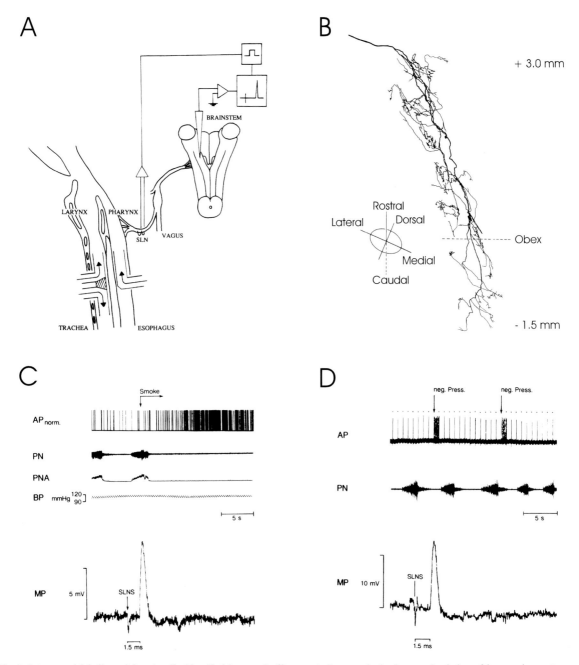

Fig. 1. Intraaxonal labeling of functionally identified laryngeal afferents. A; In anaesthetized cats, stimulation of laryngeal receptors was achieved via the rostral part of the tracheal tube, artificial ventilation was provided via the caudal tracheal tube. For discrimination of pharyngeal receptors, an additional tube was placed in the esophagus. The superior laryngeal nerve (SLN) was stimulated and laryngeal afferents were recorded intraaxonally with glass pipettes within the ipsilateral solitary tract. B, Representative serial reconstruction of a laryngeal chemoreceptor afferent, labeled intraaxonally with horseradish peroxidase. The afferent enters the solitary tract rostrally, decends within the solitary tract and sends off multiple terminal branches in distinct subnuclei of the NTS. C, Functional identification of a laryngeal chemoreceptor afferent with cigarette smoke. D, Functional identification of a laryngeal mechanoreceptor afferent with negative air pressure. AP, intraaxonal recordings of action potentials. PN, respiratory activity recorded in the phrenic nerve. PNA, integrated PN activity. MP, Membrane potential of intraaxonally recorded afferent. SLNS, electrical stimulation of the superior laryngeal nerve. Data from Schwarzacher et al. (1991).

including the dorsomedial, dorsolateral, ventromedial and ventrolateral ones. This differences could be explained by functional considerations: On one hand, chemoreceptor afferents would essentially be involved in laryngeal defense- or aspiration-reflexes, and therefore terminals would focus on the respiratory interneurons located within the ventrolateral subnucleus. On the other hand, laryngeal mechanoreceptor afferents would be involved in various reflexes that modulate breathing movements. This could explain the termination of mechanoreceptors in a greater number of subnuclei. This interpretation is supported by similar intraaxonal labeling studies of lung stretch receptor afferents revealing a comparably widespread termination in the same set of NTS subnuclei (Kalia and Richter, 1985, 1988).

As stated by several authors in the past (Spyer, 1990; Jordan, 2001), one of the most striking features of the available data on functionally identified vagal afferents is that the different subnuclei of the NTS receive input from several different primary afferent sources. This fact complicates attempts to establish a functional topography of the NTS subnuclei. On the other hand it supports hypotheses, that suggests the NTS is an area of integration of various vagal afferents.

Several reviews have summarized the information gained from neurophysiological studies of single identified afferents, and have more or less successfully tried to put the pieces of this complicated puzzle together (Spyer, 1990; Jordan, 1997, 2001; Jean, 2001; Widdicombe, 2001). Some very recent data come from elegant *in vitro* preparations that use the combination of brainstem preparations with a retained working heart and vascular system (Deuchars et al., 2000; Paton and Nolan, 2000; Paton et al., 2001). However, about one hundred years after Cajal's studies on the NTS it has to be stated, that our picture of the organization of the NTS is still far from complete. Most strikingly, it appears that Cajal's strategy of collecting many individual labeled neurons and sorting out their general morphological types remains to be a very laborious, but still the most effective method of studiying the organization of such a complex center of integration as the NTS.

Reflex mechanisms in central respiratory control

One of the most fascinating aspects of Cajal's *Histologie* are the so-called "*functional considerations*". In these sections he exhibits his ability to propose explanations of mechanisms underlying various responses known to be mediated by different nerves or groups of neurons. He writes: "*We shall not try to consider all of the reflexes associated with the IXth and Xth cranial nerves; this would be an exceedingly difficult task that is not directly relevant, and would necessarily involve many arbitrary, if not erroneous, interpretations. Our objective is simpler: We would like to illustrate, by way of several examples, how the new anatomical results may help to explain functional observations. For this, we shall choose coughing, vomiting, and inhaling. Without claiming to provide a definitive circuit, we shall indicate the possible course of neuronal activity in the production of these three responses.*" Subsequently, Cajal described the three reflex pathways and illustrated his considerations with wonderful diagrams. Much of the fascination of his figures comes from his way of abstraction, that preserves the principle anatomical relationships (Fig. 2A). His famous Fig. 313 of the *Histologie* is still used in modern neuroscience textbooks (Feldman and McCrimmon, 1999).

Cajal was obviously fascinated by the great amount of mutual integration within the NTS, due to the widespread arborization of terminal afferents and dendrites of second order neurons. Therefore, and because of his pragmatic strategy of finding the simplest explanations, he limited the integrative functions of the lower brainstem to the NTS. This view appears to be consistent with our current understanding with respect to the fast excitatory part of respiratory reflexes, that function as feedforward pathways. For example, lung stretch receptor afferents project to the ventrolateral NTS, where they end with excitatory synapses on dendrites and somata of inspiratory neurons (Anders et al., 1993). Inspiratory neurons exhibit action potential discharge during the inspiratory phase of the respiratory rhythm. The inspiratory neurons of the ventrolateral NTS form the dorsal respiratory group. These neurons exhibit an excitatory projection to respiratory motoneurons in the spinal cord, such as phrenic motoneurons (Lipski et al., 1983). Therefore, this reflexive pathway is completely excitatory, and functions in facilitating the already generated respiratory rhythm.

For Cajal and his contemporaries around 1900 the source for an inspiratory drive was "*brought about simply by a direct stimulatory effect of carbonic acid in the blood on the medullary inspiratory center*". Indeed, small increases in blood CO_2 produce large increases in

A

B

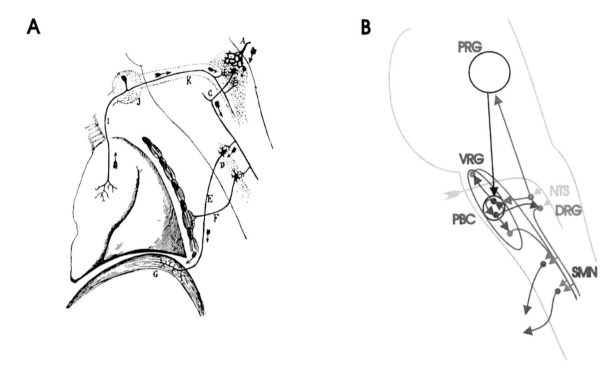

Fig. 2. A, Cajal's schematic drawing of respiratory reflexes. For explanation see text. B, schematic drawing of possible brainstem pathways of respiratory reflexes. Vagal afferents enter the medulla oblongata and terminate within the nuclei of the solitary tract (NTS). Within the NTS they form monosynaptic contacts with inspiratory neurons of the dorsal respiratory group (DRG), that directly project to spinal motoneurons (SMN). This disynaptic pathway is excitatory and can be explained as a feed forward reflex. In addition, yet unidentified NTS neurons project to the pontine respiratory group (PRG) and to the ventral respiratory group (VRG) to modulate the phases of the respiratory rhythm, that is generated within the pre-Bötzinger complex (PBC). The rhythmic output of the PBC is mediated to different types of respiratory phase related premotoneurons of the VRG and DRG, that project to brainstem and spinal motoneurons (SMN). Inhibitory interneurons that mediate inhibitory respiratory reflexes are probably localized within the VRG (see text).

breathing. The feedback for CO_2 involves peripheral chemoreceptors and central chemoreceptors. Whereas central chemoreceptors were thought for decades to be localized to the surface of the ventral medulla, more recent data provide evidence, that these receptors are likely distributed more widely in several brainstem areas, including the NTS (Nattie, 1999).

Impressed by the abundant capillaries in the commissural and medial NTS Cajal proposed this area to be the inspiratory or respiratory center (see Fig. 2A). This concept attracted many researchers over a long period of time until it was finally prooven wrong with the detection of the breathing center within the ventrolateral medulla, called the pre-Bötzinger-complex (PBC) (Smith et al., 1991). The PBC forms the kernel of a distributed network of respiratory neurons that are localized in close

vicinity to the nucleus ambiguus in the ventrolateral medulla, forming the ventral respiratory group. Smith et al. (1990) performed transsections at different rostro-caudal levels in a rhythmically active *in vitro* preparation of the brainstem and spinal cord of the neonatal rat, and could provide evidence that a transversal slice of few 100 μm just rostral to the obex was necessary for the generation of a spontaneous respiratory rhythm. This rhythm was still preserved, when the dorsal part of the medulla including the NTS was removed, and consequently the rhythmic center could be limited to a very small area in the direct vicinity of the nucleus ambiguus, the PBC, both *in vitro* and *in vivo* (Smith et al., 1990, 1991; Schwarzacher et al., 1995; see for review Rekling and Feldman, 1998; Ballanyi et al., 1998; Richter and Spyer, 2001). However, the PBC does not show any special histological characteristics. Therefore it can only be defined by cytoarchitectonic landmarks of the neighboring nuclei (Schwarzacher et al., 1995). Recent data favor the idea, that one relatively exclusive characteristic of the essential respiratory interneurons could be the expression of NK-1 receptors (Gray et al., 1999, 2001), and these observations have been partially confirmed by intracellular studies *in vivo* (Guyenet and Wang, 2001). At present it is not clear, if NK-1-receptor immunoreactivity is a selective marker for the PBC-neurons (Guyenet and Wang, 2001).

Complex reflexes and medullary reflex centers

One of the frequently studied respiratory reflexes is the Hering-Breuer reflex (Feldman and McCrimmon, 1999). It has been exploited experimentally to explore the control of timing of respiratory phases. If the lungs are prevented from emptying after normal ventilation, the subsequent expiratory period is lengthend. On the contrary, if the lungs are prevented from filling during an inspiratory period, the next inspiratory period is lengthened and the inspiratory motor activity is increased. Although the Hering-Breuer reflex is mediated by lung stretch receptor afferents terminating in the NTS, lesioning of the ventrolateral subnucleus, where the dorsal respiratory group of inspiratory neurons are located, does not affect this reflex (McCrimmon et al., 1987). Obviously, the neuronal network of the PBC and the related ventral respiratory group have to be involved. However, as the electrophysiological and neuroanatomical methods to detect and label second- and higher-order neurons still are limited, descriptions of reflexive pathways currently remain largely hypothetical. New insights come from *in vitro* preparations of the neonatal rat brainstem and spinal cord with the lungs attached and their vagal innervation retained (Mellen and Feldman, 2000). In these preparations transient lung inflation triggers off inspiratory onset and shortens the inspiratory phase, thus matching the classical inhibitory Hering-Breuer reflex. The essential inhibitory interneurons within the Hering-Breuer reflex pathway are suggested to be one special type of probably GABAergic interneurons within the ventral respiratory group (Mellen and Feldman, 2001). This would further suggest a direct projection of second-order neurons of the ventromedial subnucleus of the NTS to the ventral respiratory group.

However, functional studies provided evidence for an involvement of pontine respiratory nuclei, such as the parabrachial nuclei and the Koelliker-Fuse nucleus in complex respiratory reflexes such as the Hering-Breuer reflex (Ezure et al., 1998; Siniaia et al., 2000).

While the PBC is now well established as the primary site of respiratory rhythm and pattern generation, it remains to be questioned if there are additional central pattern generators for complex respiratory reflexes, such as sighing or coughing. In recent *in vitro* experiments two different rhythms could be demonstrated in the PBC, with striking similarities to eupeic (normal) respiration and sighs (Lieske et al., 2000). Furthermore, *in vivo* experiments in the cat revealed cough-like motor patterns (fictive cough) in several neurons in the ventral respiratory group, including the pre-Bötzinger complexes, supporting the hypothesis that the same premotor neurons help to shape motoneuron firing patterns during both eupnoea and coughing (Baekey et al., 2001). Therefore, evidence is currently increasing, that there is one general respiratory pattern generating network in the ventrolateral medulla and not multiple centers for different respiratory reflexes. In this respect, the original diagrams of Cajal can be extended by including a primary rhythm generating center, i.e. the PBC, and a closely related, if not partly identical central motor pattern forming network of respiratory interneurons, i.e. the ventral respiratory group. The output of this network is then projected to the respiratory motoneurons (Fig. 2B). A major pontine influence has to be taken into account. However, it remains to be elucidated whereas pontine respiratory centers are essential steps of complex reflectory pathways, or only indirectly involved in the control of such reflexes.

Is there a general concept of vagal reflex control?

In an attempt to generalize, it could be speculated that the concept of respiratory reflex control as illustrated in Fig. 2B could be valid for additional complex vagal reflexes. Indeed, the convergence of vagal afferents on the level of second-order neurons within the NTS, and subsequent projection to centers of motor pattern generation in the ventral medulla have been described in several reflexive systems. For example, the respiratory-related components of fictive vomiting were abolished by large lesions or kainic acid injections in the lateral medulla at the level of the retrofacial nucleus, in the cat *in vivo* (Miller et al., 1994). These results are consistent with the hypothesis that emesis is coordinated not by a unique, well-defined "vomiting-center" but rather by a distributed control system located in the medulla between the levels of the obex and the retrofacial nucleus (Miller et al., 1994,1995). Swallowing, another important and complex vagal reflex, has been extensively studied with microelectrode recordings in a variety of mammalian species. According to Jean (2001), the swallowing central pattern generator includes two main groups of neurons: a dorsal swallowing group located within the interstitial and central subnucleus of the NTS and the adjacent reticular formation, and a ventral swallowing group located in the ventrolateral medulla adjacent to the nucleus ambiguus. Despite the intriguing similarity to the localization of the dorsal and ventral respiratory groups, the dorsal swallowing center appears to contain the generator neurons involved in triggering, shaping and timing the sequential or rhythmic swallowing pattern, whereas the ventral swallowing group appears to contain the switching neurons, which distribute the swallowing drive to the various pools of motoneurons. Therefore, the grade of potential integration within the NTS proper should not be underestimated.

Conclusion

One hundred years after the publication of Cajal's *Histologie* it has to be stated, that despite the invention of important morphological and physiological methods the complex patterns of neuronal integration at the medullary level still remain hypothetical to a remarkable degree. This becomes particularly evident with respect to higher order reticular pathways. With his careful examination of individual neurons characterized only by their morphology, Cajal demonstrated a strategy, which later was successfully extended by the functional characterization of single neurons, and up to now seems to be the most laborious, but also most effective way to elucidate the complexity of neuronal networks within the reticular formation. It seems as if Cajal has compensated for the difficulties of this strategy by what appears to be a very pragmatic way of functional interpretation of his structural findings that always attempts to be as simple as possible. A good example for this pragmatic

"philosophy" might be the following sentences written in the *Histologie* on the aspect of a possible fourth-order sensory pathway proposed by other authors to exist within the reticular formation: "*Complexity of this magnitude appears unwarranted, and we hesitate to accept these conclusions because they imply that the organization of the brainstem is essentially inextricable. This is reinforced by the fact that second- and third-order sensory pathways, along with their inputs to various motor nuclei, seem apriori to be adequate for mediating all of the various reflexes and coordinated movements.*"

Acknowledgments

The author wants to thank Efrain Azmitia and Javier DeFelipe, as well as the members of the Cajal Club and Cajal Institute for organizing such an interesting and enjoyable conference, in Madrid, Spain in May, 2001.

References

Anders, K., Ohndorf, W., Dermietzel, R. and Richter, D.W. (1993) Synapses between slowly adapting lung stretch receptor afferents and inspiratory beta-neurones in the nucleus of the solitary tract of cats. *J. Comp. Neurol.*, 335: 163–172.

Ballanyi, K., Onimaru, H. and Homma, I. (1999) Respiratory network function in the isolated brainstem-spinal cord of newborn rats. *Prog. Neurobiol.*, 59: 583–634.

Beakey, D., Morris, K., Gestreau, C., Li, Z., Lindsey, B. and Shannon, R. (2001) Medullary respiratory neurones and control of laryngeal motoneurones during fictive eupnoea and cough in the cat. *J. Physiol.*, 534: 565–581.

Cajal, S.R. (1995) *Histology of the Nervous System of Man and Vertebrates.* American translation by N. Swanson and L.W. Swanson (Eds.), Oxford University Press, New York.

Deuchars, J., Li, Y.W., Kasparov, S. and Paton, J.F. (2000) Morphological and electrophysiological properties of neurones in the dorsal vagal complex of the rat activated by arterial baroreceptors. *J. Comp. Neurol.*, 417: 233–49.

Ezure, K., Tanaka, I. and Miyazaki, M. (1998) Pontine projections of pulmonary slowly adapting receptor relay neurons in the cat. *NeuroReport*, 9: 411–414.

Feldman, J.L. and McCrimmon, D.R. (1999) Neural control of breathing. In: M.J. Zigmond, F.E. Bloom, S.C. Landis, J.L. Roberts and L.R. Squire (Eds.), *Fundamental Neuroscience*, Academic Press, San Diego, pp. 1063–1090.

Gray, P.A., Rekling, J.C., Bocchiaro, C.M. and Feldman, J.L. (1999) Modulation of respiratory frequency by peptidergic input to rhythmogenic neurons in the preBötzinger complex. *Science*, 286: 1566–1568.

Gray, P.A., Janczewski, W.A., Mellen, N., Mc Crimmon, D.R. and Feldman, J.L. (2001) Normal breathing requires preBötzinger complex neurokinin-1 receptor-expressing neurons. *Nat. Neurosci.*, 4: 927–930.

Guyenet, P.G. and Wang, H. (2001) Pre-Bötzinger neurons with preinspiratory discharges *in vivo* express NK1 receptors in the rat. *J. Neurophysiol.*, 86: 438–446.

Jean, A. (2001) Brain stem control of swallowing: Neuronal network and cellular mechanisms. *Physiol. Rev.*, 81: 929–969.

Jordan, D. (1997) Central nervous control of the airways. In: D. Jordan (Ed.), *Central Nervous Control of Autonomic Function*, Harwood Academic Publishers, Chur, pp. 63–107.

Jordan, D. (2001) Central nervous pathways and control of the airways. *Respir. Physiol.*, 125: 67–81.

Kalia, M. and Mesulam, M.M. (1980) Brain stem projections of sensory and motor component of the vagus complex in the cat. II. Laryngeal, tracheobronchial, pulmonary, cardiac and gastrointestinal branches. *J. Comp. Neurol.*, 193: 467–508.

Kalia, M. and Richter, D.W. (1985) Morphology of physiologically identified slowly adapting lung stretch receptor afferents stained with intraaxonal HRP in the nucleus of the tractus solitarius of the cat I: A light microscopic analysis. *J. Comp. Neurol.*, 241: 503–520.

Kalia, M. and Richter, D.W. (1988) Rapidly adapting pulmonary receptor afferents I: arborization in the nucleus of the tractus solitarius. *J. Comp. Neurol.*, 274: 560–573.

Lieske, S.P., Thoby-Brisson, M., Telgkamp, P. and Ramiraz, J.M. (2000) Reconfiguration of the neural network controling multiple breathing patterns: eupnea, sighs and gasps. *Nat. Neurosci.*, 3: 600–607.

Lipski, J., Kubin, L. and Jodkowsi, J. (1983) Synaptic action of R-β neurons on phrenic motoneurons studied by spike-triggered averaging. *Brain Res.*, 288: 105–118.

Loewy, A.D. and Burton, H. (1978) Nuclei of the solitary tract, efferent projections to the lower brain stem and spinal cord of the cat. *J. Comp. Neurol.*, 181: 421–450.

McCrimmon, D.R., Speck, D.F. and Feldman, J.L. (1987) Role of the ventrolateral region of the nucleus of the tractus solitarius in processing respiratory afferent input from vagus and superior laryngeal nerves. *Exp. Brain. Res.*, 67: 449–459.

Mellen N.M. and Feldman, J.L. (2000) Phasic lung inflation shortens inspiration and respiratory period in the lung-attached neonate rat brain stem spinal cord. *J. Neurophysiol.*, 83: 3165–3168.

Mellen, N.M. and Feldman, J.L. (2001) Phasic vagal sensory feedback transforms respiratory neuron activity *in vitro*. *J. Neurosci.*, 21: 7363–7371.

Miller, A.D., Nonaka, S. and Jakus, J. (1994) Brain areas essential or nonessential for emesis. *Brain Res.*, 647: 255–264.

Miller, A.D., Nonaka, S., Siniaia, M.S. and Jakus, J. (1995) Multifunctional ventral respiratory group: bulbospinal expiratory neurons play a role in pudendal discharge during vomiting. *J. Auton. Nerv. Syst.*, 54: 253–260.

Nattie, E. (1999) CO2, brainstem chemoreceptors and breathing. *Prog. in Neurobiol.*, 59: 299–331.

Paton, J.F. and Nolan, P.J. (2000) Similarities in reflex control of laryngeal and cardiac vagal motor neurones. *Respir. Physiol.*, 119: 101–111.

Paton, J.F., Deuchars, J., Li, Y.W. and Kasparov, S. (2001) Properties of solitary tract neurones responding to peripheral arterial chemoreceptors. *Neuroscience.*, 105: 231–248.

Rekling, J.C. and Feldman, J.L. (1998) Pre-Bötzinger complex and pacemaker neurons: hypothesized site and kernel for respiratory rhythm generation. *Annu. Rev. Physiol.*, 60: 385–405.

Richter, D.W. and Spyer, K.M. (2001) Studying rhythmogenesis of breathing: comparison of *in vivo* and *in vivo* models. *Trends in Neurosci.*, 24: 464–472.

Sant`Ambrogio, G. and Widdicombe, J. (2001) Reflexes from airway rapidly adapting receptors. *Respir. Physiol.*, 125: 33–45.

Schwarzacher, S.W., Monschein, H., Anders, K. and Richter, D.W. (1991) Central termination of functionally identified laryngeal afferents in the cat: an ultrastructural analysis. *Ann. Anat.* 172: 300–.

Schwarzacher, S.W., Smith, J.C. and Richter, D.W. (1995) Pre-Bötzinger complex in the cat. *J. Neurophysiol.*, 73: 1452–1461.

Siniaia, M.S., Young, D.L. and Poon, C.S. (2000) Habituation and desensitization of the Hering-Breuer reflex in rat. *J. Physiol.*, 523: 479–491.

Smith, J.C., Greer, J.J., Liu, G.S. and Feldman, J.L. (1990) Neural mechanisms generating respiratory pattern in mammalian brain stem-spinal cord *in vitro*. I. Spatiotemporal patterns of motor and medullary neuron activity. *J. Neurophysiol.*, 64: 1149–1169.

Smith, J.C., Ellenberger, H.H., Ballanyi, K., Richter, D.W. and Feldman, J.L. (1991) Pre-Bötzinger complex: a brainstem region that may generate respiratory rhythm in mammals. *Science*, 254: 726–729.

Spyer, K.M. (1990) The central nervous organization of reflex circulatory control. In: A.D. Loewy and K.M. Spyer (Eds.), *Central Regulation of Autonomic Functions.* Oxford University Press, New York, pp. 168–188.

Widdicombe, J. (2001) Airway receptors. *Respir. Physiol.*, 125: 3–15.

E.C. Azmitia, J. DeFelipe, E.G. Jones, P. Rakic and C.E. Ribak (Eds.)
Progress in Brain Research, Vol. 136

CHAPTER 35

Serotonin brain circuits involved in major depression and suicide

Victoria Arango,[1,2,3,*] Mark D. Underwood[1,2] and J. John Mann[1,2]

[1]*Department of Neuroscience, New York State Psychiatric Institute,* [2]*Department of Psychiatry,*
[3]*Department of Anatomy and Cell Biology, Columbia University College of Physicians and Surgeons,*
1051 Riverside Drive, New York, NY 10032, USA

Abstract: Throughout his life and his work, Cajal realized the potential of the neurons he was so carefully studying and how, grouped in systems, they served the special senses and the maintenance and proper functioning of the organism. Over the past 25 years, major depression and suicide have come to be recognized as associated with alteration in serotonergic neurons and their target receptors. We examined whether prefrontal cortical (PFC) serotonin transporter sites (SERT) differ in major depression and suicide by quantitative receptor autoradiography. Clinical information was obtained by psychological autopsy. We found regionally distinct neurobiological correlates of major depression and suicide. A diffuse reduction of SERT binding throughout the dorsoventral extent of the PFC in major depression may reflect a widespread impairment of serotonergic function consistent with the range of psychopathology in major depression. The localized reduction in SERT binding in ventral PFC found in suicide victims may reflect reduced serotonin input to that brain region, underlying the predisposition to act on suicidal thoughts. It is conceivable that Cajal envisioned that psychiatric illness would be the result of "psychic neuron" pathophysiology. Today's informed psychiatrists will not be able to deny the role of the brain in the mental ailments that afflict their patients.

Like the entomologist in pursuit of brightly colored butterflies, my attention hunted, in the flower garden of the gray matter, cells with delicate and elegant forms, the mysterious butterflies of the soul, the beating of whose wings may someday—who knows?—*clarify the secret of mental life.*

Santiago Ramón y Cajal,
Recollections of my Life

Introduction

Throughout his life and his work, Cajal realized the potential of how the neurons he was so carefully studying, grouped in systems, served the special senses and the maintenance and proper functioning of the organism.

*Corresponding author: Tel.: (212) 543-5571; Fax: (212) 543-6017;
E-mail: varango@neuron.cpmc.columbia.edu

These same neurons were later found to manufacture neurotransmitters, be grouped into collections of neurons which use the same neurotransmitter and organized into systems within the brain. We examine the involvement of some of these systems in mental illness, such as major depression and suicide.

Over the past 25 years, major depression and suicide have come to be recognized, not by gross or microscopic changes within the brain, but by alterations in serotonin synthesizing neurons and their target receptors. Moreover, major depression and suicidal behavior appear independently related to altered indices of this key neurotransmitter, serotonin. Evidence for the "serotonergic hypothesis" for major depressive illness and suicide comes from studies in the brain, cerebrospinal fluid (CSF) and even platelets (see Mann et al., 1989, 1992, 1996a, 2000; Arango and Mann, 1992; Laruelle et al., 1993; Arango et al., 1995; Arango and

Underwood, 1997; Stoff and Mann, 1997; Flory et al., 1998; Mann, 1998).

The most widely reported serotonergic abnormality in *major* depression involves fewer platelet serotonin transporter (SERT) sites (Owens and Nemeroff, 1994). *In vivo* imaging (Malison et al., 1998; Willeit et al., 2000) and postmortem brain studies (Perry et al., 1983; Arango et al., 1995; Mann et al., 2000; Parsey et al., 2000) conducted in depressed patients suggest that SERT alterations are more widespread in the brain compared with suicides, and also includes the brainstem. We have begun to specifically investigate how serotonergic molecular abnormalities in major depression are different from those in suicides and how depression and suicide pathobiology involve different brain regions.

The prefrontal cortex

We reported in a study of suicide victims that changes in SERT binding are localized to the ventral prefrontal cortex (PFC), an area involved in behavioral inhibition (Arango et al., 1995). In contrast, major depression involves more complex psychopathology. While the full extent of the brain areas involved in depression are unknown, they appear to include areas beyond the ventral PFC. Subsequently, we published the largest postmortem study to date, assaying PFC tissue samples from 159 individuals for SERT binding (^{3}H-cyanoimipramine, Arango et al., 1995) by quantitative receptor autoradiography (Fig. 1) (Mann et al., 2000). Clinical information, including DSM-III-R axis I and axis II diagnoses, was obtained by psychological autopsy (Kelly and Mann, 1996). SERT binding was lower in the ventral PFC of suicide victims compared with controls (Figs. 2 and 3). In contrast, SERT binding in individuals with a history of major depression was lower throughout all prefrontal cortical areas studied (Figs. 2 and 4). Thus, SERT binding revealed what appear to be regionally distinct neurobiological correlates of major depression and suicide.

Cajal, as most of his contemporaries, had views towards women that would be considered to be male chauvinistic in today's society. We (and others) in the course of our studies have observed marked differences, at least in brain chemistry, between males and females, raising the possibility that Cajal's views on the differences between men and women were neurochemically

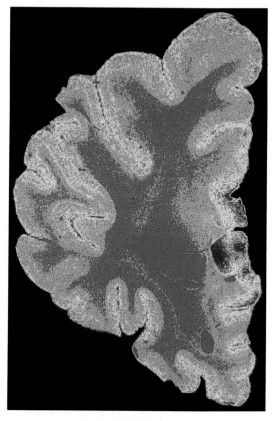

Fig. 1. Pseudocolor image of subtracted autoradiograms representing total specific serotonin transporter binding sites in human prefrontal cortex. Note that binding is higher in medial prefrontal cortex and that binding to the gray matter is much greater than that to the white matter.

and neuroanatomically correct, if not politically correct. Females have significantly lower SERT binding, compared with males, in most Brodmann areas we have studied (Fig. 5). As stated above, SERT binding to the PFC of patients with a history of major depression is significantly lower in the gyrus and sulcus of most Brodmann areas compared with those without a history of major depression (Fig. 4). Males with a history of major depression have 33% less SERT binding compared with males without depression. In contrast, depressed females have 19% less SERT binding compared with nondepressed females. In our study, more females had a history of major depression, and females had lower SERT binding than males (Mann et al., 2000). Perhaps lower SERT binding explains why females are more prone to depression compared with men.

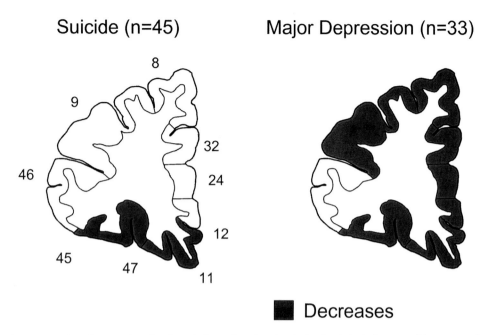

Suicide (n=45)   Major Depression (n=33)

8
9
32
46
24
12
45
47
11

■ Decreases

Fig. 2. Schematic representation of a coronal section through the prefrontal cortex at a level anterior to the genu of the corpus callosum. Shaded areas represent reductions in serotonin transporter sites (SERT). Approximate location of Brodmann areas is indicated. Note that suicide victims have reductions in SERT binding primarily in the orbital cortex. In major depression, reductions in SERT are widespread.

Effect of Suicide on SERT Binding in Prefrontal Cortex

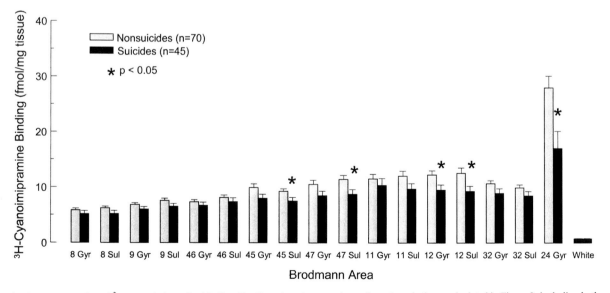

Fig. 3. Representation of ^{3}H-cyanoimipramine binding (fmol/mg tissue) across the prefrontal cortical areas depicted in Figure 2, including both the gyrus (Gyr) and sulcus (Sul). Nonsuicides (light stippling) are compared to suicide victims (dark stippling). Note that suicide victims have less binding in localized orbital regions (45, 47 and 12) and cingulated gyrus (24).

446

Effect of Major Depression on SERT Binding in Prefrontal Cortex

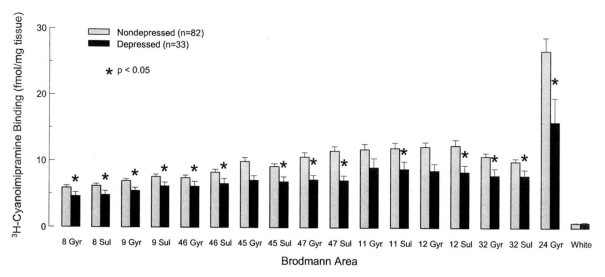

Fig. 4. Representation of ³H-cyanoimipramine binding (fmol/mg tissue) across the prefrontal cortical areas depicted in Figure 2, including both the gyrus (Gyr) and sulcus (Sul). Nondepressed individuals (light stippling) are compared to depressed individuals (dark stippling). Note that depressed individuals have less SERT binding everywhere in the prefrontal cortex.

Comparison of SERT Binding in Males and Females

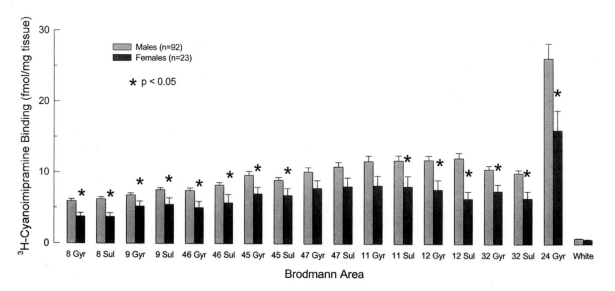

Fig. 5. Representation of ³H-cyanoimipramine binding (fmol/mg tissue) across the prefrontal cortical areas depicted in Figure 2, including both the gyrus (Gyr) and sulcus (Sul). Males (light stippling) are compared to females (dark stippling), independent of their psychiatric diagnoses. Note that females have less binding than males in multiple prefrontal cortical regions.

Not surprisingly, suicide is associated with major depression as well as with lower SERT binding. However, we observe neurochemical changes that appear to distinguish major depression and suicide. In contrast to changes in major depression, SERT binding to the PFC of suicide victims is lower only in orbital or ventral PFC (Figs. 2 and 3) compared with nonsuicides.

Because of the higher rate of suicide in cases with a history of major depression, and the association of lower SERT binding to major depression, we examined the interrelationship of major depression and suicide to SERT binding in PFC. Within the group with a history of major depression, suicides have lower SERT binding than nonsuicides. The effect of suicide on binding is also independent of sex.

A diffuse reduction of SERT binding throughout the dorsoventral extent of the prefrontal cortex in major depression may reflect a widespread impairment of serotonergic function consistent with the range of psychopathology in major depression. The cause of the diffuse reduction in SERT binding in major depression is not known. *In vivo* studies also suggest a systemic reduction in SERT sites in major depression, involving at least low SERT binding in multiple brain regions, platelets and brainstem (Owens and Nemeroff, 1994; Malison et al., 1998; Parsey et al., 2000) that would be consistent with a genetic cause or a systemic effect on gene expression. Given the elevation in cortisol levels found in some depressed patients, one could hypothesize that corticosteroids are altering SERT gene expression or binding, but animal studies do not suggest such an effect (Kuroda et al., 1994). Another possibility is an effect of prior antidepressant medication. Our cases had toxicological screenings to rule out recent exposure to SSRIs and other antidepressants. Moreover, a drug effect is unlikely to be limited to parts of the brain. Therefore, the localized reduction in SERT binding in ventral PFC found in suicide victims may reflect reduced serotonin input to that brain region, underlying the predisposition to act, or failing to inhibit acting, on suicidal thoughts. Traumatic injuries of the ventral PFC are associated with behavioral disinhibition and an increase in impulsive behaviors including aggression and suicide attempts (Damasio et al., 1994; Shallice and Burgess, 1996). Therefore, reduced serotonergic input into this brain region may underlie an impairment of behavioral inhibition or restraint, and an increased propensity for suicidal acts in patients who feel depressed or hopeless.

Cajal could not have predicted the impact or significance of how DNA, or chromatin, would be discovered and perhaps determine the phenotype, morphology or function of the brain's neurons. We examined the relationship of the serotonin transporter genotype and prefrontal SERT binding in major depression and suicide because a gene polymorphism for the SERT has been suggested to influence the amount of SERT sites in brain. This suggestion was based on the observation of differential gene expression in association with an insertion/deletion in the promoter region of the SERT gene in transformed lymphoblastoid cell lines. We found no relationship between serotonin transporter genotype and the level of SERT binding, the diagnosis of major depression, death by suicide or sex of the subject (Mann et al., 2000). Thus, in the intact organ, any effect of this variant in the 5′ flanking promoter region is offset by other homeostatic and regulatory effects. Perhaps other genetic variants are important and remain to be identified. Perhaps Cajal didn't miss the genetic revolution after all. Few studies of gene and behavior associations are replicated in the literature. Arguably, most if not all of Cajal's observations have withstood the test of time.

In conclusion, we have observed a widespread reduction in SERT binding in the PFC of deceased individuals with a history of major depression, and confirmed a reduction in SERT binding involving mainly the orbital PFC of suicide victims. A promoter region insertion/deletion in the gene for the serotonin transporter gene does not explain lower prefrontal cortical SERT binding in major depression, suicide or females.

Serotonergic neurons in the brainstem

In nonhuman primates, serotonergic innervation of the cerebral cortex and much of the forebrain is derived from serotonin-synthesizing neurons in the dorsal raphe nucleus (DRN) and in the median raphe nucleus (MRN). In the human, the DRN is a large group of neurons embedded in the ventral part of the central gray matter of the caudal mesencephalon and rostral pons. Based on topographic and cytoarchitectonic characteristics in Nissl-stained material, the DRN has been subdivided into distinct subnuclei (Baker et al., 1990). These subdivisions correspond to those observed in tissue immunoreacted with an antibody for tryptophan hydroxylase

(Törk and Hornung, 1990; Törk, 1990). The subnuclei are median (or interfascicular), ventrolateral, dorsal, lateral and caudal (Fig. 6). At present, it is not possible to verify the cortical targets of the various DRN nuclear subdivisions in the human. The projection from the DRN to cortical targets in the monkey exhibits a coarse rostro-caudal topographic relationship, as opposed to the median raphe nucleus projections which are not separated rostrocaudally (Wilson and Molliver, 1991b). The serotonergic projection to the prefrontal cortex has a very heavy component arising from cells in the rostral part of the DRN. Regarding cortical innervation in the primate, the density is highest in layer 1, except in sensory areas where the highest density is in layer IV. The serotonergic target cells in the cortex are mostly GAD-IR indicating that they are GABAergic, inhibitory neurons.

The finding of reduced serotonin transporter binding in the prefrontal cortex of suicide victims and depressed individuals raises the possibility that there is reduced serotonergic innervation to the prefrontal cortex. The functional impact of serotonergic neurons may be reduced because of less serotonin release or inadequate innervation of the target brain region reflected in a reduction in the number of serotonin transporter sites synthesized or fewer target cortical neurons. Using immunocytochemistry, we have estimated the total number and the morphometric characteristics of serotonergic neurons in the dorsal raphe nucleus (DRN) from suicide victims and a group of nonpsychiatric controls (Underwood et al., 1999). Neuron counting (and morphometry) was performed every 1000 μm throughout the rostrocaudal extent of the DRN. The distributions were examined with respect to distance from the trochlear decussation, an anatomical landmark which could be located in each case and was therefore suitable as a zero reference point.

Using a morphometric analysis, we found that suicide victims had a 35% greater density and number of serotonin neurons in the dorsal raphe nucleus compared to nonsuicide controls (Fig. 7). The total volume of the DRN did not differ in the two groups suggesting that there is a difference in the absolute number in DRN neurons because we sampled a comparable volume of DRN. We do not find any difference in neuron size or shape between groups. Finding an increase in the number and density of DRN neurons in suicide victims was the opposite of what we had predicted. On the basis of CSF and brainstem neurochemical findings (see above), we had hypothesized that reduced serotonergic activity would be associated with fewer serotonergic neurons in the DRN.

One possible explanation of the increased number of 5-HT neurons in suicide victims is abnormal neuro-development. In our study, suicide victims had a greater density of DRN 5-HT neurons across the lifespan with each group having a similar trend for an age-related rate of decline. The observation of a greater density of 5-HT neurons in the suicide group, in our youngest cases, further raises the possibility that there are greater numbers of serotonin neurons even at a young age in suicide victims. An increased number of neurons may represent a biological predisposition to suicide risk. Why there may be more neurons is unclear as serotonin function seems to be impaired as indicated by less brainstem 5-HT or 5-HIAA in suicide victims and less CSF 5-HIAA in patients surviving serious suicide attempts.

Let it be noted for posterity that, at present, many neuroanatomy journals require quantitation, particularly where group comparisons are made. Were Cajal making his observations today, perhaps many of his important findings would not be published.

SERT binding and SERT mRNA in serotonergic DRN neurons

Another potential cause for fewer SERT sites in the prefrontal cortex, and elsewhere, would be less SERT gene expression in the brainstem serotonergic neurons. Since SERT sites serve to provide reuptake of serotonin from the extracellular space back up into the neuron, they are the exclusive domain of the serotonergic neuron. SERT mRNA is therefore expressed in 5-HT neurons, the largest collection of which is in the brainstem. In rodents, nonhuman primates, and presumably humans, it is the dorsal and median raphe nuclei that provide the serotonergic innervation of the entire forebrain (Bobillier et al., 1975; Wilson and Molliver, 1991a,b).

We have examined controls and depressed suicide victims to determine whether: (1) SERT binding is reduced in the dorsal raphe nucleus; (2) alterations in SERT sites are associated with altered expression of SERT mRNA; and (3) whether 5-HT$_{1A}$ autoreceptor binding is altered in the DRN (Arango et al., 2001a).

The DRN (and MRN) are enriched with SERT sites. In addition, SERT sites are located on serotonergic axon

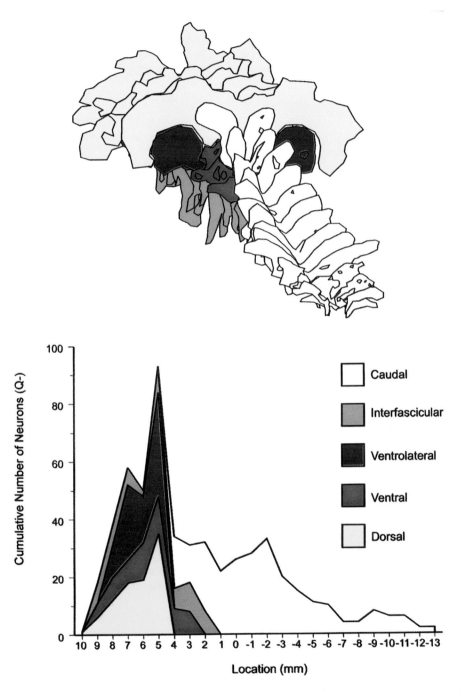

Fig. 6. Three-dimensional reconstruction of the dorsal raphe nucleus (DRN, upper) and the distribution of neurons in DRN subnuclei (lower). The DRN is comprised of component subnuclei and was reconstructed from serial sections with nuclei contours entered using a computerized pointing device and motorized microscope stage. The rostrocaudal distribution of the cumulative number of DRN neurons from each of the subnuclei from a representative case is represented in the lower panel.

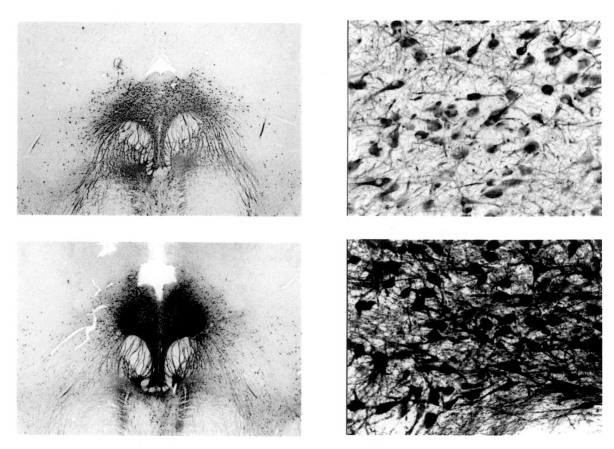

Fig. 7. Low magnification (left) and higher magnification (right) photomicrographs of brainstem sections at a rostral level of the dorsal raphe nucleus (DRN) from a representative control (upper left, upper right; 19 year old white male) and suicide victim (lower left, lower right; 15-year-old white male). Serotonin synthesizing neurons were labeled with an antibody reacting with tryptophan hydroxylase. The high power photographs were taken in the ventrolateral subnucleus of the DRN.

terminals and along serotonergic axons in nearby regions innervated by these neurons. Hence, SERT binding in the area of the raphe extends well beyond the vicinity of 5-HT cell bodies. Adjacent sections stained for Nissl substance with thionin and autoradiography of the 5-HT$_{1A}$ receptor were used to define the DRN, because there is a high degree of correspondence between the raphe as defined immunocytochemically for serotonin's synthetic enzyme tryptophan hydroxylase (PH8, Törk and Hornung, 1990) and the localization of the 5-HT$_{1A}$ receptor as defined with [^{3}H] 8-OH-DPAT autoradiography. We coined the term *"Binding Capacity"* as a novel index of the total amount of receptors in the region of interest. Data expressed in this way resemble data reported from "regions of interest" from *in vivo* imaging studies, combining both the concentration of the receptors

and the volume in which the receptors are being sampled (Arango et al., 2001a).

Doing a simple densitometric analysis of the autoradiographic images showed no differences between groups. However, when the data were analyzed using the concept of *Binding Capacity*, which we defined as total amount of binding (or mRNA) × volume of the DRN, the depressed suicide group had significantly less binding compared with the normal controls. Furthermore, when the *in situ* autoradiograms were analyzed in emulsion-coated slides using a microscope, there were 54% fewer SERT mRNA expressing neurons observed in the DRN of suicide victims compared with normal controls. We compared the characteristics of the neurons that did express the SERT gene in the two groups. SERT mRNA expression per cell in the suicide group was skewed to the right compared with controls. In suicides, a higher percentage of neurons were in the upper percentiles compared to the control group. There was no difference in the number of SERT mRNA positive neurons between males and females, but females had higher SERT mRNA grain density than males.

Similarly, total 5-HT_{1A} receptor binding in the DRN, designated as binding capacity of $[^3\text{H}]8\text{-OH-DPAT}$, was 43% lower in suicides compared with controls, and in the MRN $[^3\text{H}]8\text{-OH-DPAT}$ binding capacity was 34% lower in the suicides. These results are consistent with the *in vivo* PET finding that 5-HT_{1A} receptor binding potential (using a 5-HT_{1A} antagonist) is reduced 42% in the raphe of depressed subjects with a family history of depression, compared to controls (Drevets et al., 1999). A recent postmortem study reported a 5–30% higher 5-HT_{1A} receptor binding in the DRN of depressed suicides compared with controls (Stockmeier et al., 1998). That study examined the most rostral portion of the DRN, which may account for the different results.

If *Binding Capacity* were also applied to SERT binding, we find less SERT binding capacity in the DRN, but not the MRN of depressed suicides. This result is consistent with the *in vivo* findings of Malison et al., (Malison et al., 1998), who reported less brainstem SERT binding in patients with major depression using SPECT imaging of $[^{123}\text{I}]$ β-CIT.

We found fewer SERT mRNA expressing neurons in the DRN of depressed suicides compared to controls. Within individual sections of tissue (film), SERT mRNA per mg tissue in the DRN did not differ between suicides and controls. A similar result was reported by Little et al. (Little et al., 1997) in that the SERT mRNA levels in specific levels of the dorsal and median raphe nuclei were not different between controls and depressed suicides. However, our microscopic analysis of SERT mRNA *in situ* hybridization revealed that fewer DRN neurons express the SERT mRNA in suicide victims. Remarkably, in the subpopulation of serotonergic neurons that did express the serotonin transporter gene within the suicide group, there was evidence of elevated expression relative to the controls.

In light of our report that suicides do not have fewer, but more, tryptophan hydroxylase containing neurons in the DRN compared to controls (Underwood et al., 1999), the question arises why there are fewer SERT mRNA containing neurons if both SERT mRNA and tryptophan hydroxylase are located in the same neurons.

Mechanistically, the biosynthetic enzyme tryptophan hydroxylase and the mRNA for the SERT are functionally related, yet distinct. One possibility is that increasing the amount of the biosynthetic enzyme, reducing the amount of SERT mRNA, and reducing the amount of 5-HT_{1A} inhibitory autoreceptors are homeostatic mechanisms consistent with our overall hypothesis of a serotonergic deficit. There are two possible interpretations of these results. The first is that reduced serotonergic function or release in suicide victims and lower CSF 5-HIAA in the CSF of suicide attempters and depressed patients (Mann et al., 1996b), leads to a compensatory reduction in expression of the gene for the serotonin transporter, resulting in fewer transporter sites and an amplification of the effect of serotonin release by reduced reuptake. An alternative explanation is that the failure of expression of the transporter gene represents a broader failure of expression of key serotonergic genes, related to the dysfunction in the serotonin system that underlies the predisposition to suicidal behavior or to mood disorders. Future studies should examine the regulation of gene expression of other genes in the serotonergic neurons and whether there is a more general impairment of expression of serotonin-related genes. Separate analysis of suicide victims without a major depressive episode and depressed patients dying from causes other than suicide is required to determine whether the observed effects are associated with depression or suicide.

Neuron density in ventral prefrontal cortex

As a birthday present to Cajal, we include in this chapter preliminary observations we have made in the cerebral cortex (Arango et al., 2001b). Possible cytoarchitectonic alterations may explain the changes in receptor binding we have observed in the ventral PFC in suicide. We used 3-D unbiased stereology to estimate the density of neurons in the same areas of orbital prefrontal cortex (Brodmann area 45) where the receptor binding was measured (Arango et al., 2001b). Combining receptor binding and neuron density, we calculated an index of receptor binding per neuron: (fmol/mg tissue)/(neurons/mm^3). We have found neuron density is lower in suicides. Consistent with our previous observations, binding to the 5-HT transporter is lower in the suicide group. However, since binding and neuron density are both reduced, SERT binding per neuron is not different.

Postsynaptic 5-HT$_{1A}$ binding (^{3}H-8-0H-DPAT) is 27% higher in the suicide group, making the binding per neuron over 50% higher compared to controls. 5-HT$_{2A}$ binding (^{3}H-Ketanserin) is not different between groups, but the 5-HT$_{2A}$ binding per neuron is also higher in the suicide group, consistent with some previous reports.

We believe this is the first report of decreased neuronal density in the orbital cortex of suicide victims, most of whom were depressed. It appears that suicide victims have decreased serotonergic innervation from the brainstem raphe nuclei, but due to the lower neuronal density, the binding per neuron is statistically comparable to controls. Higher postsynaptic 5-HT$_{1A}$ and 5-HT$_{2A}$ binding per neuron in ventral prefrontal cortex in suicides suggests receptor upregulation.

Conclusions

It is hard to know whether Cajal envisioned that psychiatry would finally begin to develop as a scientific field and focus on the brain, its components and connections, in order to unveil many of the mysteries of mental illness. This union began a very short time ago and yet the results are profound and promising. Today's informed psychiatrist will not be able to deny the role of the brain in the mental ailments of his/her patients.

Acknowledgments

This work was supported by PHS grants MH40210, MH62185, AA09004, AA11293, the American Foundation for Suicide Prevention, the Stanley Foundation, the Diane Goldberg Foundation and the National Alliance for Research in Schizophrenia and Affective Disorders. We thank the families who participated in our studies and the staff from the Coroner's Office of Allegheny County and the New York City Medical Examiner's Office. Drs. Andrew J. Dwork, Thomas Kelly, Sara Oppenheim and Maura Boldrini contributed with neuropathology, psychological autopsies and brainstem analysis. Victor V. Arkhipov, Mihran J. Bakalian, Suham A. Kasssir, Yung-yu Huang, Virginia L. Johnson, Zachariah Mathai, Renata Kouchner, Alfia Khaibulina, Andrew Moran and Emily Le provided expert technical help.

This work is dedicated to the thousands of victims of the terrorist attack to the World Trade Center in New York City, which occurred while the authors were still writing this chapter.

References

Arango, V. and Mann, J.J. (1992) Relevance of serotonergic post-mortem studies to suicidal behavior. *Int. Rev. Psychiatry*, 4: 131–140.

Arango, V. and Underwood, M.D. (1997) Serotonin Chemistry in the brain of suicide victims. In: R. Maris, M. Silverman and S. Canetto (Eds.), *Review of Suicidology*, First. [9] Guilford Press, New York, pp. 237–250.

Arango, V., Underwood, M.D., Boldrini, M., Tamir, H., Kassir, S.A., Hsiung, S., Chen, J.-X. and Mann, J.J. (2001a) Serotonin 1A receptors, serotonin transporter binding and serotonin transporter mRNA expression in the brainstem of depressed suicide victims. *Neuropsychopharmacology*, 25(6): 892–903.

Arango, V., Underwood, M.D., Gubbi, A.V. and Mann, J.J. (1995) Localized alterations in pre- and postsynaptic serotonin binding sites in the ventrolateral prefrontal cortex of suicide victims. *Brain Res.*, 688(1,2): 121–133.

Arango, V., Underwood, M.D., Le, E., Johnson, V.L., Kassir, S.A. and Mann, J.J. (2001b) Suicide victims have lower neuronal density, decreased 5-HT innervation and higher 5-HT$_{1A}$ and 5-HT$_{2A}$ receptor binding per neuron than controls in orbital prefrontal cortex. *ACNP 40th Annual Meeting* .

Baker, K.G., Halliday, G.M. and Törk, I. (1990) Cytoarchitecture of the human dorsal raphe nucleus. *J. Comp. Neurol.*, 301: 147–161.

Bobillier, P., Petitjean, F., Salvert, D., Ligier, M. and Seguin, S. (1975) Differential projections of the nucleus raphe dorsalis and nucleus raphe centralis as revealed by autoradiography. *Brain Res.*, 85: 205–210.

Damasio, H., Grabowski, T., Frank, R., Galaburda, A.M. and Damasio, A.R. (1994) The return of Phineas Gage: Clues about the brain from the skull of a famous patient. *Science*, 264: 1102–1105.

Drevets, W.C., Frank, E., Price, J.C., Kupfer, D.J., Holt, D., Greer, P.J., Huang, Y., Gautier, C. and Mathis, C. (1999) PET imaging of serotonin 1A receptor binding in depression. *Biol. Psychiatry*, 46: 1375–1387.

Flory, J.D., Mann, J.J., Manuck, S.B. and Muldoon, M.F. (1998) Recovery from major depression is not associated with normalization of serotonergic function. *Biol. Psychiatry*, 43: 320–326.

Kelly, T.M. and Mann, J.J. (1996) Validity of DSM-III-R diagnosis by psychological autopsy: a comparison with antemortem diagnosis. *Acta Psychiatr. Scand.*, 94: 337–343.

Kuroda, Y., Watanabe, Y., Albeck, D.S., Hastings, N.B. and McEwen, B.S. (1994) Effects of adrenalectomy and Type I or Type II glucocorticoid receptor activation on 5-HT$_{1A}$ and 5-HT$_2$ receptor binding and 5-HT transporter mRNA expression in rat brain. *Brain Res.*, 648: 157–161.

Laruelle, M., Abi-Dargham, A., Casanova, M.F., Toti, R., Weinberger, D.R. and Kleinman, J.E. (1993) Selective abnormalities of prefrontal serotonergic receptors in schizophrenia: a postmortem study. *Arch. Gen. Psychiatry*, 50(10): 810–818.

Little, K.Y., McLauglin, D.P., Ranc, J., Gilmore, J., Lopez, J.F., Watson, S.J., Carroll, F.I. and Butts, J.D. (1997) Serotonin transporter binding sites and mRNA levels in depressed persons committing suicide. *Biol. Psychiatry*, 41: 1156–1164.

Malison, R.T., Price, L.H., Berman, R., Van Dyck, C.H., Pelton, G.H., Carpenter, L., Sanacora, G., Owens, M.J., Nemeroff, C.B., Rajeevan, N., Baldwin, R.M., Seibyl, J.P., Innis, R.B. and Charney, D.S. (1998) Reduced brain serotonin transporter availability in major depression as measured by [^{123}I]-2b-carbomethoxy-3b-(4-iodophenyl)tropane and single photon emission computer tomography. *Biol. Psychiatry*, 44: 1090–1098.

Mann, J.J. (1998) The neurobiology of suicide. *Nature Med.*, 4(1): 25–30.

Mann, J.J., Arango, V., Marzuk, P.M., Theccanat, S. and Reis, D.J. (1989) Evidence for the 5-HT hypothesis of suicide: a review of post-mortem studies. *Br. J. Psychiatry*, 155 (Suppl. 8): 7–14.

Mann, J.J., Henteleff, R.A., Lagattuta, T.F., Perper, J.A., Li, S. and Arango, V. (1996a) Lower ^{3}H-paroxetine binding in cerebral cortex of suicide victims is partly due to fewer high-affinity, nontransporter sites. *J. Neural. Transm.*, 103: 1337–1350.

Mann, J.J., Huang, Y., Underwood, M.D., Kassir, S.A., Oppenheim, S., Kelly, T.M., Dwork, A.J. and Arango, V. (2000) A serotonin transporter gene promoter polymorphism (5-HTTLPR) and prefrontal cortical binding in major depression and suicide. *Arch. Gen. Psychiatry*, 57(8): 729–738.

Mann, J.J., Malone, K.M., Diehl, D.J., Perel, J., Cooper, T.B. and Mintun, M.A. (1996b) Demonstration *in vivo* of reduced serotonin responsivity in the brain of untreated depressed patients. *Am. J. Psychiatry*, 153(2): 174–182.

Mann, J.J., McBride, P.A., Brown, R.P., Linnoila, M., Leon, A.C., DeMeo, M.D., Mieczkowski, T.A., Myers, J.E. and Stanley, M. (1992) Relationship between central and peripheral serotonin indexes in depressed and suicidal psychiatric inpatients. *Arch. Gen. Psychiatry*, 49(6): 442–446.

Owens, M.J. and Nemeroff, C.B. (1994) Role of serotonin in the pathophysiology of depression: focus on the serotonin transporter. *Clin. Chem.*, 40(2): 288–295.

Parsey, R.V., Arango, V., Simpson, N., Huang, Y., Dwork, A.J., Laruelle, M., Underwood, M.D. and Mann, J.J. (2000) Serotonin transporter changes associated with major depression and suicide. *ACNP 39th Annual Meeting, San Juan, Puerto Rico*, 300.

Perry, E.K., Marshall, E.F., Blessed, G., Tomlinson, B.E. and Perry, R.H. (1983) Decreased imipramine binding in the brains of patients with depressive illness. *Br. J. Psychiatry*, 142: 188–192.

Shallice, T. and Burgess, P. (1996) The domain of supervisory processes and temporal organization of behaviour. *Phil. Trans. R.Soc. Lond.*, 351(1346): 1405–1412.

Stockmeier, C.A., Shapiro, L.A., Dilley, G.E., Kolli, T.M., Friedman, L. and Rajkowska, G. (1998) Increase in serotonin-1A autoreceptors in the midbrain of suicide victims with major depression—Postmortem evidence for decrease serotonin activity. *J. Neurosci.*, 18(18): 7394–7401.

Stoff, D.M. and Mann, J.J. (1997) The Neurobiology of Suicide. From the Bench to the Clinic. Stoff, D.M. and Mann, J.J. *Ann. N.Y. Acad. Sci.* (836), 1–365. New York, The New York Academy of Sciences.

Törk, I. (1990) Anatomy of the serotonergic system. *Ann. N.Y. Acad. Sci.*, 600: 9–35.

Törk, I. and Hornung, J.-P. (1990) Raphe nuclei and the serotonergic system. In: G. Paxinos (Ed.), *The Human Nervous System*. [30] Academic Press, San Diego, pp. 1001–1022.

Underwood, M.D., Khaibulina, A.A., Ellis, S.P., Moran, A., Rice, P.M., Mann, J.J. and Arango, V. (1999) Morphometry of the dorsal raphe nucleus serotonergic neurons in suicide victims. *Biol. Psychiatry*, 46(4): 473–483.

Willeit, M., Praschak-Rieder, N., Neumeister, A., Pirker, W., Asenbaum, S., Vitouch, O., Tauscher, J., Hilger, E., Stastny, J., Brücke, T. and Kasper, S. (2000) [123I]-beta-CIT SPECT imaging shows reduced brain serotonin transporter availability in drug-free depressed patients with seasonal affective disorder. *Biol. Psychiatry*, 47(6): 482–489.

Wilson, M.A. and Molliver, M.E. (1991a) The organization of serotonergic projections to cerebral cortex in primates: regional distribution of axon terminals. *Neuroscience*, 44: 537–553.

Wilson, M.A. and Molliver, M.E. (1991b) The organization of serotonergic projections to cerebral cortex in primates: retrograde transport studies. *Neuroscience*, 44: 555–570.

E.C. Azmitia, J. DeFelipe, E.G. Jones, P. Rakic and C.E. Ribak (Eds.)
Progress in Brain Research, Vol. 136

CHAPTER 36

Structural changes in the normally aging cerebral cortex of primates

Alan Peters*

Department of Anatomy and Neurobiology, Boston University School of Medicine, 715 Albany Street, Boston, MA 02118-2526, USA

Abstract: During normal aging humans exhibit some cognitive decline, but it is difficult to determine the underlying causes of this decline, because information about cognitive status is rarely available and preservation of the brain is usually inadequate for detailed cytological examination. One solution to this problem is to use a nonhuman primate model, such as the rhesus monkey, which exhibits age-related cognitive decline similar to humans, and can be cognitively tested before the brains are preserved for detailed examination. It is now known that cognitive decline in human and nonhuman primates is not due to loss of cortical neurons and there is no correlation between the frequency of senile plaques and cognitive status. Indeed apart from layer 1, neurons of cerebral cortex show few signs of aging, although there may be some loss of synapses throughout cortex. In contrast, both microglia and astrocytes come to contain phagocytosed material, but its origin is unknown. There is also loss of white matter, which is accompanied by some breakdown of myelin sheaths and alterations in oligodendrocytes. It is suggested that the myelin changes alter conduction velocities along axons. This would alter timing in neuronal circuits, contributing to cognitive decline.

Introduction

Santiago Ramón y Cajal's basic interests were in the circuitry and function of the mature nervous system and in the dynamics of development. He knew that lipofuscin in neurons increases with age (Cajal, 1911), and he was aware of Alzheimer's (1906, 1907) account of the presence of neurofibrillary tangles and senile plaques in the brains of senile humans. But Cajal had little to say about the neurofibrillary tangles which had been demonstrated by Bielschowsky and Brodmann, using silver staining (Cajal, 1911), although he did have some comments about senile plaques. Thus, at the end of volume II of "Degeneration and Regeneration of the Nervous System" there is a discussion of the meaning of senile plaques (plates), which had been first recognized by Marinesco in

1898, and later described in more detail by Fischer (1907), Beilschowsky (1911) and Lafora (1914), using silver staining. However, Cajal's interest in senile plaques was not in terms of their role in dementia. He was more interested in the possibility that plaques are regenerative, and occupied by colonies of newly growing nerve fibers (Cajal, 1928). In more recent years, of course, the structure and distribution of senile plaques and neurofibrillary tangles and their relationship with dementia have been the focus of a great deal of research, so far with little success in curing, or halting the progress of Alzheimer's disease.

Our interest is in the effects of normal aging on the brain, and this is a field of research with a very recent history, because it is only in the past 15 years or so that the pitfalls that can affect these studies have been realized. And although studies of the normally aging brain have taken second place to studies of dementia, an understanding of the effects of age on the normally aging brain is important if we are to counteract the cognitive

---
*Corresponding author: Tel.: 617 638 4235; Fax: 617 638 4216;
E-mail: apeters@cajal-1.bu.edu

456

decline that accompanies normal aging. This becomes urgent because the number of aging individuals in our society is gradually increasing, and many more individuals age normally than become demented. It is also important to realize that the alterations that occur as a consequence of normal aging are the canvas upon which the changes produced by dementia are superimposed, making it increasingly necessary to understand the nature of the alterations that occur in normal aging, and to differentiate them from the changes that bring about dementia.

Neuron counts in the human cerebral cortex

As far as humans and the cerebral cortex are concerned, the first studies of the effects of normal aging were carried out by Brody (1950, 1970). He examined the cortices of humans between the ages of 19 and 95 and based on cell counts he concluded that there is a progressive reduction of between 29 and 50% in neuronal density with age. Over the next fifteen years or so, Brody's studies were followed by those of others (see Peters et al., 1998; Peters, 1999) who basically reached the same conclusion, leading to a general and popular acceptance that there is a loss of cortical neurons with age and that this is the basis of the forgetfulness shown by many older individuals. That this may be an erroneous conclusion was not seriously considered until the studies of Haug and his colleagues (e.g. Haug, 1984, 1985; Haug et al., 1984) and of Terry et al. (1987). Haug and his colleagues concluded that the reported neuronal losses with age were due to the fact that during processing, tissue from younger individuals shrinks more than that from older individuals, in which the tissue is probably stabilized by the increase in myelin. The consequence was that when cell counts were made on tissue sections the neuronal density was higher in young than in old cortices. After corrections had been made to compensate for this shrinkage, Haug and his colleagues concluded that there is no significant loss of neurons from the human cerebral cortex with age. Terry et al. (1987) found that neuronal density does not change with age, but because they encountered a slight thinning of cortex they concluded that there might be some overall neuronal loss, but of a magnitude much less that that reported by previous investigators. Terry et al. (1987) also suggested that some of the earlier studies reporting significant

neuronal losses with age in humans might have reached that conclusion because brains of some early stage Alzheimer patients were included in the material being studied. In Alzheimer's disease there is a significant loss of neurons.

Almost coincidental with the awareness that it is important to ensure brains of Alzheimer's patients are not included in studies of normal brain aging, Gundersen (Sterio, 1984) and his colleagues caused a stir in the scientific community by introducing the new, so-called, unbiased methods for estimating volume and cell numbers. This led to a re-evaluation of how neuronal counts are made. The consequence is that there is mounting evidence that while there may (e.g. Pakkenberg and Gundersen 1997), or may not (e.g., Leuba and Kraftsik, 1994b Gómez-Isla et al., 1997) be some loss of cortical neurons during normal aging (see Peters et al, 1998), any loss is at most not more than a few percent.: nowhere as great as the loss that occurs in the brains of Alzheimer's patients (e.g. Terry and Hansen, 1988; Leuba and Kraftsik, 1994a; Gómez-Isla, et al., 1997).

The cerebral cortex of the monkey

Other problems in dealing with the effects of normal aging on the human brain are that the cognitive status of the individuals from whom the brains are obtained is not usually known and the preservation of the brains is rarely of good quality. This led to a search for a model system in which such problems could be avoided and one obvious choice is to study the effects of normal aging using the brain of a nonhuman primate such as the rhesus monkey. Rhesus monkeys live to about 30 years of age and if they are from a primate colony their life histories are well documented and their cognitive status can be assessed. Like humans, rhesus monkeys exhibit cognitive decline as they age (e.g. Killiany et al., 2000), and although their brains can accumulate some senile plaques after about 25 years of age, the frequency of these plaques is usually low and does not correlate with the cognitive dysfunction observed in elderly monkeys (Sloane et al., 1997). But unlike humans, monkeys do not get neurofibrillary tangles and they show no signs of Alzheimer type dementia. Most importantly, after the cognitive status of a monkey has been determined the brain can be well preserved, so that correlations can be made between age, cognitive status and structural changes.

The first studies of the effects of age on neuronal numbers in the cortices of monkeys were made by Brizzee and his colleagues (e.g. Brizzee, 1973; Brizzee et al., 1975) and as with the early human studies, they concluded that there is a loss of neurons with age. No other studies were carried out until 1989, when Vincent et al. (1989) examined the effects of age on primary visual cortex and concluded that there is no significant age-related loss of neurons from this cortical area. Other studies of the effects of age on primary visual cortex (e.g., Peters and Sethares, 1993; Kim et al., 1997; Hof et al., 2000) have come to the same conclusion, as have studies of the effects of age on motor (Tigges et al., 1990), prefrontal (Peters et al., 1994) cortices, and entorhinal and hippocampal cortices (Amaral, 1993; Rosene, 1993; Gazzaley et al., 1997; Merrill et al., 2000) of the monkey. And apart from neurons such as the Betz cells in motor cortex, few neurons in the cerebral cortex of old monkeys even show extensive accumulations of lipofuscin. One point of interest, however, is that in the monkey age pigment becomes more prominent in the cell bodies of nonpyramidal neurons than in pyramidal neurons, which might indicate that inhibitory neurons are more affected by age than excitatory ones.

Dendrites and spines

If cognitive decline in normal aging cannot be attributed to a significant loss of cortical neurons, can it be due to the effects of age on the processes of the neurons? At present the data are sparse, since only few useful studies have been carried out on primates. Cupp and Uemura (1980) examined Golgi impregnated preparations from the prefrontal gyrus of rhesus monkey and concluded that with age entire branches or segments are lost from the apical dendritic tufts of pyramidal cells, while Uemura (1980) counted the visible spines on dendrites and concluded that with age some 25% of dendritic spines are lost. Similar results have been obtained by Jacobs et al. (1997) in Golgi impregnation studies of the effects of age on the basal dendritic trees of pyramidal neurons in areas 10 and 18 of human cortex. They found the decrease in spine numbers to be almost as great as 50%. Results consistent with these have been obtained in our studies of the effects of age on layer 1 in areas 46 (Peters et al., 1998) and 17 (Peters et al., 2001a) of

rhesus monkey cortex. In both these areas there are obvious age-related changes in layer 1. In brains from old monkeys the profiles of dendrites of layer 1 show swelling and the layer becomes thinner. Primarily these changes appear to be due to a loss of branches from the apical tufts of pyramidal cells that occupy layer 1, and this is accompanied by a loss of dendritic spines and their synapsing axon terminals, so that compared to young monkeys the numerical density of synapses in old monkeys is reduced by between 30 and 60%. The reason for these layer 1 changes is not known, but they are accompanied by a thickening of the glial limiting membrane, and by hypertrophy of the astrocytes. There is also some degeneration of layer 1 neurons, although the number of neurons lost appears to be minimal (unpublished data).

In both areas 17 and 46, there is a correlation between the thinning of layer 1 and age, and in area 46 there is also a correlation between impairment in cognition, and both the thinning of the layer and the decrease in the numerical density of synapses. In contrast, in area 17 there is no correlation between cognitive decline and either the thinning of layer 1, or the numerical density of its synapses. It is suggested that this difference between the two cortical areas might reflect the fact that prefrontal cortex has a greater role than primary visual cortex in subserving cognition.

Since Golgi studies indicate that there is an age-related loss of dendritic spines throughout the primate cortex, and these are the main receptors for synapsing axon terminals, it is reasonable to assume that with age there is a loss of some of the synaptic input to cortical neurons. However, the origins of the presynaptic components of the lost synapses, and whether the inhibitory inputs are more affected than the excitatory ones are not known. But if there is a severe loss of synapses it can be expected to affect the response properties of cortical neurons, and indications of this come from studies such as the recent one by Schmolesky et al. (2000). These investigators compared the stimulus selectivity of neurons in primary visual cortex of young and old monkeys and found a significant degradation of orientation and direction selectivity in old monkeys. It is of interest that in a comprehensive study done on the rat, in which whole cell patch clamp recordings were combined with morphological analyses of layer 5 pyramidal neurons, Wong et al. (2000) found that although neurons lost basal dendritic branches and spines with age, the neurons compensated for this loss, so that they showed no dramatic loss of spontaneous activity with age.

Astrocytes and microglia

When sections of cerebral cortex are examined, the most obvious difference between young and old cortices is seen not in the neurons, but in the neuroglial cells. With age each of the three neuroglial cell types accumulate inclusions in their cell bodies, and in electron micrographs it is obvious that the inclusions are characteristic for each cell type (Peters et al., 1991). The astrocytes and microglial cells probably acquire their inclusions by phagocytosis, and in both of them some inclusions are electron dense and patchy, so that they contain dense granular material intermixed with paler areas. Other inclusions consist of a mainly pale, often flocculent material that has the appearance of lipids. However, the inclusions in the microglial cells, which are usually considered to be the primary phagocytes, are more diverse in structure and can be much larger than those in astrocytes. Indeed some of the microglial cell inclusions are so large that they are surrounded by only a thin rim of cytoplasm, with the microglial cell nucleus pushed to one side.

Counts indicate that in the cortex astrocytes account for about 50% of the total population of glial cell body profiles that contain nuclei, and that their numbers do not increase with age (Peters et al., 1991). However, astrocytes do hypertrophy, leading to an increased number of processes that also become thicker and contain more prominent bundles of filaments. An example of this is seen in the age-related thickening of the glial limiting membrane. In addition, some of the processes of astrocytes in old monkeys swell and become filled with a flocculent material, so that they resemble corpora amylacea.

Although microglia only account for 7.6% of the neuroglial cell profiles in young monkeys, as they become activated and phagocytic, their numbers increase significantly to about 9.4% in the cortices of older monkeys. But as will be considered later, the increase in numbers of activated microglia is most obvious in white matter (e.g., Sloane et al., 1999).

What is being phagocytozed by the astrocytes and microglia as the cortex ages is not known, but presumably the phagocytozed material is derived from the breakdown of components of neurons and their sheaths.

Oligodendrocytes

Oligodendrocytes also show changes with age (Peters et al., 1991; Peters, 1996). They develop bulbous processes that are filled with characteristic inclusions resembling lipofuscin, and similar inclusions also accumulate in the cell bodies (Figs. 1 and 3). In addition, whereas the oligodendrocytes in young monkeys generally occur singly, in old monkeys it is common to find oligodendrocytes in groups and rows (Figs. 2 and 4). This suggests that some of these cells, or their precursors, have undergone division to generate clones of oligodendrocytes, as has been shown to occur in adult rat neocortex (Levison et al., 1999). Indeed, in recent years there has been an increasing awareness of the existence of oligodendritic precursors in the mature brain. The precursors become especially evident when the nervous system is damaged, since this causes them to become activated and to proliferate (see Levine et al., 2001). Since the main role of oligodendrocytes in the central nervous system is to produce myelin, these observations raise the question of what happens to myelin with age that necessitates additional oligodendrocytes.

Myelin sheath alterations

As we have shown in the vertical bundles of myelinated fibers that pass through primary visual cortex of the monkey (Peters et al., 2000), myelin is significantly altered by age and the alterations can be categorized as being of four basic kinds. The most common alteration is a splitting of sheaths at the major dense line to accommodate dense cytoplasm that is derived from the oligodendrocytes (Fig. 5). The dense cytoplasm can occupy several splits in the sheaths, so it can be quite voluminous, in which case it is not uncommon to find lysosomes and vacuoles within the dense cytoplasm (Fig. 5: N_4). A less common, but more dramatic alteration, is one in which a myelin sheath splits at the intraperiod line and balloons out to produce an almost spherical, fluid-filled blister, or balloon (Feldman and Peters, 1998). Such myelin balloons can be as large as 10 μm in diameter, about the same size as the cell body of a neuron. Other age-related alterations are the formation of sheaths composed of redundant myelin, such that the sheath is much too large for the enclosed axon, and the formation of splits within thick sheaths. These splits can be so extensive that they give the spurious appearance of a double sheath, in which

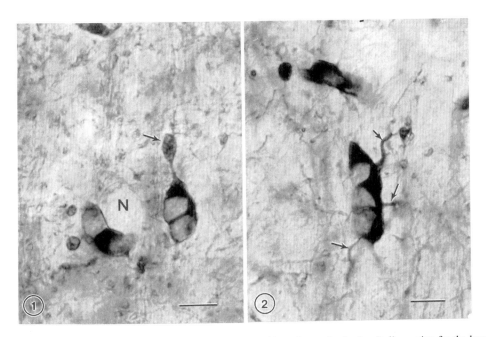

Figs. 1. and 2. Preparation of area 17 of cerebral cortex from a 29 year old monkey stained using Perl's reaction for the location of iron-containing compounds. This reaction is a useful light microscope stain for oligodendrocytes. Differential interference light microscopy. Scale bars = 10 μm.
Fig. 1. This oligodendrocyte in layer 4B has an ascending process that expands into a large bulb (arrow). To the left is another oligodendrocyte that is lying next to a cell body of a neuron (N).
Fig. 2. A row of oligodendrocytes in layer 3. There are three oligodendrocytes in the row and a number of thick processes (arrows) can be seen to extend from them.

an outer set of compact lamellae surrounds, but is separated from, an inner set. Such complete splits become more common with age, as nerve fibers with thick sheaths become more common (Peters et al., 2001b).

In electron micrographs of cross sections through the myelin bundles in monkey primary visual cortex, as many as 5% of the nerve fiber profiles show age-related alterations in the structure of their sheaths and in longitudinal sections several defects can be seen to occur in succession along individual nerve fibers. Thus, these age-related alterations are quite common, but what proportion of the internodal lengths of myelin are affected by these alterations is not known, although it is suspected that most of the internodal lengths along each axon have some alterations in myelin. However, despite these alterations in myelin sheaths in primary visual cortex, there is little evidence for degeneration of nerve fibers in the vertical bundles (Nielsen and Peters, 2000).

These age-related alterations in myelin are probably ubiquitous, because they have been found to occur in other areas of cortex and in the corpus callosum, as well

as white matter in the cerebral hemispheres, and there is a significant correlation between the percentage of myelin sheath profiles affected by age in each location. However, in the optic nerve the age-related myelin alterations are overlain by some degeneration of nerve fibers (Sandell and Peters, 2001). Similar changes may occur throughout white matter, because there is evidence that the volume of white matter in the cerebral hemispheres of both humans and monkeys is reduced with age (e.g. Albert, 1993; Lai et al., 1995; Double et al., 1996).

In monkey primary visual cortex, the frequency of age-related alterations in myelin sheaths correlates not only with age, but also with the impairments in cognition showed by individual monkeys (Peters et al., 2000). And this correlation between impairment in cognition and myelin sheath defect frequency even hold true if only the old monkeys, that are between 25 and 33 years old, are considered as a group. This raises the question of why such a correlation exists, and it is suggested that the correlation occurs because of the role that myelin plays in determining speed of nerve fiber conduction in the brain.

460

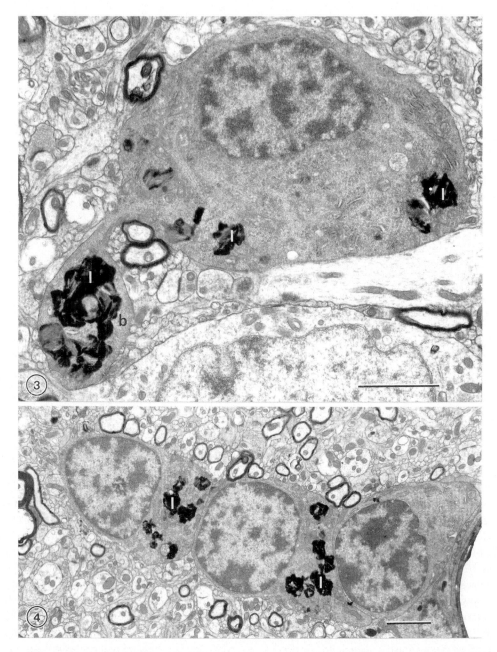

Fig. 3. Electron micrograph of an oligodendrocyte in layer 4B of the primary visual cortex of a 35 year old monkey. The process that extends from the cell body of the oligodendrocyte expands into a bulbous enlargement (b) that contains an irregular dense and laminar inclusion (I). This bulbous enlargement is like the one seen in Fig. 1. There are also similar inclusions (I) in the perikaryon of the oligodendrocyte. Scale bar = 2 μm.

Fig. 4. A row of oligodendrocytes in layer 4B of a 27 year old monkey. Two of the oligodendrocytes have dense inclusions (I) in their perikarya. Scale bar = 2 μm.

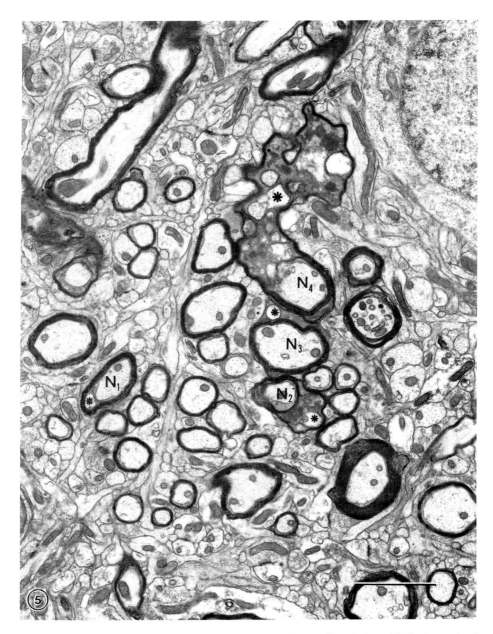

Fig. 5. An electron micrograph of a transversely sectioned bundle of myelinated nerve fibers in layer 4C of primary visual cortex. From a 27 year old monkey. While most of the nerve fibers have sheaths that appear normal, four of them (N_1–N_4) have splits in their sheaths where dense cytoplasm is present (asterisks). In one case (N_4) the splitting is very extensive so that the sheath has expanded out to one side to accommodate a significant amount of dense cytoplasm that contains vesicles and lysosomes. Scale bar = 2 μm.

Conduction velocities and age

While conduction rates along nerve fibers have not yet been compared in young and old monkeys, there is relevant information from studies carried out on cats. Thus, Xi et al. (1999) compared the conduction velocities of axons in the pyramidal tracts of young and old cats and found that overall, old cats show a 43% decrease in median conduction velocity, and that there are some 50% fewer fast conducting fibers than in young cats. Morales et al. (1987) have also shown that there is a decrease in the conduction velocities of lumbar neurons in old cats. Similarly, in rats Aston-Jones et al. (1985) found that the conduction latencies from nucleus basalis to frontal cortex are about 30% slower in old, as compared to young rats. Further, it is known that decreases in conduction rates commonly occur in demyelinating disorders (see Waxman et al., 1995). Consequently, it seems likely that alterations in myelin sheaths in monkeys do cause reductions in conduction velocities.

It is suggested that the reason for the correlation between myelin sheath alterations and cognitive decline is because the age-related reductions in conduction velocities, brought about by alterations in myelin, affect the timing in neuronal circuits. This would appear to affect memory, or the retrieval of stored information.

Speculation

To pursue this thesis further, a number of questions need to be answered. For example, are the age-related myelin alterations an indication that myelin sheaths are degenerating in older primates? It is usually assumed that dark cytoplasm of the type that frequently occurs within the myelin sheaths of old monkeys is a sign of degeneration, especially when the cytoplasm contains lysosomes (see Fig. 5). The source of this dark cytoplasm must be the oligodendrocytes forming those myelin sheaths, because the dark cytoplasm is contained in spaces formed by splits of the major dense line, and it is possible that the altered sheaths are connected to the oligodendrocytes that have swollen processes and contain dense bodies (see Fig. 3). Oligodendrocytes with similar swellings along their processes occur in the twitcher mouse mutant, which is regarded as being a model for globoid cell leukodystrophy, and LeVine and Torres (1992) suggest that oligodendrocytes with these features are degenerating. So far, however, we have seen no oligodendrocytes degenerating, dying, or undergoing apoptosis in the cortices of aging monkeys.

If oligodendrocytes are not degenerating as a consequence of the aging process, why are new oligodendrocytes being generated in the adult animal (e.g. Levison, et al., 1999; Levine et al., 2001)? At present the answer is not known, but it is possible that while oligodendrocytes

are not dying some of them are being affected in a way that causes myelin sheaths to degenerate, leading to some axons being demyelinated. Perhaps the new oligodendrocytes are required to remyelinate the axons that become denuded. On the other hand the newly generated oligodendrocytes may be necessary to carry out some function that has yet to be elucidated (Levine et al., 2001).

If some myelin sheaths are degenerating, we would expect to see microglial cells in the cerebral cortex engulfing the degenerating myelin, as they do in the optic nerve, in which there is frank degeneration of myelin sheaths (Sandell and Peters, 2001). But so far microglial cells with engulfed myelin in their cytoplasm have not been seen in the cortices of old monkeys. It is possible, however, that so few myelin sheaths are degenerating at any one point in time that the microglial cells are not extensively activated, as they are when significant numbers of axons and their myelin sheaths are degenerating simultaneously (e.g. Sandell and Peters, 2001). Nevertheless, with age the numbers of microglial cells that contain phagocytozed material increases, and some of them contain large amounts of debris. Astrocytes also come to contain large amounts of phagocytozed material, and a few of them have been seen to contain myelin figures, so the astrocytes might be the neuroglial cells principally involved in phagocytozing myelin that is degenerating as a consequence of the aging process. It is unfortunate that in general, the phagocytosed material inside microglial cells and astrocytes has such an amorphous appearance that it gives no clue as to its origins.

Obviously there are many questions yet to be answered about what happens to oligodendrocytes and myelin sheaths as a consequence of normal aging in the cerebral cortex.

Interestingly, what happens in white matter with aging might be somewhat different from the effects of aging on nerve fibers passing through gray matter. Thus, there is evidence from MRI scans of both humans (e.g., Albert, 1993; Double et al., 1996) and monkeys (Lai et al., 1995) that white matter is lost from the cerebral hemispheres with age. Using stereology Pakkenberg and Gundersen (1997) have also shown that there is a decrease in the volume of white matter from the human brain with age. This is corroborated by Tang et al. (1997), who have demonstrated that there is a significant age-related decrease in the total length of nerve fibers in the white matter of human cerebral hemispheres, and that the decrease is largely due to a loss of small diameter nerve fibers. Concomitant with these alterations there is significantly increased microglial activation in the white matter of the hemispheres in aging monkeys (Sheffield and Berman, 1998; Sloane et al., 1999). Taken together, these data suggest that in white matter not only is there an age-related breakdown of myelin, but there is a loss, and therefore a degeneration of nerve fibers. This would cause microglial cells to become activated to phagocytoze the degenerating axons and their myelin sheaths, as occurs in the optic nerve (Sandell and Peters, 2001).

Conclusion

Obviously, there is much more to be learned about the effects of normal aging on the neurons and neuroglial cells of the primate cerebral cortex, and how age-related changes in these cells and their processes may affect cognition. But based upon the morphological studies that have been carried out thus far, one promising lead to follow is to learn more about the age-related alterations that affect myelinated nerve fibers. There seems little doubt that nerve fibers are lost from white matter, but nothing is known about what brings about this loss and which neurons are losing axons or branches of axons. In grey matter the loss of nerve fibers may be less marked, but the age-related changes in myelin appear to be ubiquitous. We do not know what brings about these changes in myelin, how they affect the functioning of neuronal circuits, and whether there is a continuous breakdown and renewal of myelin sheaths with age but, hopefully, answers will emerge as research on normal aging in primates continues.

Acknowledgments

Supported by NIH grant P01 AG 00001 from the National Institute on Aging.

References

Albert, M. (1993) Neuropsychological and neurophysiological changes in healthy humans across the age range. *Neurobiol. Aging*, 14: 623–625.

Alzheimer, A (1906) Über einen eigenartigen schweren Krankheitsprozess der Hirnrinde. *Neurologisches Centalblatt*, 25: 1134.

Alzheimer, A. (1907) Über eine eigenartigen schweren Krankheitsprozess der Hirnrinde. *Centrablatt für Nervenheilkunde und Psychiatrie*, 30: 177–179.

Amaral, D.G. (1993) Morphological analysis of the brains of behaviorally characterized aged nonhuman primates. *Neurobiol. Aging*, 14: 671–672.

Aston-Jones, G., Rogers, J., Shaver, R.D., Dinan, T.G. and Moss, D.E. (1985) Age-impaired impulse flow from nucleus basalis to cortex. *Nature*, 318: 462–464.

Bielschowsky, M. (1911) Zur Kennitniss der Alzheimerschen Krankheit (präsenile Demenz mit Herdsymtomen). *J. Psychol. Neurol.*, 18: 273–292.

Brizzee, K.R. (1973) Quantitative studies on aging changes in cerebral cortex of rhesus monkeys and albino rat, with notes on effects of prolonged low-dose radiation in the rat. *Progr. Brain Res.*, 40: 141–160.

Brizzee, K.R., Klara, P. and Johnson, J. (1975) Changes in microanatomy and fine structure with aging. In: J.M. Ordy and K.R. Brizzee, (Eds.), *Neurobiology of Aging*, Plenum Press, New York, pp. 574–594.

Brody, H.D. (1950) Organization of the cerebral cortex III. A study of aging in the human cerebral cortex. *J. Comp. Neurol.*, 102: 511–556.

Brody, H.D. (1970) Structural changes in the aging nervous system. *Interdisc. Top. Gerentol.*, 7: 9–21.

Cajal, S.R. (1911) *Histologie du système nerveuse de l'homme et des vertébrés*. Translated by L. Azoulay, Maloine, Paris

Cajal, S.R. (1928) *Degeneration and Regeneration of the Nervous System*. Translated and edited by R.M. May, Oxford University Press, London

Cupp, C.J. and Uemura, E. (1980) Age-related changes in prefrontal cortex of Macaca mulatta: quantitative analysis of dendritic branching patterns. *Exptl. Neurol.*, 69: 143–163.

Double, K.L., Halliday, G.M., Kril, J.J., Harasty, J.A., Cullen, K., Brooks, K., Creasey, W.S., and Broe, G.A. (1996) Topography of brain atrophy during normal aging and Alzheimer's disease. *Neurobiol. Aging*, 17: 513–521.

Feldman, M.L. and Peters, A. (1998) Ballooning of myelin sheaths in normally aged macaques. *J. Neurocytol.*, 27: 605–614.

Fischer, O. (1907) Miliare Nekrosen mit drusigen Wucherungen der Neurofibrillen, eine regelmässige Veränderung der Hirnrinde bei seniler Demenz. *Monatschr. Psychiatr Neurol.*, 22: 361–372.

Gazzaley, A.H. Thakker, M.M., Hof, P.R., and Morrison, J.H. (1997) Preserved number of entorhinal cortex layer II neurons in aged macaque monkeys. *Neurobiol. Aging*, 18: 549–554.

Gómez-Isla, T., Hollister, R., West, H, Mui, S., Growden, J.H., Petersen, R.C., Paris, J.E. and Hyman, B.T. (1997) Neuronal loss correlates with, but exceeds neurofibrillary tangles in Alzheimer's disease. *Ann. Neurol.*, 41: 17–24.

Haug, H. (1984) Macroscopic and microscopic morphometry of the human brain and cortex. A survey in the light of new results. *Brain Pathol.*, 1: 123–149.

Haug, H. (1985) Are neurons of the cerebral cortex really lost during aging? A morphometric evaluation. In: J. Traber and W.H. Gispen (Eds.), *Senile dementia of the Alzheimer type,* Springer, Berlin, pp. 150–163

Haug, H., Kuhl, S., Mecke, E., Sass, N.-L., and Wasner, K. (1984) The significance of morphometric procedures in the investigation of age changes in cytoarchitectonic structures of human brain. *J. Hirnforsch.*, 25: 353–374.

Hof, R.P., Nimchinsky, E.A., Young, W. and Morrison, J.H. (2000) Numbers of Meynert and layer IVB cells in area V1; stereological analysis in young and aged macaque monkeys. *J. Comp. Neurol.*, 420: 113–126.

Jacobs,B., Driscoll, L. and Schall, M. (1997) Life-span dendritic and spine changes in areas 10 and 18 of human cortex: a quantitative Golgi study. *J. Comp. Neurol.*, 386: 661–680.

Killiany, R.J., Moss, M.B., Rosene, D.L. and Herndon, J. (2000) Recognition memory function in early senescent monkeys. *Pyschobiol.*, 28 : 45–56.

Kim, C.B.Y., Pier, L.P. and Spear, P.D. (1997) Effects of aging on numbers and sizes of neurons in histochemically defined subregions of monkey striate cortex. *Anat. Rec.*, 247: 119–128.

Lafora, G.A. (1914) Neuronal dendritic neoformations and neurological alterations in the senile dog. *Trajabos Lab. Invest. Biol. Univ. Madrid*, 12: 39–53.

Lai, Z.C., Rosene, D.L., Killiany, R.J., Pugliese, D., Albert, M.S., and Moss. M.B. (1995) Age-related changes in the brain of the rhesus monkey: MRI changes in white matter but not gray matter. *Soc. Neurosci. Abstr.*, 21: 1564.

Leuba,G. and Kraftsik, R. (1994a) Visual cortex in Alzheimer's disease: occurrence of neuronal death and glial proliferation and correlation with pathological landmarks. *Neurobiol. Aging*, 15: 29–43.

Leuba, G. and Kraftsik, R. (1994b) Changes in volume, surface estimate, three dimensional shape and total number of neurons of the human primary cortex from midgestation until old age. *Anat. Embryol.*, 190: 351–366.

Levine, J.M., Reynolds, R. and Fawcett, J.W. (2001) The oligdendrocyte precursor cell in health and disease. *Trends Neurosci.*, 24: 39–47.

LeVine, S.M. and Torres, M.V. (1992) Morphological features of degenerating oligodendrocytes in twitcher mice. *Brain Res.*, 587: 348–352.

Levison, S.W., Young, G.M. and Goldman, J.E. (1999) Cycling cells in the adult rat neocortex preferentially generate oligodendroglia. *J. Neurosci Res.*, 57: 435–446.

Merrill, D.A., Roberts, J.A. and Tuszynski, M.H. (2000) Conservation of neuron number and size in entorhinal cortex layers II, III, and V/VI of aged primates. *J. Comp. Neurol.*, 422: 396–401.

Morales, F.R., Boxer, P.A., Fung, S.J. and Chase, M.H. (1987) Basic electrophysiological properties of spinal cord motoneurons during old age in the cat. *J. Neurophysiol.*, 58 : 180–194.

Nielsen, K. and Peters, A. (2000) The effect of aging on the frequency of nerve fibers in rhesus monkey striate cortex. *Neurobiol. Aging*, 21: 621–628.

Pakkenberg, B. and Gundersen, H.J.G. (1997). Neocortical neuron number in humans: effect of sex and age. *J. Comp. Neurol.*, 384: 312–320.

Peters, A. (1996) Age-related changes in oligodendrocytes in monkey cerebral cortex. *J. Comp. Neurol.*, 371: 153–163.

Peters, A. (1999). Normal aging in the cerebral cortex of primates. In: A. Peters and J.H. Morrison, (Eds.), *Neurodegenerative and Age-related Changes in Structure and Function of Cerebral Cortex*. Cerebral Cortex Vol. 14, Kluwer Academic/Plenum publishers, New York, pp. 49–80.

Peters, A., Josephson, K. and Vincent, S.L. (1991) Effects of aging on the neuroglial cells and pericytes with area 17 of the rhesus monkey cerebral cortex. *Anat. Rec.*, 229: 384–398.

Peters, A., Leahu, D., Moss, M.B. and McNally, K.J. (1994) The effects of aging on area 46 of frontal cortex of the rhesus monkey. *Cereb. Cortex*, 5: 621–635.

Peters, A., Morrison, J.H., Rosene,. D.L. and Hyman, B.T. (1998) Are neurons lost from the primate cerebral cortex during normal aging? *Cereb. Cortex*, 8: 295–300.

Peters, A., Moss, M.B. and Sethares, C. (2000) Effects of aging on myelinated nerve fibers in monkey primary visual cortex. *J. Comp. Neurol.*, 419: 364–376.

Peters, A., Moss, M.B. and Sethares, C. (2001a) The effects of aging on layer 1 of primary visual cortex in the rhesus monkey. *Cereb. Cortex*, 11: 93–103.

Peters, A. and Sethares, C. (1993). Aging and the Meynert cells in rhesus monkey primary visual cortex. *Anat. Rec.*, 236: 721–729.

Peters, A., Sethares,C. and Killiany, R.J. (2001b). Effects of age on the thickness of myelin sheaths in monkey primary visual cortex. *J. Comp. Neurol.*, 435: 241–248.

Peters, A., Sethares, C. and Moss., M.B. (1998) The effects of aging on layer 1 in area 46 of prefrontal cortex in the rhesus monkey. *Cereb. Cortex*, 8: 671–684.

Rosene, D.L. (1993) Comparing age-related changes in the basal forebrain and hippocampus of the rhesus monkey. *Neurobiol. Aging*, 14: 669–670.

Sandell, J.H. and Peters, A. (2001) Effect of age on nerve fibers in the rhesus monkey optic nerve. *J. Comp. Neurol.*, 429: 541–553.

Schmolesky, M.T., Wang, Y., Pu, M. and Leventhal, A.G. (2000) Degradation of stimulus selectivity of visual cortical cells in senescent rhesus monkeys. *Nature Neurosci.*, 3: 384–390.

Sheffield, L.G. and Berman, N.E.J. (1998) Microglial expression of MCH class II increases in normal aging of nonhuman primates. *Neurobiol. Aging*, 19: 47–55.

Sloane, J.A., Hollander, W. Moss, M.B., Rosene, D.L. and Abraham, C.R. (1999) Increased microglial activation and protein nitration in white matter of aging monkey. *Neurobiol. Aging*, 20: 395–405.

Sloane, J.A., Pietropaolo, M.F., Rosene, D.L., Moss, M.B., Peters, A., Kemper, T. and Abraham, C.R. (1997) Lack of correlation between plaque burden and cognition in the aged monkey. *Acta Neuropathol.*, 94: 471–478.

Sterio, D.C. (1984) The unbiased estimation of number and sizes of arbitrary particles using the disector. *J. Microsc.*, 134: 127–136.

Tang, Y., Nyengaard, J.R., Pakkenberg, B. and Gundersen, H.J.G. (1997) Age-induced white matter changes in the human brain; a stereological investigation. *Neurobiol. Aging*, 18: 609–615.

Terry, R.D., Deteresa, R. and Hansen, L.A. (1987). Neocortical cell counts in normal human adult aging. *Ann. Neurol.*, 21: 530–539.

Terry, R.D. and Hansen, L.A. (1988). Some morphometric aspects of Alzheimer's disease and of normal aging. In: R.D. Terry (Ed.), *Aging and the Brain.*, Raven Press, New York, pp. 47–59.

Tigges, J., Herndon, J.G. and Peters, A. (1990) Neuronal population in area 4 during the life span of the rhesus monkey. *Neurobiol. Aging*, 11: 201–208.

Uemura, E (1980) Age-related changes in prefrontal cortex of Macaca mulatta: synaptic density. *Exptl. Neurol.*, 69: 164–172.

Vincent, S., Peters, A. and Tigges, J. (1989). Effects of aging on the neurons within area 17 of rhesus monkey cerebral cortex. *Anat. Rec.*, 223: 329–341.

Waxman, S.G., Kocsis, J.D. and Black, J.A. (1995). Pathophysiology of demyelinated axons. In: S.G. Waxman, J.D. Kocsis and P.K. Stys (Eds.), *The Axon: Structure, Function, and Pathophysiology.* Oxford University Press, New York, pp. 438–461.

Wong, T.P., Marchese, G., Casu, M.A., Ribeiro-da-Silva, A., Cuello, A.C. and De Koninck, Y. (2000). Loss of presynaptic and postsynaptic structures accompanied by compensatory increase in action potential-dependent synaptic input to layer V neocortical pyramidal neurons in aged rats. *J. Neurosci.*, 20: 8596–8606.

Xi, M.-C., Liu, R.-H., Engelhardt, K.K., Morales, F.R. and Chase, M.H. (1999) Changes in the axonal conduction velocity of pyramidal tract neurons in the aged cat. *Neuroscience*, 92: 219–225.

E.C. Azmitia, J. DeFelipe, E.G. Jones, P. Rakic and C.E. Ribak (Eds.)
Progress in Brain Research, Vol. 136
© 2002 Elsevier Science B.V. All rights reserved

CHAPTER 37

Selective vulnerability of corticocortical and hippocampal circuits in aging and Alzheimer's disease

John H. Morrison[1,2,3,*] and Patrick R. Hof[1,2,3,4]

[1]*Kastor Neurobiology of Aging Laboratories,* [2]*Fishberg Research Center for Neurobiology,*
[3]*Department of Geriatrics and Adult Development, and* [4]*Department of Ophthalmology,*
Mount Sinai School of Medicine, One Gustave L. Levy Place, New York, NY 10029, USA

Abstract: Alzheimer's disease (AD), a classic neurodegenerative disorder, is characterized by extensive yet selective neuron death in the neocortex and hippocampus that leads to dramatic decline in cognitive abilities and memory. Crucial subsets of pyramidal cells and their projections are particularly vulnerable. A more modest disruption of memory occurs often in normal aging, yet such functional decline does not appear to be accompanied by significant neuron death. However, the same circuits that are devastated through degeneration in AD are vulnerable to sublethal age-related biochemical and morphologic shifts that alter synaptic transmission, and thereby impair function. For example, in the monkey neocortex, pyramidal cells that are homologous to those that degenerate in AD do not degenerate with aging, yet they lose spines, suggesting that an age-related synaptic disruption has occurred. Such age-related synaptic alterations have also been reported in hippocampus. For example, NMDA receptors are decreased in certain hippocampal circuits with aging. NMDA receptors are also responsive to circulating estrogen levels, thus interactions between reproductive senescence and brain aging may also affect excitatory synaptic transmission in the hippocampus. Thus, the aging synapse may be the key to age-related memory decline, whereas neuron death is the more prominent and problematic culprit in AD.

Introduction

Based largely on morphologic criteria, Cajal developed the essential vocabulary of cell typology in the central nervous system (Fig. 1). Cell typology bears a strong relationship to the important concept of *selective vulnerability* in aging and neurodegenerative disorders, yet selective vulnerability incorporates two critical elements that were not available to Cajal; connectivity and neurochemical phenotype. The nature of selective vulnerability in aging and Alzheimer's disease (AD) will be discussed from the perspective of this broadened notion of cell and circuit specificity. AD is characterized by neuritic plaque and neurofibrillary tangle formation, and extensive yet selective neuron death in the neocortex and hippocampus that leads to dramatic decline in cognitive abilities and memory. Crucial subsets of pyramidal cells and their projections are particularly vulnerable. A more modest disruption of memory referred to as age-associated memory impairment (AAMI) occurs often in the context of normal aging, yet unlike AD, neuron death is unlikely to underlie AAMI. In AD, the perforant path connecting the entorhinal cortex and the hippocampus is devastated, as are corticocortical circuits that interconnect association regions. While the death of these neurons is minimal in normal aging, these same circuits are vulnerable to sublethal age-related shifts in morphology, neurochemical phenotype and synaptic alterations that might

*Corresponding author: Tel.: 1-212-659-5985; Fax: 212-849-2510;
E-mail: John.Morrison@mssm.edu

468

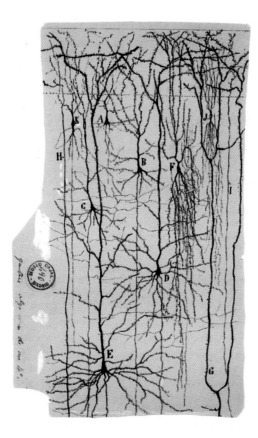

Fig. 1. An original drawing by Santiago Ramón y Cajal of several cortical cell types as visualized with the Golgi stain. Neurons A–E are all pyramidal cells, yet they display a wide variation in laminar location, size, and dendritic arbor typical of this cell class. F, J, and K represent three distinct classes of nonpyramidal cells that Cajal also analyzed and categorized in great detail.

impair function. For example, in the aged monkey neocortex, the pyramidal cells that interconnect prefrontal and temporal association cortex do not degenerate, yet they lose spines, suggesting that an age-related synaptic disruption has occurred. Such subtle age-related synaptic alterations have been reported in hippocampus as well. Biochemical alterations of the synapse may also contribute to memory impairment, particularly in nonhuman primates, where we have demonstrated that NMDA receptors are decreased in certain hippocampal circuits. NMDA receptors are also responsive to circulating estrogen levels, thus critical interactions between reproductive senescence and brain aging may affect excitatory synaptic transmission in the hippocampus as well. In fact, we have demonstrated that the nature of the estrogen-induced

synaptic plasticity differs fundamentally across age groups. Thus, the aging synapse may be the key to age-related memory decline, whereas the missing circuit is the more prominent and problematic culprit in AD.

Selective vulnerability in Alzheimer's disease

The pathogenetic events that lead to AD are not fully understood, although the current knowledge of the pathological changes that occur in AD suggests that structurally and functionally AD is predominantly a disease of the cerebral cortex that involves only certain populations of neurons displaying specific regional and laminar distribution and connectivity patterns, whereas other neuron types are spared. Thus, differential neuronal vulnerability exists in AD that can be related to the morphologic and biochemical characteristics of identifiable neuronal populations and cortical connections. In this section, we provide an overview of the relationships between the distribution of pathologic changes in AD and the localization of specific elements of the cortical circuitry that are affected by these alterations. Also, we will discuss observations that relate the neurochemical characteristics of particular neuronal types to their relative vulnerability or resistance to the degenerative process. It is possible that through such morphologic and molecular analyses, correlations will emerge between distribution of cellular pathologic changes, neurochemical characteristics related to vulnerability, and cortical circuits at risk. Such correlations may be useful for the development of preventative or protective interventions against the specific neuronal degenerative events that occur during the progression of the dementing illness.

Neocortical pathology in AD

Lesion types and cortical distribution

Alzheimer's disease is a neurodegenerative disorder classically characterized by the presence of two major types of histopathologic alterations in the cerebral cortex, neurofibrillary tangles (NFT) and senile plaques (SP) (Fig. 2). The distribution and density of NFT and SP have been analyzed in great detail and constitute the basis of the neuropathologic diagnosis of AD (Mirra et al., 1993). NFT are characterized by the accumulation of abnormal components of the neuronal cytoskeleton that form paired

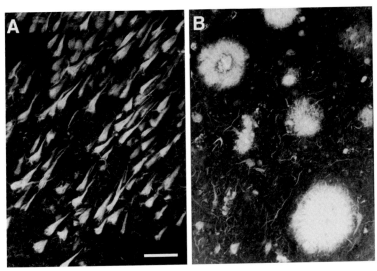

Fig. 2. Examples of NFT (**A**) and SP (**B**) from the hippocampus of a severe AD case. Note the flame-shape morphology of NFT and the more variable features of SP. In (**B**), a classical plaque with a central amyloid core and a rim of degenerating neurites, an isolated dense amyloid core, a predominantly neuritic plaque, and a few small diffuse deposits are visible. Scale bar = 50 μm.

helical filaments, whereas SP are composed of dystrophic neurites and glial elements with or without a central amyloid core (Hof et al., 1999). These lesions are consistently observed throughout the brain and are predominant in the cerebral cortex, where NFT are located in the perikaryon of large pyramidal neurons, and SP are distributed throughout the cortical regions, but are particularly numerous in association areas (Arnold et al., 1991; Hof et al., 1999).

These visible reflections of pathology are important markers of AD, but the critical issue is the degree to which each of them reflects neuron or synapse loss that amounts to circuit disruption leading to dementia. A considerable degree of neuronal loss occurs in the association regions of the neocortex in AD, leaving primary sensory and motor areas relatively spared (Morrison and Hof, 1997). There are strong correlations between the distribution patterns of SP, NFT, and neuron loss in identifiable regions and layers of the cerebral cortex, and the presumed neurons of origin of certain long corticocortical and hippocampal projections (Pearson et al., 1985; Rogers and Morrison, 1985; Hyman et al., 1986; Lewis et al., 1987; Hof et al., 1990; Hof and Morrison, 1990). Overall, the distribution and severity of neuron loss follows closely that of NFT in the neocortex (Gómez-Isla et al., 1996, 1997; Morrison and Hof, 1997). Regionally, NFT are more numerous in the temporal cortex than in other cortical regions, the frontal

cortex displays intermediate NFT densities followed by the parietal cortex and the occipital cortex, and certain cortical regions, such as the posterior cingulate cortex, exhibit substantial case-to-case variability (Vogt et al., 1990, 1998). NFT are found primarily within layers III and V in the neocortex, though the relative distribution across layers varies considerably among cortical regions, with primary sensory and motor regions having much fewer NFT than association areas (Pearson et al., 1985; Lewis et al., 1987; Hof and Morrison, 1990; Arnold et al., 1991). For example, when comparing the primary visual cortex (area 17) to the secondary visual cortex (area 18), there is an approximately 20-fold increase in the density of NFT in area 18, and regions in the inferior temporal cortex that comprise high-order visual association areas are characterized by a further doubling of NFT densities (Lewis et al., 1987). Similar differences are found between the primary auditory cortex and auditory association areas which display a 10-fold increase in NFT density (Lewis et al., 1987). Considerable differences in laminar NFT distribution exist among neocortical regions. In areas 17 and 18, the majority of NFT are located in layer III, whereas in the inferior temporal cortex only 40% of the NFT are found in layer III. A more striking difference exists in the auditory association cortex where only 27% of the NFT are observed in the supragranular layers (Lewis et al., 1987).

470

In contrast to NFT, SP show a relatively homogeneous distribution among cortical areas (Lewis et al., 1987; Arnold et al., 1991), although the frontal and anterior cingulate cortex contain more SP than temporal cortices (Rogers and Morrison, 1985). In the neocortex, SP are generally more numerous in layers II to IV than in layers V and VI (Rogers and Morrison, 1985). Also, synapse loss may represent an early marker of the dementing process. In fact, a strong association between loss of neocortical synapses estimated on the basis of synaptophysin immunoreactivity and cognitive impairment has been documented (Terry et al., 1991), which was stronger than that between NFT and cognitive deficit, indicating that synapse loss might be a more accurate neuropathologic indicator of dementia (Fig. 3).

Alzheimer's disease affects specific elements of the cortical circuits

The preferential distribution of NFT in layers III and V indicates that elements of feedforward, lateral and feedback projections are likely to be affected by the degenerating process of AD (Fig. 4). The fact that layer V contains generally higher NFT densities than layer III in association areas suggests that feedback as well as lateral projections may be at higher risk in AD than feedforward systems. Interestingly, most of the projection neurons from the occipital and temporal association cortex to the frontal and from the occipital cortex to the temporal

cortex are located in layer III. However, the ratio of the densities of projection neurons in layer III to layer V progressively decreases from the occipital to inferior temporal and further to superior temporal regions (Barbas, 1986), and this change in laminar distribution is paralleled by a progressive shift of NFT densities from supragranular layers to infragranular layers (Lewis et al., 1987). In severe AD cases, only feedforward projections are affected in areas 17 and 18, as NFT predominate in layer III which contains most of the efferent cortico-cortical neurons in these areas (Fig. 4). The regional and laminar distribution of SP suggests that they may be related to NFT formation. It has been proposed that, in fact, SP reflects the degeneration of the terminations of projections from neurons that contain NFT (Pearson et al., 1985), and that the slightly higher incidence of SP in the supragranular layers and in layer IV in the association cortex reflects the involvement of feedforward projections (Lewis et al., 1987).

The degeneration of presumed corticocortical circuits within the neocortex appears therefore to be the necessary factor for the clinical expression of AD dementia (Morrison and Hof, 1997). Elderly individuals can maintain a high level of cognitive performance while sustaining significant compromise of hippocampal circuits, and they may rely more on neocortical than on hippocampal circuits for memories essential for daily activities (Albert, 1996). Compared to patients with early AD, healthy elders retain the new information after a delay, whereas patients with mild cognitive impairment

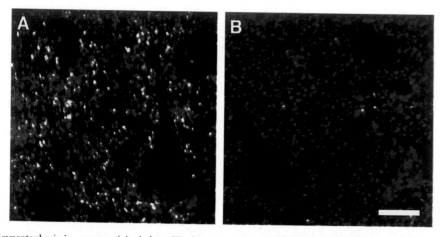

Fig. 3. Patterns of synaptophysin immunoreactivity in layer III of area 9 in a control case (**A**) and a CDR 3.0 case (**B**). The glow scale on these laser scanning confocal microscope images reveals the intensity of the immunolabeling. Note the much lower synapse density and staining intensity in the AD case. Scale bar (on B) = 20 μm.

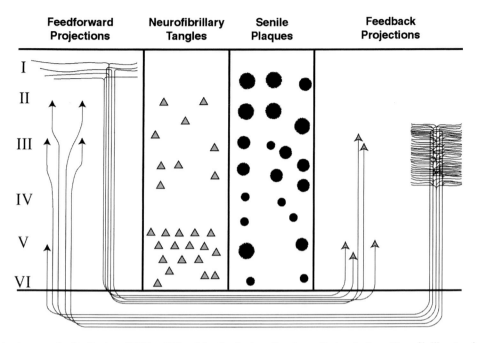

Fig. 4. Correlation between the distribution of NFT and SP and the distribution of corticocortical projections. Neurofibrillary tangles are located in the same layers as the neurons of origin of forward and feedback corticocortical projections. The NFT tend to be more numerous in the deep layers suggesting a stronger correlation with feedback projections. Senile plaques are observed in higher densities in the zone of termination of forward projection (layer IV and lower two-third of layer III).

retain little of it (Albert, 1996). This impairment in information retention that characterizes the very early stages of AD is correlated to neuronal loss in the entorhinal cortex and to volumetric changes in the temporal lobe (Albert, 1996; Gómez-Isla et al., 1996, 1997). Increases in the volume of the temporal horn of the lateral ventricle may selectively reflect the loss of projections from the entorhinal cortex. Normal aging can thus be defined by intact cognitive abilities in spite of the presence of scarce neurofibrillary pathology in the entorhinal cortex, that can be referred to as aging-related asymptomatic AD-like neurofibrillary pathology (Fig. 5).

Neurofilament protein is a marker of neuronal vulnerability in Alzheimer's disease

Certain pyramidal neurons in the neocortex of both human and monkeys have been shown to be enriched in neurofilament protein (Campbell and Morrison, 1989; Hof et al., 1990; Hof and Morrison, 1990, 1995). Neurofilament protein immunoreactivity in the primate neocortex is restricted to the perikaryon and dendrites of

a subpopulation of large pyramidal neurons and is more concentrated in the cell body and dendrites of the largest of these neurons. Interestingly, neurofilament protein as well as other cytoskeletal proteins have been implicated in NFT formation (Morrison et al., 1987; Trojanowski et al., 1993; Morrison and Hof, 1997; Hof et al., 1999), and pyramidal cells with a high content of nonphosphorylated neurofilament protein emerge as a neuron type highly susceptible to NFT formation.

Detailed descriptions of the cellular, laminar, and regional characteristics of neurofilament protein-containing cells in many frontal, cingulate, temporal and occipital areas of the macaque monkey and human neocortex have revealed that extensive regional heterogeneity exists in the size, density and laminar distribution of neurofilament protein-containing neurons (Campbell and Morrison, 1989; Hof et al., 1990, 1995, 1996, 1997; Hof and Morrison, 1990, 1995; Campbell et al., 1991; Nimchinsky et al., 1995, 1996, 1997). The distribution of neurofilament protein-containing neurons corresponds to the distribution of corticocortically projecting cells as demonstrated by transport studies in the macaque

472

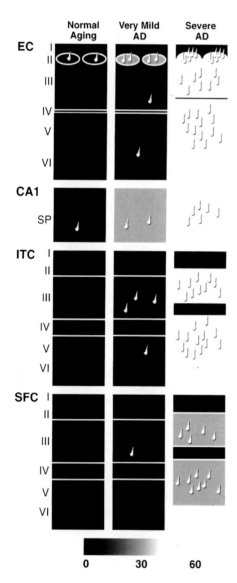

Fig. 5. Schematic representation of regional and laminar NFT formation and neuronal loss in normal aging and AD. The flame-shaped structures represent a semi-quantitative assessment of NFT densities. An estimate of the percent of neuronal loss is shown by the grayscale. In normal aging, a few NFT are consistently observed in layer II of the entorhinal cortex (EC) and rare NFT are found in the CA1 field (SP, stratum pyramidale). The inferior temporal cortex (ITC) and superior frontal cortex (SFC) remain devoid of NFT. There is no measurable neuronal loss in normal aging. In contrast, very early AD cases exhibit higher NFT densities in the entorhinal cortex and CA1, and NFT are consistently observed in layer III of the inferior temporal cortex. Rare NFT are present in superior frontal cortex. The neocortical areas still do not display measurable neuronal loss, but a significant degree of neuronal loss is present in layer II of the entorhinal cortex and in the CA1 field. In severe AD cases, NFT are found in very high densities in layer II of the entorhinal cortex, CA1 field, and in layers III and V–VI of the inferior temporal cortex, with moderately high density in superior frontal cortex as well. The degree of neuronal loss parallels NFT densities in these regions, although NFT numbers alone cannot account for the total loss of neurons indicating that not all dying neurons necessarily undergo NFT formation. The size of the cortical boxes reflects a certain degree of tissue shrinkage in severe AD. (Adapted from Morrison and Hof, 1997.)

monkey cortex (Campbell et al., 1991; Hof et al., 1995, 1996, 1997; Nimchinsky et al., 1996). Of direct relevance to AD, we have shown that in the macaque monkey, many long association corticocortical projections originate from neurofilament protein-containing neurons, and that in some of them, 90–100% of the neurons of origin of the projection contain neurofilament protein (Hof et al., 1995). This is particularly the case for projections from the temporal to the prefrontal and parietal neocortex that are known to be involved in networks subserving many aspects of cognition (Goldman-Rakic, 1988), and are likely devastated in AD.

Furthermore, we have observed that in AD neurofilament protein-containing neurons in certain neocortical and hippocampal areas are dramatically affected and die through NFT formation (Morrison et al., 1987; Hof et al., 1990; Hof and Morrison, 1990; Vickers et al., 1992, 1994, 2000; Morrison and Hof, 1997; Vickers et al., 1997). The laminar distribution of neurofilament protein-containing neurons in visual association, prefrontal, and anterior cingulate in human cerebral cortex is very similar to the distribution of NFT. Furthermore, the layers that have high NFT density in an AD brain no longer contain a high density of neurofilament protein-immunoreactive neurons (Hof et al., 1990, 1999; Hof and Morrison, 1990). A comparable situation exists in the hippocampal formation where layers II, III and V of entorhinal cortex and the pyramidal neurons of the subiculum have a very high density of neurofilament protein-immunoreactive neurons in the normally aging human brain and present with a dramatic loss of these neurons in AD (Fig. 5) (Vickers et al., 1992, 1994; Morrison and Hof, 1997).

These observations demonstrate that neurofilament protein-containing neurons are highly vulnerable in AD, and quantitative analyses have demonstrated a severe loss of neurofilament protein-containing neurons in layers III and V in the inferior temporal and superior frontal cortex. The severity of the loss correlates with the size of these neurons in that the neurofilament protein-containing neurons larger than 6,000 μm^3 of perikaryal volume are the most affected with up to 60% cell loss, while the smaller size neurons are not affected (Hof et al., 1990). In addition to regional distribution and relationship to connectivity, NFT identified by thioflavine S stain or immunohistochemistry using antibodies to neurofilament protein and microtubule-associated protein tau have revealed dynamic cellular alterations in vulnerable neuronal populations during normal aging. For instance, layer II of the entorhinal cortex contains neurofilament protein-immunoreactive neurons that also display immunoreactivity to tau protein and thioflavine S-positive materials, suggesting the existence of transitional forms of NFT (Fig. 6) (Vickers et al., 1992;

Morrison and Hof, 1997). In such cases, very rare NFT are seen in the frontal cortex which contains preserved neurofilament protein-immunoreactive neurons in layers III and V. However, in AD cases, most NFT in the entorhinal cortex progress to an end-stage and are no longer immunoreactive to tau and neurofilament protein but are stained only with thioflavine S. At this stage, transitional forms of NFT are observed in the frontal cortex indicating that a time-dependent process takes place in the formation of NFT in certain neurofilament protein-containing neurons (Vickers et al., 1992, 1994, 2000; Morrison and Hof, 1997; Vickers, 1997; Hof et al., 1999) (Fig. 6). Moreover, the presence of high levels of neurofilament protein appears to be a prerequisite for the formation of NFT, because certain neurons, such as the pyramidal neurons of the CA1 field, that do not normally express detectable levels of this protein in young adults

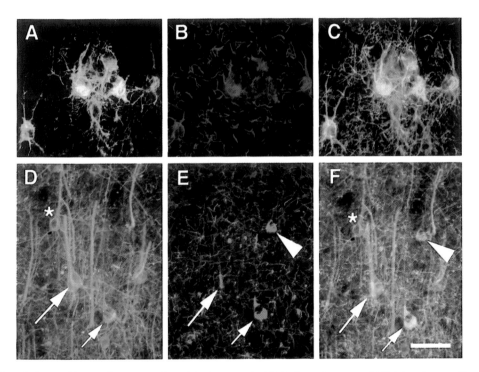

Fig. 6. Progression of changes in neurofilament protein-enriched neurons in AD. In the early stages of AD, intensely neurofilament protein-immunoreactive neurons in layer II of the entorhinal cortex (**A**) begin to form NFT as demonstrated by the presence of hyperphosphorylated tau protein (**B**). At this stage most of the layer II neurons are affected by NFT formation but still retain neurofilament protein immunoreactivity (double labeling, **C**). As AD progresses, these neurons will eventually lose neurofilament protein immunoreactivity. In a more advanced AD case, transitional forms can be observed in layer III of the superior frontal cortex (**D–F**). Several neurons contain both neurofilament protein (**D**) and tau (**E**) immunoreactivity (arrows on **F**), while a few have lost their neurofilament protein immunoreactivity and contain only an NFT labeled by the anti-tau antibody (arrowhead, **E**, **F**). Also, some healthy neurons are still visible that do not yet contain a tau immunoreactivity (asterisk, **D**, **F**). Scale bar (on **F**) = 80 μm. (Taken from Morrison and Hof, 1997, as adapted from Vickers et al., 1992.)

yet are prone to NFT formation in AD, begin to show increasing levels of neurofilament protein immunoreactivity during aging (Vickers et al., 1994).

Dynamic neuronal changes during aging and AD

If the monkey data are considered within the context of the distribution of neurofilament protein-containing neurons and NFT in human, it is likely that the human homologues of the neurofilament protein-containing, corticocortically projecting neurons of the macaque monkey are those that are highly vulnerable in AD. Thus, one of the neurochemical characteristics of the vulnerable neurons in AD is the presence of high somatic and dendritic concentrations of nonphosphorylated neurofilament proteins, although this may clearly represent only part of the neurochemical phenotype associated with selective vulnerability. To test this correlation more directly in human aging and AD, we have initiated sterological analyses targeting these neurons in neocortex and hippocampus (see below).

Existing stereologic data on the neuronal alterations in AD consist almost exclusively of total neuron counts based on the Nissl stain or of NFT counts. Both of these measurements may be misleading because they do not take into account a large and dynamic population of transitional alterations described above that can be identified by several neurochemical markers such as neurofilament proteins or modified tau proteins (Morrison and Hof, 1997; Vickers, 1997; Vickers et al., 2000) (Fig. 6). In addition, most available studies do not take into consideration the very high variability in neuron numbers that exists among human brains, and generally do not provide accurate estimates of numbers in cytoarchitecturally defined regions in the neocortex or rely on density measurements. We have analyzed two sets of projection neurons, layer II of ERC and layer III of area 9 as a focus for quantitative analysis in which neuron counts are correlated with clinical assessment as reflected in the Clinical Dementia Rating Scale (CDR), where a rating of 0.5 amounts to mild cognitive impairment (MCI), 1 reflects probable AD, 2 is early AD, 3 is moderate AD, and 5 is severe AD. The most recent data obtained indicate that in area 9, neurofilament protein-containing pyramidal cells already undergo notable neuronal loss in CDR 2 cases, whereas a more dramatic loss of neurons overall occurs in CDR 3 cases. This result suggests that

CDR 2 may be considered as the clinical transition stage at which considerable development of AD degenerative changes takes place in the prefrontal cortex.

Hippocampal pathology in AD

It has been known for a long time that layer II of the entorhinal cortex, the subiculum, and the CA1 field of the hippocampus represent particularly vulnerable cortical domains that consistently display very high NFT densities in AD, and that the most consistent observation in AD cases is the presence of large numbers of NFT in layers II and V of the entorhinal cortex (Hyman et al., 1984) (Fig. 5). In the hippocampus, the most severely affected zones are the CA1 and subiculum, while the presubiculum, CA2, CA3 fields and dentate hilus are much less affected. The distribution of SP in the hippocampal formation is variable, with certain zones displaying high SP densities, such as layer III of the entorhinal cortex, the molecular layer of the dentate gyrus and the superficial layer of the subiculum (Hyman et al., 1990).

The distribution of NFT and SP in the hippocampal formation also parallels specific projections (Hyman et al., 1990). Thus, the perforant pathway that projects from layers II and III of the entorhinal cortex is severely and early involved in AD, and the presence of NFT in the neurons of origin of this pathway and its termination in the dentate gyrus is correlated with high densities of SP in the molecular layer of the dentate gyrus (Hyman et al., 1984). Similarly, in the hippocampal formation, the large pyramidal efferent neurons in layers II, III and V of the entorhinal cortex and of the CA1 field and subiculum are all severely affected. However, other cellular characteristics than these are also linked to vulnerability to the degenerative process, because certain large efferent neurons, such as the principal cells in the CA3 field and the large neurons of the dentate hilus are generally relatively resistant to degeneration in AD. In addition, CA1 neurons have a low level of neurofilament in young human brain, and only after a dramatic age-related increase in somato-dendritic levels of neurofilament protein occurs, do the neurons transition to NFT (Vickers et al., 1994).

It is important to draw a distinction between the neurobiological events underlying the dementia of AD and those that we suspect underlie age-related memory impairment. In AD, and for that matter neurodegenerative disorders in general, neuron death occurs that results in circuit disruption leading to a profound impairment of the neural functions dependent on the degenerating circuits. In contrast to the selective but extensive neuron loss reflective of AD, neuron death is minimal in the regions classically associated with cognition and memory in the normal course of aging. The lack of significant hippocampal and neocortical neuron death in normal aging has been demonstrated now in human, monkey, and rat, (West et al., 1993; Gómez-Isla et al., 1996; Gazzaley et al., 1997).

However, a lack of quantifiable neuron loss does not necessarily mean that no degenerative changes are occurring in a given brain region and it does not negate non-degenerative changes that lead to compromised function. The entorhinal cortex is a particularly instructive case in this regard. It appears that the neurons within layer II of entorhinal cortex that serve as a neocortical conduit to the hippocampus are likely to be the single most vulnerable class of neurons in the brain with respect to both aging and AD. While these neurons are clearly devastated early in AD, their status in cognitively normal aged individuals and those with mild cognitive impairment (MCI) has been more difficult to pinpoint. Neuron counts in neurologically normal individuals suggest that there is no neuron loss in entorhinal cortex (Gómez-Isla et al., 1996) however, analyses of neurofibrillary tangles (NFT), the classic reflection of a degenerating neuron in AD, suggest that virtually all humans over the age of 55 have some NFT in layer II of entorhinal cortex (Bouras et al., 1994). How does one reconcile these two findings and draw a distinction between age-related degenerative events in the entorhinal cortex that are progressive and those that are not? While the answer to this question continues to be elusive, one approach that we have found to be particularly valuable is the use of finer biochemical refinement in the entorhinal cortex in order to distinguish and quantify transitional events that can be correlated with the CDR scale. This has led to a particular focus on patients with a CDR of 0.5 that have mild cognitive impairment (MCI) where it is unclear whether their condition represents early AD or a more stable condition that might be referred to as age-associated memory impairment or AAMI. The key to reconciling the presence of NFT in this region with the fact that there does not appear to be neuron loss is that the various profile counts that have been done have not taken into consideration "transitional neurons," i.e., neurons that are still intact and included in an analysis of total neuron counts, yet have transitional

intraneuronal pathology resembling an NFT (Perl et al., 2000). When neurons in layer II of entorhinal cortex and prefrontal cortex are counted in three categories—ghost tangles, transitional neurons, and healthy neurons—the data are far more revealing with respect to early pathologic events in layer II of entorhinal cortex, and it is quite clear that there might be significant pathology in neurologically normal individuals in the absence of quantifiable neuron death and in the absence of massive NFT formation (Fig. 7). These estimates of neuron number in three classes can also be related to each other as ratios in a given case, establishing a case-by-case "Index of neurodegeneration" in several brain areas (Fig. 7) (Perl et al., 2000). It will be very important to continue to pursue patients with a CDR of 0.5, and to try to determine whether this pathology is a precursor to overt AD or a level of pathology that can be sustained and stabilized over a long period of time without cascading to a more extensive hippocampal and neocortical degeneration that would lead to the dementia of AD. However, even a more precise delineation of the events surrounding degeneration will not provide a full understanding of the vulnerability of this circuit, since as described below, this circuit displays age-related changes short of degeneration that would also impact function.

A synthetic neuronal phenotype of vulnerability and resistance in the neocortex

Selective neuronal vulnerability is a hallmark of all of the major neurodegenerative disorders and is apparent not only at the level of affected brain regions, subregions or layers, but also at the level of specific neuron populations (Hof et al., 1990, 1999a; Arnold et al., 1991; Morrison and Hof, 1997). The notion of differential vulnerability can be best understood in the context of a broad, yet integrative definition of neuronal typology that includes morphology, regional and laminar location, connectivity, and neurochemical phenotype. This approach is useful to delineate the cellular organization of neocortex as well as the cellular pathologic changes in diseases such as AD, as it takes into consideration the complex relationships among these morphofunctional parameters. In a very general sense, the most vulnerable group of cortical neurons includes large pyramidal cells, and more specifically those providing long corticocortical projections between association neocortical areas and hippocampal

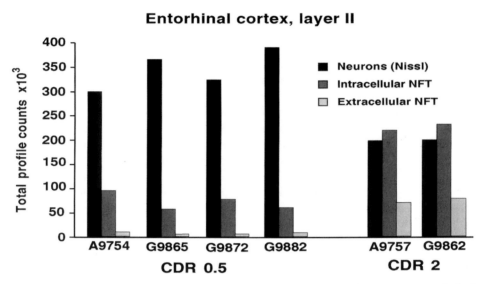

Fig. 7. Total number of neurons in layer II of the entorhinal cortex in CDR 0.5 and CDR 2 cases. Neuron counts were obtained stereologically and have been subdivided into normal neurons revealed by Nissl stain, neurons containing an intracellular NFT (i.e., a Nissl-stained cell labeled with an antibody to hyperphosphorylated tau protein), and extracellular ghost NFT. Note that a significant proportion of the neurons demonstrate transitional pathology in the CDR 0.5 cases, but that the majority remains unaffected by NFT formation. However, in the CDR 2 cases, the majority of neurons has progressed to NFT formation as revealed by the higher proportion of intra- and extracellular NFT.

projections. These systems utilize glutamate and are driven by glutamatergic inputs. However, not all cortico-cortical projections are equally vulnerable, short projections from primary sensory to adjacent secondary sensory areas being resistant to degeneration. It is therefore likely that the specific neurochemical and morphologic phenotype of certain pyramidal neurons may predispose them to degeneration as well as NFT formation. In contrast, quantitative analyses of the superior frontal (area 9) and inferior temporal (area 20) in AD have demonstrated that several classes of GABAergic interneurons containing the calcium-binding proteins parvalbumin, calbindin and calretinin are largely resistant to the degenerative process, even in severe cases displaying very high densities of NFT and SP (Hof et al., 1991, 1993; Hof and Morrison, 1991; Sampson et al., 1997).

The relevance and impact of pathologic changes in AD have to be understood within the context of organized systems that underlie neocortical function. For instance, integrated processing in a given sensory modality such as vision involves the simultaneous activity of numerous separable visual areas that have extensive highly ordered interconnections that establish a distributed system subserving the proper integration of the visual information. Similarly, cognition and language, that are not

modality-specific functions, presumably depend strongly on the complex communication among neocortical regions provided by the corticocortical circuits which are the particular projections that degenerate in AD, leading in turn to a global neocortical disconnection syndrome that presents clinically as dementia (Morrison and Hof, 1997). Clearly, other degenerative processes occur in AD, and they may also contribute to the clinical characteristics of the disease, but the generalized loss of long corticocortical projections emerges functionally as the most devastating component of AD, and the most directly related to dementia. Importantly in this context, the cells that provide these projections appear to be highly specialized neurons that share identifiable morphological and neurochemical features.

This interpretation of the pathological features of AD suggest that the debilitating dementia results from changes restricted to the association neocortex, whereas extensive hippocampal alterations can exist in the absence of neocortical involvement and with only minor disruptions in activities of daily living of the individual, whose memory deficits could be revealed by formal testing, but are not compatible with the diagnosis of dementing illness. As the elements of the biochemical and anatomical phenotype that are linked to differential cellular vulnerability in AD are increasingly recognized, it will be hopefully possible to develop therapeutic interventions to protect or rescue the neurons that are at higher risk in AD. The protection of these neurons appears to be an attractive strategy for the management of AD, that may have the advantage of being more achievable than the development of a cure.

Age-associated memory impairment: functional decline without neuron loss

While NFT and SP are also present in the brains of humans without clinical AD, their presence is not associated with measurable neuron loss, with the possible exception of some loss in layer II of entorhinal cortex. In fact, while layer II of entorhinal cortex shows some pathology in virtually all humans over 55 years old (Bouras et al., 1993), CA1 and other hippocampal fields as well as neocortex do not display significant neuron loss in normal aging (Fig. 5), and even in entorhinal cortex, the loss does not appear to be dramatic enough to account for the common occurrence of AAMI that primarily affects memory in elderly people, in the absence of progressive cognitive impairment reflective of AD. If neuron loss cannot account for memory loss with aging in this population, then what is the neurobiological complement of such functional decline? Insight on this issue has been gained from animal studies of aging, where AAMI can be analyzed without the potential confound of early AD. Studies from both nonhuman primates and rodents have illuminated both neocortical and hippocampal changes associated with aging. These studies (reviewed below) essentially all suggest that age-related changes in key excitatory synaptic connections in the absence of frank circuit degeneration may be the primary neurobiological correlate of decline in memory performance.

The aging synapse: nonhuman primate studies

Neocortex

Morphologic analyses of corticocortical circuits

As described above, a distinct subpopulation of neurons forming long corticocortical projections in the association neocortex is highly vulnerable to the degenerative

process in AD (Hof et al., 1990; Morrison and Hof, 1997). However, the degree to which age-related molecular and morphologic alterations of these same circuits might lead to functional decline has not been determined. No neuronal loss in neocortex is observed in the course of normal aging in nonhuman primates, although significant cognitive changes can be observed in animals older than 19 years of age (Gallagher and Rapp, 1997). In this context, it is worth noting that recent studies of the prefrontal cortex and primary visual cortex in behaviorally tested old macaque monkeys have generally failed to reveal any objective age-related alteration at the light microscopic level. However, electron microscopic investigations have demonstrated consistent pathological changes in oligodendrocyte and axonal myelin sheath morphology in aged nonhuman primates (Peters et al., 1996, 1998, 2000), pointing to the possible involvement of certain cortical projection systems in aging. Several studies indicate that the cognitive processes mediated by the prefrontal cortex are impaired during the normal aging processes (Peters et al., 1996; Rapp and Gallagher, 1997; O'Donnell et al., 1999). In particular, old macaque monkeys show consistently lower performance in delayed response and delayed nonmatching to sample tasks that test prefrontal cortex function, when compared to young animals (Rapp and Gallagher, 1997). These and other data indicate that age-related cognitive deficits in nonhuman primates may be a consequence of abnormalities in cortical circuits that clearly do not include loss of neurons but rather involve subcellular compartments of the neurons at risk. We have now quantified age-related morphological changes at the single cell level in identified populations of corticocortically-projecting neurons in the Patas monkey, a cercopithecine species closely related to the macaques (Page et al., 2002).

Neurons furnishing long corticocortical projections from parietal and temporal regions to area 46 in prefrontal cortex were targeted for these studies. These neurons were targeted through retrograde transport of fluorescent dyes following injections in area 46, followed by intracellular filling and 3-dimensional reconstruction of the retrogradely filled neurons (Fig. 8). Through such an approach we were able to develop detailed quantitative data on the dendritic arbor and spine density of the precise corticocortically projecting neurons that we hypothesize to be vulnerable to AD in human cortex. Based on the 3-dimensional reconstructions of these neurons, few differences in dendritic morphology could be

478

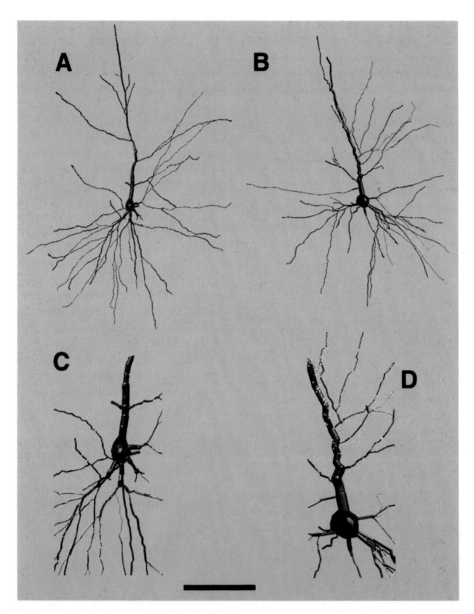

Fig. 8. Examples of retrogradely traced neurons, filled with Lucifer Yellow, and reconstructed in 3-dimensions. Neuron **A** is from layer III of the temporal cortex from a 24 year old animal and neuron **B** from the same region of a 12 year old animal. Note that some differences in the complexity of the apical dendrites are visible. Higher magnification views centered on the soma of the same neurons as in **A** and **B** are shown in **C** and **D**. Age-related differences in spine numbers are apparent at this magnification (yellow dots; compare **A–C** with **B–D**). Scale bar = 150 μm (**A, B**), and 60 μm (**C, D**). (Adapted from Page et al., 2002.)

observed between the age groups. The total length of the dendrites in the basal and apical domains was not different in old animals compared to the young ones, and the number of dendritic branches did not change in aging in either type of projections, even though qualitatively some neurons appeared less complex in old than in young animals. The most consistent finding in aged animals was a reduction in dendritic spine numbers and densities along the dendritic branches (Fig. 8). Depending on the neuron analyzed, the total number of spines decreased by 28–37% in the basal and apical dendrites of aged animals compared to young ones (Page et al., 2002). The spine densities per mm of dendritic length decreased by about 23% overall and was consistent across the entire dendritic arborization after the second order of dendritic branching.

These data demonstrate that a significant decrease in the density of dendritic spines occurs during aging in neurons forming long corticocortical projections from the temporal to the prefrontal cortex in a nonhuman primate (Page et al., 2002). A certain impoverishment of the complexity of dendritic arborizations may also occur in old animals, although additional morphometric tools will be necessary to quantify these differences appropriately (Henry et al., 2002). The observed change in spine numbers may lead to a potential deficit in the excitatory drive on the neurons that receive these inputs. Such a change in synaptic inputs to these neurons could lead to cognitive deficits such as those described in aged monkeys in the absence of neuron loss.

Neurochemical analyses of corticocortical circuits

Previous data on the distribution of neurofilament protein-containing neurons in the human neocortex in Alzheimer's disease have revealed that these neurons are prone to neurofibrillary tangle formation and suffer a dramatic loss in the course of the dementing process (Hof et al., 1990; Morrison and Hof, 1997). Additional data from tract-tracing studies have demonstrated that the neurons of origin of long association corticocortical pathways, such as those connecting the superior temporal cortex and the prefrontal cortex, are particularly enriched in neurofilament protein, suggesting that these pathways have a neurochemical phenotype that may render them vulnerable to age-related pathology (Hof et al., 1990; Morrison and Hof, 1997). In addition, there exist age-related shifts in the expression of neurofilament protein and other molecules, such as ionotropic glutamate receptors (GluRs) (Vickers et al., 1992, 1994; Gazzaley et al., 1996; Morrison and Hof, 1997), that may represent attributes of a general profile of vulnerability and may render certain neuronal types prone to neurodegeneration, leading to the functional compromise observed in AD. We analyzed the glutamate receptor profile of these circuits in young and aged monkeys as well as neurofilaments, to determine whether circuit-specific age-related changes in cytoskeletal profile and/or glutamate receptors were underway that might suggest that degenerative changes or neurochemical shifts that might contribute to cognitive decline in aged monkeys. To do this, we performed retrograde tract-tracing of cortical projections in young and aged individuals between the prefrontal, parietal, and temporal cortices in combination with immunohistochemistry using specific monoclonal antibodies to neurofilament protein, GluR2, and NR1 (Hof et al., 2002). The immunohistochemical characteristics of corticocortical projection neurons forming short (e.g., within prefrontal area 46) and long connections (e.g., projections from the superior temporal cortex to area 46) were compared, and the effects of aging on these neurochemical markers were quantified. Changes in neurofilament labeling would have suggested potential degenerative changes were underway, and because we do not think these circuits degenerate in aged monkey, we did not anticipate changes in the cytoskeletal phenotype reflected by neurofilaments. In contrast, since we did see spine alterations as described above in these same circuits, we hypothesized that the key excitatory receptors on spines, AMPA and NMDA receptors, might show alterations in neurochemical phenotype in these targeted neurons. GluR2 was chosen as the marker for AMPA receptors, because it is a functionally dominant subunit, in that when present in the receptor complex it renders the AMPA receptor calcium-impermeable, consistent with the properties of AMPA receptors on pyramidal cell spines. NR1 was chosen because it is the obligatory subunit for NMDA receptors, and thus the best reflection of overall NMDA receptor presence.

As anticipated, age had no significant effects on the distribution of neurofilament protein among these projections, but a notable down-regulation in the expression of NMDAR1 and GluR2 was observed in most of the projections (Hof et al., 2002). These effects were particularly robust for GluR2 in the prefrontal cortex in both macaque and patas monkeys. There were substantial reductions in NR1 immunoreactivity in all of the long corticocortical projections, but the short projections within area 46 did not demonstrate a statistically significant reduction in the proportion of double labeled neurons. This indicates that GluRs have a differential distribution among different corticocortical circuits and that their expression patterns in the neurons of origin of these pathways is variably influenced by the aging process.

These results are particularly illuminating when viewed in the context of the comparison of normal aging with AD. In normal aging, we suspect that the major focus of functionally relevant alterations is the excitatory synapse (see discussion of hippocampus below, as well), which is compromised in the absence of frank degeneration of circuits. In AD, key pyramidal neurons, their circuits, and their synaptic terminations degenerate, and in some cases (e.g., perforant path connection from entorhinal cortex to dentate gyrus), the degeneration is nearly complete. As discussed above, neurofilament proteins and their alteration in these neurons are a marker of vunerability for degeneration in AD. The fact that neurofilament abundance and distribution was not altered in corticocortically projecting neurons in these two monkey species is entirely consistent with the fact that they do not degenerate in aging, unlike their homolgues in human during AD. In contrast, the GluRs are synaptic proteins, and their decreased abundance is consistent with the loss of spines and related decrease in the requirement for such synaptic proteins following from the loss of spines in precisely these same neurons described above. While additional studies are needed to assess the quantitative distribution of NR1 and GluR2 at the subcellular level in neurons participating in these subsets of corticocortical connections, these data in two monkey species suggest that during aging, cortical neurons furnishing long and short corticocortical projections display a differential and considerable decrease in the cellular expression of certain GluRs. These observations support the notion that aging alters synaptic properties, and point to the fact that different neuronal populations in the primate neocortex can be characterized not only according to morphological and hodological criteria but also based on their intrinsic neurochemical phenotype.

Circuit-specific shifts in NMDA receptors in hippocampus of aged monkeys

Spatial memory is particularly vulnerable to aging (Gallagher and Rapp, 1997), and is also disrupted by pharmacological blockade of NMDA receptor function (Kentros et al., 1998) or hippocampal knockout of NR1 (Tsien et al., 1996). NMDA-receptor mediated functions such as maintenance and induction of long-term potentiation and maintaining stability of spatial information coding by "place cells" are compromised in aging (Barnes et al., 1997). At the regional level, receptor binding studies have been used to study potential age-related changes in hippocampal GluRs (Wenk and Walker, 1991; Magnusson and Cotman, 1993; Le Jeune et al., 1996). However, in studying age-related changes in synaptic proteins such as receptors, it is particularly important to be able to take the analysis from the regional level to that of cell classes, circuits, individual neuronal compartments and synapses, because the changes are very likely to be cell, circuit, and synapse-specific and therefore difficult to resolve at the regional level. In addition, because subunit composition is a crucial determinant of the functional characteristics of GluRs (Hollman and Heinemann, 1994), the analyses should be carried to the level of individual subunits.

In 1996, we reported age-related shifts in NR1, the obligatory subunit of the NMDA receptors, in the molecular layer of the dentate gyrus (Gazzaley et al., 1996). The projection from entorhinal cortex to the dentate gyrus is strictly confined to the outer molecular layer (OML), i.e., to the distal dendrites of granule cells, whereas other excitatory inputs terminate in a nonoverlapping fashion in the inner molecular layer (IML), on the proximal dendrites. This quantitative analysis demonstrated that aged monkeys, compared to young adult monkeys, exhibit a decrease in the fluorescence intensity for NR1 in the OML of the dentate gyrus as compared to the IML (Fig. 9). Given the tight laminar organization of these circuits, this suggested that the decreased NR1 levels primarily affect the input from the entorhinal cortex, pointing to the entorhinal cortex input to the hippocampus as a key element in age-related changes. Parallel qualitative and quantitative studies with antibodies to AMPA and kainate subunits demonstrated that the intradendritic alteration in NR1 occurs without a similar alteration of nonNMDA receptor subunits. Further analyses, using markers for presynaptic terminals and dendritic markers demonstrated that the circuit is not grossly interrupted in these aged animals. These findings suggested that the intradendritic distribution of a neurotransmitter receptor is modified in an age-related and circuit-specific manner.

While these results were compelling, in that they represented a particularly high level of both molecular and anatomic specificity for age-related shifts in circuit attributes, they were limited in that the animals were not behaviorally characterized, so these neurobiological changes could not be directly linked to functional change. However, we recently carried out studies of GluRs in

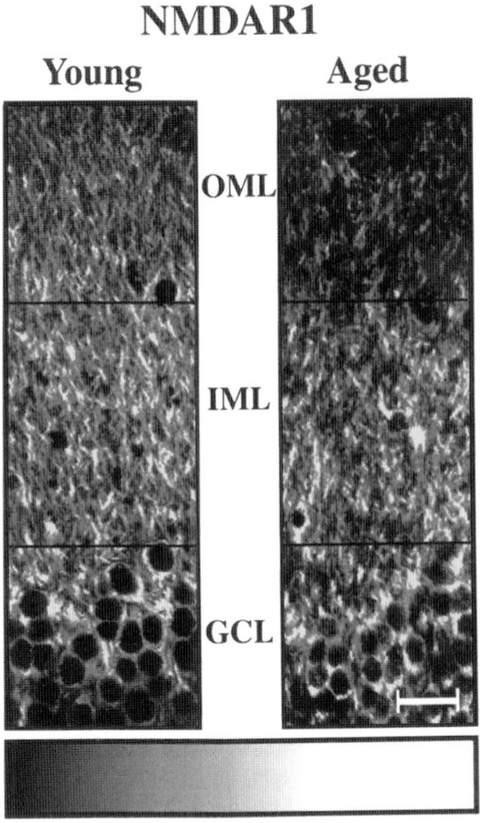

NMDAR1

Young   Aged

Fig. 9. Age-related changes in NR1 fluorescence intensity in the perforant path terminal zone of the macaque monkey. In aged macaque monkey there is a consistent decrease in immunofluo rescent staining intensity for the NR1 subunit restricted to the outer molecular (OML) layer of the dentate gyrus compared to young animals, while no such changes are visible in the inner molecular (IML) and granule cell (GCL) layers. Quantitative analyses demonstrated that the decrease in the ratio of OML/IML is approximately 30% in aged monkeys as compared to young monkeys. This decrease is qualitatively apparent in this figure where relative fluorescence intensity is reflected by the gray scale. See text for details regarding the lack of any structural perturbation of these dendrites. (Adapted from Gazzaley et al., 1996.) Scale bar = 25 μm.

hippocampus of behaviorally characterized aged monkeys, and while they are not yet complete, the data on NR1 confirm our previous observations on the dentate gyrus molecular layer, and extend those findings to an involvement of CA3 as well. In addition, these NR1 deficits correlate strongly with an age-related deficit in hippocampus-dependent memory in these monkeys, again demonstrating the power of such interdisciplinary analyses (Rapp, Mao, Adams, and Morrison, unpublished observations).

Age-related changes in rat hippocampus

While neuroanatomic data sets and behavioral data sets can be compared across experiments, it is most powerful when the neuroanatomic and cellular analyses are done in the same animals that have been behaviorally characterized. This has been particularly powerful in the hands of investigators that behaviorally screen aged animals so that the behaviorally impaired aged animals can be considered as a distinct group from those that are not behaviorally impaired (Gallagher and Rapp, 1997; Peters et al., 1998). In addition, when the neurobiological data are quantitative and derived from behaviorally characterized animals, direct correlations can be drawn in individual subjects between a given neurobiological index (e.g., synapse number) and behavioral performance (Rapp and Gallagher, 1996; Peters et al., 1998). This interdisciplinary approach has been applied with great success to the rat hippocampus and aging, and has led to the conclusion that just as in AD in humans and aging in monkeys, the projection from entorhinal cortex to the dentate gyrus (i.e., the perforant path) is highly vulnerable to aging and directly linked to age-related memory defects.

In 1996, a key negative finding was reported on hippocampus and aging using behaviorally characterized rats. Rapp and Gallagher (1996) carried out a careful stereological analysis of neuron number in numerous hippocampal fields in behaviorally characterized young and aged rats, and found that neuron number was equivalent in all hippocampal fields in young, aged-impaired and aged-unimpaired rats. This finding represented key evidence that neuron loss could not explain age-related decrements in hippocampal-dependent memory tasks, and as such, it reinforced the notion that the cause of such decrements was likely to be subtle changes in circuit and synapse characteristics, not degeneration, similar to the evolving picture in monkey hippocampus (Gazzaley et al., 1996, 1997). Recently, an interdisciplinary team carried out a comprehensive analysis of several neurochemical indices in the hippocampus of behaviorally characterized young and aged rats, and used quantitative immunohistochemical procedures to examine the hypothesis that changes in the connectional organization of the hippocampus contribute to age-related learning impairment (Smith et al., 2000; Adams et al., 2001). Immunohistochemical markers were used for key pre- and postsynaptic proteins as well as structural proteins, such as MAP2, that would reveal the degree to which the circuits were affected by shifts in protein distribution as differentiated from frank degeneration. Young and aged rats were tested on a hippocampal-dependent version of the Morris water maze that reveals substantial variability in spatial learning ability among aged rats (Gallagher and Rapp, 1997). A quantitative confocal method was used to quantify changes in immunofluorescence staining for the presynaptic vesicle glycoprotein, synaptophysin, which is an established marker for presynaptic terminals and is required for synaptic release. The intensity of specific immunoreactivity was measured in inner, middle and outer portions of the dentate gyrus molecular layer, stratum lucidum and stratum lacunosum-moleculare of CA3, and CA1 stratum radiatum and stratum lacunosum-moleculare, such that terminal zones for all three major excitatory hippocampal circuits were sampled, and in particular, multiple sites of termination of the entorhinal input to hippocampus were assessed. Comparisons based on chronological age alone failed to reveal a reliable difference in synaptophysin staining intensity in any region examined, however, individual differences in spatial learning capacity correlated with levels of synaptophysin staining in three of the regions examined; the OML and MML of the dentate gyrus, and CA3 stratum lacunosum-molecular (Fig. 10). These changes in relative synaptophysin levels occur in the absence of any evidence of structural degeneration of the innervated dendrites, and thus would impact synaptic transmission perhaps though compromised glutamate release rather than degeneration of pre- or postsynaptic elements. Most importantly, all three of the regions displaying decreased levels of

synaptophysin receive a major projection from layer II of entorhinal cortex, offering further evidence that this circuit is exquisitely sensitive to aging. These findings suggest that circuit-specific alterations in glutamate release in the hippocampus may contribute to the effects of aging on learning and memory, in the absence of frank degeneration.

In these same animals, the AMPA receptor subunit, GluR2, and the NMDA receptor subunit NR1 were investigated as well, to determine whether or not postsynaptic shifts in receptors such as those observed in monkey (Gazzaley et al., 1996) might also be occurring in the context of aging that would further impact the functional status of the entorhinal inputs to the dentate gyrus and CA3 (Adams et al., 2001). Interestingly, there was no statistically significant decrease in NR1 directly associated with age-related memory impairment in rat hippocampus. However, there was a positive correlation between performance on the Morris water maze and NR1 fluorescence intensity levels regardless of age, and this correlation was present only in CA3 (Adams et al., 2001). AMPA receptors did not show such a correlation. Could performance on a memory task be so clearly linked to one particular GluR in a small subset of hippocampal circuits? Clearly, it is difficult to draw any definitive conclusions from these light microscopic data, however, transgenic mouse experiments support the notion of a direct relationship between the NMDA receptor proteins and memory performance. First, mice that have the NR1 gene knocked out in a manner that is confined to the hippocampus have impaired learning and memory performance (Tsien et al., 1996). In addition,

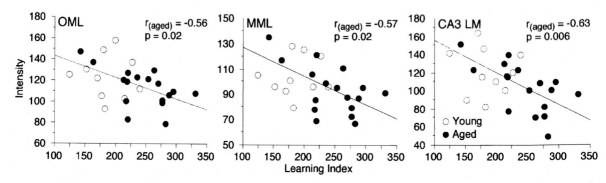

Fig. 10. Scatter plots relating individual spatial learning index scores to levels of hippocampal synaptophysin-immunoreactive (SYN-IR) in aged rats. Lower learning index scores, indicative of better learning, correlated with higher SYN-IR intensity values selectively in the dentate gyrus MML, OML, and CA3-LM. Regression lines and correlation coefficients refer to the relationship between individual differences in spatial learning and SYN-IR for the aged subjects alone. (Taken from Smith et al., 2000.)

mice which have a different NMDA receptor subunit, NR2B, overexpressed in the forebrain display enhanced memory and learning in several behavioral paradigms (Tang et al., 1999). While these studies require extensive ultrastructural analysis to confirm the synaptic nature of the receptor changes, it appears that both pre- and postsynaptic proteins (including GluRs) in specific circuits can be correlated with performance under many conditions, including decrements in performance associated with aging.

Interactions between neural and endocrine senescence

One of the most difficult challenges for research on brain aging over the next several decades will be to determine the critical points of interaction and influence between neural senescence and the aging of other systems. For example, it is particularly critical that we understand the interaction of reproductive senescence with the aging of the nervous system. At the turn of the century, the life expectancy of American women was roughly equivalent to the average age of onset of menopause. Currently, there is a thirty year discrepancy between these two demographic indices, with a life expectancy of approximately 80 years and the average onset of menopause remaining in the early fifties, making the issue of endocrine senescence particularly relevant to human aging.

The role of estrogen in controlling the reproductive axis at the level of the hypothalamus has been studied for many years and characterized in great detail (Fink, 1986). However, estrogens also impact synaptic communication in brain regions involved in cognitive processing, such as the hippocampus (Woolley, 1998), and these effects may be of particular importance in the context of aging when both circulating estrogen levels change and hippocampal-dependent functions decline (Sherwin, 2000). However, our current understanding of estrogen effects on synaptic plasticity in the hippocampus is based primarily on data from young animals. For example, dendritic spine density in CA1 pyramidal cells is sensitive to naturally occurring estrogen fluctuations in young animals (Woolley et al., 1990), as well as experimentally-induced estrogen depletion and replacement (Gould et al., 1990; Woolley and McEwen, 1992, 1993; Woolley et al., 1996).

These effects of estrogen on hippocampal circuitry are NMDA receptor-dependent (McEwen et al., 2001), and estrogen replacement directly increases NMDAR1 levels in CA1 dendrites and somata (Gazzaley et al., 1996b). Using quantitative postembedding immunogold electron microscopy, a recent study investigated estrogen's effects on axospinous synapse density and the synaptic distribution of the NMDA receptor subunit, NR1, within the context of aging (Adams et al., 2001). While estrogen induced an increase in axospinous synapse density in young animals, it did not alter the synaptic representation of NR1 at this age, in that the amount of NR1 per synapse was equivalent across groups. Estrogen replacement in aged female rats failed to increase axospinous synapse density. However, estrogen upregulated synaptic NR1 compared to aged animals not receiving estrogen. Therefore, the young and aged hippocampus react differently to estrogen replacement, with the aged animals unable to mount a plasticity response generating additional synapses, yet responsive to estrogen with respect to additional NMDA receptor content per synapse (Fig. 11).

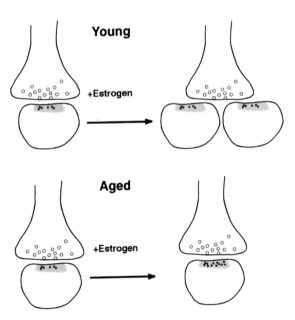

Fig. 11. A schematic of estrogen-induced plasticity in young and aged animals. Estrogen treatment increases NR1 expression per synapse in aged hippocampus, whereas it increases spine number but not synaptic NR1 in young female rat hippocampus. Small black dots represent immunogold particles labeling NR1 associated with the postsynaptic density, and open circles are synaptic vesicles. The gray zone indicates the postsynaptic density. (Taken from Adams et al., 2001.)

These data demonstrate that the effects of estrogen on CA1 synapses must be viewed in the context of brain aging. The synaptic scenario most conducive to NMDA receptor-mediated effects in CA1 is that of the young female with estrogen treatment, in that this condition results in the highest synaptic density and the synapses have a representation of NR1 equivalent to or higher than all the other groups (Adams et al., 2001). With age there is a loss of axospinous synapses in CA1, and this loss is not reversible or apparently even impacted by the presence of estrogen in this paradigm. However, aged animals without estrogen display an additional compromise in NMDA receptor-mediated CA1 synapses: their synapses exhibit a low synaptic representation of NMDA receptors. Thus, while estrogen impacts the aged CA1 synapse in a manner that might enhance hippocampal function, it does so in the context of a synaptic density compromised by age.

References

Adams, M.M., Shah, R.A., Janssen, W.G.M. and Morrison, J.H. (2001a) Different modes of hippocampal plasticity in response to estrogen in young and aged female rats. *Proc. Natl. Acad. Sci. USA*, 98: 8071–8076.

Adams, M.M., Smith, T.D., Moga, D., Gallagher, M., Wang, Y., Wolfe, B.B., Rapp, P.R. and Morrison, J.H. (2001b) Hippocampal dependent learning ability correlates with *N*-methyl-D-aspartate (NMDA) receptor levels in CA3 neurons of young and aged rats. *J. Comp. Neurol.*, 432: 230–243.

Albert, M.S. (1996) Cognitive and neurobiologic markers of early Alzheimer's disease. *Proc. Natl. Acad. Sci. USA*, 93: 13547–13551.

Arnold, S.E., Hyman, B.T. and Van Hoesen, G.W. (1994) Neuropathologic changes in the temporal pole in Alzheimer's disease and Pick's disease. *Arch. Neurol.*, 51: 145–150.

Arnold, S.E., Hyman, B.T., Flory, J., Damasio, A.R. and Van Hoesen, G.W. (1991) The topographical and neuroanatomical distribution of neurofibrillary tangles and neuritic plaques in the cerebral cortex of patients with Alzheimer's disease. *Cereb Cortex*, 1: 103–116.

Barbas, H. (1986) Pattern in the laminar origin of corticocortical connections. *J. Comp. Neurol.*, 252: 415–422.

Barnes, C.A., Suster, M.S., Shen, J. and McNaughton, B.L. (1997) Multistability of cognitive maps in the hippocampus of old rats. *Nature*, 388: 272–275.

Bouras, C., Hof, P.R. and Morrison, J.H. (1993) Neurofibrillary tangle densities in the hippocampal formation in a nondemented population define subgroups of patients with differential early pathologic changes. *Neurosci. Lett.*, 153: 131–135.

Bouras, C., Hof, P.R., Giannakopoulos, P., Michel, J.P. and Morrison, J.H. (1994) Regional distribution of neurofibrillary

tangles and senile plaques in the cerebral cortex of elderly patients: a quantitative evaluation of a one-year autopsy population from a geriatric hospital. *Cereb. Cortex*, 4: 138–150.

Brion, J.P. (1990) Molecular pathology of Alzheimer amyloid and neurofibrillary tangles. *Semin. Neurosci.*, 2: 89–100.

Campbell, M.J. and Morrison, J.H. (1989) A monoclonal antibody to neurofilament protein (SMI-32) labels a subpopulation of pyramidal neurons in the human and monkey neocortex. *J. Comp. Neurol.*, 282: 191–205.

Campbell, M.J., Hof, P.R. and Morrison, J.H. (1991) A subpopulation of primate corticocortical neurons is distinguished by somatodendritic distribution of neurofilament protein. *Brain Res.*, 539: 133–136.

Fink, G. (1986) The endocrine control of ovulation. *Sci. Prog.*, 70: 403–423.

Gallagher, M. and Rapp, P.R. (1997) The use of animal models to study the effects of aging on cognition. *Annu. Rev. Psychol.*, 48: 339–370.

Gazzaley, A.H., Siegel, S.J., Kordower, J.H., Mufson, E.J. and Morrison, J.H. (1996) Circuit-specific alterations of *N*-methyl-D-aspartate subunit 1 in the dentate gyrus of aged monkeys. *Proc. Natl. Acad. Sci. USA*, 93: 3121–3125.

Gazzaley, A.H., Thakker, M.M., Hof, P.R. and Morrison, J.H. (1997) Preserved number of entorhinal cortex layer II neurons in aged macaque monkeys. *Neurobiol. Aging*, 18: 549–553.

Gazzaley, A.H., Weiland, N.G., McEwen, B.S. and Morrison, J.H. (1996) Differential regulation of NMDAR1 mRNA and protein by estradiol in the rat hippocampus. *J. Neurosci.*, 16: 6830–6838.

Goldman-Rakic, P.S. (1988) Topography of cognition: parallel distributed networks in primate association cortex. *Annu. Rev. Neurosci.*, 11: 137–156.

Gómez-Isla, T., Price, J.L., McKeel, Jr. D.W., Morris, J.C., Growdon, J.H. and Hyman, B.T. (1996) Profound loss of layer II entorhinal cortex neurons occurs in very mild Alzheimer's disease. *J. Neurosci.*, 16: 4491–4500.

Gómez-Isla, T., Hollister, R., West, H., Mui, S., Growdon, J.H., Petersen, R.C., Parisi, J.E. and Hyman, B.T. (1997) Neuronal loss correlates with but exceeds neurofibrillary tangles in Alzheimer's disease. *Ann. Neurol.*, 41: 17–24.

Gould, E., Woolley, C.S., Frankfurt, M. and McEwen, B.S. (1990) Gonadal steroids regulate dendritic spine density in hippocampal pyramidal cells in adulthood. *J. Neurosci.*, 4: 1286–1291.

Henry, B.I., Hof, P.R., Rothnie, P. and Wearne, S.L. (2002) Fractal analysis of aggregates of nonuniformly sized particles: an application to macaque monkey cortical pyramidal neurons. *Fractals*, in press.

Hof, P.R. and Morrison, J.H. (1990) Quantitative analysis of a vulnerable subset of pyramidal neurons in Alzheimer's disease: II. Primary and secondary visual cortex. *J. Comp. Neurol.*, 301: 55–64.

Hof, P.R. and Morrison, J.H. (1991) Neocortical neuronal subpopulations labeled by a monoclonal antibody to calbindin exhibit differential vulnerability in Alzheimer's disease. *Exp. Neurol.*, 111: 293–301.

Hof, P.R. and Morrison, J.H. (1995) Neurofilament protein defines regional patterns of cortical organization in the macaque monkey visual system: a quantitative immunohistochemical analysis. *J. Comp. Neurol.*, 352: 161–186.

Hof, P.R., Bouras, C. and Morrison, J.H. (1999) Cortical neuropathology in aging and dementing disorders: neuronal typology, connectivity, and selective vulnerability. In: A. Peters and J.H. Morrison (Eds.), *Cerebral Cortex, Neurodegenerative and Age-Related Changes in Cerebral Cortex*, Vol. 14, Kluwer Academic-Plenum, New York, pp. 175–312.

Hof, P.R., Cox, K. and Morrison, J.H. (1990) Quantitative analysis of a vulnerable subset of pyramidal neurons in Alzheimer's disease: I. Superior frontal and inferior temporal cortex. *J. Comp. Neurol.*, 301: 44–54.

Hof, P.R., Cox, K., Young, W.G., Celio, M.R., Rogers, J. and Morrison, J.H. (1991) Parvalbumin-immunoreactive neurons in the neocortex are resistant to degeneration in Alzheimer's disease. *J. Neuropathol. Exp. Neurol.*, 50: 451–462.

Hof, P.R., Nimchinsky, E.A., Celio, M.R., Bouras, C. and Morrison, J.H. (1993) Calretinin-immunoreactive neocortical interneurons are unaffected in Alzheimer's disease. *Neurosci. Lett.*, 152: 145–149.

Hof, P.R., Nimchinsky, E.A. and Morrison, J.H. (1995) Neurochemical phenotype of corticocortical connections in the macaque monkey: quantitative analysis of a subset of neurofilament protein-immunoreactive projection neurons in frontal, parietal, temporal, and cingulate cortices. *J. Comp. Neurol.*, 362: 109–133.

Hof, P.R., Ungerleider, L.G., Webster, M.J., Gattass, R., Adams, M.M., Sailstad, C.A. and Morrison, J.H. (1996) Neurofilament protein is differentially distributed in subpopulations of corticocortical projection neurons in the macaque monkey visual pathways. *J. Comp. Neurol.*, 376: 112–127.

Hof, P.R., Ungerleider, L.G., Adams, M.M., Webster, M.J., Gattass, R., Blumberg, D.M. and Morrison, J.H. (1997) Callosally-projecting neurons in the macaque monkey V1/V2 border are enriched in nonphosphorylated neurofilament protein. *Vis. Neurosci.*, 14: 981–987.

Hof, P.R., Duan, H., Page, T.L., Einstein, M., Wicinski, B., He, Y., Erwin, J.M. and Morrison, J.H. (2002) Age-related changes in GluR2 and NMDAR1 glutamate receptor subunit protein immunoreactivity in corticocortically projecting neurons in macaque and patas monkeys. *Brain Res.*, 928: 175–186.

Hollmann, M. and Heinemann, S. (1994) Cloned glutamate receptors. *Annu. Rev. Neurosci.*, 17: 31–108.

Hyman, B.T., Damasio, A.R., Van Hoesen, G.W. and Barnes, C.L. (1984) Alzheimer's disease: cell specific pathology isolates the hippocampal formation. *Science*, 225: 1168–1170.

Hyman, B.T., Van Hoesen, G.W., Kromer, L.J. and Damasio, A.R. (1986) Perforant pathway changes and the memory impairment of Alzheimer's disease. *Ann. Neurol.*, 20: 472–481.

Hyman, B.T., Van Hoesen, G.W. and Damasio, A.R. (1990) Memory-related neural systems in Alzheimer's disease: an anatomic study. *Neurology*, 40: 1721–1730.

Kentros, C., Hargreaves, E.L., Hawkins, R.D., Kandel, E.R., Shapiro, M. and Muller, R.V. (1998) Abolition of long-term stability of new hippocampal place cell maps by NMDA receptor blockade. *Science*, 280: 2121–2126.

Le, Jeune, H., C'cyre, D., Meaney, M.J. and Quirion, R. (1996) Ionotropic glutamate receptor subtypes in the aged memory-impaired and unimpaired Long-Evans rat. *Neuroscience*, 74: 349–363.

Lewis, D.A., Campbell, M.J., Terry, R.D. and Morrison, J.H. (1987) Laminar and regional distribution of neurofibrillary tangles and neuritic plaques in Alzheimer's disease: a quantitative study of visual and auditory cortices. *J. Neurosci.*, 7: 1799–1808.

Magnusson, K.R. and Cotman, C.W. (1993) Age-related changes in excitatory amino acid receptors in two mouse strains. *Neurobiol. Aging*, 14: 197–206.

McEwen, B.S., Akama, K., Alves, S., Brake, W.G., Bulloch, K., Lee, S., Li, C., Yuen, G. and Milner, T.A. (2001) Tracking the estrogen receptor in neurons: implications for estrogen-induced synapse formation. *Proc. Natl. Acad. Sci. USA*, 98: 7093–7100.

Mirra, S.S., Hart, M.N. and Terry, R.D. (1993) Making the diagnosis of Alzheimer's disease—A primer for practicing neuropathologists. *Arch. Pathol. Lab. Med.*, 117: 132–144.

Morrison, J.H. and Hof, P.R. (1997) Life and death of neurons in the aging brain. *Science*, 278: 412–419.

Morrison, J.H., Lewis, D.A., Campbell, M.J., Huntley, G.W., Benson, D.L. and Bouras, C. (1987) A monoclonal antibody to nonphosphorylated neurofilament protein marks the vulnerable cortical neurons in Alzheimer's disease. *Brain Res.*, 416: 33–336.

Nimchinsky, E.A., Vogt, B.A., Morrison, J.H. and Hof, P.R. (1995) Spindle neurons of the human anterior cingulate cortex. *J. Comp. Neurol.*, 355: 27–37.

Nimchinsky, E.A., Hof, P.R., Young, W.G. and Morrison, J.H. (1996) Neurochemical, morphologic and laminar characterization of cortical projection neurons in the cingulate motor areas of the macaque monkey. *J. Comp. Neurol.*, 374: 136–160.

Nimchinsky, E.A., Vogt, B.A., Morrison, J.H. and Hof, P.R. (1997) Neurofilament and calcium-binding proteins in the human cingulate cortex. *J. Comp. Neurol.*, 384: 597–620.

O'Donnell, K.A., Rapp, P.R. and Hof, P.R. (1999) The volume of prefrontal cortex area 46 is preserved during aging in macaque monkeys. *Exp. Neurol.*, 160: 300–310.

Page, T.L., Einstein, M., Duan, H., He, Y., Flores, T., Rolshud, D., Erwin, J.M., Wearne, S.L., Morrison, J.H. and Hof, P.R. (2002) Morphological alterations in neurons forming corticocortical projections in the neocortex of aged patas monkeys. *Neurosci. Lett.*, 317: 37–41.

Pearson, R.C.A., Esiri, M.M., Hiorns, R.W., Wilcock, G.K. and Powell, T.P.S. (1985) Anatomical correlates of the distribution of the pathological changes in the neocortex in Alzheimer disease. *Proc. Natl. Acad. Sci. USA*, 82: 4531–4534.

Perl, D.P., Good, P.F., Bussière, T., Morrison, J.H., Erwin, J.M. and Hof, P.R. (2000) Practical approaches to stereology in the setting of aging- and disease-related brain banks. *J. Chem. Neuroanat.*, 20: 7–19.

Peters, A., Sethares, C. and Moss, M.B. (1998a) The effects of aging on layer 1 in area 46 of prefrontal cortex in the rhesus monkey. *Cereb. Cortex*, 8: 671–684.

Peters, A., Morrison, J.H., Rosene, D. and Hyman, B.T. (1998b) Are neurons lost from the primate cerebral cortex during normal aging? *Cereb. Cortex*, 8: 295–300.

Peters, A., Moss, M.B. and Sethares, C. (2000). Effects of aging on myelinated nerve fibers in monkey primary visual cortex. *J. Comp. Neurol.*, 419: 364–376.

Peters, A., Rosene, D., Moss, M., Kemper, T., Abraham, C., Tigges, J. and Albert, M. (1996) Neurobiological bases of age-related cognitive decline in the rhesus monkey. *J. Neuropathol. Exp. Neurol.*, 55: 861–874.

Rapp, P.R. and Gallagher, M. (1996) Preserved neuron number in the hippocampus of aged rats with spatial learning deficits. *Proc. Natl. Acad. Sci. USA*, 93: 9926–9930.

Rapp, P.R. and Gallagher, M. (1997) Toward a cognitive neuroscience of normal aging. *Adv. Cell Aging Gerontol.*, 2: 1–21.

Rogers, J. and Morrison, J.H. (1985) Quantitative morphology and regional and laminar distributions of senile plaques in Alzheimer's disease. *J. Neurosci.*, 5: 2801–2808.

Sampson, V.L., Morrison, J.H. and Vickers, J.C. (1997) The cellular basis for the relative resistance of parvalbumin and calretinin immunoreactive neocortical neurons to the pathology of Alzheimer's disease. *Exp. Neurol.*, 154: 295–302.

Sherwin, B.B. (2000) Oestrogen and cognitive function throughout the female lifespan. *Novartis Found. Symp.*, 230: 188–196.

Smith, T.D., Adams, M.M., Gallagher, M., Morrison, J.H. and Rapp, P.R. (2000) Circuit-specific alterations in hippocampal synaptophysin immunoreactivity predict spatial learning impairment in aged rats. *J. Neurosci.*, 20: 6587–6593.

Tang, Y.P., Shimizu, E., Dube, G.R., Rampon, C., Kerchner, G.A., Zhuo, M., Liu, G. and Tsien, J.Z. (1999) Genetic enhancement of learning and memory in mice. *Nature*, 401: 63–69.

Terry, R.D., Masliah, E., Salmon, D.P., Butters, N., DeTeresa, R., Hill, R., Hansen, L.A. and Katzman, R. (1991) Physical basis of cognitive alterations in Alzheimer's disease: synapse loss is the major correlate of cognitive impairment. *Ann. Neurol.*, 30: 572–580.

Trojanowski, J.Q., Schmidt, M.L., Shin, R.W., Bramblett, G.T., Rao, D. and Lee, V.M.Y. (1993) Altered tau and neurofilament proteins in neurodegenerative diseases: diagnostic implications for Alzheimer's disease and Lewy body dementias. *Brain Pathol.*, 3: 45–54.

Tsien, J.Z., Herta, P.T. and Tonegawa, S. (1996) The essential role of hippocampal CA1 NMDA receptor-dependent synaptic plasticity in spatial memory. *Cell*, 87: 1327–1338.

Vickers, J.C. (1997) A cellular mechanism for the neuronal changes underlying Alzheimer's disease. *Neuroscience*, 78: 629–639.

Vickers, J.C., Delacourte, A. and Morrison, J.H. (1992) Progressive transformation of the cytoskeleton associated with normal aging and Alzheimer's disease. *Brain Res.*, 594: 273–278.

Vickers, J.C., Dickson, T.C., Adlard, P.A., Saunders, H.L., King, C.E. and McCormack, G. (2000) The cause of neuronal degeneration in Alzheimer's disease. *Prog. Neurobiol.*, 60: 139–165.

Vickers, J.C., Riederer, B.M., Marugg, R.A., Buée-Scherrer, V., Buée, L., Delacourte, A. and Morrison, J.H. (1994) Alterations in neurofilament protein immunoreactivity in human hippocampal neurons related to normal aging and Alzheimer's disease. *Neuroscience*, 62: 1–13.

Vogt, B.A., Van Hoesen, G.W. and Vogt, L.J. (1990) Laminar distribution of neuron degeneration in posterior cingulate cortex in Alzheimer's disease. *Acta Neuropathol.*, 80: 581–589.

Vogt, B.A., Vogt, L.J., Vrana, K.E., Meadows, R.S., Challa, V.R., Hof, P.R. and Van Hoesen, G.W. (1998) Neuropathological subtypes of Alzheimer's disease: laminar patterns of neurodegeneration in posterior cingulate cortex. *Exp. Neurol.*, 153: 8–22.

Wenk, G.W. and Walker, L.C. (1991) Loss of NMDA, but not GABA-A, binding in the brains of aged rats and monkeys. *Neurobiol. Aging*, 12: 93–98.

West, M.J. (1993) Regionally specific loss of neurons in the aging human hippocampus. *Neurobiol. Aging*, 14: 287–293.

Woolley, C.S. (1998) Estrogen-mediated structural and functional synaptic plasticity in the female rat hippocampus. *Horm. Behav.*, 34: 140–148.

Woolley, C.W., Gould, E., Frankfurt, M. and McEwen, B.S. (1990) Naturally occurring fluctuations in dendritic spine density on adult hippocampal pyramidal neurons. *J. Neurosci.*, 10: 4035–4039.

Woolley, C.S. and McEwen, B.S. (1992) Estradiol mediates fluctuations in hippocampal synapse density during the estrous cycle in the adult rat. *J. Neurosci.*, 12: 2549–2554.

Woolley, C.S. and McEwen, B.S. (1993) Roles of estradiol and progesterone in regulation of hippocampal dendritic spine density during the estrous cycle in the rat. *J. Comp. Neurol.*, 336: 293–306.

Woolley, C.S., Wenzel, H.J. and Schwartzkroin, P.A. (1996) Estradiol increases the frequency of multiple synapse boutons in the hippocampal CA1 region of the adult female rat. *J. Comp. Neurol.*, 373: 108–117.

Subject index